Evaluations of
Drug Interactions

Evaluations of Drug Interactions

Arthur F. Shinn, Pharm.D.

Director, Medical Affairs,
Professional Drug Systems, Inc.;
Staff Consultant, Clinical Pharmacology,
Department of Medicine, Faith Hospital,
St. Louis, Missouri

Robert P. Shrewsbury, Ph.D.

Assistant Professor of Pharmaceutics,
University of North Carolina, School of Pharmacy,
Chapel Hill, North Carolina;
Consultant, MEDICOM™ Consulting Group,
Professional Drug Systems, Inc.,
St. Louis, Missouri

THIRD EDITION

The C. V. Mosby Company

ST. LOUIS • TORONTO • PRINCETON   1985

MOSBY

A TRADITION OF PUBLISHING EXCELLENCE

Editors: Thomas A. Manning, Chester L. Dow
Editing supervisor: Peggy Fagen
Manuscript editors: Daphna Gregg, Jerie Jordan
Book design: Jeanne Genz
Cover design: Kathleen A. Johnson
Production: Barbara Merritt

First two editions published by the American Pharmaceutical Association

Printed in the United States of America

The C. V. Mosby Company
11830 Westline Industrial Drive, St. Louis, Missouri 63146

Library of Congress Cataloging in Publication Data
Main entry under title:

Evaluations of drug interactions.

   Includes bibliographical references and index.
   1. Drug interactions. 2. Drugs—Side effects. I. Shinn,
Arthur F. II. Shrewsbury, Robert P. [DNLM: 1. Drug Interactions—
handbooks. QV 39 E92]
RM302.E94 1985   615'.7045   84-18894
ISBN 0-8016-4602-2

TS/VH/VH 9 8 7 6 5 4 3 2 1   04/C/563

Consulting Contributors

Marie A. Abate, Pharm.D
Assistant Professor of Clinical Pharmacy,
Assistant Director, Drug Information Center,
School of Pharmacy, West Virginia University,
Morgantown, West Virginia

C. Jelleff Carr, Ph.D.
Consultant, Toxicology and Pharmacology,
Columbia, Maryland

Ernest A. Daigneault, Ph.D.
Chairman and Professor,
Department of Pharmacology,
East Tennessee State University,
Quillen-Dishner College of Medicine,
Johnson City, Tennessee

John M. Fischer, Pharm.D.
Associate Professor of Pharmacy Practice,
Director, Drug Information Center,
University of Pittsburgh School of Pharmacy,
Pittsburgh, Pennsylvania

Richard J. Fleck, Pharm.D.
Clinical Research Scientist,
Clinical Pharmacokinetics/Dynamics Section,
Medical Division,
Burroughs Wellcome Co.,
Research Triangle Park, North Carolina

George E. Francisco, Jr., Pharm.D.
Assistant Professor of Pharmacy Practice,
University of Georgia School of Pharmacy,
Athens, Georgia

Gary R. Gallo, M.S., R.Ph.
Director, Drug Information Services,
University of Minnesota Hospitals
    and College of Pharmacy;
Assistant Professor, College of Pharmacy,
University of Minnesota,
Minneapolis, Minnesota

Michael R. Halbert, B.Sc., Pharm.D.
Clinical Pharmacist, McKennan Hospital,
Assistant Professor of Pharmacy Practice,
South Dakota State University,
College of Pharmacy,
Sioux Falls, South Dakota

Linda L. Hart, Pharm.D.
Associate Clinical Professor,
Director, Drug Information Analysis Services,
University of California,
School of Pharmacy,
Division of Clinical Pharmacy,
San Francisco, California

Susan M. Hatfield, Pharm.D.
Clinical Coordinator,
Harper-Grace Hospitals;
Adjunct Assistant Professor,
Clinical Pharmacy,
Wayne State University,
Detroit, Michigan

Steven K. Hebel, B.S., R.Ph.
Research Assistant,
Professional Drug Systems, Inc.,
St. Louis, Missouri

v

Mark J. Hogan, Pharm.D.
Manager, Research and Development,
Professional Drug Systems, Inc.,
St. Louis, Missouri

Arthur I. Jacknowitz, Pharm.D.
Professor of Clinical Pharmacy,
Director, Drug Information Center,
School of Pharmacy, West Virginia University,
Morgantown, West Virginia

Paul L. Jeffrey, Pharm.D.
Assistant Director for Clinical Affairs,
Director, Drug Information Services,
University of Maryland Hospital;
Clinical Assistant Professor,
University of Maryland, School of Pharmacy,
Baltimore, Maryland

John H. Loomis, Jr., Pharm.D.
Director, Drug Information Services,
Turner Drug Information Center,
University of Houston,
College of Pharmacy,
Houston, Texas

David L. Lourwood, Jr., Pharm.D.
Clinical Pharmacist in Obstetrics
    and Gynecology,
Department of Pharmacy Services,
Cook County Hospital;
Adjunct Assistant Professor of
    Pharmacy Practice,
University of Illinois-Chicago,
Chicago, Illinois

William A. Parker, Pharm.D., M.B.A.
Clinical Pharmacist and Consultant,
Departments of Pharmacy and
    Family Medicine,
Halifax Infirmary;
Coordinator and Associate Professor,
    Clinical Pharmacy,
Dalhousie University,
College of Pharmacy,
Halifax, Nova Scotia

Timothy A. Robert, Ph.D.
Assistant Professor,
Department of Pharmacology,
Quillen-Dishner College of Medicine,
East Tennessee State University,
Johnson City, Tennessee

William T. Sawyer, M.S.
Director of Pharmacy Education,
Area Health Education Center,
Charlotte Memorial Hospital and
    Medical Center,
Charlotte, North Carolina;
Associate Professor of Clinical Pharmacy,
School of Pharmacy,
Clinical Assistant Professor of
    Family Medicine,
School of Medicine,
University of North Carolina,
Chapel Hill, North Carolina

Terrence L. Schwinghammer, Pharm.D.
Associate Professor of Pharmacy Practice,
University of Pittsburgh School of Pharmacy,
Pittsburgh, Pennsylvania

Walter F. Stanaszek, Ph.D.
Associate Professor of Clinical Pharmacy,
University of Oklahoma College of Pharmacy,
Oklahoma City, Oklahoma

William A. Wargin, Ph.D.
Research Scientist,
Department of Medicinal Biochemistry,
Burroughs Wellcome Co.,
Research Triangle Park, North Carolina

Interdisciplinary Review Panel

John R. Sharp, M.D., FACP
Assistant Clinical Professor of Medicine,
Uniformed University of the Health Sciences;
Hospital Commander,
USAF Hospital Plattsburgh,
Plattsburgh Air Force Base,
Plattsburgh, New York

Fred A. Richeda, D.D.S.
Private Family Practice,
Richeda-Brace Family Dental Associates, Inc.,
St. Louis, Missouri

Ellen J. Hoops, R.N., B.S.N.
Coordinator, Nursing Education,
St. Luke's Episcopal Hospital,
Texas Childrens Hospital,
Texas Heart Institute,
Houston, Texas

American Pharmaceutical Association Scientific Review Panel

Foreword

Health professionals know that pharmaceutical products often have a dramatic beneficial impact in patient care and treatment. Many times, drugs represent the crucial difference between life and death.

Health professionals also are acutely aware that pharmaceutical products can be "double-edged swords." They can be subject to abuse; they can deteriorate to toxic degradation products because of inherent instability; they can be taken in overdose; they can be taken at improper times or with incorrect frequency; they can cause severe allergic reactions; and so on.

Approximately 20 years ago, pharmacists and other health care practitioners began to recognize another drug-related problem. This new hazard came to be known or identified as "drug interactions"—a phenomenon in which a patient taking two drugs concurrently has a response that is significantly different from that which would have been anticipated from the two drugs individually.

The pharmacy profession was in the forefront in recognizing this new problem and in attempting to manage it. Pharmacists authored articles for pharmacy and medical publications in order to alert their colleagues to the problem. Also, individual pharmacists prepared charts and tabulations for their personal use in monitoring drugs prescribed for their patients. Some of these charts were reproduced for distribution to their fellow pharmacists. But the American Pharmaceutical Association (APhA) considered these well-intended efforts to fall short of the authoritative information that pharmacists needed to deal with this serious drug interaction problem.

Accordingly, APhA developed a solution embodying a unique approach: a reference book entitled *Evaluations of Drug Interactions* (EDI). Several things made EDI different from other available sources of drug interaction information, whether in chart form or in book form: (1) broadly based panels of experts were constituted to deal with each pharmacologic drug class, thereby providing both special expertise and a group consensus; (2) interactions were covered in monograph format with all related drugs appropriately discussed; (3) clinical significance was carefully weighed and described; (4) suggestions were offered as to alternate therapy or other suitable routes to best manage the interaction; (5) only carefully culled, original literature references were utilized and, after documentation, were cited in the monograph; and (6) for ease of identification, drug trade names were listed and cross referenced for all nonproprietary drug names in the monographs. APhA also enlisted the cooperation of related organizations of health care professionals and included on its panels individual experts from medicine, dentistry, nursing, and other areas of the health sciences.

The publication (EDI) was well received within pharmacy as well as by the health care community at large. APhA was gratified with the highly favorable reception and subsequently produced an extensive supplement, then an entirely new edition, and then a major supplement to that second edition.

But technology advanced in giant steps during those years, and the need to computerize the information in EDI became increasingly apparent—both for keeping the information database itself up-to-date and for efficient utilization at the user level. As a consequence, APhA sought out a potential partner with strong experience, know-how, and capabilities in the field of computerized drug information, as well as a serious commitment and dedication to maintaining the integrity and high standard of quality of APhA's EDI information base.

Such a partner was found in Professional Drug Systems, Inc. (PDS). Their willingness to establish and maintain the staff and outside consultant expertise needed to accomplish the task of producing a high-quality new edition of EDI was a crucial consideration from APhA's viewpoint. They have admirably met and even exceeded that commitment.

Indeed, they have brought into the partnership an added benefit. From PDS came a computerized database backed up with over 6 years of experience in the active practice of pharmacy. That database used EDI as a primary source of drug interaction information. In addition, it had been used to analyze several million prescription orders for hundreds of thousands of patients. This experience offered the background necessary for developing an information bank that combines a sophisticated, comprehensive database with a practical easy-to-use format that is readily adapted to most pharmacy practices.

For the past 2 years, PDS has worked diligently to update and expand EDI and to convert its resource information into forms and formats that would be convenient to use by pharmacists and other practitioners. APhA staff and an APhA appointed and administered Scientific Review Panel have closely monitored the efforts and products emanating from Professional Drug Systems' operation relative to the EDI database and to the software and hard-copy publications derived from the database.

On the basis of its monitoring and review activity, APhA is pleased to extend its full endorsement regarding the overall scientific quality of the technical content of these PDS produced products. Moreover, the APhA-PDS joint commitment is planned to be an on-going one, with future updates, supplements, and new editions all derived in a similar, carefully developed manner.

Before closing, APhA wishes to recognize the many, many people who collectively joined together in working to make and keep EDI a highly credible and invaluable resource. For EDI's third edition these people include the Professional Drug Systems' Contributors, the APhA Scientific Review Panel, and key scientific and professional staff people at PDS and APhA. Their names may be found elsewhere in this publication.

It is our fervent hope that this new EDI will play a significant part in helping to control the overall drug interaction problem and in reducing the level of those unfortunate deaths and hospitalizations.

John F. Schlegel, Pharm.D.
President
American Pharmaceutical Association

Acknowledgments

The preparation of the third edition of *Evaluations of Drug Interactions* could not have been possible without the efforts of many individuals. Space does not permit us to acknowledge each person separately. Nevertheless, we want to express our appreciation to all those who have helped in the development of this book, for without each one of them this publication would have been impossible.

We would especially like to express our appreciation to Mr. Stuart L. Bascomb, Chief Operating Officer of Professional Drug Systems, the late Dr. William S. Apple, Past President of APhA, and Dr. Norman A. Campbell, J.D., Ph.D., Professor of Pharmacy Administration, University of Rhode Island, whose work and perseverance lead to the relationship that allowed EDI-3 to be developed.

Special appreciation is also given to Dr. John F. Schlegel, APhA President, Dr. Edward G. Feldmann, APhA Vice President for Scientific Affairs, and Dr. Richard P. Penna, APhA Vice President for Professional Affairs, for their support, advice, and review of this publication. We would also like to acknowledge the individuals who worked with and for the APhA and were involved in the previous editions of EDI. In a very real sense, they set a foundation upon which we were able to develop this project.

We are deeply indebted to Mr. M. Gale Fridley, B.S., R.Ph., who gave professional and scientific support to this project during many tiring hours.

We acknowledge the generous cooperation and expertise of all Consulting Contributors, Interdisciplinary Review Panel members, and the APhA Scientific Review Panel. The names of these individuals are listed elsewhere in this book.

We would also like to thank Mrs. Lynn M. Riddle and Mrs. Linda S. Poehlein, who worked so diligently and gave so much of their time in typing and other secretarial duties pertaining to this project.

We would like to give a special note of appreciation to Tom Manning, publisher, Chet Dow, editor, Peggy Fagen, book editor, and Mike Riley, publisher, all of The C. V. Mosby Co., for their encouragement and assistance in the completion of this project.

Finally we wish to express our appreciation to our wives and families—Peggy and Kara, Laura and Steve—who gave us love, motivation, and the understanding that was necessary in completing this project.

Arthur F. Shinn
Robert P. Shrewsbury

Contents

Detailed Contents

2 Anesthetic and Neuromuscular Blocking Agents' Drug Interactions, 62

*indicates drug or combination not available in the U.S.

3   Antiarrhythmic Drug Interactions, 111

4   Anticoagulant Drug Interactions, 131

5 Anticonvulsant Drug Interactions, 211

6 Antidepressant Drug Interactions, 279

9   Antineoplastic Drug Interactions, 407

10   Antipsychotic and Antianxiety Drug Interactions, 425

11   Beta-Adrenergic Blocking Agents' Drug Interactions, 469

Introduction

There has been an increasing awareness of the possibility of drug interactions among health care practitioners. Because of the growing number of available drugs, both prescription and nonprescription, and the great amount of literature dealing with the subject, it is becoming increasingly difficult for the health care professional to effectively evaluate drug interactions. EDI provides the clinician a concise evaluation of the literature in a comprehensive, easy-to-use format.

A drug interaction is defined as occurring whenever the effects of one drug are modified in or on the body by the prior or concurrent administration of another pharmacologically active substance. Drug interactions included in this book are those that, when they occur, may result in an antagonistic, synergistic, or unexpected response.

All attempts have been made to include drug interactions that have occurred in humans. When necessary, supportive medical literature discussing animal or in vitro studies have been included to clarify mechanisms, related drugs, or the drug interactions themselves.

When evaluating the various drug interactions, one must address numerous considerations. Most interactions are quite complex and variable, depending on different "patient-specific parameters" such as disease states, weight, age, sex, and renal excretion. These parameters are certainly a concern to the health professional, and these patient variables need to be considered since they may further affect the drug interaction significance. It is important to remember that what is of minor clinical significance with one patient could be a major problem to another patient, and vice versa, if history applies (e.g., renal failure, hepatic function problems, duration of therapy).

The editors, consulting contributors, interdisciplinary review panel, and members from the MEDICOM™ consulting group have reviewed the known and pertinent medical documentation and developed a meaningful monograph for the user regarding each particular drug interaction. This group of professionals has analyzed each drug interaction monograph and has assigned a significance code (see User's Guide). This coding is intended to give an immediate and firsthand referencing guide to the particular drug interaction. The user may then combine the medical information in the monograph with his or her own professional judgment to develop a final decision and course of action. This third edition of *Evaluations of Drug Interactions* is to be considered as one tool available to a health care practitioner making a drug therapy decision and not as a substitute for professional judgment.

The contents of each chapter is divided into two sections: summary tables and detailed monographs.

The *summary tables* include a brief description of each individual drug interaction in a condensed tabular format. Included are statements of potential pharmacologic effects and recommendations as well as the significance code pertaining to that specific drug interaction. This section is intended to provide the user with a readily accessible, concise review of the drug interactions involving the therapeutic class of drugs pertinent to that chapter.

The *detailed monographs* are arranged as follows:

1. *Title of the Interacting Drugs by Generic Name.* The generic names of the drug interaction pair that appear in the title of the monograph relate to those agents that have the greatest degree of documentation in the medical literature and/or those that are most often used in clinical practice. Combinations like multiple metal ions found in antacid preparations are listed in the heading as a group of interacting agents when it is not ascertained in the literature which particular agents may be involved. Oral contraceptive agents are handled in a similar manner in that most dosage forms are in combination and assessment of the causative agent is difficult to document. Refer to the User's Guide for a discussion of chapter assignments and significance coding.

2. *Summary.* This pertains to the overall effect of the interaction.

3. *Related Drugs.* This section broadens the scope of the monograph and includes a discussion of those agents that are either pharmacologically, pharmacokinetically, or chemically related to either of the drugs appearing in the monograph title. If any of these related agents is specifically implicated by the mechanism of action of the primary drug interaction, a statement discussing this involvement appears in the related drug section of the monograph.

   If more than three agents exist in that particular class, only three representative agents are listed in parenthesis followed by [see Appendix]. The user may refer to the Appendix of Related Drugs, which will contain a complete list of other agents in a related drug class.

   Agents that are no longer commercially available in the United States have not been included in this edition unless it was necessary to discuss a noteworthy drug interaction, in which case it is noted by an asterisk that the agent is not commercially available in the United States. An agent that is currently in research or one that is soon to be marketed has been included within the monograph if medical literature and documentation are available.

4. *Mechanism.* This is a discussion of the proposed or postulated mechanism for the drug interaction.

5. *Recommendations.* Suggested management to be considered by the practitioner in regard to the specific drug interaction is given here.

6. *References.* These have been footnoted numerically in order of appearance within the monograph. Other reference sources that have been reviewed but not specifically cited within the monograph are not included.

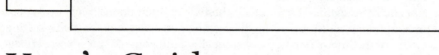

User's Guide

CHAPTER ASSIGNMENTS

In an attempt to uniformly classify the drug-to-drug interaction monographs by their categories, eighteen chapters have been devised. Each monograph is assigned a chapter depending upon classification and pharmacologic effect. Criteria used for this assignment are:

1. The first drug listed in the monograph heading designates its alphabetical chapter assignment. This will be the drug whose pharmacologic effect is altered by the second drug in the combination. However, if the affected drug does not have a chapter cited (other than the miscellaneous chapter), the above does not apply. Instead, the monograph is placed alphabetically in the therapeutic chapter of the other agent.

2. For the drug interactions where neither of the two involved agents has an assigned chapter, the monographs are listed in the Miscellaneous Drug Interaction chapter (Chapter 18) and are listed in alphabetical order by the drug whose pharmacologic action is altered.

It is intended by the editors that this classification will enable the user to more efficiently identify those agents that may alter the desired effects of the patient's prescribed regimen.

SIGNIFICANCE CODING

Each drug-drug interaction has been assigned a significance code based on three major factors: (1) potential harm to the patient, (2) frequency and predictability of occurrence, and (3) degree and quality of documentation.

The editors, consulting contributors, and the interdisciplinary review panel have applied these factors to each drug interaction and assigned a significance code to each monograph heading. The significance code is to be considered applicable only to the agents that appear in the header of the monograph. The related drugs that are mentioned or discussed in the monograph are not given a significance code.

Code 1. *Highly clinically significant:* includes drug interactions that are of great potential harm to the patient, are predictable or occur frequently, and are well documented.

Code 2. *Moderately clinically significant:* drug interactions that are of moderate potential harm to the patient, are less predictable or occur less frequently, or lack complete documentation.

Code 3. *Minimally clinically significant:* drug interactions that are of little potential harm to the patient, have variable predictability or occur infrequently, or have little documentation.

Code 4. *Not clinically significant:* although these drug interactions may occur, documentation may be based on theoretical considerations or the resulting effects of the interactions are not clinically significant and no adverse effects would be anticipated to occur.

NOTICE

AN OVERVIEW

Basic Principles of Drug Interactions

General Considerations
    Transport processes, rationale of plasma level studies, rate constants and elimination half-life, volume of distribution, reversible and irreversible processes, clearance

Interactions Affecting Drug Absorption
    Clinical considerations, rate and amount of drug absorbed, disintegration and dissolution, gastric emptying, ionization, presystemic metabolism, site specific absorption, malabsorption, adsorption, complexing agents

Interactions Affecting Drug Elimination
    Clinical considerations, interactions affecting drug metabolism, interactions affecting urinary excretion

Interactions Affecting Drug Distribution
    Clinical considerations, tissue distribution, plasma protein binding

Interactions at Site of Action
    Competition for site, alteration of receptor, alteration of other receptor site components, effect on a different biologic system

Clinical Considerations Regarding Interactions
    Physiologic and pathologic characteristics of patients

The great variation in chemical structures, physical properties, and pharmacologic effects of the numerous compounds used as therapeutic agents suggests that any two drugs administered concurrently might interact in a number of ways. However, experimental findings and clinical experience have shown that the great majority of interactions occur by a small number of basic mechanisms.

An understanding of the mechanism involved with a particular interaction is essential in interpreting, preventing, and treating specific interactions. Such an understanding may also be useful in predicting the possibility of previously unreported interactions by virtue of the drug's characteristics that are similar to other known interacting drugs. However, the present predictive capability is not sufficiently advanced to permit generalizations in most cases. The practitioner is still dependent on future reports in the literature to extend this knowledge base.

A background for entry into the original literature and to better understand some of the more technical aspects of the monographs is presented in this introduction. Several quantitative relationships and terms that are used frequently—half-life, volume of distribution, protein binding constant, rate constant for elimination, and total body clearance—are discussed.

GENERAL CONSIDERATIONS

The increase in the potency and number of new drugs has contributed immeasurably to modern drug therapy, but this has also created new problems. A matter of increasing concern is the greater incidence of adverse effects when two or more drugs are given concurrently.

It is clear that either the therapeutic or toxic effects of a drug can be greatly modified by interactions with other drugs, foods, environmental substances (e.g., aromatic hydrocarbons from smoking and insecticides) or endogenous substances (e.g., hormones, neuronal transmitters, and vitamins). Serious crises, even death, have been reported in some interactions. Many others are less dramatic but clinically significant. Drugs can also interact outside the body. Chemical and physical interactions of drugs in intravenous fluids may negate pharmacologic effects before the drug is ever given. Drugs and their metabolites in blood or urine may interfere with the clinical laboratory analysis of endogenous substances (e.g., glucose or 17-ketosteroids), which may lead to serious misdiagnosis. Because these in vitro interactions involves different principles than in vivo drug interactions, the former will not be considered here.

It is difficult to estimate how often drug interactions have contributed to increased toxicity or decreased therapeutic efficacy. A possible correlation would be expected between a significant increase in adverse effects and the use of multiple drug therapy. Unfortunately, only very dramatic effects are usually observed, and many clinically significant interactions no doubt have been overlooked. There are many reports on potential drug interactions and long lists of such interactions have been compiled. However, many of these reports are based on insufficient data, questionable study design, a limited number of patients, or animal data alone.

There are several basic problems in interpreting and using existing information to reduce the incidence and severity of drug interactions. These include: (1) evaluation of the validity and clinical significance of the reported drug interactions; (2) detection and prevention of drug interactions that are known to be potentially hazardous; (3) determination of the significance of a reported drug interaction for a specific patient; and (4) recognition of previously unreported interactions.

Most drug interactions in humans that result in either increased toxicity or decreased therapeutic effects are detected by qualitative observations during the clinical use of several drugs concurrently. To determine the mechanisms involved in the observed clinical effects, subsequent definitive studies usually involve quantitative measurements on: (1) pharmacologic response which can be easily quantitated such as prothrombin times, serum glucose levels, blood pressure, electrocardiograms, or (2) the time course of serum levels of the active drug and metabolites.

Transport Processes

Basically, the events that determine the onset, duration, and intensity of a drug effect and the sites involved in drug interactions can be divided into the following two categories:

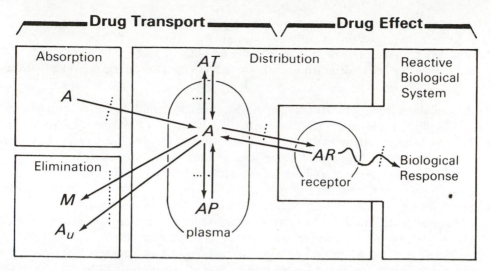

Fig. 1. Schematic diagram of some mechanisms involved in drug action and potential sites of drug interactions (designated by dotted lines). Key: A, free (unbound) active species; M, drug eliminated by drug-metabolizing enzymes; $A\mu$, drug elimination by excretion of unchanged drug (e.g., urinary, fecal, or pulmonary excretion); AP, drug reversibly bound to plasma proteins; AT, drug reversibly distributed into tissue (e.g., fat, muscle, and organs); AR, drug reversibly bound to some part of the reactive biologic system that initiates the biologic effect, usually referred to as the "receptor site."

1. The transport processes that deliver and remove the drug molecules to and from the site of action including absorption, metabolism, excretion, and tissue distribution (i.e., ADME processes).
2. The effect of the drug on the organism after the drug molecules reach the site of action or receptor site, i.e., that component of the reactive biological system that interacts with the drug to initiate the biological response. The total biological response also may involve an additional sequence of biochemical events or homeostatic mechanisms which may or may not be dependent on the initial drug effect at the receptor site. These factors and potential sites of interaction are shown in Fig. 1.

The effect of a drug or substance on the onset, duration, and intensity of the pharmacologic effect of a second drug is usually through an increase or decrease of one of the events in these two categories. Viewed in this way, most drug actions and interactions can be seen as variations on a few basic themes, differing quantitatively but essentially following a few recurring patterns.

The basic factors affecting transport to and from the receptor site that can be altered by drug interactions can be summarized:

Factors affecting transport of active drug to the site of action:
- The rate and extent of drug absorption into the systemic circulation
- Distribution of the active drug to the site of action
- Metabolism of an inactive drug to a biologically active metabolite

Factors affecting removal of active drug from the site of action:
- Distribution from site of action to other tissues
- Metabolism of active drug to inactive metabolite
- Excretion of active drug from the body (e.g., urinary, fecal, or pulmonary excretion)

It is apparent that a small fraction of the drug available binds to the receptor site and elicits the pharmacologic effect. This fraction is the result of a dynamic equilibrium established between many rate processes: absorption, elimination (metabolism and excretion), reversible plasma protein binding, and tissue distribution.

Quantitative concepts describing the rates and dynamic equilibrium of the various processes have been developed (pharmacokinetics). These estimates are most frequently derived from serum/plasma concentration time data. Analysis of serum levels yields the following parameters that can be used, together with measurements of pharmacologic effects, to deduce mechanisms of interactions: (1) rate constant for absorption; (2) amount of drug absorbed; (3) rate constant for metabolism; (4) rate constant for urinary excretion; (5) overall elimination rate constant and elimination half-life; (6) total body clearance, renal clearance, and metabolic clearance; (7) extent of tissue distribution and apparent volume of distribution; and (8) plasma protein binding affinity constant and fraction bound to plasma proteins.

Rationale of Plasma Level Studies

The value of plasma drug concentrations in determining the time course of the pharmacologic effect or the pharmacokinetics of the drug is apparent from inspection of Fig. 1. The concentration of free drug in plasma is central to all events and is the common denominator reflecting changes in the reversible processes of plasma protein binding, tissue distribution, and drug receptor binding. It also directly reflects the amount of drug entering the body by absorption and eliminated from the body through metabolism and excretion.

If a series of plasma (or serum) drug concentrations are determined at different times after an oral dose of the drug had been administered, a plasma concentration–time curve could be constructed as illustrated in Fig. 2. The general shape of the curve is the result of all the simultaneous influences that occur in the body while the drug is undergoing the various ADME processes.

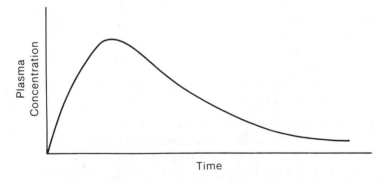

Fig. 2. A plasma concentration–time curve following oral administration.

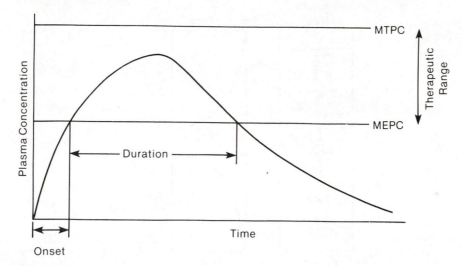

Fig. 3. Time course between plasma concentration and pharmacologic effect after oral administration.

If a therapeutic range for the drug is known, the plasma concentration–time curve can be related to the time course of the pharmacologic effect as illustrated in Fig. 3. A minimum effective plasma concentration (MEPC) must be attained to elicit the pharmacologic effect. The effect will be seen when the plasma concentration reaches that particular plasma concentration. The time between the administration of the drug and the appearance of the pharmacologic effect is called the "onset" or "lag" time. The duration of the pharmacologic effect will be the time interval that the plasma concentration remains above the MEPC. The therapeutic range also would have a minimum toxicity plasma concentration (MTPC), above which toxicity would be expected to be seen.

It should be recognized that not all drugs have a direct relationship between their pharmacologic effect and the time course of their plasma concentrations. For example, if the drug produced an active metabolite, attempting to correlate the plasma concentration of the parent drug with the pharmacologic effect would underestimate the effect. Such would be true with prodrugs such as diazepam, hetacillin, aspirin, etc. Some drugs such as cocaine and warfarin produce pharmacologic effects only after a time delay following administration. In these cases, the effect may appear after the drug's plasma concentrations have disappeared.

Rate Constants and Elimination Half-Life

Besides providing a correlation between the pharmacologic effect and time, plasma concentrations are useful to describe a rate process. The rate of transfer of an amount of drug from one location to another location (e.g., drug in the body transferred to the urine by urinary excretion) or from one chemical form to another (e.g., metabolism of active drug to inactive drug) can often be described by the first-order rate expression:

$$R = -kA$$

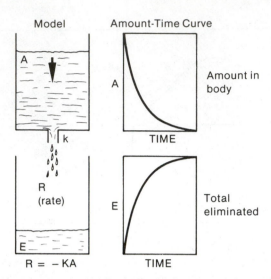

Fig. 4. Hydrodynamic model illustrating the relationships among the rate of transfer *(R)*, the amount of drug available for transfer *(A)*, the rate constant of transfer *(k)*, and the amount of drug eliminated *(E)*. Corresponding amount-time curves are shown at the right.

where A is the amount of drug available for transfer, k is a rate constant that describes the proportional relationship between the rate of transfer and A, and R is the rate of transfer. The expression contains a negative sign since as the rate of transfer proceeds, there will be less of A to be transferred. Thus, as A changes, the rate (R) will also change by a proportional amount, which is governed by the rate constant (k).

A simple but useful analogy in visualizing these relationships is to imagine a container of water with an opening in the bottom through which the water flows. The rate that the water leaves the container is dependent on the amount (A) of water, which is changing, in the container and the size of the opening, which is constant (k). The water represents the drug in the body, and the size of the opening represents the rate constant for the process (Fig. 4).

This rate constant is a valuable tool because it permits a transfer process to be characterized by a single number that gives the rate of transfer corresponding to any amount of drug present. Determination of a rate constant allows quantitative comparison of two different rate processes such as metabolism by two different pathways or a comparison of the same pathway in two different groups of patients.

A single transfer process is usually represented:

$$A_{body} \xrightarrow{k_u} A_{urine}$$

where the rate constant (k_u) designates the specific process involved, such as the urinary excretion rate constant as in this case. A series of consecutive rate processes such as the absorption of drug into the body (k_a) followed by elimination from the body by urinary excretion (k_u) can be expressed:

$$A_{gut} \xrightarrow{k_a} A_{body} \xrightarrow{k_u} A_{urine}$$

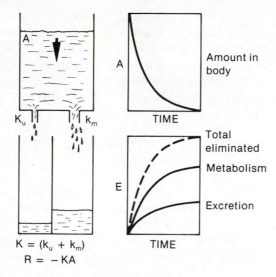

Fig. 5. Hydrodynamic model illustrating elimination by two pathways, metabolism and urinary excretion, and the relationship of the overall elimination rate constant (K) to the individual rates $(k_m$ and $k_u)$.

Often a drug is simultaneously removed from the body by more than one process (e.g., by metabolism and urinary excretion), each process being governed by its own rate constant:

$$A_b \underset{k_m}{\overset{k_u}{\rightleftharpoons}} \begin{array}{l} A_u \\ M \end{array}$$

When this occurs, the overall elimination rate of removal is the sum of the individual rates of removal:

Rate of total elimination = Rate of metabolism + Rate of excretion

The rate constant to describe the rate of total elimination is the sum of all individual rate constants and is represented by the symbol K:

$$K = k_m + k_u$$

This relationship can again be visualized by the simple hydrodynamic analogy shown in Fig. 5. The rates of removal by each of the pathways are proportional to the amount of water in the container (analogous to the amount of drug in the body) and the individual sizes of the openings (analogous to the rate constants for metabolism, k_m, and urinary excretion, k_u). The rate of removal of water would be the same if one larger opening was substituted for the two openings (analogous to K). The additive contribution of each individual process to the total elimination of drug is particularly important in understanding drug interactions. Many interactions affect only metabolism or only urinary excretion. Thus, the contribution of the remaining pathways to the overall disposition of the drug is important in determining the significance of the interaction.

The overall rate constant (K) is expressed in units of reciprocal time and can be interpreted as an approximation of the fraction of the amount of drug in the body that will be eliminated per unit time. For example, a rate constant value of $0.1\ hr^{-1}$ means that approximately one-tenth (or 10%) of the amount of drug present in the body at any given time will be eliminated per hour. More frequently, the rate of elimination is described by the elimination half-life. The overall elimination rate constant (K) of a drug is related to the elimination half-life ($t_{1/2}$) through the equation:

$$t_{1/2} = \frac{0.693}{K}$$

The elimination half-life is the time for 50% of the drug in the body to be eliminated by all pathways. It is one of the most frequently altered parameters involved in drug interactions and may be a quantitative parameter in relating plasma drug levels to pharmacologic effects. The clinical significance of changes in $t_{1/2}$ caused by drug interactions will be discussed in a later section on drug interactions affecting drug elimination.

Volume of Distribution

Plasma concentrations can also provide a quantitative estimate of the extent of tissue distribution using a parameter termed the apparent volume of distribution (V). When some drugs are injected intravenously, there is a rapid decline of the plasma levels caused by the predominate distribution of the drug to the tissues (called the distributive phase). This rapid decline is followed by a slower decline that represents the elimination of drug from the body and a dynamic equilibrium between the drug in the plasma and the drug in the tissues. After the distributive phase, the ratio of drug in plasma and tissue is essentially constant, and the total amount of drug in the body at a given time (A_b) can be related to the plasma concentration (C) by a proportionality constant, which is called the apparent volume of distribution (V):

$$A_b = (V)(C)$$

This relationship is the basis for using plasma levels to determine the amount of total drug eliminated from the body. Drug interactions that change the ratio of drug in plasma to drug in tissues will be reflected by changes in the volume of distribution.

Reversible and Irreversible Reactions

When the transfer of a drug by a particular process is essentially unidirectional, it can be considered an irreversible process. Absorption, metabolism, and excretion are essentially unidirectional and can often be conveniently considered as irreversible processes. Other transfer processes such as tissue distribution, protein binding, and binding at the receptor site are bidirectional rate processes characterized by both the forward and reverse rates and are considered reversible processes. For example, binding of drugs with plasma proteins can be expressed as:

$$A + P \underset{k_2}{\overset{k_1}{\rightleftharpoons}} AP$$

where A is the unbound drug concentration in plasma, P is the plasma protein concentration, and AP is the concentration of drug bound to plasma protein.

If the processes described by k_1 and k_2 are sufficiently rapid compared with other competing rate processes, an apparent equilibrium may be reached that can be described by an affinity constant. In most cases, the ratio of A to AP (or the fraction of drug that is bound) is constant over a range of plasma concentrations. Competing drugs that change this ratio may also affect the relative fractions of bound and unbound drug at the receptor site and reversible sites of distribution in the tissues. The degree to which each reversible process is affected depends on the relative values of the affinity and rate constants.

Clearance

Total body clearance is defined as the product of the apparent volume of distribution (V) and the overall elimination rate constant (K). However, total body clearance has been used as the process which relates the rate of drug elimination to the plasma concentration:

$$\text{Rate of drug elimination} = \text{Total body clearance} \times \text{Plasma concentration}$$

If the total body clearance is altered as the result of a drug interaction, the rate of drug elimination is altered, which will influence how fast the plasma concentrations will decline.

Since total body clearance reflects the combined effect of all processes eliminating the drug from the body, it is the summation of all individual clearances. Thus,

$$\text{Total body clearance} = \text{Urinary clearance} + \text{Hepatic clearance} + \text{Other clearances}$$

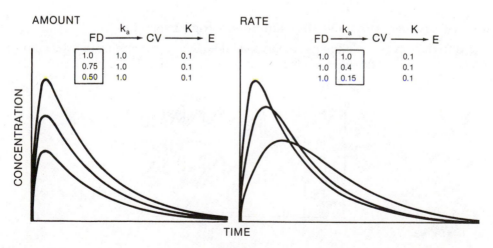

Fig. 6. Effects of changes in the rate constant of absorption (k_a) and fraction absorbed (F) on plasma levels after a single dose. In the left graph only F is changed; in the right graph, only k_a is changed. (Adapted with permission from W.H. Barr: Drug Inform. Bull. **3**:27, 1969.[1])

9

INTERACTIONS AFFECTING DRUG ABSORPTION
Clinical Considerations of Interactions Affecting the Rate and Amount of Drug Absorbed

Interactions during the absorptive phase result in one or both of the following potentially clinically significant effects:

1. Increase or decrease in the relative rate of absorption (k_a)
2. Increase or decrease in the amount of drug absorbed (F)

Fig. 6 shows the effect of these changes on plasma levels.

A decrease in the fraction of drug absorbed is equivalent to a decrease in the dose given, with the obvious clinical implications. Although a drug may eventually be completely absorbed, it may be absorbed so slowly that (1) effective plasma levels are never reached; (2) the onset of the pharmacologic effect may be greatly delayed when prompt relief of acute symptoms is needed; or (3) the formulation acts as a sustained release product and unduly prolongs an effect.

It is important to distinguish between drug interactions in which decreased rates of absorption are clinically significant and those in which this type of interaction may occur but is of no concern. As a general rule, a decreased rate of absorption is most often important for drugs that are given as a single dose in clinical situations requiring a rapid onset of activity (e.g., analgesics such as aspirin and hypnotics such as flurazepam).

The rate of absorption is usually not important for compounds that are given in multiple dose regimens to achieve a constant plasma level such as antibiotics, sedatives, or tranquilizers. The reason is that the average steady-state plasma levels in a multiple dose regimen are affected by the fraction of drug absorbed (F) but not usually by the relative rate of absorption (k_a). The effects of changes in the rate and amount of drug absorbed on multiple dose plasma levels are shown in Fig. 7.

There are several ways in which the rate and amount of absorption of a drug can be modified. Like other types of drug interactions, most drug interactions during absorption are simple alterations of one of the steps involved in absorption. These events and the potential sites of drug interactions are shown in Fig. 8.

Effect Of Disintegration and Dissolution on Drug Absorption

Drugs that are orally administered as solid dosage forms (capsules or tablets) must be released from the dosage form before absorption can begin. The physicial breaking

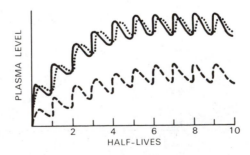

Fig. 7. Effects of changes in the relative rate of absorption (k_a) and fraction absorbed (F) on steady-state plasma levels during multiple dosing. Key:———, normal; . . ., absorption rate decreased; and - - -, amount absorbed decreased.

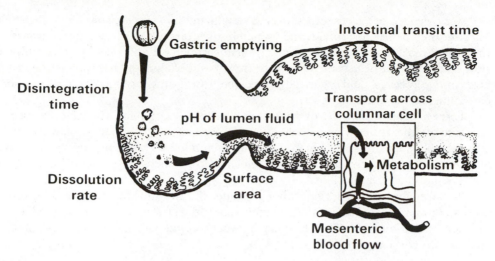

Fig. 8. Potential sites of drug interactions during drug absorption. (Adapted with permission from W.H. Barr: Am. J. Pharm. Ed. **32:**958, 1968.[2])

apart of the tablet or the eroding away of the capsule shell is termed disintegration. When released from the dosage form, the drug is generally still embedded in a granulated particle. The drug must dissolve out of that particle and into the lumen contents, a process called dissolution. For many drugs, dissolution is the slowest (rate limiting) step in the absorption processes.

The rate of dissolution in gastric and intestinal fluids is influenced by several factors:

- Physicochemical properties of the drug such as its solubility, salt or ester form, polymorphic form, hydrate form, particle size of drug
- Characteristics of the dosage form such as particle size of drug granulation, type and thickness of dosage form coating, excipients used in the formulation, manufacturing procedures
- Conditions at the site of dissolution such as pH, volume of luminal fluid, presence of interfering substances such as surfactants, enzymes, food
- Residence time at sites where dissolution can occur

Effect of Gastric Emptying and Intestinal Transit Time on Drug Absorption

The rate at which a drug or drug product is emptied from the stomach can significantly affect the overall absorption process. If gastric emptying is slow, drugs will have a longer time to dissolve in the gastric contents and should have improved absorption when emptied into the small intestine. However, if they are acid labile drugs such as benzyl penicillin or methicillin, slow gastric emptying time will result in a decreased amount of active drug available to be absorbed.

If gastric emptying is rapid, the drug or drug product will be emptied into the small intestine sooner and will have a quicker onset of absorption if the drug has had sufficient time to dissolve. However, dissolution may be slowed in the small intestine by the increasing pH found descending the tract.

Some drugs, such as ferrous salts and riboflavin, have specific sites along the small intestine where their absorption predominately takes place. If the drug is not dissolved by the time it reaches that absorption site, drug absorption is diminished. If transit time is slow enough for the drug to dissolve by the time its site of absorption is reached, a normal absorption process should occur. Therefore, the transit time through the small intestine can influence the extent of absorption.

There are many examples of drugs that alter gastric emptying affecting the absorption rate of other drugs. Propantheline reduces the absorption rate of riboflavin,[3] sulfamethoxazole,[4] and acetaminophen.[5] Intramuscular administration of meperidine causes a delay in acetaminophen absorption.[6] Metoclopramide increases the absorption rate of tetracycline[7] and pivampicillin.[8]

Propantheline and metoclopramide also alter the intestinal transit time. Propantheline causes an increased absorption of hydrochlorothiazide,[9] nitrofurantoin,[10] and digoxin.[11] Metoclopramide significantly alters digoxin absorption leading to decreased steady-state serum concentrations.[11]

Effect of Ionization on Drug Absorption

Once the drug is dissolved in the gastrointestinal contents, the degree of drug ionization plays a substantial role in the absorption process. A basic principle is that the rate of passive transport of a drug across biologic membranes is proportional to the lipid solubility of the drug.[12,13] For weak acids and bases, the un-ionized species has greater lipid solubility and can pass through biologic membranes preferential to the ionized species. Thus the ionization tendency of the drug, indicated by the pKa of the drug and the pH of the aqueous environment, affect the rate of transport by influencing the fraction of the drug which is unionized. Transfer of acids across biologic membranes will be favored by low pH, and transfer of bases will be favored by high pH (Fig. 9). The pH of the gastrointestinal (GI) lumen fluids increases from stomach (pH = 1 to 2) to colon (pH = 6 to 8), which may affect the transport of drugs with pKa's between 3 and 8.

Even though a large amount of the drug in solution is ionized, the rate of reversible proton transfer is so rapid that as soon as part of the un-ionized fraction in solution is absorbed it is immediately replenished by protonation of an ionic molecule. When the drug is in contact with the absorbing site this reversible process continues until all drug is absorbed, passes its site of absorption, or is removed from the site by other mechanisms.

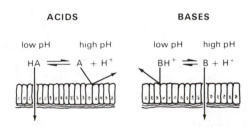

Fig. 9. Effect of pH on the fraction of an acidic or basic drug that is un-ionized and able to pass across biologic membranes.

Additional Physiologic Factors Affecting Drug Absorption

Metabolism of the drug before or during absorption would affect the amount of active drug ultimately absorbed. Acid hydrolysis occurs with some drugs and has already been mentioned. Drugs can undergo extensive enzymatic metabolism since enzymes may be found in the gastrointestinal fluids as well as the gastrointestinal membrane. Such is the case with flurazepam, levodopa, and phenacetin.

Presystemic metabolism may also occur when the drug enters the liver directly from the gastrointestinal tract. This so-called "first pass effect" has been demonstrated for many drugs including propranolol, propoxyphene, lidocaine, and imipramine.

Metabolism before absorption is a positive process when giving prodrugs. Prodrugs generally are esters of the drug that must be hydrolyzed to liberate the active drug. The hydrolysis may occur in the gastrointestinal fluid or membrane or in the liver. Examples of prodrugs that hydrolyze presystemically are clorazepate, chloramphenicol palmitate or stearate, and erythromycin estolate or ethylsuccinate.

There appear to be many absorption sites in the intestinal tract that are specific for certain drugs. Riboflavin and some ferrous salts have already been mentioned. Many amino acids and monosaccharides also have these absorption sites, which generally involve carrier-mediated processes such as active transport or facilitated transport. Competition between two drugs that are absorbed by the same transport process could inhibit the absorption of one or both drugs. Penicillamine, an amino acid analog, has decreased absorption in the presence of some amino acids, presumably resulting from competition for the same amino acid system.[14]

A drug requiring an active transport system may have decreased absorption when used with an agent such as sodium fluoride. This agent interrupts normal cell metabolism, which leads to an inhibition of energy to the active transport system.

Drug absorption may be altered when the normal physiologic state of the gastrointestinal tract is disrupted by disease or drugs; such absorption is termed malabsorption. Drug-induced malabsorption has been observed after the administration of many drugs. Examples are neomycin, phenytoin, aminosalicylic acid, and methotrexate. 5-Fluorouracil enhances the absorption of tobramycin presumably by destroying the integrity of the gastrointestinal mucosa.[15]

Studies of drug absorption in patients with malabsorption have been limited. The results of many such studies have shown little difference between these subjects and controls. For example, isoniazid, chloramphenicol, aspirin, and cycloserine absorption in patients with villous atrophy was similar to control subjects.[16] Similar studies with digoxin in radiation-induced malabsorptive patients[17] and propranolol in untreated celiac disease patients[18] have been published.

Surgical resection of the small bowel appears to alter drug absorption by reducing the surface area available for transport. Digoxin bioavailability has been reduced in these patients[19] as well as the absorption of hydrochlorothiazide[20] and phenytoin.[21]

Physicochemical Interactions that Influence Drug Absorption

Several drugs can be adsorbed or complexed to other drugs or endogenous substances, which would lead to altered absorption. Kaolin is a known adsorbent of lincomycin[22]; charcoal adsorbs promazine[23] as well as many other drugs. Cholestyramine, a

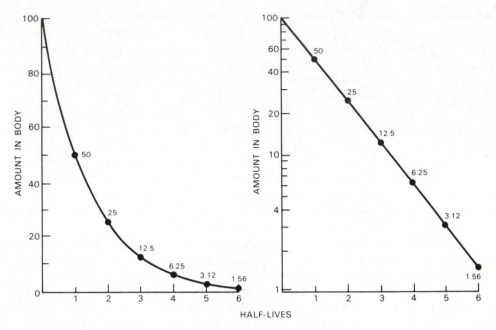

Fig. 10. Plots of the amount of drug in the body at each half-life. When the amount is plotted on a cartesian scale *(left)*, an exponential decline is observed. When the amount is plotted on a logarithmic scale *(right)*, a straight line is observed that is used to determine the half-life.

quaternary ion exchange resin used to bind intestinal salts and reduce serum cholesterol levels, also binds thyroxine[24] and warfarin.[25]

Antacids containing polyvalent cations (aluminum, calcium, or magnesium) complex with tetracycline resulting in decreased antibiotic absorption. Chelation is also involved in the reduction of serum levels of various tetracycline analogs when small doses of ferrous sulfate are given. It has been speculated that streptomycin and dihydrostreptomycin complex with intestinal mucus causing the poor absorption of both these antibiotics. Bile salts in the small intestine form insoluble, nonabsorbable complexes with tubocurarine, neomycin, and kanamycin.[26,27]

Complexing agents may be part of the pharmaceutical dosage form. Amphetamine forms a poorly soluble complex with carboxymethylcellulose that leads to reduced amphetamine absorption.[22] Phenobarbital undergoes a similar interaction with polyethylene glycol 4000.[28]

INTERACTIONS AFFECTING DRUG ELIMINATION
Clinical Considerations of Changes in Rate of Drug Elimination and Elimination Half-Life

Elimination of drugs usually occurs by metabolism and excretion (i.e., renal or fecal). Although these processes are dissimilar in the mechanisms involved and the factors affecting them, they both result in changes in the elimination rate constant and the elimination half-life. The elimination half-life of a drug provides the following information:

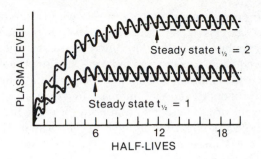

Fig. 11. Effect of a change in half-life on the steady-state plasma levels and the time to reach steady-state plasma levels.

1. The half-life quantitates the overall rate of elimination and the amount of drug remaining in the body at a given time. The elimination half-life is the time for one-half of the drug present in the body to be eliminated from the body. For example, if 100 mg of drug is present at a given time and the half-life of the drug is 4 hours, 50 mg will be eliminated in the first 4 hours. In the second 4 hours, 50% of the remaining amount will be eliminated (25 mg); in the third half-life, 50% of the remaining drug will be eliminated (12.5 mg), and so on. After 6 half-lives, elimination of the drug is over 98% complete (see Fig. 10). It can be seen that the decline of drug in the body is exponential. If the amount in the body or corresponding plasma levels is plotted on semilog paper, a straight line results from which the half-life can be easily determined. Half-lives of drugs vary from a few minutes to months.

2. The half-life influences the average plasma concentration at steady-state during multiple dosing as shown by[29]:

$$C_{ss} = \frac{1.44\ (FD)\ (t_{1/2})}{V}$$

where C_{ss} is an average plasma level at steady state, D is the dose given, F is the fraction of the dose absorbed, V is the apparent volume of distribution, and $t_{1/2}$ is the half-life of the drug. It can be seen that a drug interaction that doubles the half-life will double the average steady-state plasma level (Fig. 11). Drug interactions that decrease the half-life by 50% will reduce the steady-state plasma levels to one-half their original value.

3. The time to reach steady-state during multiple dosing is about 6 half-lives if doses are given at intervals close to the half-life. For drugs with very long half-lives, it would take several weeks before steady-state levels are reached.

Interactions Affecting Drug Metabolism

A large number of drugs are chemically altered in the body to produce metabolites that are generally more water soluble than the parent compound. Drugs are metabolized by a variety of phase I pathways including oxidation, reduction, hydroxylation, dealkylation, and deacetylation and by phase II or conjugating pathways such as glucuronidation. These biotransformations take place principally in the smooth endoplasmic reticulum (microsomal fraction) of the hepatic cell. These processes have been shown to be age-dependent and are poorly developed in the neonate and reduced in the elderly.

Induction of drug metabolism. It has been shown in animals that many drugs in virtually all pharmacologic classes can induce an increase in the size and enzyme content of the endoplasmic reticulum and, therefore, increase the rate of metabolism of other drugs.[30,31] The most frequently encountered inducers in humans are barbiturates, rifampin, and phenytoin as well as ethanol and the polycyclic aromatic hydrocarbons of tobacco smoke.[32,33] These compounds cause an increase in a drug's metabolism often necessitating an increase in the drug's dosage to maintain the same therapeutic plasma concentrations. A danger occurs when the inducer is withdrawn. Metabolism returns to normal and plasma levels increase and may reach toxic levels unless the dosage is reduced.

Phenobarbital has been the most frequently studied enzyme inducing agent. Phenobarbital stimulates a wide variety of metabolic pathways and appears to be a potent inducer in most species studied. Phenobarbital has reduced warfarin levels and anticoagulant effect within 6 days.[34] Oral contraceptive agent steroid levels have also been reduced by phenobarbital induction.[35] Secobarbital[36] and pentobarbital[37] also show enzyme inducing properties.

In addition to drugs already mentioned, carbamazepine has been shown to induce the metabolism of clonazepam.[38] Some dietary factors induce the metabolism of some drugs in humans: low carbohydrate–high protein diets and antipyrine[39]; brussels sprouts and cabbage and phenacetin[40]; and charcoal-broiled beef and phenacetin, antipyrine, and theophylline.[41,42] Some insecticides (mixtures of Lindane and DDT) have been shown to induce antipyrine metabolism.[43] The half-life of antipyrine in normal subjects averaged 13.1 hours with a large range (5.2 to 35 hours), whereas the half-lives in subjects exposed to the insecticide mixture averaged 7.7 hours with a smaller range (2.7 to 11.7 hours) (see Fig. 12).

Inhibition of drug metabolism. There are many clinically significant examples of inhibition of drug metabolism in humans. Such inhibition leads to a reduction in the rate of metabolism and an increased elimination half-life of the compound being affected.

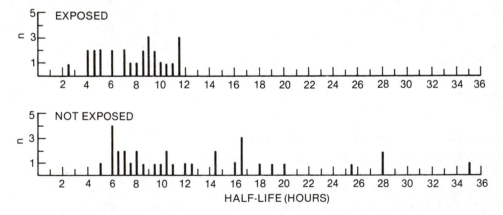

Fig. 12. Distribution of antipyrine half-lives in workers exposed to insecticides and unexposed subjects. (Adapted with permission from B. Kolmodin and others: Clin. Pharmacol. Ther. **10:**638, 1969.[43])

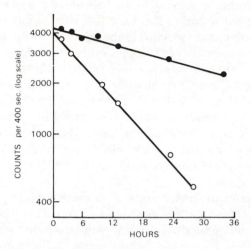

Fig. 13. Increase in half-life of phenytoin by dicumarol resulting from inhibition of metabolism. Key: ○, before dicumarol administration (half-life = 9 hours); ●, after dicumarol administration (half-life = 36 hours). (Adapted with permission from J.M. Hansen and others: Lancet **2**:265, 1966.[44])

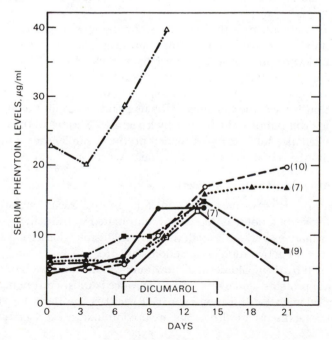

Fig. 14. Effect of dicumarol on steady-state serum levels of phenytoin in 6 subjects. The numbers in parentheses indicate the peak serum level of dicumarol. (Adapted with permission from J.M. Hansen and others: Lancet **2**:265, 1966.[44])

This often leads to serious adverse effects since the affected compound may accumulate in the body resulting in toxic concentrations.

The results of a dramatic increase in the half-life of phenytoin caused by pretreatment with dicumarol are shown in Fig. 13.[44] It is worthwhile to consider the clinical consequences of this one-fourth reduction in the expected rate of metabolism by applying the multiple dose relationships described previously. It would be expected that average steady-state serum levels would increase 4-fold, but it would take 6 half-lives to reach the new level (9 days). Fig. 14 shows that multiple dose serum levels actually increased from 5 to about 15 μg/ml during the 7 days that dicumarol was administered.

Chloramphenicol has been found to be a potent inhibitor of tolbutamide, phenytoin, and dicumarol biotransformation.[45] Sulfinpyrazone potentiates the effects of oral anticoagulants, phenytoin, and tolbutamide via enzyme inhibition.[46] Chlorpromazine decreases the presystemic clearance of propranolol, which results in a 70% increase in propranolol steady-state levels.[47]

Valproic acid inhibits the metabolism of phenobarbital, requiring a phenobarbital dosage reduction of 40% to 50%.[48] It also has a similar effect on another anticonvulsant, ethosuximide.[49] Cimetidine binds through its imidazole ring structure to cytochrome P-450, thereby inhibiting the metabolism of warfarin.[50] Cimetidine also inhibits the metabolism of benzodiazepines undergoing phase I metabolism but not phase II pathways.[51]

The metabolic pathways, including glycine, glucuronide, and sulfate conjugation, can also be inhibited. Glycine conjugation of salicylic acid is decreased by aminobenzoic acid.[52] Salicylamide appears to block glucuronide conjugation of acetaminophen and salicylic acid.[53,54]

Inhibition of metabolism is the basis for some therapeutics. For example, the therapeutic effect of the monoamine oxidase inhibitors (e.g., isocarboxazid, pargyline, phenelzine, and tranylcypromine) results in part from their ability to inhibit the enzyme monoamine oxidase, which metabolizes sympathomimetic amines in tissues. The ability of these drugs to inhibit enzymes does not appear to be limited to monoamine oxidase. Another drug that is used therapeutically for its ability to inhibit a specific enzyme is disulfiram. This drug inhibits aldehyde dehydrogenase, leading to the accumulation of acetaldehyde when alcohol is ingested, which produces unpleasant symptoms. Disulfiram also impairs the metabolism of antipyrine,[55] warfarin,[56] and phenytoin.[57]

Interactions Affecting Urinary Excretion

Interactions that affect urinary excretion of drugs are clinically significant only when the drug or its active metabolite is appreciably eliminated by the urinary route. Drugs are eliminated by urinary excretion through three mechanisms: glomerular filtration, tubular reabsorption, and active tubular secretion (Fig. 15).

Glomerular filtration. Glomerular filtration is an ultrafiltration of drug that is not bound to plasma proteins. Renal creatinine clearance is most commonly used clinically to evaluate the glomerular filtration rate (GFR) and is the basis for dosage regimen adjustments in renal disease for drugs that are predominantly excreted unchanged in the urine.

Renal excretion of a drug is dependent on the degree of plasma protein binding when glomerular filtration accounts for the major portion of renal excretion. This is because

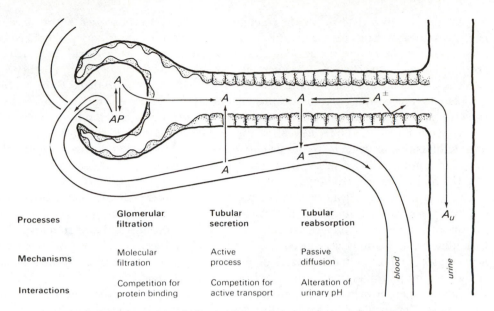

Fig. 15. Mechanisms of renal elimination and potential sites of drug interactions.

the free fraction of the drug in the blood is filtered through the glomerulus. Such a relationship has been found with several tetracyclines.[58] Therefore, drugs that would displace one of these tetracyclines by competitive plasma protein binding would promote the excretion of tetracycline.

Furosemide decreases the rate of glomerular filtration in healthy subjects. These changes in GFR decreased the renal clearance of practolol, gentamicin, and cephaloridine.[59]

Active secretion. Many drugs are transported from the blood across the proximal tubular cell into the tubular urine against a concentration gradient by an active process. There are apparently two systems that actively transport drugs across the tubular epithelium, one for acidic drugs and one for basic drugs. The mechanisms involved in tubular secretion are rather complex and are not completely understood.

Interactions can occur by competition of these agents for tubular transport.[60] The effect of probenecid on increasing serum levels of penicillins, cephalosporins, dapsone, rifampin, sulfonamides, and thiazide diuretics is well known.[61] Such a mechanism is also thought to be responsible in part for the decreased renal clearance of digoxin with concomitant quinidine.[62] Similar digoxin results have been seen with verapamil[63] and amiodarone.[64]

Tubular reabsorption. Drug delivered to tubular urine by glomerular filtration and tubular secretion is concentrated as water is reabsorbed. The reabsorption of water increases the concentration gradient between the drug in urine and the drug in blood. If the drug possesses sufficient lipid solubility, it will passively diffuse into the blood. Very lipid soluble drugs may be completely reabsorbed.

The reabsorption of weak electrolytes can be influenced greatly by the pH of the tubular urine, which determines the fraction un-ionized and subsequently transferred. Half-lives of some drugs can be greatly changed by alterations in urinary pH induced by alkalizers such as sodium bicarbonate or acetazolamide and urinary acidifiers such as ammonium chloride. These drugs generally have the following properties[65]: (1) they are weak acids (pKa 3 to 7) or weak bases (pKa 7 to 11); (2) the un-ionized form is lipid soluble (high oil–water partition coefficient); and (3) they are eliminated appreciably (>20%) by urinary excretion. An increase in urinary pH increases the tubular reabsorption of weak bases, therefore decreasing the urinary excretion and increasing the half-life. Acidification of urine increases urinary excretion of bases and decreases their half-lives.[65] The magnitude of these effects can be significant.

The half-life of amphetamine, a weak base, is doubled when urinary pH is increased from 5 to 8, which may lead to sleepless nights for a person taking the drug during the day.[66,67] Clearances of quinidine and its optical isomer quinine are greatly affected by urinary pH, resulting in changes in electrocardiogram recordings and potential toxicities. Quinidine renal clearance is reduced to one-tenth the level seen when urine pH below 6.0 is increased to 7.5.[68] Other bases that may show pH dependence are amitriptyline, ephedrine, imipramine, meperidine, and methamphetamine.[65]

Acidification of urine increases and alkalinization decreases the half-life of some weak acids. The renal clearance of sulfisoxazole was increased when urine pH changed from 5.3 to 7.4.[69] Other sulfonamides (e.g., sulfaethidole,[70] sulfalene, sulfasymazine,[71] and sulfamethoxazole[72]) have urinary pH dependent elimination. Steady-state salicylate levels were reduced approximately 50% when urinary pH was increased one pH unit with sodium bicarbonate.[73]

Long-term administration of therapeutic doses of common antacids can also affect urine pH. Magnesium hydroxide and calcium carbonate increase urine pH by about 0.5 units, while aluminum–magnesium hydroxide suspension increases pH by 0.9 units.[74] Such changes in urinary pH are also expected to affect the excretion of the before mentioned drugs.

INTERACTIONS AFFECTING DRUG DISTRIBUTION
Clinical Considerations of Changes in Drug Distribution and Protein Binding

As was shown in Fig. 1, drugs are reversibly bound to tissue proteins, plasma proteins, and the receptor. The ratio of free drug to bound drug at each of these sites depends on the properties of the drug, the properties of the binding proteins, and the presence of other competing substances. Where a drug distributes is influenced by many factors such as pH-partitioning, relative lipid solubility, active transport systems, and macromolecular binding such as protein binding.

Distribution to Tissues

Drug distribution to various tissues is governed by three major factors: the blood flow to tissues, the mass of the tissue, and the affinity of the tissue for the drug. A drug is more rapidly equilibrated with tissues having high blood flow (e.g., brain, liver, and kidney) than with tissues having lower blood flow, even though they may have a higher affinity for the drug. For example, the hypnotic effect of thiopental is terminated as the cerebrospinal fluid levels of the lipid-soluble drug rapidly decline while thiopental is more slowly but preferentially distributed to fat tissue.[75]

Many drugs are highly localized in specific tissues. The concentration of the anti-malarial drug quinacrine is 22,000 times greater in the liver than in the serum after 14 days of treatment. When a second antimalarial drug, pamaquine, is administered even months after quinacrine was given, toxic effects of pamaquine may occur because a decreased number of tissue binding sites are available since some are still occupied by quinacrine.[76]

The increased activity of the neuromuscular blocker, hexafluorenium bromide, in the presence of cyclopropane and other "inert" lipid soluble compounds has been attributed to their abilities to displace hexafluorenium from nonspecific tissue storage sites.[77]

Pharmacokinetic evidence indicates that probenecid increases serum levels of penicillins by decreasing the volume of distribution as well as inhibiting renal secretion.[78] This mechanism has been suggested for other interactions.

Plasma Protein Binding

Most drugs and many endogenous compounds (e.g., bilirubin and hormones) are reversibly bound in varying degrees by proteins circulating in the plasma. The fraction of total drug bound to plasma protein is a function of the concentration of drug in the plasma, the concentration of the plasma protein, the number of binding sites on the protein, and the equilibrium affinity constant between the drug and the protein. A decrease in plasma protein concentration will generally be significant only for drugs that are highly plasma protein bound (>90% bound). This effect is easily appreciated by considering the examples of warfarin, which is 95% bound, and phenobarbital, which is

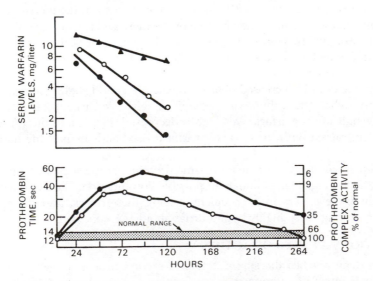

Fig. 16. Serum levels of warfarin (dose of 1.5 mg/kg) and anticoagulant effect when given alone and with phenylbutazone. Key: ▲, after phenylbutazone administration (uncorrected values); ○, before phenylbutazone administration; and ●, after phenylbutazone administration (corrected values). (Adapted with permission from P.M. Aggeler and others: N. Engl. J. Med. **276**:496, 1967.[79])

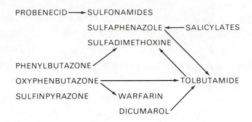

Fig. 17. Some pairs of drugs that are reported to compete for plasma protein binding sites. Drug at arrow tail will displace drug at arrow head.

50% bound. If 5% of warfarin is displaced, the concentration of free warfarin available to diffuse to the site of action is increased 2-fold, from 5% to 10%. If 5% of phenobarbital is displaced, the increase of free phenobarbital is only 10% (from 50% to 55%), which is probably inconsequential.

The unbound fraction may be increased by a second drug that also binds at the same site. The competitive binding would depend on the relative concentrations and affinity constants of the two drugs. Displacement might increase, decrease, or have no effect on the amount of drug at the receptor site, depending on the relative rates of tissue distribution and elimination of the drug. For example, an increase in the fraction of unbound drug in plasma would generally increase the fraction of drug at the tissue receptor, leading to increased pharmacologic effects. The ratio of drug in tissue to drug in plasma would be increased, resulting in an increased apparent volume of distribution. However, the relative rate of elimination may be increased as a result of the increased amount of drug available in the liver to be metabolized or the increased fraction of unbound drug in plasma to be excreted by glomerular filtration. The net result of these effects is that the biologic action may be increased but the total plasma concentration (both bound and unbound drug) is decreased.

An example of both increased pharmacologic effect and slightly increased elimination occurred when phenylbutazone was given with warfarin (97% plasma protein bound). The half-life of warfarin was slightly decreased (Fig. 16). In this example, phenylbutazone interfered with the assay of warfarin used and the half-life had to be corrected.[79]

Several pairs of drugs compete for plasma protein binding sites, leading to increased biological effects (Fig. 17). Although all possible combinations have not been tested, it appears that there is very little specificity among these drugs, and the possibility of competition among these highly bound drugs should be considered.

INTERACTIONS AT SITE OF ACTION

Once a drug reaches the site of action, a second drug may modify the ultimate pharmacologic effect by altering the site of action in several ways including: (1) competition for the receptor site; (2) alteration of the receptor; (3) alteration of other components at the site of action; and (4) effects on a different biologic system that has similar or opposite effects and may augment or diminish the total biologic response. Understanding these types of interactions usually depends on a thorough knowledge of each biologic system involved.

Competition of one agent for another at the receptor site is a well-known phenomenon. Many therapeutic agents such as atropine, propranolol, and tubocurarine can occupy a receptor and block the effects of an active substance such as acetylcholine or epinephrine.[14] Receptor site competition provides one explanation for the increased mortality in patients taking isoproterenol by inhalation. Isoproterenol is metabolized to 3-methylisoproterenol, a weak blocker of the beta-adrenergic receptor site, which blocks the effects of the parent compound and also increases airway obstruction. Increased use of isoproterenol leads to greater accumulation of 3-methylisoproterenol, leading to progressive deterioration of the asthmatic condition.[80] An even more serious consequence of the beta-adrenergic blockade may occur if epinephrine is given parenterally for an acute asthmatic attack. Since epinephrine can stimulate both the alpha- and beta-adrenergic receptors, an exaggerated effect may occur, leading to death.[81,82]

Other agents may interact with the active site to modify the intensity of the response through noncompetitive processes. Thyroxine increases the anticoagulant effect of warfarin in this manner. Potassium depletion by diuretics sensitizes the heart to the pharmacologic effects of the digitalis glycosides.

Modification of other components involved at the site of action can occur by blocking specific metabolizing enzymes at the site of action (e.g., acetylcholinesterase and monoamine oxidase) or by blocking uptake or facilitating release of norepinephrine from storage sites.

Enhancement of effects, elicited by drugs that act at different sites of the same system or different systems with similar biological response, is well known. Sedation may be increased by any combination of alcohol, some antihistamines, barbiturates, benzodiazepines, narcotic analgesics, and phenothiazines, all of which probably have different sites of action. The small amount of blood loss caused by the direct effect of aspirin on gastric mucosa is usually benign but may be exacerbated when anticoagulants are administered.

CLINICAL CONSIDERATIONS REGARDING INTERACTIONS

Not all drug interactions are hazardous. In fact, many types of interactions have been used to therapeutic advantage. Enzyme induction by phenobarbital has been used to reduce bilirubin levels in neonatal hyperbilirubinemia or excessive cortisol levels in patients with increased adrenocortical activity (Cushing's syndrome). Displacement of penicillin from plasma proteins by salicylates or inhibition of renal secretion by probenecid may increase serum and tissue antibacterial levels. Alteration of urinary pH to increase urinary drug excretion is frequently useful in the treatment of drug overdose of phenobarbital or aspirin.

The potentially deleterious interactions may be classified by the severity and the frequency of occurrence. Several interactions are severe and occur almost always when the two drugs are given concurrently. In these cases, the course of action is clear. Surveillance systems must be established to prevent their concurrent use.

Interactions between drugs that are neither frequent nor severe are also manageable. The two drugs are usually administered with the knowledge that dosage adjustments may be necessary. Unfortunately, many interactions fall in the less predictable class that may be severe but occur only in a few patients depending on the dosage regimen of each drug, the age, physiologic and pathologic conditions of the patient, and a host of other unknown variables. In these cases, value judgments must usually be made on the total information available (which is often incomplete), and the course of therapy must be monitored closely.

A good example of the variation that occurs between different individuals can be obtained from the data given in Fig. 14. Five of the subjects receiving phenytoin (300 mg/day) averaged serum levels of 5 μg/ml, which is below the levels usually associated with toxicity (about 20 μg/ml). The sixth subject attained serum levels of 23 μg/ml. When dicumarol was given, this subject's serum level reached the toxic level of 40 μg/ml, whereas the serum levels of the other 5 individuals increased to only 15 μg/ml. Unless previous serum levels of each subject was available, one would be hard pressed to explain why a toxic effect might occur in only one subject. If the initial maintenance dose was doubled in the other 5 subjects, the steady-state serum levels would still be below usual toxic levels. Addition of dicumarol at this dosage level might increase the serum levels sufficiently to result in toxic effects in all 5 patients. Thus, dose and individual variation can be extremely important factors.

Duration of therapy also is a critical factor. Enzyme induction requires several days to take effect and therefore may not occur at all unless a drug is taken over a long period. Inhibition of metabolism usually occurs rapidly. An increase in the half-life may not be immediately apparent until a new steady-state plateau is reached, which requires 6 half-lives. Likewise, an interaction that involves competition for plasma protein binding occurs immediately and is a transient effect, disappearing when the second drug is removed[83] or in some cases during long-term therapy.

There are some general guidelines that indicate the types of patients and drugs most likely to be involved in drug interactions. The age of the patient is apparently one of the most critical factors in determining the potential severity of an interaction. Examination of a large number of interactions that were fatal or nearly fatal shows that in the majority of cases the subject was more than 50 years old. Infants, because of decreased metabolic and renal excretory functions, are also particularly susceptible to drug interactions.

Several disease states such as glaucoma, hypertension, ulcer, renal insufficiency, and diabetes predispose a patient to adverse reactions in general. Patients taking long-term medication including corticosteroids, oral contraceptives, sedatives, and tranquilizers or who are alcoholics are more susceptible, as are those taking inherently toxic agents such as methotrexate at the upper limit of the dosage range. Drugs that must be titrated to the individual such as anticoagulants, anticonvulsants, digitalis, hypoglycemics, quinidine, and theophylline are involved frequently in drug interactions.

References

1. Barr, W.H.: Factors involved in the assessment of systemic or biological availability of drug products, Drug Inform. Bull. **3**:27, 1969.
2. Barr, W.H.: Principles of biopharmaceutics, Am. J. Pharm. Ed. **32**:958, 1968.
3. Levy, G., and others: Effect of an anticholinergic agent on riboflavin absorption in man, J. Pharm. Sci. **61**:798, 1972.
4. Antonioli, J.A., and others: Effect of gastrectomy and of an anticholinergic drug on the gastrointestinal absorption of sulfonamide in man, Int. J. Clin. Pharmacol. **5**:212, 1971.
5. Nimmo, J., and others: Pharmacological modification of gastric emptying: effects of propantheline and metoclopramide on paracetamol absorption, Br. Med. J. **1**:587, 1973.
6. Nimmo, W.S., and others: Inhibition of gastric emptying and drug absorption by narcotic analgesics, Br. J. Clin. Pharmacol. **2**:509, 1975.

7. Nimmo, J.: The influence of metoclopramide on drug absorption, Postgrad. Med. J. **49** (suppl):25,28, 1973.

8. Gothoni, G., and others: Absorption of antibiotics: influence of metoclopramide and atropine on serum levels of pivampicillin and tetracycline, Ann. Clin. Res. **4:**228, 1972.

9. Beermann, B., and Groschinsky-Grind, M.: Enhancement of the gastrointestinal absorption of hydrochlorothiazide by propantheline, Eur. J. Clin. Pharmacol. **13:**385, 1978.

10. Jaffe, J.M.: Effects of propantheline on nitrofurantion absorption, J. Pharm. Sci. **64:**1729, 1975.

11. Manninen, V., and others: Altered absorption of digoxin in patients given propantheline and metoclopramide, Lancet **1:**398, 1973.

12. Schanker, L.W.: Physiological transport of drugs. In Harper, N.J., and Simmonds, A.B., editors: Advances in drug research series, vol. 1, London, 1964, Academic Press.

13. Crouthamel, W.G., and others: Drug absorption IV: influence of pH on absorption kinetics of weakly acidic drugs, J. Pharm. Sci. **60:**1160, 1971.

14. Wass, M., and Evered, D.F.: Transport of penicillamine across mucosa of the rat small intestine, in vitro, Biochem. Pharmacol. **19:**1287, 1970.

15. Siber, G.R., and others: Increased gastrointestinal absorption of large molecules in patients after 5-fluorouracil therapy for metastatic colon carcinoma, Cancer Res. **40:**3430, 1980.

16. Mattila, J.J., and others: Drug absorption in patients with intestinal villous atrophy, Arzneimittelforsch. **23:**583, 1973.

17. Jusko, W.J., and others: Digoxin absorption from tablets and elixir: the effect of radiation-induced malabsorption, J.A.M.A. **230:**1554, 1974.

18. Sandle, G.I., and others: Propranolol absorption in untreated coeliac disease, Clin. Sci. **63:**81, 1982.

19. Gerson, C.D., and others: Bioavailability of digoxin tablets in patients with gastrointestinal dysfunction, Am. J. Med. **69:**43, 1980.

20. Backman, L., and others: Malabsorption of hydrochlorothiazide following intestinal shunt surgery, Clin. Pharmacokinet. **4:**63, 1979.

21. Kennedy, M.C.V., and Wade, D.N.: Phenytoin absorption in patients with ileojejunal bypass, Br. J. Clin. Pharmacol. **7:**515, 1979.

22. Wagner, J.G.: Biopharmaceutics: absorption aspects, J. Pharm. Sci. **50:**539, 1961.

23. Sorby, D.L.: Effect of adsorbents on drug absorption. I. Modification of promazine absorption by activated attapulgite and activated charcoal, J. Pharm. Sci. **54:**677, 1965.

24. Northcutt, R.C., and others: The influence of cholestyramine on thyroxine absorption, J.A.M.A. **208:**1857, 1969.

25. Robinson, D.S., and others: Interaction of warfarin and non-systemic gastrointestinal drugs, Clin. Pharmacol. Ther. **12:**491, 1971.

26. Mahfouz, M.: Fate of tubocurarine in the body, Br. J. Pharmacol. **4:**295, 1949.

27. Faloon, W.W., and others: Effect of neomycin and kanamycin on intestinal absorption, Ann. N.Y. Acad. Sci. **132:**879, 1966.

28. Singh, P., and others: Effect of inert table ingredients on drug absorption. I. Effect of PEG 4000 on intestinal absorption of four barbiturates, J. Pharm. Sci. **55:**63, 1966.

29. Wagner, J.G., and others: Blood levels of drug at the equilibrium state after multiple dosing, Nature **207:**1301, 1965.

30. Conney, A.H.: Pharmacological implications of microsomal enzyme induction, Pharmacol. Rev. **19:**317, 1967.

31. Levine, R.R.: Pharmacology: drug actions and reactions, 2nd edition, Boston, 1978, Little, Brown and Company.

32. Jusko, W.J.: Role of tobacco in pharmacokinetics, J. Pharmacokinet. Biopharm. **6:**7, 1979.

33. Jusko, W.J.: Influence of cigarette smoking on drug metabolism in man, Drug Metab. Rev. **9:**221, 1979.

34. Breckenridge, A.M., and Orme, M. L'E.: Clinical implications of enzyme induction, Ann. N.Y. Acad. Sci. **179:**421, 1971.

35. Hempel, E., and Klinger, W.: Drug stimulated biotransformation of hormonal steroid contraceptives: clinical implications, Drugs **12:**442, 1976.

36. Udall, J.A.: Clinical implications of warfarin interactions with five sedatives, Am. J. Cardiol. **35:**67, 1975.

37. Alvan, G., and others: Effect of pentobarbital on the disposition of alprenolol, Clin. Pharmacol. Ther. **22:**316, 1977.
38. Lai, A.A., and others: Time course of interaction between carbamazepine and clonazepam in normal man, Clin. Pharmacol. Ther. **24:**316, 1978.
39. Kappas, A., and others: Influence of dietary protein and carbohydrate on antipyrine and theophylline metabolism, Clin. Pharmacol. Ther. **20:**643, 1976.
40. Pantuck, E.J., and others: Stimulatory effect of brussels sprouts and cabbage in human drug metabolism, Clin. Pharmacol. Ther. **25:**88, 1979.
41. Conney, A.H., and others: Enhanced phenacetin metabolism in human subjects fed charcoal-broiled beef, Clin. Pharmacol. Ther. **20:**633, 1976.
42. Kappas, A., and others: Effect of charcoal-broiled beef on antipyrine and theophylline metabolism, Clin. Pharmacol. Ther. **23:**445, 1978.
43. Kolmodin, B., and others: Effect of environmental factors on drug metabolism: decreased plasma half-life of antipyrine in workers exposed to chlorinated hydrocarbon insecticides, Clin. Pharmacol. Ther. **10:**638, 1969.
44. Hansen, J.M., and others: Dicoumarol-induced diphenylhydantoin intoxication, Lancet **2:**265, 1966.
45. Christensen, L.K., and Skousted, L.: Inhibition of drug metabolism by chloramphenicol, Lancet **2:**1397, 1969.
46. Pedersen, A.K., and others: Clinical pharmacokinetics and potentially important drug interactions of sulphinpyrazone, Clin. Pharmacokinet. **7:**42, 1982.
47. Vestal, R.E., and others: Inhibition of propranolol metabolism by chlorpromazine, Clin. Pharmacol. Ther. **25:**19, 1979.
48. Wilder, B.J., and Cramer, J.A.: Valproic acid: interaction with other anticonvulsant drugs, Neurology **28:**892, 1978.
49. Mattson, R.H., and Cramer, J.A.: Valproic acid and ethosuximide interaction, Ann. Neurol. **7:**583, 1980.
50. Serlin, M.J., and others: Cimetidine interactions with oral anticoagulants in man, Lancet **2:**317, 1979.
51. Somogyi, A., and Gugler, R.: Drug interactions with cimetidine, Clin. Pharmacokinet. **7:**23, 1982.
52. Levy, G., and Amsel, L.P.: Kinetics of competitive inhibition of salicylic acid conjugation with glycine in man, Biochem. Pharmacol. **15:**1033, 1966.
53. Levy G., and Procknal, J.: Drug biotransformation interactions in man. I. Mutual inhibition in glucuronide formation of salicylic acid and salicylamide in man, J. Pharm. Sci. **57:**1330, 1968.
54. Levy, G., and Yamada, H.: Drug biotransformation interactions in man. III. Acetaminophen and salicylamide, J. Pharm. Sci. **60:**215, 1971.
55. Vesell, E.S., and others: Impairment of drug metabolism by disulfiram in man, Clin. Pharmacol. Ther. **12:**785, 1971.
56. O'Reilly, R.A.: Interaction of disulfiram (Antabuse) in man, Ann. Intern. Med. **78:**73, 1973.
57. Svendsen, T.L., and others: The influence of disulfiram on the half-life and metabolic clearance rate of diphenylhydantoin and tolbutamide in man, Eur. J. Clin. Pharmacol. **9:**439, 1976.
58. Kunin, C.M., and others: Distribution and excretion of four tetracycline analogues in normal young men, J. Clin. Invest. **38:**1950, 1959.
59. Tilstone, W.J., and others: Effects of furosemide on glomerular filtration rate and clearance of practolol, digoxin, cephaloridine, and gentamicin, Clin. Pharmacol. Ther. **22:**389, 1977.
60. Weiner, I.M., and Mudge, G.H.: Renal tubular mechanisms for excretion of organic acids and bases, Am. J. Med. **36:**743, 1964.
61. Offerhaus, L.: Drug interactions at excretory mechanisms, Pharmacol. Ther. **15:**69, 1981.
62. Leahey, E.B., and others: Interaction between quinidine and digoxin, J.A.M.A. **240:**533, 1978.
63. Pedersen, K.E., and others: Digoxin-verapamil interaction, Clin. Pharmacol. Ther. **30:**311, 1981.
64. Moysey, J.O., and others: Amiodarone increases plasma digoxin concentrations, Br. Med. J. **282:**272, 1981.
65. Milne, M.D.: Influence of acid-base balance on efficacy and toxicity of drugs, Proc. R. Soc. Med. **58:**961, 1965.
66. Beckett, A.H., and Rowland, M.: Urinary excretion kinetics of amphetamine in man, J. Pharm. Pharmacol. **17:**628, 1965.

67. Asatoor, A.M., and others: The excretion of dextroamphetamine and its derivatives, Br. J. Pharmacol. Chemother. **24:**293, 1965.
68. Kostenbauder, H.B., and others: Quinidine excretion in aciduria and alkaluria, Ann. Intern. Med. **71:**927, 1969.
69. Cohen, M., and Pocelinko, R.: Renal transport mechanisms for the excretion of sulfisoxazole, J. Pharmacol. Exp. Ther. **185:**703, 1973.
70. Kostenbauder, H.B., and others: Control of urine pH and its effect on sulfaethidole excretion in humans, J. Pharm. Sci. **51:**1084, 1962.
71. Dettli, L., and others: The influence of alkali administration on the biological half-life of two sulfon-amides in human blood serum, Int. J. Clin. Pharmacol. **2:**130, 1967.
72. Vree, T.B., and others: Pharmacokinetics of sulfamethoxazole in man: effects of urinary pH and urine flow on metabolism and renal excretion of sulfamethoxazole and its metabolite N_4-acetylsulfame-thoxazole, Clin. Pharmacokinet. **3:**319, 1978.
73. Levy, G., and Leonards, J.R.: Urine pH and salicylate therapy, J.A.M.A. **217:**81, 1971.
74. Gibaldi, M., and others: Effects of antacids on pH of urine, Clin. Pharmacol. Ther. **16:**520, 1974.
75. Brodie, B.B.: Displacement of one drug by another from carrier or receptor sites, Proc. R. Soc. Med. **58:**946, 1965.
76. Brodie, B.B.: Physicochemical factors in drug absorption. In Binns, T.B., editor: Absorption and distribution of drugs, Edinburgh, 1964, E. & S. Livingstone, Ltd.
77. Cavallito, C.J., and others: Influence of anesthesia on the neuromuscular blocking activity of mylaxen, Anesthesiology **17:**547, 1956.
78. Gibaldi, M., and Schwartz, M.A.: Apparent effect of probenecid on the distribution of penicillins in man, Clin. Pharmacol. Ther. **9:**345, 1968.
79. Aggeler, P.M., and others: Potentiation of anticoagulant effect of warfarin by phenylbutazone, N. Engl. J. Med. **276:**496, 1967.
80. Paterson, J.W., and others: Isoprenaline resistance and the use of pressurised aerosols in asthma, Lancet **2:**426, 1968.
81. McManis, A.G.: Deaths following IV epinephrine in patients using isoproterenol, Med. J. Aust. **2:**76, 1964.
82. Refshauge, W.D.: Deaths due to epinephrine and self administered isoproterenol, Med. J. Aust. **1:**93, 1965.
83. Koch-Weser, J., and Sellers, E.M.: Drug interactions with coumarin anticoagulants, N. Engl. J. Med. **285:**487,547, 1971.

CHAPTER ONE

Analgesic Drug Interactions: Narcotics, Nonnarcotics, Nonsteroidal Anti-inflammatory Agents, and Agents for Gout

*Not available in the U.S.

TABLE 1. Analgesic Drug Interactions

Drug Interaction	Significance Code	Potential Effects	Recommendations	See Page
Allopurinol–Probenecid	3	Probenecid may decrease the effectiveness of allopurinol. Allopurinol may prolong the half-life of probenecid. Inhibition of uric acid production may be decreased.	Concurrent use need not be avoided. However, use cautiously in patients with impaired renal function because of the danger of precipitation of urate or urate precursors in the kidney.	33
Aspirin–Alcohol, Ethyl	2	Alcohol potentiates the erosive effects of aspirin, increases fecal blood loss, and may prolong bleeding time related to aspirin.	Although this combination does not appear to present a significant problem in normal subjects, avoid in those with predisposition to gastrointestinal disease.	34
Aspirin–Aluminum Hydroxide, Magnesium Hydroxide	2	Antacids decrease serum levels of aspirin to varying degrees and cause premature release of enteric-coated aspirin.	Antacids should be used cautiously with high dose aspirin therapy and should not be ingested simultaneously with enteric-coated aspirin.	36
Aspirin–Hydrocortisone	3	Hydrocortisone may increase the renal clearance of aspirin. Discontinuing or tapering steroid therapy may increase serum levels of aspirin.	Concurrent use need not be avoided. Aspirin dosage may need to be decreased when steroid therapy is discontinued.	38
Indomethacin–Aspirin	3	Aspirin may decrease the absorption, increase enterohepatic circulation and biliary excretion, and in large doses decrease serum levels of indomethacin.	Since these drugs have similar pharmacologic activity and aspirin-induced changes are generally small, this interaction is of minimal significance and concomitant use need not be avoided.	39
Indomethacin–Phenylpropanolamine	2	A single report of serious hypertension after concurrent use of these agents has been published.	Monitor blood pressure frequently during the first hour after administration. If a hypertensive episode should occur, phentolamine has been used to reduce the blood pressure.	41
Indomethacin–Probenecid	2	Probenecid may reduce plasma clearance and elevate plasma levels of indomethacin, and probenecid may also induce a reduction in nonrenal clearance of indomethacin.	Reduced indomethacin dosage may need to be considered.	42
Meperidine–Chlorpromazine	2	Chlorpromazine potentiates the sedative, hypotensive, and respiratory depressant properties of meperidine.	Meperidine dose may need to be reduced.	43

Abbreviations: CNS, central nervous system; GI, gastrointestinal.

TABLE 1. Analgesic Drug Interactions—cont'd

Drug Interaction	Significance Code	Potential Effects	Recommendations	See Page
Meperidine–Phenelzine	1	Concurrent use may cause excitatory and depressant effects on the CNS leading to deep coma and death. This interaction may occur several weeks after discontinuation of phenelzine.	Avoid concomitant use, substituting a noninteracting narcotic (i.e., morphine, methadone) after a small test dose.	44
Meperidine–Phenytoin	3	Phenytoin may cause increased systemic clearance as well as decreased elimination half-life and bioavailability of meperidine. Analgesia may be decreased and toxicity may increase because of increased plasma levels of the metabolite normeperidine.	Intravenous rather than oral doses of meperidine may be preferable, as well as more frequent and larger doses.	46
Methadone–Diazepam	4	No apparent alteration occurs in methadone serum levels, urinary excretion, or plasma protein binding after concurrent diazepam.	Concurrent use need not be avoided.	47
Methadone–Rifampin	2	Narcotic withdrawal symptoms may occur following concurrent therapy.	Methadone dosage may need to be increased. If methadone is being used to treat narcotic withdrawal, clonidine may be substituted since it has been effective in averting withdrawal symptoms.	48
Morphine–Cimetidine	2	Concurrent use of these agents may lead to serious CNS side effects such as apnea, confusion, disorientation, and respiratory depression.	The dose of morphine may need to be decreased or discontinued if CNS effects develop. Naloxone has reversed these effects.	49
Oxyphenbutazone–Methandrostenolone*	3	Methandrostenolone may elevate oxyphenbutazone levels by approximately 50%. Phenylbutazone is unaffected by methandrostenolone.	Monitor closely for oxyphenbutazone toxicity.	50
Phenylbutazone–Cholestyramine	4	Although not documented in vivo, cholestyramine may delay or decrease absorption of phenylbutazone based on in vitro studies.	Administer phenylbutazone 1 hour before or 4-6 hours after cholestyramine to avoid possible interaction.	51

*Not available in the U.S.

TABLE 1. Analgesic Drug Interactions—cont'd

Drug Interaction	Significance Code	Potential Effects	Recommendations	See Page
Phenylbutazone–Desipramine	3	Desipramine may cause reduced plasma levels of phenylbutazone, probably by delaying GI absorption because of its anticholinergic effect.	Patients may be monitored for possible decreased phenylbutazone effects. However, since only the rate of phenylbutazone absorption is affected, the clinical significance may be minor.	52
Phenylbutazone–Phenobarbital	3	Phenobarbital may reduce the half-life of phenylbutazone, and this may continue for several days after discontinuation of phenobarbital.	Monitor patients for a decreased response to phenylbutazone; a higher dose of phenylbutazone may be necessary.	53
Probenecid–Clofibrate	3	Probenecid may reduce the renal and metabolic clearance of clofibric acid (the deesterified active form of clofibrate), which may increase toxic and therapeutic effects of clofibrate, although this has not been documented.	A lower dose of clofibrate may be necessary.	54
Propoxyphene–Alcohol, Ethyl	2	Alcohol may increase systemic availability and lower minimum lethal blood concentration of propoxyphene, resulting in respiratory and CNS depression and death.	Although moderate amounts of alcohol with usual doses of propoxyphene may not present problems, patients should be warned against excessive use of either agent.	55
Propoxyphene–Amphetamine	3	Amphetamine may increase the seizure potential of propoxyphene when used to treat CNS depression from propoxyphene overdose.	It is not recommended that CNS depression from propoxyphene overdose be treated with amphetamine.	56
Propoxyphene–Orphenadrine	4	Interaction between these agents cannot be substantiated, since similar CNS effects are seen with either drug alone.	Concurrent use need not be avoided, although it may be prudent to be aware of a possible interaction and reduce the dose or discontinue one or both drugs.	57
Sulfinpyrazone–Aspirin	2	Aspirin antagonizes uricosuric activity and may also decrease the antiplatelet effect of sulfinpyrazone. Sulfinpyrazone may also inhibit the uricosuria that follows large doses of aspirin.	Avoid concomitant use, especially aspirin in large doses.	58
Sulfinpyrazone–Niacin	3	The concurrent use of these agents may inhibit the uricosuric activity of sulfinpyrazone.	Discontinue niacin if decreased uricosuric activity of sulfinpyrazone occurs.	60
Sulfinpyrazone–Probenecid	4	Probenecid blocks the renal tubular secretion of sulfinpyrazone, and thus concurrent use may increase uric acid secretion.	Avoid concurrent use since the possible benefits would be negligible.	61

Allopurinol–Probenecid

3

Summary: Concurrent use of allopurinol and probenecid may decrease the effectiveness of allopurinol. However, the clinical significance of this effect has not been established, and concurrent therapy may be useful in therapeutic situations requiring both a maximum reduction in uric acid production and a maximum increase in uric acid excretion (e.g., congenital overproduction of uric acid).

Related Drugs: Sulfinpyrazone can be expected to have an effect similar to that of probenecid.[1,2] There are no drugs related to allopurinol.

Mechanism: Various mechanisms have been proposed for the allopurinol-probenecid interaction. Allopurinol may inhibit the metabolism of probenecid, thereby prolonging the half-life of probenecid.[3,4] Probenecid may increase the renal excretion of oxypurinol (alloxanthine), the active metabolite of allopurinol, resulting in a decrease in the overall inhibition of uric acid production.[5]

Recommendations: The concurrent administration of allopurinol and probenecid need not be avoided. However, this regimen should be used cautiously in patients with impaired renal function because of the danger of urate or urate precursors forming in the kidney. Fluid intake should be maintained at a level of 3 liters/day in all patients taking these drugs. Alkalinization of the urine may also be desirable as a means of promoting and ensuring adequate uric acid clearance through the kidney.[6]

References

1. Yu, T.F., and Gutman, A.B.: Effect of allopurinol (4-hydroxypyrazolo [3,4-d] pryimidine) on serum and urinary uric acid in primary and secondary gout, Am. J. Med. **37:**885, 1964.
2. Goldfinger, S., and others: The renal excretion of oxypurines, J. Clin. Invest. **44:**623, 1972.
3. Tjandramaga, T.B., and others: Observations on the disposition of probenecid in patients receiving allopurinol, Pharmacology **8:**259, 1972.
4. Yu, T.F.: In Gutman, A.B., editor: Gout, Research Triangle Park, N.C. 1971, Medcom, Burroughs-Wellcome.
5. Elion, G.B., and others: Metabolic studies of allopurinol, an inhibitor of xanthine oxidase, Biochem. Pharmacol. **15:**863, 1966.
6. Rastegar, A., and Thier, S.O.: The treatment of hyperuricemia in gout, Ration. Drug. Ther. **8:**1, 1974.

Aspirin–Alcohol, Ethyl

2

Summary: Either aspirin or alcohol alone will disrupt the gastric mucosal barrier,[1-4] and alcohol potentiates the erosive effects of aspirin resulting in increased fecal blood loss.[4-7] It has also been recently reported that alcohol enhances the prolongation of bleeding time produced by aspirin ingestion.[8] Although these interactions occur in nearly all persons, there is only indirect evidence that the combination results in increased morbidity.[9,10] Considering that this combination must be widely employed by much of the population, it would seem that this interaction is only significant in patients with predisposing risk factors such as gastrointestinal bleeding or those receiving anticoagulant therapy.

Related Drugs: Buffered salicylate products do not produce increased gastrointestinal blood loss when combined with alcohol[4,11,12] and may actually protect against alcohol-induced irritation of gastric mucosa.[4] Alcohol plus choline salicylate did not affect bleeding time.[4] Other salicylates (e.g., salicylamide, salsalate, sodium salicylate, [see Appendix]) do not inhibit platelet aggregation as does aspirin, but they do affect clotting factor synthesis and are irritating to the gastric mucosa.[13] Therefore, alcohol may be expected to interact with these salicylates in a manner similar to aspirin regarding the potentiation of the erosive effects on the gastric mucosa. There was no significant effect on fecal blood loss when alcohol was coadministered with diflunisal.[7]

Mechanism: Un-ionized aspirin breaks down the normal gastric mucosal barrier against back diffusion of hydrogen ions and leakage of other ions, which results in injury to the submucosal capillaries, necrosis, and bleeding.[2,14,15] Alcohol is also irritating to the gastrointestinal mucosa[3,15] and potentiates the mucosal effects of aspirin.[15]

Aspirin affects hemostasis by inhibiting platelet function and depressing clotting factor synthesis in large doses.[16] By an unknown mechanism, alcohol potentiates the prolonged bleeding time associated with aspirin therapy.[8]

Recommendations: The combination of alcohol and aspirin should be avoided in patients predisposed to gastrointestinal disease. Concurrent use does not appear to present a significant problem in normal subjects. Predisposed patients requiring an analgesic may use acetaminophen or buffered aspirin. Patients receiving aspirin for its hematologic (antiplatelet) effects should be cautioned about the potential hazards of concurrent alcohol use.

References

1. Geall, M.G., and others: Profile of gastric potential difference in man: effects of aspirin, alcohol, bile and endogenous acid, Gastroenterology **58:**437, 1970.
2. Flower, R.J., and others: Analgesic-antipyretics and anti-inflammatory agents: drugs employed in the treatment of gout. In Gilman, A.G., Goodman, L.S., and Gilman, A., editors: The pharmacological basis of therapeutics, New York, 1980, MacMillan Publishing.
3. Ritchie, J.M.: The aliphatic alcohols. In Gilman, A.G., Goodman, L.S., and Gilman, A., editors: The pharmacological basis of therapeutics, New York, 1980, MacMillan Publishing.

4. Murray, H.S., and others: Effect of several drugs on gastric potential differences in man, Br. Med. J. **1:**19, 1974.
5. Goulston, K., and Cooke, A.R.: Alcohol, aspirin and gastrointestinal bleeding, Br. Med. J. **4:**664, 1968.
6. DeSchepper, P.J., and others: Gastrointestinal blood loss after diflunisal and after aspirin: effect of ethanol, Clin. Pharmacol. Ther. **23:**669, 1978.
7. DeSchepper P.J., and others: Diflunisal versus aspirin: a comparative study of their effect on faecal blood loss in the presence and absence of alcohol, Curr. Med. Res. Opin. **5:**520, 1978.
8. Deykin, D., and others: Ethanol potentiation of aspirin-induced prolongation of the bleeding time, N. Engl. J. Med. **306:**852, 1982.
9. Needham, C.D., and others: Aspirin and alcohol in gastrointestinal hemorrhage, Gut **12:**819, 1971.
10. Caranasos, G.J., and others: Drug-induced illness leading to hospitalization, J.A.M.A. **228:**713, 1974.
11. Bouchier, I.A.D., and Williams, H.S.: Determination of faecal blood loss after combined alcohol and sodium acetylsalicylate intake, Lancet **1:**178, 1969.
12. Leonards, J.R.: Faecal blood loss after sodium acetylsalicylate taken with alcohol, Lancet **1:**943, 1969.
13. Bowman, W.C., and Rand, M.J.: Textbook of Pharmacology, London, 1980, Blackwell Publication.
14. Leonards, J.R., and Levy, G.: Gastrointestinal blood loss during prolonged aspirin administration, N. Engl. J. Med. **289:**1020, 1973.
15. Smith, B.M., and others: Permeability of the human gastric mucosa: alteration by acetylsalicylic acid and ethanol, N. Engl. J. Med. **285:**716, 1971.
16. Rothschild, B.M.: Hematologic perturbations associated with salicylate, Clin. Pharmacol. Ther. **26:**145, 1979.

Aspirin–Aluminum Hydroxide, Magnesium Hydroxide

2

Summary: Decreased serum salicylate levels have been reported following the concurrent administration of a combination antacid preparation containing aluminum hydroxide and magnesium hydroxide with aspirin. Concomitant dosing of aluminum hydroxide and magnesium hydroxide plus aspirin caused serum salicylate levels to decrease 30% to 70% in a study involving 3 children who were receiving other medications.[1] Aluminum hydroxide alone was given with enteric-coated aspirin and resulted in an enhanced salicylate renal excretion rate[2] in one case, while the administration of preparations containing aluminum hydroxide showed that the peak salicylate excretion time is decreased approximately 2 hours.[3] However, studies in healthy subjects indicate no antacid-induced change in aspirin bioavailability, only an increased renal clearance.[1,3,4]

Related Drugs: Magnesium trisilicate[2] and sodium bicarbonate[5,6] have been shown to have a similar influence on salicylate levels or excretion. It is anticipated that a similar effect would be seen with calcium carbonate since it is capable of alkalinizing the urinary pH about one-half pH unit.[7] There is one report in which aluminum hydroxide and dihydroxyaluminum aminoacetate suspension had no effect on urinary pH.[7] It has not been documented whether these formulations will change serum salicylate concentrations. Decreased salicylate concentrations were seen when choline salicylate was coadministered with a preparation containing aluminum hydroxide and magnesium hydroxide. One study found a significant decrease in serum choline salicylate concentration only in subjects who developed serum levels above 10 mg/dl. This would suggest that patients with serum levels less than 10 mg/dl will have minimal changes in serum choline salicylate levels when antacids are simultaneously administered.[4] Other salicylate preparations (e.g., salsalate, sodium salicylate, salicylamide [see Appendix]) would be expected to undergo a similar interaction due to pharmacological similarity. Two studies indicate that the bioavailability, plasma concentration, and urinary excretion of diflunisal (a salicylate derivative) are reduced by concurrent aluminum hydroxide.[8,9] Another report describes a reduced absorption and excretion of diflunisal when administered with an aluminum–magnesium hydroxide antacid combination.[10] However, one study states that magnesium hydroxide actually increased the early plasma concentration and area-under-curve of diflunisal while having no effect on urinary excretion, whereas a combination of aluminum–magnesium hydroxide had no effect on diflunisal when administered after eating.[8]

Mechanism: The decreased serum salicylate concentration is attributed to an increase in urine alkalinity from the presence of the magnesium ion, resulting in an increase in renal salicylate clearance.[1,4] With enteric-coated products, the increased gastric pH from antacid administration may result in delivery of the salicylate to the gastric area or a decreased gastric transit time, either of which could account for the enhanced salicylate excretion rate.[3,4]

Recommendations: Patients should be counseled before initiating, switching, or discontinuing antacid use while on high dose salicylate therapy, since different antacids affect salicylate levels to varying degrees because of differing extents of urinary alkalinization. Patients using enteric-coated products should be advised not to ingest antacids simultaneously to avoid premature drug release from this particular dosage form.

References

1. Levy, G., and others: Decreased serum salicylate concentrations in children with rheumatic fever treated with antacid, N. Engl. J. Med. **293:**323, 1975.
2. Strickland-Hodge, B., and others: The effects of antacids on enteric-coated salicylate preparations, Rheumatol. Rehabil. **15:**148, 1976.
3. Feldman, S., and Carlstedt, B.C.: Effect of antacid on absorption of enteric-coated aspirin, J.A.M.A. **227:**660, 1974.
4. Hansten, P.D., and Hayton, W.L.: Effect of antacid and ascorbic acid on serum salicylate concentration, J. Clin. Pharmacol. **24:**326, 1980.
5. Levy, G., and Leonards, J.R.: Urine pH and salicylate therapy, J.A.M.A. **217:**81, 1971.
6. Prescott, L.F., and others: Diuresis or urinary alkalinization for salicylate poisoning, Br. Med. J. **285:**1383, 1982.
7. Gibaldi, M., and others: Effect of antacids on pH of urine, Clin. Pharmacol. Ther. **16:**520, 1974.
8. Tobert, J.A., and others: Effect of antacids on the bioavailability of diflunisal in the fasting and postprandial states, Clin. Pharmacol. Ther. **30:**385, 1981.
9. Verbeck, R., and others: Effect of aluminum hydroxide on diflunisal absorption, Br. J. Clin. Pharmacol. **7:**519, 1979.
10. Holmes, G.I., and others: Effects of Maalox on the bioavailability of diflunisal, Clin. Pharmacol. Ther. **25:**229, 1979.

Aspirin–Hydrocortisone

3

Summary: Corticosteroids, including hydrocortisone, may increase the renal clearance of salicylates during concurrent therapy. Conversely, discontinuation or tapering of steroid therapy may result in a corresponding increase in serum salicylate levels.[1] Aspirin and hydrocortisone may theoretically exert combined deleterious effects on the gastric mucosa, but this remains unsupported by clinical evidence.

Related Drugs: Two patients stabilized on choline salicylate and prednisone had a 3- to 10-fold increase in serum salicylate levels when prednisone therapy was decreased and ultimately discontinued. Other corticosteroids (e.g., betamethasone, dexamethasone, triamcinolone [see Appendix]) and salicylates (e.g., sodium salicylate, salicylamide, salsalate [see Appendix]) may be expected to produce similar results due to pharmacologic similarity, although no documentation exists.

Mechanism: When both agents are used chronically, steroids may increase free salicylate clearance primarily through an increase in glomerular filtration rate. Altered renal tubular transport mechanisms and extrarenal metabolism have also been suggested as possible reasons for enhanced salicylate excretion, although no evidence exists to support this.[1] Both aspirin and corticosteroids can adversely affect the gastric mucosa by different mechanisms. Aspirin use results in exfoliation of mucosal cells without an accompanying increase in renewal rate, deterioration of the hydrogen ion barrier, decreased mucous production, and retardation of connective tissue repair.[2-4] Steroids are thought to delay the process of wound healing, possibly by decreased epithelial cell renewal.[5,6] Steroids also increase gastric acid secretion and reduce mucous secretion.[2] Ulcerogenesis attributable to steroids, however, has been disputed.[7] No carefully controlled studies have demonstrated an increased incidence of peptic ulceration in humans when steroids and salicylates are given together.

Recommendations: Concurrent administration of aspirin and hydrocortisone need not be avoided, but patients receiving both should be observed closely for adverse gastrointestinal effects. It may also be necessary to reduce the salicylate dosage when steroid therapy is discontinued.

References

1. Klinenberg, J.R., and Miller, F.: Effect of corticosteroids on blood salicylate concentration, J.A.M.A. **194:**131, 1965.
2. Ivey, K.J., and others: Effect of prednisolone and salicylic acid on ionic fluxes across the human stomach, Aust. N. Z. J. Med. **5:**408, 1975.
3. Hunt, T.K.: Injury and repair in acute gastroduodenal ulceration, Am. J. Surg. **125:**12, 1973.
4. Bolton, J.P., and Cohen, M.M.: Effect of repeated aspirin administration on the gastric mucosal barrier and cell turnover, J. Surg. Res. **23:**251, 1977.
5. Croft, D.N.: Cell turnover and loss and the gastric mucosal barrier, Dig. Dis. Sci. **22:**383, 1977.
6. Eastwood, G.L., and others: Effects of chronic steroid ingestion on gastroduodenal epithelial renewal in the rat, Tissue Kinet. **14:**405, 1981.
7. Conn, H.O., and Blitzer, B.L.: Nonassociation of adrenocorticosteroid therapy and peptic ulcer, N. Engl. J. Med., **294:**473, 1976.

Indomethacin–Aspirin

Summary: Concurrent administration of indomethacin and large doses of aspirin (3 to 4 g/day) have been shown to decrease the serum levels of indomethacin.[1-5] In one study, mean plasma levels of indomethacin were reduced by 20% after a single 1200 mg dose of aspirin, by smaller amounts after multiple dosing, and not at all after intravenous indomethacin administration.[5] Buffered aspirin either increases[6] or does not change[7,8] indomethacin absorption. Because these drugs have similar pharmacologic activity, and aspirin-induced changes in indomethacin blood levels are generally small, this interaction is of minimal clinical significance.[9] Salicylate accumulation is not affected by concurrent use of indomethacin.[5]

Related Drugs: Sodium salicylate has also been shown to interact with other nonsteroidal anti-inflammatory agents (NSAIAs).[10] Documentation is lacking regarding an interaction between indomethacin and other salicylates (e.g., choline salicylate, salicylamide, salsalate [see Appendix]), although two reports suggest the salicylate moiety, rather than aspirin itself, is probably responsible for the interaction.[5,11]

Decreased serum levels of several other nonsteroidal anti-inflammatory agents have also been reported with concurrent aspirin use, including fenoprofen,[2,12,13] ibuprofen,[14-16] meclofenamate,[17] tolmetin,[18,19] and naproxen.[20-23] Although the interaction results in decreased serum levels of the nonsteroidal anti-inflammatory agent, the postulated mechanism differs from that proposed for indomethacin.

Mechanism: The mechanism has not been fully elucidated. However, aspirin decreases the bioavailability of oral but not intravenous[5] or rectal[24] indomethacin. The interaction may therefore be explained by aspirin's ability to decrease indomethacin absorption and increase its enterohepatic circulation and biliary excretion.[5,11]

The postulated mechanism for the other NSAIAs involves aspirin causing a slight decrease in NSAIA plasma levels caused by displacement from plasma protein binding sites. This results in increased metabolism and renal clearance of the free fraction of the NSAIA.[17,18,20-23,25-27]

Recommendations: Because concurrent administration of these agents offers no therapeutic advantage over higher doses of either drug alone, concurrent use is not recommended. However, the clinical significance of this interaction appears to be minimal, and concomitant use need not be avoided.

References

1. Jeremy, R., and Towson, J.: Interaction between aspirin and indomethacin in the treatment of rheumatoid arthritis, Med. J. Aust. **2:**127, 1970.
2. Rubin, A., and others: Interactions of aspirin with nonsteroidal anti-inflammatory drugs in man, Arthritis Rheum. **16:**635, 1973.
3. Moller, P.W.: Proceedings: anti-inflammatory drugs and their interactions, N.Z. Med. J. **76:**78, 1973.
4. Kaldestad, E., and others: Interaction of indomethacin and acetylsalicylic acid as shown by serum concentrations of indomethacin and salicylate, Eur. J. Clin. Pharmacol. **9:**199, 1975.
5. Kwan, K.C., and others: Effects of concomitant aspirin administration on the pharmacokinetics of indomethacin in man, J. Pharmacokinet. Biopharm. **6:**451, 1978.

6. Garnham, J.C., and others: The effect of buffered aspirin on plasma indomethacin, Eur. J. Clin. Pharmacol. **8:**107, 1975.
7. Brooks, P.M., and others: Indomethacin-aspirin interactions: a clinical appraisal, Br. Med. J. **3:**69, 1975.
8. Champion, G.D., and others: The effect of aspirin on serum indomethacin, Clin. Pharmacol. Ther. **13:**239, 1972.
9. Miller, D.R.: Combination use of nonsteroidal anti-inflammatory drugs, Drug Intell. Clin. Pharm. **15:**3, 1981.
10. Ezer, E., and others: Antagonism of the gastrointestinal ulcerogenic effect of some nonsteroidal anti-inflammatory agents by sodium salicylate, J. Pharm. Pharmacol. **28:**655, 1976.
11. Yesair, D.W., and others: Comparative effects of salicylic acid, phenylbutazone, probenecid, and other anions on the absorption, metabolism, distribution, and excretion of indomethacin by rats, Biochem. Pharmacol. **19:**1591, 1970.
12. Warrick, P., and Rubin, A.: Interactions in rats between the nonsteroidal anti-inflammatory drugs; aspirin and fenoprofen, Proc. Soc. Exp. Biol. Med. **147:**599, 1974.
13. Gruber, C.M.: Clinical pharmacology of fenoprofen: a review, Scand. J. Rheumatol. **2**(suppl.):8, 1976.
14. Kaiser, D.G., and Glenn, E.M.: Aspirin-ibuprofen interaction in the adjuvant-induced polyarthritic rat, Res. Commun. Chem. Pathol. Pharmacol. **9:**583, 1974.
15. Greenan, D.M., and others: The aspirin-ibuprofen interaction in rheumatoid arthritis, Br. J. Clin. Pharmacol. **8:**497, 1979.
16. Kimberly, R.P., and others: Apparent acute renal failure associated with therapeutic aspirin and ibuprofen administration, Arthritis Rheum. **22:**281, 1979.
17. Barger, F.D., and Smith, T.C.: Drug interactions with sodium meclofenamate (Meclomen®), Curr. Ther. Res. **23:**S-51, 1978.
18. Cressman, W.A., and others: Absorption and excretion of tolmetin in man, Clin. Pharmacol. Ther. **19:**224, 1975.
19. Chalers, A., and others: A double-blind study comparing the use of ASA and tolmetin with ASA and placebo in the treatment of rheumatoid arthritis, Curr. Ther. Res. **24:**517, 1978.
20. Segre, E., and others: Interaction of naproxen and aspirin in the rat and in man, Scand. J. Rheumatol. **2**(suppl.):37, 1973.
21. Willkens, R.F., and Segre, E.J.: Combination therapy with naproxen and aspirin in rheumatoid arthritis, Arthritis Rheum. **19:**677, 1976.
22. Chaplin, M.D.: Lowering of plasma concentrations of (+)-6-methoxy-alpha-methyl-2-naphthalenacetic acid (naproxen) by aspirin in rats, Biochem. Pharmacol. **22:**1589, 1973.
23. Segre, E.J., and others: Naproxen-aspirin interactions in man, Clin. Pharmacol. Ther. **15:**374, 1973.
24. Lindquist, B., and others: Effect of concurrent administration of aspirin and indomethacin on serum concentrations, Clin. Pharmacol. Ther. **15:**247, 1974.
25. Runkel, R., and others: Naproxen-metabolism, excretion, and comparative pharmacokinetics, Scand. J. Rheumatol **2**(suppl.):29, 1973.
26. Willis, J.V., and others: A study of the effect of aspirin on the pharmacokinetics of oral and intravenous diclofenac sodium, Eur. J. Clin. Pharmacol. **18:**415, 1980.
27. Williams, R.L., and others: Ketoprofen-aspirin interactions, Clin. Pharmacol. Ther. **30:**226, 1981.

Indomethacin–Phenylpropanolamine

2

Summary: A patient regularly taking a preparation containing phenylpropanolamine developed serious hypertension within 30 minutes after taking a single 25 mg dose of indomethacin.[1] The patient had no hypertensive episode with either agent alone.

Related Drugs: There is no documented interaction between indomethacin and other sympathomimetics (direct-acting: e.g., norepinephrine; indirect-acting: e.g., amphetamine; mixed-acting: e.g., metaraminol).

No documented reports are available involving phenylpropanolamine and other nonsteroidal anti-inflammatory agents (e.g., ibuprofen, naproxen, sulindac [see Appendix]). Because of the postulated mechanism of the interaction, it may be possible that other sympathomimetics (direct, indirect, and mixed-acting) and other nonsteroidal anti-inflammatory agents may also interact similarly.

Mechanism: Although undocumented, the following mechanism has been postulated. Phenylpropanolamine is an indirect-acting sympathomimetic amine possessing vasoconstrictive activity and has produced hypertension on its own.[2-4] Indomethacin suppresses the synthesis of the prostaglandins (prostacyclin, PGA, and PGE), which normally reduce blood pressure by vasodilatation. Therefore, theoretically, the vasopressor activity of phenylpropanolamine is unopposed, leading to a sharp rise in blood pressure.

Recommendations: This one isolated case does not indicate that these agents cannot be used concomitantly. However, one may wish to use alternative agents which have no such reports of interactions.

If indomethacin and a product containing phenylpropanolamine are to be used together, the patient's blood pressure should be monitored frequently within the first hour after both agents are administered. If a hypertensive episode should occur, phentolamine has been used to successfully reduce the blood pressure.[1]

References

1. Lee, K.Y., and others: Severe hypertension after ingestion of an appetite suppressant (phenylpropanolamine) with indomethacin, Lancet **1:**1110, 1979.
2. Livingston, P.H.: Transient hypertension and phenylpropanolamine, J.A.M.A. **196:**1159, 1966.
3. Duvernoy, W.F.C.: Positive phentolamine test in hypertension induced by a nasal decongestant, N. Engl. J. Med., **280:**877, 1969.
4. Shapiro, S.R.: Hypertension due to anorectic agent, N. Engl. J. Med. **280:**1363, 1969.

Indomethacin–Probenecid

2

Summary: The administration of probenecid during indomethacin therapy can reduce the plasma clearance and elevate the plasma levels of indomethacin.[1] Patients may experience increased therapeutic and toxic effects.[2]

The uricosuric effect of probenecid is not affected by indomethacin administration.[1]

Related Drugs: Although sulfinpyrazone is a uricosuric drug pharmacologically similar to probenecid, it is unknown whether sulfinpyrazone interacts similarly with indomethacin. It is also undocumented whether other nonsteroidal anti-inflammatory agents (e.g., ibuprofen, naproxen, sulindac [see Appendix]) will interact similarly with probenecid; however, because of a similar metabolic fate, an interaction may be expected to occur.

Mechanism: Earlier studies indicated that probenecid inhibited renal tubular secretion of indomethacin.[1] However, recent studies in which more specific assay methods were used suggests that probenecid reduces nonrenal (possibly biliary) clearance of indomethacin, resulting in elevation of indomethacin serum levels, reduction of the volume of distribution, and no significant change in indomethacin half-life.[3]

Recommendations: Indomethacin dosage reductions should be considered when probenecid is added to indomethacin therapy.

References

1. Skeith, M.D., and others: The renal excretion of indomethacin and its inhibition by probenecid, Clin. Pharmacol. Ther. **9:**89, 1968.
2. Brooks, P.M., and others: The clinical significance of indomethacin-probenecid interaction, Br. J. Pharmacol. **1:**287, 1974.
3. Baber, N., and others: Clinical studies of the interaction between indomethacin and probenecid, Br. J. Clin. Pharmacol. **5:**364, 1978.

Meperidine–Chlorpromazine

2

Summary: Chlorpromazine potentiates the sedative, hypotensive, and respiratory depressant effects of meperidine, requiring a reduction in the meperidine dose.

Related Drugs: There are numerous reports of similar interactions between meperidine and other phenothiazine derivatives. The hypotensive and sedative effects of morphine and meperidine have long been recognized to be potentiated by chlorpromazine.[1-3] Prochlorperazine,[4] promethazine,[5] and propiomazine[6,7] have all been reported to interact with meperidine. Other phenothiazines (e.g., promazine, thioridazine, trifluoperazine [see Appendix]), thioxanthenes (chlorprothixene and thiothixene), as well as the butyrophenone (haloperidol), dihydroindolone (molindone), and dibenzoxazepine (loxapine) may also be expected to interact with meperidine because of pharmacologic similarity. Other narcotics that have been reported to interact with phenothiazines include fentanyl, hydromorphone, and oxymorphone.[5,8] There is no documentation regarding an interaction with the other narcotics (e.g., codeine, levorphanol, opium [see Appendix]), although they may be expected to interact similarly because of pharmacologic similarity.

Mechanism: Chlorpromazine increases the rate of appearance of normeperidine, a toxic metabolite of meperidine.[8] This may explain the increased respiratory depression seen when meperidine plus chlorpromazine was compared with each agent used alone.[9] It has also been proposed that promethazine decreases the metabolism and prolongs the half-life of narcotic analgesics.[5]

Recommendations: The combination of meperidine and chlorpromazine is widely used as an operative premedicant.[10] The dose of meperidine should be reduced by 25% to 50% when given with phenothiazines.[11]

References

1. Sadove, M.S., and others: Chlorpromazine and narcotics in the management of pain of malignant lesions, J.A.M.A. **155:**626, 1954.
2. Dripps, R.D., and others: Use of chlorpromazine in anesthesia and surgery, Ann. Surg. **142:**774, 1955.
3. Dobkin, A.B., and others: Chlorpromazine: review and investigation as premedicant in anesthesia, Anesthesiology **17:**135, 1956.
4. Steen, S.N., and Yates, M.: The effects of benzquinamide and prochlorperazine, separately and combined, on the human respiratory center, Anesthesiology **36:**519, 1972.
5. Keeri-Szanto, M.: The mode of action of promethazine in potentiating narcotic drugs, Br. J. Anaesth. **46:**918, 1974.
6. Hoffman, J.C., and Smith, T.C.: The respiratory effects of meperidine and propiomazine in man, Anesthesiology **32:**325, 1970.
7. Reier, C.E., and Johnstone, R.E.: Respiratory depression: narcotic versus narcotic-tranquilizer combinations, Anesth. Analg. (Cleve.) **49:**119, 1970.
8. Stambaugh, J.E., and Wainer, I.W.: Drug interaction: meperidine and chlorpromazine, a toxic combination, J. Clin. Pharmacol. **21:**140, 1981.
9. Lambertsen, C.L., and others: The separate and combined respiratory effects of chlorpromazine and meperidine in normal men controlled at 46 mm Hg alveolar Pco_2, J. Pharmacol. Exp. Ther. **131:**381, 1961.
10. McGee, J.L., and Alexander, M.R.: Phenothiazine analgesia—fact or fantasy? Am. J. Hosp. Pharm. **36:**633, 1979.
11. Demerol, Product information, Winthrop Laboratories, New York, N.Y., 1983.

Meperidine–Phenelzine

1

Summary: Concomitant use of meperidine and phenelzine may result in excitatory and depressant effects on the central nervous system (CNS), leading to deep coma and death.[1-4] An animal study showed similar results.[5] This interaction may occur for several weeks after discontinuation of phenelzine, a monoamine oxidase (MAO) inhibitor.

Related Drugs: Several other MAO inhibitors have also been reported to interact with meperidine. These include pargyline,[6,7] tranylcypromine,[8-10] and isocarboxazid.[11,12] Furazolidone and procarbazine, an antibacterial and an antineoplastic with MAO inhibitory activity, may also be expected to interact with meperidine.

Dextromethorphan, the d-isomer of the codeine analog of levorphanol having antitussive but no analgesic activity, is available in nonprescription products and has interacted with phenelzine with death resulting.[13] Nalorphine has reportedly enhanced the depression caused by a combination injection of meperidine-levallorphan in a patient receiving phenelzine.[2] Whether the administration of nalorphine added to the preexisting interaction of phenelzine and the other narcotics is not clear.

Morphine[8,14] and methadone[14] have also been studied in relation to a potential interaction with phenelzine and have been shown to be relatively devoid of this effect. While full experimental data do not exist for this and other narcotic analgesics (e.g., codeine, hydromorphone, oxycodone, [see Appendix]), all narcotics should be used cautiously in the presence of MAO inhibitors.

Mechanism: Although not specifically known, the combination of meperidine and MAO inhibitors have been shown to result in increases in serotonin (5-hydroxytryptamine, 5-HT).[5,7,14-20] Another proposed mechanism involves the ability of MAO inhibitors to act as enzyme inhibitors and thus reduce the rate of meperidine's N-demethylation or hydrolysis (or both) to inactive metabolic products, thus allowing accumulation of toxic levels of the agent.[10,21,22]

Recommendations: The clinical literature indicates the potential for a small number of patients receiving MAO inhibitors to experience reactions to meperidine. This interaction is unpredictable and has the potential to be life-threatening because of the extreme rapidity of onset within the CNS. Based on these facts, meperidine should not be used in patients receiving MAO inhibitors, and other narcotics should be utilized only with extreme caution. If this interaction should occur, intravenously administered corticosteroids may be beneficial to reverse the effects. If narcotic analgesia is deemed necessary, one should consider that the clinical effects of the MAO inhibitors lasts for several days and that the use of morphine or methadone may be preferable. Monitoring patient response to small doses of the narcotic analgesic in patients receiving phenelzine would be prudent prior to initiating therapeutic dosages.

References

1. Palmer, H.: Potentiation of pethidine (letter), Br. Med. J. **2**:944, 1960.
2. Cocks, D.P., and Passmore-Rowe, A.: Dangers of monoamine oxidase inhibitors (letter to the editor), Br. Med. J. **2**:1545, 1962.
3. Reid, N.C.R.W., and Jones, D.: Pethidine and phenelzine (letter), Br. Med. J. **1**:408, 1962.
4. Meyer, D., and Halfin, V.: Toxicity secondary to meperidine in patients on monoamine oxidase inhibitors: a case report and critical review, J. Clin. Psychopharmacol. **1**:319, 1981.
5. Brownlee, G., and Williams, G.W.: Potentiation of amphetamine and pethidine by monoamine oxidase inhibitors (letter), Lancet **1**:669, 1963.
6. Vigran, I.M.: Dangerous potentiation of meperidine hydrochloride by pargyline hydrochloride, J.A.M.A. **187**:953, 1964.
7. Gong, S.N.C., and Rogers, K.J.: Role of brain monoamines in the fatal hyperthermia induced by pethidine or imipramine in rabbits pretreated with pargyline, Br. J. Pharmacol. **42**:646P, 1971.
8. Evans-Prosser, C.D.G.: The use of pethidine and morphine in the presence of monoamine oxidase inhibitors, Br. J. Anesth. **40**:279, 1968.
9. London, D.R., and Milne, M.D.: Dangers of monoamine oxidase inhibitors, Br. Med. J. **2**:1752, 1962.
10. Eade, N.R., and Renton, K.W.: The effect of phenelzine and tranylcypromine on the degradation of meperidine, J. Pharmacol. Exp. Ther. **173**:31, 1970.
11. Shee, J.C.: Dangerous potentiation of pethidine by iproniazid, and its treatment, Br. Med. J. **2**:507, 1960.
12. Mitchell, R.S.: Fatal toxic encephalitis occurring during iproniazid treatment in pulmonary tuberculosis, Ann. Intern. Med. **55**:447, 1955.
13. Rivers, N., and Horner, B.: Possible lethal reaction between nardil and dextromethorphan (letter), Can. Med. Assoc. J. **103**:85, 1970.
14. Carlsson, A., and Lindquist, M.: Central and peripheral monoaminergic membrane pump blockade by some addictive analgesics and antihistamines, J. Pharm. Pharmacol. **20**:460, 1969.
15. Rogers, K.J.: Role of brain monoamines in the interaction between pethidine and tranylcypromine, Eur. J. Pharmacol. **14**:86, 1971.
16. Sinclair, J.G., and Lo, G.F.: The blockade of serotonin uptake and the meperidine-monoamine oxidase inhibitor interaction, Proc. West. Pharmacol. Soc. **20**:373, 1977.
17. Fuller, R.W., and Snoddy, H.D.: Inhibition of serotonin uptake and the toxic interaction between meperidine and monoamine oxidase inhibitors, Toxicol. Appl. Pharmacol. **32**:129, 1975.
18. Gessner, P., and Soble, A.G.: A study of the tranylcypromine-meperidine interaction: effects of p-chlorophenylalanine and 1-5-hydroxytryptophan, J. Pharmacol. Exp. Ther. **186**:276, 1973.
19. Penn, R.G., and Rogers, K.J.: Comparison of the effects of morphine, pethidine, and pentazocine in rabbits pretreated with a monoamine oxidase inhibitor, Br. J. Pharmacol. **42**:485, 1971.
20. Rogers, K.J., and Thorton, J.A.: The interaction between monoamine oxidase inhibitors and narcotic analgesics in mice, Br. J. Pharmacol. **36**:1470, 1969.
21. Clark, B.: The in vitro inhibition of the N-demethylation of pethidine by phenelzine (phenethylhydrazine), Biochem. Pharmacol. **16**:2369, 1967.
22. Eade, N.R., and Renton, K.W.: Effect of monoamine oxidase inhibitors on the N-demethylation and hydrolysis of meperidine, Biochem. Pharmacol. **19**:2243, 1970.

Meperidine–Phenytoin

3

Summary: In one study involving 4 healthy subjects, the concurrent use of meperidine (oral and intravenous) and phenytoin resulted in an increased systemic clearance of meperidine as well as a decreased elimination half-life and bioavailability. The volume of distribution, renal clearance, and protein binding of meperidine did not change. The plasma concentrations of normeperidine, a metabolite of meperidine, were also increased. Because analgesia relates to meperidine blood concentrations, the effectiveness of meperidine may be decreased during concomitant use with phenytoin, and toxicity may increase because of increased normeperidine levels.[1]

Related Drugs: Documentation is lacking regarding an interaction between meperidine and the other hydantoin anticonvulsants (ethotoin and mephenytoin), although because they are related pharmacologically a similar interaction may be expected. In a study involving 5 patients maintained on methadone, the concurrent use of phenytoin resulted in moderately severe withdrawal symptoms and a decreased methadone area-under-curve. Methadone plasma concentration returned to baseline levels 2 to 3 days after discontinuation of phenytoin.[2] There is also a lack of documentation regarding a similar interaction with the other narcotic analgesics (e.g., codeine, hydromorphone, morphine [see Appendix]); however, because of a similar metabolic fate, an interaction may be expected to occur.

Mechanism: Because the renal clearance of meperidine was not altered by phenytoin, the probable mechanism of the increased elimination of meperidine is enhancement of metabolism by phenytoin.[1] The same mechanism has been suggested in the methadone study.[2]

Recommendations: Oral doses of meperidine generate greater amounts of normeperidine then equal analgesic intravenous (IV) doses. Therefore, IV doses may be preferable to oral dosing in those receiving phenytoin. Also, to gain satisfactory analgesia, patients on long-term phenytoin therapy may require more frequent and larger doses of meperidine when phenytoin is being used concurrently.

References

1. Pond, S.M., and Kretschzmas, K.M.: Effect of phenytoin on meperidine clearance and normeperidine formation, Clin. Pharmacol. Ther. **30:**680, 1981.
2. Tong, T.G., and others: Phenytoin-induced methadone withdrawal, Ann. Intern. Med. **94:**349, 1981.

Methadone–Diazepam

4

Summary: Four patients who were maintained on methadone were given 2 oral doses of diazepam 1 and 5 hours after the daily maintenance dose of methadone. According to pharmacokinetic studies, there were no alterations in blood levels, urinary excretion, or plasma protein binding of methadone in any of the patients. However, 1 patient did have a higher area-under-curve of the pyrrolidine metabolite of methadone.[1]

Related Drugs: There is no documentation whether a similar effect would occur between the other narcotic analgesics (e.g., codeine, meperidine, morphine [see Appendix]) and the other benzodiazepines (e.g., chlordiazepoxide, flurazepam, triazolam [see Appendix])

Mechanism: The mechanism of this interaction is unknown. Since the opiate effects that occurred during concurrent therapy appeared to be similar to the effects of methadone alone, methadone's effects do not appear to be enhanced by kinetic interactions with diazepam.[1]

Recommendations: The concurrent use of methadone and diazepam need not be avoided.

Reference

1. Pond, S.M.: Lack of effect of diazepam on methadone metabolism in methadone-maintained addicts. Clin. Pharm. Ther. **31:**139, 1982.

Methadone–Rifampin

2

Summary: Patients receiving methadone and antituberculosis medications that included rifampin developed narcotic withdrawal symptoms while those receiving similar medications without rifampin did not.[1-6] Subsequently, it was determined that methadone plasma concentrations were decreased 33% to 68% in patients receiving concomitant rifampin compared with patients on non-rifampin regimens.[1,3-6]

Related Drugs: There are no drugs related to rifampin. Documentation is lacking regarding a similar interaction with other narcotics (e.g., codeine, hydromorphone, morphine [see Appendix]); however, because of pharmacologic similarity, an interaction may be expected to occur.

Mechanism: Rifampin decreased methadone plasma concentrations and increased the urinary excretion of methadone's major metabolite.[1] These results suggest that rifampin induces the hepatic metabolism of methadone. However, there was no consistent change in the methadone half-life, indicating that other mechanisms may be involved.

Recommendations: In those patients receiving methadone, antituberculosis therapy with isoniazid should be well tolerated. However, rifampin alone or rifampin plus isoniazid may offer desirable therapeutic benefits. In those cases, methadone dosage may need to be increased within several days of beginning co-therapy. Clonidine has also been effective in averting narcotic withdrawal symptoms. However, rifampin did not significantly change clonidine disposition in one report[7] (see Clonidine-Rifampin, p. 315). In light of the possible noninteraction of rifampin and clonidine, clonidine might be a suitable alternative for methadone when used for narcotic withdrawal.

References

1. Kreek, M.J., and others: Rifampin-induced methadone withdrawal, N. Engl. J. Med. **294:**1104, 1976.
2. Bending, M.R., and Skagel, P.O.: Rifampin and methadone withdrawal, Lancet **1:**1211, 1977.
3. Garfield, J.W., and others: Rifampin-methadone relationship. 1. The clinical effects of rifampin-methadone interaction, Am. Rev. Resp. Dis. **3:**926, 1975.
4. Kreek, M.J., and others: Rifampin-methadone relationship. 2. Rifampin effects on plasma concentration, metabolism, and excretion of methadone, Am. Rev. Resp. Dis. **3:**926, 1975.
5. Garfield, J.W.: Surprising side effect of rifampin, Med. World News **16**(16):60, 1975.
6. Kreek, M.J.: Medical complications in methadone patients, Ann. N.Y. Acad. Sci. **311:**110, 1978.
7. Affrime, M.B., and others: Failure of rifampin to induce the metabolism of clonidine in normal volunteers, Drug Intell. Clin. Pharm. **15:**964, 1981.

Morphine–Cimetidine

2

Summary: The concurrent administration of cimetidine and intramuscular morphine has been reported to lead to serious central nervous system (CNS) side effects including apnea, confusion, disorientation and respiratory depression in 1 patient.[1] Similar effects were reported in 2 studies involving cimetidine and either morphine or methadone.[2,3] A specific cause and effect relationship was not determined in any of these cases.

Related Drugs: In the report involving cimetidine and morphine, the same effects were seen in this patient after concurrent administration of opium alkaloids.[1] Although documentation is lacking, a similar interaction may be expected to occur between cimetidine and the other narcotic analgesics (e.g., codeine, hydromorphone, oxycodone [see Appendix]), because of a similar metabolic fate. Documentation is lacking regarding an interaction between morphine and the other H_2 receptor antagonist (ranitidine). However, if the mechanism only involves hepatic enzyme inhibition ranitidine would not be expected to interact similarly.

Mechanism: The mechanism is unknown. It has been suggested that cimetidine may reduce the metabolism of morphine, either by inhibition of hepatic microsomal enzymes[3] or by reducing hepatic clearance and blood flow.[2] However, pharmacokinetic evaluation from one study suggests that cimetidine did not appreciably alter hepatic blood flow.[4]

Recommendations: Since no cause and effect relationship has been established, these agents need not be avoided. However, it is prudent to be aware of a possible severe or fatal interaction, and if respiratory depression or other CNS side effects develop, the narcotic dose may need to be decreased or the drug may need to be discontinued. In one report, naloxone successfully reversed the CNS effects.[3]

References

1. Fine, A., and Churchill, D.N.: Potentially lethal interaction of cimetidine and morphine, Can. Med. Assoc. J. **124**:1434, 1981.
2. Lam, A.M.: Potentially lethal interaction of cimetidine and morphine, Can. Med. Assoc. J. **125**:820, 1981.
3. Sorkin, E.M., and others: Cimetidine potentiation of narcotic action, Drug Intell. Clin. Pharm. **17**:60, 1983.
4. Mojaverian, P., and others: Does cimetidine alter the pharmacokinetics of morphine in man? Clin. Pharmacol. Ther. **31**:251, 1982.

Oxyphenbutazone–Methandrostenolone*

Summary: When oxyphenbutazone and methandrostenolone (which is no longer available in the United States) are administered concurrently in humans, serum oxyphenbutazone levels may be elevated approximately 50%.[1-4] Although a greater incidence of untoward effects from increased serum oxyphenbutazone levels may be expected in the presence of methandrostenolone, no adverse effects have been reported. Additionally, there are no studies showing that a clinical response to lower doses of oxyphenbutazone is attained when methandrostenolone is administered concurrently.

Related Drugs: Phenylbutazone is unaffected by concurrent administration of methandrostenolone.[1] Because of conflicting results, it is difficult to determine whether an interaction would occur between sulfinpyrazone, another pyrazoline derivative, and methandrostenolone.

Although documentation is lacking, other anabolic steroids (e.g., fluoxymesterone, methyltestosterone, nandrolone [see Appendix]), because of pharmacologic similarity, would probably also increase serum oxyphenbutazone levels.

Mechanism: The mechanism of this interaction is not known. Inhibition of oxyphenbutazone metabolism has been suggested but the half-life[2] or urinary recovery[5] of oxyphenbutazone was unaffected by methandrostenolone. Displacement of oxyphenbutazone from its binding site on serum albumin has also been proposed.[2,6] Phenylbutazone, which is partially metabolized to oxyphenbutazone, may be unaffected by androgens because of stronger binding to albumin than oxyphenbutazone and apparently is not displaced. The metabolism of phenylbutazone is also unaffected by methandrostenolone.[1]

Recommendations: When oxyphenbutazone is administered concurrently with methandrostenolone, and possibly other anabolic steroids, the resulting increased serum oxyphenbutazone levels may increase the risk of adverse reactions. Patients receiving both agents should be monitored closely for oxyphenbutazone-induced toxicity.

References

1. Hvidberg, E.F., and others: Studies of the interaction of phenylbutazone, oxyphenbutazone, and methandrostenolone in man, Proc. Soc. Exp. Biol. Med. **129:**438, 1968.
2. Weiner, M., and others: Effect of steroids on disposition of oxyphenbutazone in man, Proc. Soc. Exp. Biol. Med. **124:**1170, 1967.
3. Dayton, P.G., and others: Interaction of phenylbutazone, oxyphenbutazone, and methandrostenolone in man, Fed. Proc. **27:**531, 1968.
4. Weiner, M., and others: Drug interactions: the effect of combined administration on the half-life of coumarin and pyrazolone drugs in man, Fed. Proc. **24:**153, 1965.
5. Perel, J.M., and others: A study of structure-activity relationships in regard to species differences in the phenylbutazone series, Biochem. Pharmacol. **13:**1305, 1964.
6. Brodie, B.B.: Displacement of one drug by another from carrier to receptor sites, Proc. Roy. Soc. Med. **58:**946, 1965.

*Not available in the U.S.

Phenylbutazone–Cholestyramine

4

Summary: Cholestyramine binds weak acids such as phenylbutazone in vitro. Absorption studies in rats imply a delay rather than a decrease in absorption of phenylbutazone.[1] Substantiation of clinical consequences in humans is lacking.

Related Drugs: No evidence documents delayed or decreased oxyphenbutazone absorption when given with cholestyramine, although it may be expected to be bound in a similar manner. There is no documentation of an interaction between phenylbutazone and the other anion exchange resin (colestipol), although because of similar pharmacologic activity an interaction may be expected to occur.

Mechanism: Cholestyramine is an anion exchange resin that binds bile acids when given orally. It is reported that anionic agents, such as phenylbutazone, may be bound to cholestyramine forming an unabsorbable drug-resin complex. Results from studies in rats suggest that the resin delayed phenylbutazone absorption.[1]

Recommendation: An interaction between cholestyramine and phenylbutazone has not been documented in humans. Any potential interaction can be avoided by administering phenylbutazone at least 2 hours before or 4 to 6 hours after administration of cholestyramine.[1,2]

References

1. Gallo, D.G., and others: The interaction between cholestyramine and drugs, Proc. Soc. Exp. Biol. Med. **120:**60, 1965.
2. Schwandt, P.: Drug interactions and side effects of hypolipidemic drugs, Int. J. Clin. Pharmacol. Biopharm. **17:**351, 1979.

Phenylbutazone–Desipramine

3

Summary: Concurrent administration of phenylbutazone and desipramine has resulted in reduced plasma levels of phenylbutazone in animal[1,2] and human[3] studies. Diminished therapeutic effect of phenylbutazone may result from the delayed absorption caused by desipramine.

Related Drugs: Oxyphenbutazone[1-3] absorption is also decreased by desipramine; however, clinical studies show simultaneous administration of desmethylimipramine did not affect the half-life of oxyphenbutazone.[4] Imipramine[1,3] has been shown to decrease phenylbutazone absorption. It is unknown whether the other tricyclic antidepressants (e.g., amitriptyline, nortriptyline, protriptyline [see Appendix]) or the tetracyclic antidepressant (maprotiline) produce the same effect as desipramine on phenylbutazone absorption, but agents with significant anticholinergic effect may be expected to exert a similar effect.

Mechanism: Gastrointestinal absorption of phenylbutazone is inhibited or delayed by both short- and long-term treatment with desipramine, apparently from an anticholinergic inhibition of gastric emptying.[2] The metabolism of phenylbutazone does not seem to be affected.[5]

Recommendations: Data on the clinical effects of this interaction are not available. Since both drugs are normally administered on a long-term basis and since only the rate, rather than the extent of phenylbutazone absorption, seems to be affected, the clinical significance may be minor. Patients may be monitored for possible decreased phenylbutazone effect if concurrent tricyclic antidepressant therapy is indicated.

References

1. Consolo, S.: An interaction between desipramine and phenylbutazone, J. Pharm. Pharmacol. **20:**574, 1968.
2. Consolo, S., and Garattini, S.: Effect of desipramine on intestinal absorption of phenylbutazone and other drugs, Eur. J. Pharmacol. **6:**322, 1969.
3. Prescott, L.F.: Pharmacokinetic drug interactions, Lancet **2:**1239, 1969.
4. Hammer, W., and others: A comparative study of the metabolism of desmethylimipramine, nortriptyline and oxyphenylbutazone in man, Clin. Pharmacol. Ther. **10:**44, 1969.
5. Consolo, S, and others: Delayed absorption of phenylbutazone caused by desmethylimipramine in humans, Eur. J. Pharmacol. **10:**239, 1970.

Phenylbutazone–Phenobarbital

Summary: The concurrent use of phenylbutazone and phenobarbital may reduce the half-life of phenylbutazone by approximately one-third as has been reported in patients with sickle cell anemia and in healthy subjects.[1-3] This reduced half-life appears to be more pronounced in those who show a longer initial phenylbutazone half-life.[1] The effects of this interaction may continue for several days after discontinuation of phenobarbital.[3] The clinical significance of this interaction (i.e., decreased action of phenylbutazone) was not determined in these studies.

Related Drugs: Although documentation is lacking a similar interaction may be expected to occur between oxyphenbutazone and the other barbiturates (e.g., amobarbital, butabarbital, secobarbital [see Appendix]) because of similar activity on hepatic microsomal enzymes.

Mechanism: It has been suggested that phenobarbital may increase the metabolism of phenylbutazone by inducing the hepatic microsomal enzymes responsible for its metabolism.[1]

Recommendations: Patients should be monitored for a decreased response to phenylbutazone during concurrent use of these agents. A higher dose of phenylbutazone may be necessary.

References

1. Whittaker, J.A., and Price Evans, D.A.: Genetic control of phenylbutazone metabolism in man, Br. Med. J. **4:**323, 1970.
2. Anderson, K.E., and others: Oxidative drug metabolism and inducibility of phenobarbital in sickle cell anemia, Clin. Pharmacol. Ther. **22:**580, 1977.
3. Levi, J.A., and others: Phenylbutazone and isoniazid metabolism in patients with liver disease in relation to previous drug therapy, Lancet **1:**1275, 1968.

Probenecid–Clofibrate

3

Summary: A study involving 4 healthy subjects found that concurrent use of probenecid and clofibrate caused a reduction in renal and metabolic clearance of clofibric acid (chlorphenoxyisobutyric acid, the deesterified active form of clofibrate which is present after intestinal absorption). There was a doubling of mean clofibric acid plasma concentrations and a 4-fold increase in mean free clofibric acid concentration.[1] The clinical significance of this interaction was not determined; however, the therapeutic and toxic effects of clofibrate may be increased.

Related Drugs: There are no drugs related to clofibrate. There is no documentation regarding an interaction between clofibrate and the other uricosuric agent, sulfinpyrazone; however, because of pharmacologic similarity, an interaction may be expected to occur.

Mechanism: The decrease in clofibric acid binding during probenecid administration may be caused by mechanisms other than direct displacement from plasma protein binding sites. Metabolites of probenecid or the effect of probenecid on the composition of plasma may contribute to this effect. It has also been suggested that probenecid inhibits the active tubular secretion of clofibric acid glucuronide, leading to accumulation of the glucuronide in the plasma with subsequent hydrolysis to clofibric acid. Also, probenecid may inhibit the formation of clofibric acid glucuronide. This may occur by competitive inhibition.[1]

Recommendations: Although the clinical significance was not determined, it is important to monitor patients and use a lower dose of clofibrate when necessary.

Reference

1. Veenendaal, J.R., and others: Probenecid-clofibrate interaction, Clin. Pharmacol. Ther. **29:**351, 1981.

Propoxyphene–Alcohol, Ethyl

2

Summary: Concurrent ingestion of propoxyphene and alcohol, especially when one or both are taken in excessive quantities, may result in dangerous respiratory and central nervous system (CNS) depression.[1-6]

Related Drugs: Based on similar pharmacologic properties an interaction may be expected to occur between alcohol and the other narcotic analgesics (e.g., codeine, meperidine, morphine [see Appendix]); however, documentation is lacking.

Mechanism: Alcohol has been shown to increase the systemic availability of propoxyphene in rats[1] and to lower the minimum lethal blood concentration of propoxyphene in humans.[2] Toxic doses of propoxyphene alone may cause coma, respiratory depression, and apnea.[3-5] In most reported cases of fatal propoxyphene overdoses, the victim had also ingested alcohol[2,6] in excessive quantities.

Recommendations: It is unlikely that moderate amounts of alcohol and the usual doses of propoxyphene will result in a serious adverse reaction. However, patients should be advised about the dangers associated with concurrent ingestion of therapeutic doses of propoxyphene and large amounts of alcohol or excessive amount of propoxyphene with any amount of alcohol. Naloxone has been used successfully to reverse propoxyphene-induced respiratory depression.[7,8]

References

1. Oguma, T., and Levy, G.: Acute effect of ethanol on hepatic first-pass elimination of propoxyphene in rats, J. Pharmacol. Exp. Ther. **219:**7, 1981.
2. Christensen, J.: Dextropropoxyphene and norpropoxyphene in blood, muscle, liver and urine in fatal poisoning, Acta Pharmacol. Toxicol. **40:**298, 1977.
3. Robbins, E.B.: The pharmacologic effects of a new analgesic alpha-4-dimethylamino-1, 2-diphenyl-3-methyl-4-propionyloxybutane, J. Am. Pharm. Assoc. (Sci. Ed.) **44:**497, 1955.
4. Cann, H.M., and Verhulst, H.L.: Convulsions as a manifestation of acute dextropropoxyphene intoxication, Am. J. Dis. Child. **99:**380, 1960.
5. Frasier, S.D., and others: Dextropropoxyphene hydrochloride poisoning in two children, J. Pediatr. **63:**158, 1963.
6. Sturner, W.Q., and Garriott, J.C.: Deaths involving propoxyphene: a study of 41 cases over a two year period, J.A.M.A. **223:**1125, 1973.
7. Fiut, R.E., and others: Antagonism of convulsive and lethal effects induced by propoxyphene, J. Pharm. Sci. **55:**1085, 1966.
8. Vlasses, P.M., and Fraher, T.: Naloxone for propoxyphene overdosage, J.A.M.A. **229:**1167, 1974.

Propoxyphene–Amphetamine

3

Summary: Amphetamines, which may be used to treat the central nervous system (CNS) depression resulting from propoxyphene overdoses, may increase the seizure potential of propoxyphene, although this has not been documented.

Related Drugs: Based on similar pharmacologic activity other indirect-acting sympathomimetics (e.g., ephedrine, methamphetamine, methylphenidate [see Appendix]) may also interact similarly with propoxyphene. Although undocumented, the other narcotic analgesics (e.g., codeine, meperidine, morphine [see Appendix]) may interact in a like manner with amphetamine because of pharmacologic similarity.

Mechanism: Convulsive seizures have been reported in cases of propoxyphene overdose;[1-3] however, the mechanism of this effect has not been studied. Amphetamines produce CNS stimulation by indirectly increasing the release of norepinephrine and possibly by impeding its neuronal reuptake.[4] Toxic doses of amphetamine can result in convulsions and coma.[5]

Recommendations: The use of amphetamines and other indirect acting sympathomimetics for the treatment of propoxyphene-induced CNS depression is not recommended. Naloxone, a narcotic antagonist, has been shown to be effective in controlling both respiratory depression and convulsive seizures following propoxyphene overdoses[3,6-8] and has not been shown to have proconvulsant activity.

References

1. Karliner, J.S.: Propoxyphene hydrochloride poisoning: report of a case treated with peritoneal dialysis, J.A.M.A. **199:**1006, 1967.
2. McCarthy, W.H., and Keenan, R.L.: Propoxyphene hydrochloride poisoning, report of the first fatality, J.A.M.A. **187:**460, 1964.
3. Cann, H.M., and Verhulst, H.L.: Convulsions as a manifestation of acute dextropropoxyphene intoxication, Am. J. Dis. Child. **99:**380, 1960.
4. Hollister, L.E.: Clinical use of psychotherapeutic drugs II: Antidepressant and antianxiety drugs and special problems in the use of psychotherapeutic drugs, Drugs **4:**361, 1972.
5. Weiner, N.: Norepinephrine, epinephrine and the sympathomimetic amines. In Gilman, A.G., Goodman, L.S., and Gilman, A., editors: The pharmacological basis of therapeutics, New York, 1980, MacMillan Publishing.
6. Fraiser, S.D., and others: Dextropropoxyphene hydrochloride poisoning in two children, J. Pediatr. **63:**158, 1963.
7. Gary, N.E., and others: Acute propoxyphene hydrochloride intoxication, Arch. Intern. Med. **121:**453, 1968.
8. Fiut, R.E., and others: Antagonism of convulsive and lethal effects induced by propoxyphene, J. Pharm. Sci. **55:**1085, 1966.

Propoxyphene–Orphenadrine

4

Summary: An alleged interaction with the concurrent use of these agents[1,2] cannot be substantiated.[3-5] The central nervous system (CNS) effects observed (e.g., tremors, mental confusion, and anxiety) were similar to those reported for either agent alone. Some of the previously reported cases had received twice the recommended dose of orphenadrine.

Related Drugs: Based on similar pharmacologic properties a lack of interaction may also be expected between orphenadrine and the other narcotic analgesics (e.g., codeine, meperidine, morphine, [see Appendix]), as well as between propoxyphene and the other antiparkinsonian anticholinergics (e.g., benztropine, biperiden, procyclidine [see Appendix]).

Mechanism: The mechanism is unknown because of lack of documentation regarding the interaction. One possibility, if a drug interaction actually does occur, is the combined effect on the central nervous system by both drugs.

Recommendations: Although it may be prudent to be aware of a possible interaction, the concurrent use of these agents need not be avoided. If CNS effects do occur, they are probably caused by either agent alone or by an additive effect and may require a reduction in the dose or discontinuation of one or both agents.

References

1. Renforth, W.: Orphenadrine and propoxyphene, N. Engl. J. Med. **283:**998, 1970.
2. Pearson, R.E., and Salter, F.J.: Drug interaction?—orphenadrine with propoxyphene, N. Engl. J. Med. **282:**1215, 1970.
3. Puckett, W.H., and Visconit, J.A.: Orphenadrine and propoxyphene, N. Engl. J. Med. **283:**544, 1970.
4. Parkes, J.D.: Adverse effects of antiparkinsonian drugs, Drugs **21:**341, 1981.
5. Cooper, T.B.: Plasma monitoring of antipsychotic drugs, Clin. Pharmacokinet. **3:**14, 1978.

Sulfinpyrazone–Aspirin

2

Summary: Aspirin antagonizes the uricosuric activity of sulfinpyrazone.[1] Sulfinpyrazone-induced uric acid excretion may be significantly inhibited or abolished by large doses of aspirin. Sulfinpyrazone may also inhibit the uricosuria that follows large doses of aspirin.

Although sulfinpyrazone, like aspirin, has antiplatelet activity, no statistically significant interaction of either synergy or antagonism has been detected between the two drugs regarding this pharmacologic effect.[2] However, one study showed that aspirin significantly increased the plasma clearance of sulfinpyrazone, suggesting the antiplatelet effect of sulfinpyrazone may be decreased during concurrent use.[3]

Related Drugs: Sodium salicylate has been shown to interact in a similar manner with sulfinpyrazone.[4-6] Although data are lacking, other salicylates (e.g., choline salicylate, salicylamide, salsalate [see Appendix]) may have the same effect based on their similar pharmacologic activity.

Phenylbutazone, which is structurally related to sulfinpyrazone, has been shown to block the uricosuric action of large amounts of aspirin and vice versa.[7] Although not documented, oxyphenbutazone may be expected to interact with aspirin because of pharmacologic similarity.

Aspirin (3 g/day) has also been shown to decrease the uricosuric effect of probenecid. Probenecid may also raise salicylate blood levels by decreasing the excretion of aspirin.[5,8,9]

Mechanism: Sulfinpyrazone and salicylates compete for common binding sites on plasma proteins. In addition, salicylates appear to block the inhibitory effect of sulfinpyrazone on the renal tubular reabsorption of uric acid, causing urate retention.[4-5] Aspirin has been shown to enhance the binding of phenylbutazone to serum albumin and may thereby prevent it from reaching its site of action.[10]

Recommendations: Aspirin and other salicylates, especially in high doses, should be avoided in patients taking sulfinpyrazone for its uricosuric effect.

References

1. Kersley, G.D., and others: Value of uricosuric agents and in particular of G28315 in gout, Ann. Rheum. Dis. **17:**326, 1958.
2. Canadian Cooperative Study Group: A randomized trial of aspirin and sulfinpyrazone in threatened stroke, N. Engl. J. Med. **299:**53, 1978.
3. Buchanan, M.R., and others: The effect of aspirin on the pharmacokinetics of sulfinpyrazone in man, Thromb. Res. Suppl. IV:145, 1983.
4. Yu, T.F., and others: Mutual suppression of the uricosuric effects of sulphinpyrazone and salicylate: a study in interactions between drugs, J. Clin. Invest. **42:**1330, 1963.
5. Seegmiller, J.E., and Grayzel, A.: Use of the newer uricosuric agents in the management of gout, J.A.M.A. **173:**1076, 1960.
6. Stockley, I.H.: Drug interactions with sulphinpyrazone, Pharm. J. **230:**163, 1983.
7. Oyer, J.H., and others: Suppression of salicylate-induced uricosuria by phenylbutazone, Am. J. Med. Sci. **251:**1, 1966.

8. Pascale, L.R.: Inhibition of uricosuric action of Benemid by salicylate, J. Lab. Clin. Med. **45:**771, 1955.
9. Brooks, C.D., and others: Effect of ibuprofen or aspirin on probenicid-induced uricosuria, J. Int. Med. Res. **8:**283, 1980.
10. Chignell, C.F., and Starkweather, D.K.: Optical studies of drug-protein complexes. V. The interaction of phenylbutazone, flufenamic acid, and dicoumarol with acetylsalicyclic acid-treated human serum albumin, Mol. Pharmacol. **7:**229, 1971.

Sulfinpyrazone–Niacin

3

Summary: One report indicated that the concurrent use of sulfinpyrazone and niacin may inhibit the uricosuric action of sulfinpyrazone.[1]

Related Drugs: There are no drugs related to niacin. Although documentation is lacking, an interaction may be expected to occur between niacin and probenecid based on similar pharmacologic activity.

Mechanism: It is not know if niacin interferes with the mechanism of action of sulfinpyrazone or if it is from the hyperuricemia that is a common side effect of niacin.[1]

Recommendations: Patients should be monitored for a possible decrease in the uricosuric activity of sulfinpyrazone. Niacin may need to be discontinued if this occurs.

Reference

1. Gershon, S.L., and Fox, I.H.: Pharmacologic effects of nicotinic acid on human purine metabolism, J. Lab. Clin. Med. **84:**179, 1974.

Sulfinpyrazone–Probenecid

4

Summary: The concurrent use of sulfinpyrazone and probenecid may produce an increase in uric acid secretion when compared with either drug alone.[1,2] However, well controlled studies have documented that the renal clearance of sulfinpyrazone is reduced, but the uricosuria is not altered.

Related Drugs: There is no documentation of a similar interaction between probenecid and phenylbutazone or its metabolite oxyphenbutazone.

Mechanism: Probenecid blocks the renal tubular secretion of sulfinpyrazone and its major active metabolite.[3]

Recommendations: The data concerning this drug interaction are inconclusive; therefore, no particular action need be taken. However, concurrent use might be avoided because the possible benefits of such therapy would be negligible.

References

1. Seegmiler, J.E., and Grayzel, A.I.: Use of the newer uricosuric agents in the management of gout, J.A.M.A. **173**:1076, 1960.
2. Yu, T.F., and Gutman, A.B.: Renal interaction of drugs affecting urate excretion in man, Pharmacologist **1**:53, 1959.
3. Perel, J.N., and others: Studies of interactions among drugs at the renal level: probenecid and sulfinpyrazone, Clin. Pharmacol. Ther. **10**:834, 1969.

CHAPTER TWO

Anesthetic and Neuromuscular Blocking Agents' Drug Interactions

TABLE 2. Anesthetic and Neuromuscular Blocking Agents' Drug Interactions

Drug Interaction	Significance Code	Potential Effects	Recommendations	See Page
Ether– Neomycin	1	Enhanced respiratory depression or prolonged neuromuscular blockade directly related to the dose of neomycin may result.	IV use of neostigmine, calcium, and possibly sodium bicarbonate may reverse the blockade in some patients. Otherwise, supportive care and ventilatory assistance are necessary.	67
Gallamine– Diazepam	3	One study reported IV diazepam increased the neuromuscular blockade of gallamine and decreased that of succinylcholine; this is unconfirmed by others who report no effect.	Concurrent use need not be avoided, but changes in response to neuromuscular blocking agents should be monitored.	69
Halothane– Epinephrine	1	Concurrent use may lead to serious ventricular arrhythmias, particularly when epinephrine is given IV.	The interaction may be less severe and occur less frequently by avoiding the IV route of epinephrine and by providing adequate ventilation and limiting the epinephrine dose with subcutaneous or intramuscular routes.	70
Halothane– Phenytoin	3	Phenytoin may increase the potential hepatoxicity of halothane, which may reduce the clearance of phenytoin resulting in phenytoin toxicity.	If signs of hepatitis appear after concurrent use, monitor for phenytoin levels and signs of toxicity. The phenytoin dose may need to be adjusted.	72
Halothane– Rifampin	2	Two studies reported serious or near-fatal hepatoxicity following concurrent use; however, no clear-cut cause and effect relationship could be determined.	Use cautiously and only when necessary.	73
Ketamine– Diazepam	2	Pretreatment with diazepam prior to ketamine anesthesia results in less initial tachycardia and hypertension, as well as lower steady-state plasma concentration and longer half-life of ketamine.	A lower dose of ketamine may be necessary.	74
Ketamine– Halothane	2	Concurrent use may lead to a rapid increase in arteriolar peripheral resistance and a decrease in cardiac output, stroke volume, and blood pressure.	Use cautiously and carefully; the monitor patients for hypotension.	75
Ketamine– Thyroid	3	Ketamine may cause marked hypertension and tachycardia in patients receiving thyroid hormone replacement.	Propranolol may control the heart rate and reduce the blood pressure if this interaction occurs.	76

Abbreviations: CNS, central nervous system; IM, intramuscular; IV, intravenous.

TABLE 2. Anesthetic and Neuromuscular Blocking Agents' Drug Interactions—cont'd

Drug Interaction	Significance Code	Potential Effects	Recommendations	See Page
Methoxyflurane–Secobarbital	2	Secobarbital causes increased production of methoxyflurane toxic metabolites, which increases the incidence of nephrotoxicity.	The concomitant use of these drugs should be avoided.	77
Methoxyflurane–Tetracycline	2	Because tetracycline induces prerenal azotemia and methoxyflurane has nephrotic potential, nephrotoxicity may result from concurrent use.	Renal status must be carefully monitored if concurrent use is unavoidable. Doxycycline may be a suitable alternative for tetracycline.	78
Pancuronium–Aminophylline	2	Aminophylline may cause resistance to the neuromuscular blockade produced by pancuronium. One study reported supraventricular tachycardia during concomitant use.	Monitor patients closely and increase the pancuronium dose if needed.	79
Pancuronium–Azathioprine	3	Azathioprine may antagonize the neuromuscular blocking action of pancuronium.	Avoid concurrent use if possible; however, the pancuronium dose may need to be increased if concomitant use is necessary.	80
Pancuronium–Clindamycin	2	Clindamycin may prolong the neuromuscular blockade produced by pancuronium.	Use with caution and only if necessary.	81
Pancuronium–Hydrocortisone	3	Hydrocortisone may lead to partial recovery of the neuromuscular blockade produced by pancuronium.	The dose of pancuronium may need to be increased.	82
Pancuronium–Lithium Carbonate	3	Concurrent use of these agents may enhance or prolong the neuromuscular blockade produced by pancuronium, although a conflicting report did not find similar results.	Use pancuronium cautiously in patients on lithium. Monitor closely and provide ventilatory assistance as necessary.	83
Pancuronium–Nitroglycerin	3	Nitroglycerin increases the duration and possibly the depth of neuromuscular blockade in animal studies.	Noninteracting neuromuscular blocking agents such as succinylcholine may be advisable. Neostigmine can be used to reverse this effect.	84
Pancuronium–Thiotepa (Triethylenethiophosphoramide)	3	One patient developed rapid and prolonged respiratory depression after concurrent use of these agents, although myasthenia gravis may have been the predisposing factor in this interaction since it does not appear to be an additive or synergistic effect.	Use these agents cautiously; ventilatory assistance should be available.	85

TABLE 2. Anesthetic and Neuromuscular Blocking Agents' Drug Interactions—cont'd

Drug Interaction	Significance Code	Potential Effects	Recommendations	See Page
Succinylcholine–Cyclophosphamide	2	Cyclophosphamide may potentiate the neuromuscular blockade, resulting in prolonged respiratory depression.	Determine pseudocholinesterase levels before concurrent use, or substitute another neuromuscular blocking agent.	86
Succinylcholine–Dexpanthenol	4	Dexpanthenol may prolong respiratory depression induced by succinylcholine.	The possibility of this interaction is unlikely at the usual doses of these agents.	87
Succinylcholine–Isoflurane	2	Isoflurane may potentiate phase II (desensitizing) neuromuscular blockade. The tachyphylaxis that occurs with prolonged succinylcholine administration is followed by a decreased requirement of this drug during isoflurane anesthesia.	Monitor patients and decrease the succinylcholine dose if needed.	88
Succinylcholine–Lidocaine	2	Large doses of lidocaine may prolong and intensify the neuromuscular blockade and duration of apnea produced by succinylcholine.	Monitor patients to determine the need for artificial ventilation.	89
Succinylcholine–Neostigmine	2	Neostigmine may either antagonize phase I (depolarizing) or enhance phase II (desensitizing) neuromuscular blockade produced by succinylcholine.	Avoid concomitant use during phase I and use cautiously if at all in phase II blockade.	91
Succinylcholine–Procainamide	3	Procainamide may prolong and intensify the neuromuscular blockade produced by succinylcholine.	Monitor patients to determine the need for artificial ventilation.	93
Succinylcholine–Promazine	2	Concurrent use of these agents may lead to total muscle relaxation and prolonged apnea.	Use promazine cautiously. Ventilatory assistance should be available.	94
Succinylcholine–Trimethaphan	2	Concurrent use of these agents may increase neuromuscular blockade characterized by prolonged apnea. Trimethaphan alone has caused respiratory paralysis and may have some neuromuscular blocking activity itself.	Use these agents cautiously. Ventilatory assistance should be available.	95
Thiopental–Morphine	2	Concurrent use may increase respiratory depression greater than that seen with either agent alone, possibly because of an additive synergistic effect.	Monitor patients closely. If the morphine dose cannot be lowered, ventilatory assistance should be available.	96

TABLE 2. Anesthetic and Neuromuscular Blocking Agents—cont'd

Drug Interaction	Significance Code	Potential Effects	Recommendations	See Page
Thiopental–Probenecid	3	Probenecid may prolong the anesthesia of thiopental. However, arterial blood pressure, heart rate, recovery time, pain tolerance, and frequency of apnea are not altered.	If prolonged anesthesia is not desired, discontinue probenecid before administering thiopental.	97
Thiopental–Reserpine	2	Reserpine may enhance presurgical CNS depression caused by thiopental, resulting in hypotension and bradycardia. Barbiturates may cause autonomic nervous system depression, which may add to reserpine's effects.	Withdrawal of reserpine before surgery is not mandatory, but it is important to be aware of the possibility of hypotension and bradycardia.	98
Thiopental–Sulfisoxazole	2	IV sulfisoxazole immediately before anesthesia induction with thiopental shortens awakening time.	Smaller, more frequent doses of thiopental should be given to patients using sulfisoxazole.	100
Tubocurarine–Chlorothiazide	3	The change in extracellular potassium levels that may occur with chlorothiazide may result in an enhanced neuromuscular blockade of tubocurarine.	Determine serum potassium and correct if tubocurarine is used in a patient on chlorothiazide or other potassium-depleting diuretics.	101
Tubocurarine–Gentamicin	1	Gentamicin, an aminoglycoside antibiotic, produces neuromuscular blockade which may prolong the respiratory depressant and muscle relaxant properties of tubocurarine.	Alternative antibiotics should be used whenever possible if a neuromuscular blocking agent is used.	102
Tubocurarine–Ketamine	2	A single IV dose of ketamine may augment the neuromuscular blocking properties of tubocurarine.	Patients should be carefully monitored during concurrent use of these agents.	105
Tubocurarine–Morphine	2	IV or IM morphine augments the neuromuscular blockade produced by tubocurarine. Since both agents reduce blood pressure, hypotension may occur with concurrent use.	Interaction may be avoided by giving morphine after the effects of tubocurarine have dissipated. If used concurrently, monitor respiration. Small intermittent doses of each agent may minimize hypotension.	106
Tubocurarine–Propranolol	2	Propranolol has been reported to prolong the neuromuscular blocking action of tubocurarine.	Monitor patients for respiratory depression, apnea, and hypotension.	107
Tubocurarine–Quinidine	2	Parenteral quinidine given shortly after or simultaneously with tubocurarine may enhance the neuromuscular blockade, resulting in prolonged or intensified respiratory depression and apnea.	Monitor the patient for increased respiratory depression.	109

Ether–Neomycin

1

Summary: Depression of neuromuscular transmission can be produced independently with ether or neomycin[1-10] Concurrent administration of these drugs may enhance respiratory depression or may prolong neuromuscular blockade. The extent of the depressed neuromuscular transmission can be directly related to the dose of neomycin administered and the resulting serum level of drug achieved.[10,11]

Related Drugs: Inhalation anesthetic agents such as cyclopropane,[3,4] halothane,[1] methoxyflurane,[1] and nitrous oxide[1] have been reported to interact with neomycin. Although not documented, based on similar pharmacologic activity other inhalation anesthetics (e.g., enflurane, ethylene, isoflurane [see Appendix]) may interact with neomycin in a similar manner.

Other aminoglycoside antibiotics such as kanamycin[1,12] and streptomycin[1,13] are known to have neuromuscular blocking activity and to interact with ether. Gentamicin[2,14-16] in humans and amikacin[15] and tobramycin[15] in animals have been shown to have a neuromuscular blocking activity similar to neomycin and may be expected to interact with ether and related agents (e.g., cyclopropane, halothane, methoxyflurane, and nitrous oxide). There is no documentation of an interaction between ether and the other aminoglycosides (netilmicin and paromomycin), although one may be expected to occur because of pharmacologic similarity.

Other nonaminoglycoside antibiotics such as colistin,[2] bacitracin,[2] polymyxin,[2] oxytetracycline,[2] and clindamycin[17] have neuromuscular blocking activity and may be expected to interact with ether in a similar manner.

Mechanism: Ether primarily blocks neuromuscular action by depressing depolarization at the neuromuscular junction or end plate site.[18] The neuromuscular blockade of nemycin and other aminoglycosides is directly related to the dose and probably results from a combination of the reduced sensitivity of the postjunctional membrane and interference with transmitter release.[10,19] Therefore, this interaction may be from a synergistic effect of the neuromuscular blocking properties of both agents.

Recommendations: It is important to be prepared to treat the neuromuscular and respiratory depression that is frequently produced by this interaction, particularly if the aminoglycoside is administered intraperitoneally.

If neuromuscular blockade and respiratory depression are encountered, the intravenous use of neostigmine (0.2 to 2.5 mg), calcium (1 g), and possibly sodium bicarbonate (dose not reported), either alone or concurrently, may be helpful in reversing the blockade[1-5] in some but not all patients. The administration of analeptic agents (e.g., doxapram and nikethamide) is of no value.[1] Supportive care and ventilatory assistance should be administered and continued until the neuromuscular blockade has passed. Vital signs should be monitored because secondary circulatory collapse may occur, and volume replacement should be administered as necessary.[1,5]

References

1. Pittinger, C.B., and others: Antibiotic-induced paralysis, Anesth. Analg. (Cleve.) **49:**487, 1970.
2. Pittinger, C., and Adamson, R.: Antibiotic blockade of neuromuscular function, Ann. Rev. Pharmacol. **12:**169, 1972.
3. Webber, B.M.: Respiratory arrest following intraperitoneal administration of neomycin, Am. Med. Assoc. Arch. Surg. **75:**174, 1957.
4. Jones, W.P.G.: Calcium treatment for ineffective respiration resulting from administration of neomycin, J.A.M.A. **170:**943, 1959,
5. Wright, E.A., and McQuillen, M.P.: Antibiotic-induced neuromuscular blockade, Ann. N. Y. Acad. Sci. **183:**358, 1971.
6. Foldes, F.F., and others: Prolonged respiratory depression caused by drug combinations, J.A.M.A. **183:**672, 1963.
7. McQuillen, M.P., and others: Myasthenia syndrome associated with antibiotics, Arch. Neurol. **18:**402, 1968.
8. Pittinger, C.B., and others: The neuromuscular blocking action of neomycin: a concern of the anesthesiologist, Anesth. Analg. (Cleve.) **37:**276, 1958.
9. Pridgen, J.E.: Respiratory arrest thought to be due to intraperitoneal neomycin, Surgery, **40:**571, 1956.
10. Corrado, A.P., and others: Neuromuscular blockade by neomycin potentiation by ether anesthesia and d-tubocurarine and antagonism by calcium and prostigmine, Arch. Int. Pharmacodyn. Ther. **121:**380, 1959.
11. Markalous, P.: Respiration and the intraperitoneal application of neomycin and neolymphin, Anaesthesia **17:**427, 1962.
12. Brady, J.P., and Williams, H.C.: Magnesium intoxication in a premature infant, Pediatrics **40:**100, 1967.
13. Levanen, J., and Nordman, R.: Complete respiratory paralysis caused by a large dose of streptomycin and its treatment with calcium chlóride, Ann. Clin. Res. **7:**47, 1975.
14. Warner, W.A., and Sanders, E.: Neuromuscular blockade associated with gentamicin therapy, J.A.M.A. **215:**1153, 1971.
15. L'Hommedieu, C.S., and others: Potentiation of magnesium sulfate-induced neuromuscular weakness by gentamicin, tobramycin, and amikacin, J. Pediatr. **102:**629, 1983.
16. Holtzman, J.L.: Gentamicin and neuromuscular blockade, Ann. Intern. Med. **84:**55, 1976.
17. Fodgall, R.P., and Miller, R.D.: Prolongation of a pancuronium-induced neuromuscular blockade by clindamycin, Anesthesiology **41:**407, 1974.
18. Waud, B.E., and Waud, D.R.: Comparison of the effects of general anesthetics on the end-plate of skeletal muscle, Anesthesiology **43:**540, 1970.
19. Brazil, O.V., and Prado-Franceschi, J.: The nature of the neuromuscular blockade produced by neomycin and gentamicin, Arch. Int. Pharmacodyn. Ther. **1:**179, 1969.

Gallamine–Diazepam

3

Summary: Much controversy exists in the literature regarding an interaction between diazepam and the depolarizing and nondepolarizing neuromuscular blocking agents.[1] Results from a study on human subjects suggest that intravenous administration of diazepam increased the magnitude of the neuromuscular block resulting from gallamine and decreased the blockade induced by succinylcholine.[2] Other researchers have not been able to confirm these results and report no interaction between the neuromuscular blocking agents (depolarizing and nondepolarizing) and diazepam.[3-7]

Related Drugs: Other benzodiazepines that are pharmacologically related to diazepam (e.g., chlordiazepoxide, flurazepam, triazolam [see Appendix]) might be expected to interact with the other nondepolarizing neuromuscular blocking agents (e.g., atracurium, pancuronium, tubocurarine [see Appendix]) in a manner similar to diazepam. However, there is no documentation to support this suggestion.

Mechanism: Because of insufficient data, the mechanism for this interaction is unknown. However, it has been postulated that diazepam may exert a peripheral action at the neuromuscular junction involving direct muscle depression.[4,6] This peripheral effect was demonstrated only at high concentrations of diazepam and did not account for the other observed actions.

Recommendations: Until further clinical evidence is available, patients receiving both diazepam and a neuromuscular blocking agent should be monitored closely for signs of any unusual changes in the response to the neuromuscular blocking agent. Because data are inconsistent the concomitant use need not be avoided.

References

1. Sharma, K.K., and Sharma, U.C.: Influence of diazepam on the effect of neuromuscular blocking agents, J. Pharm. Pharmacol. **30:**64, 1978.
2. Feldman, S.A., and Crawley, B.E.: Interactions of diazepam with the muscle-relaxant drugs, Br. Med. J. **2:**336, 1970.
3. Fahmy, N.R., and others: Diazepam prevents some adverse effects of succinylcholine, Clin. Pharmacol. Ther. **26:**395, 1979.
4. Dretchen, K., and others: The interaction of diazepam with myoneural blocking agents, Anesthesiology **34:**463, 1971.
5. Webb, S.N., and Bradshaw, E.G.: Diazepam and neuromuscular blocking drugs, Br. Med. J. **3:**690, 1971.
6. Bradshaw, E.G., and Maddison, S.: Effect of diazepam at the neuromuscular junction, Br. J. Anaesth. **51:**955, 1979.
7. Stovner, J., and Endrosen, R.: Diazepam in intravenous anesthesia, Lancet **2:**1298, 1965.

Halothane–Epinephrine

1

Summary: The parenteral, primarily intravenous, administration of epinephrine during halothane anesthesia may lead to serious ventricular arrhythmias.[1-12]

Related Drugs: Levarterenol (norepinephrine) has been shown to interact with halothane in a manner similar to epinephrine.[13] Although not documented, isoproterenol causes similar effects on the heart[14] and would probably interact with halothane in a similar manner. The indirect acting sympathomimetics (e.g., amphetamine, ephedrine, methylphenidate, [see Appendix]) affect the heart indirectly by releasing endogenous catecholamines[14] and may also interact with halothane in a similar manner.

Other inhalation anesthetics that reduce the arrhythmogenic dose of epinephrine include cyclopropane,[1,15-17] chloroform,[14] methoxyflurane,[14] and enflurane.[6] There is no documentation of an interaction between epinephrine and the other inhalation anesthetics (e.g., ethylene, isoflurane, nitrous oxide [see Appendix]), although because pharmacologic activity is similar an interaction may be expected to occur.

Mechanism: Although the exact mechanism for this interaction is unknown, the anesthetics produce conduction changes that increase impulse reentry into the myocardial tissue.[13] The anesthetics' ability to precipitate arrhythmias is enhanced by elevated arterial blood pressure, tachycardia, hypercapnia, and/or hypoxia, events that stimulate the release of endogenous catecholamines.[13]

Recommendations: Intravenous use of epinephrine during surgery with halothane and related halogenated general anesthetics should be strongly discouraged. When intravenous epinephrine is necessary, nitrous oxide anesthesia supplemented with ether, muscle relaxants, or narcotics should be used instead of halothane.[5,7]

Epinephrine may safely be used subcutaneously with the following precautions: the patient is adequately ventilated to prevent hypoxia or respiratory acidosis; the total dose of epinephrine is limited to 100 μg/10 minute period or 300 μg/hour in adults, 3.5 μg/kg in infants, 2.5 μg/kg in children up to 2 years of age, and 1.45 μg/kg in children over 2 years of age; a minimum effective concentration of anesthetic is maintained; the drugs are not coadministered in patients with hypertension or other cardiovascular disorders; and the cardiac rhythm is continuously monitored during and after injection.[2,4,5,7,16,18-21]

If arrythmias occur after the administration of the epinephrine, the drugs of choice are lidocaine or propranolol, depending on the type of arrhythmia.[13]

When administration of a sympathetic brochodilator is necessary in patients receiving halogenated anesthetics, one should use an agent with a beta$_2$ adrenergic receptor specificity for bronchial smooth muscle (e.g., terbutaline and salbutamol).[13]

References

1. Katz, R.L., and Katz, G.J.: Surgical infiltration of pressor drugs and their interaction with volatile anaesthetics, Br. J. Anaesth. **38:**712, 1966.
2. Andersen, N., and Johansen, S.H.: Incidence of catecholamine-induced arrhythmias during halothane anesthesia, Anesthesiology **24:**51, 1963.
3. Forbes, A.M.: Halothane, adrenaline and cardiac arrest, Anaesthesia **21:**22, 1966.
4. Hirshom, W.I., and others: Arrhythmias produced by combinations of halothane and small amounts of vasopressor, Br. J. Oral Surg. **2:**131, 1964-1965.
5. Katz, R.L., and others: The injection of epinephrine during general anesthesia with halogenated hydrocarbons and cyclopropane in man. 2. Halothane, Anesthesiology **23:**597, 1962.
6. Reisner, L.S., and Lippman, P.: Ventricular arrhythmias after epinephrine injection in enflurane and halothane anesthesia, Anesth. Analg. (Cleve.) **54:**468, 1975.
7. Johnstone, M.: Adrenaline and noradrenaline during anesthesia, Anaesthesia **8:**32, 1953.
8. Ikezono, E., and others: Effects of propranolol on epinephrine-induced arrhythmias during halothane anesthesia in man and cats, Anesth. Analg. (Cleve.) **48:**598, 1969.
9. Ueda, W., and others: Appraisal of epinephrine administration to patients under halothane anesthesia for closure of cleft palate, Anesthesiology **58:**574, 1983.
10. Kaufman, L.: Cardiac arrhythmias in dentistry, Lancet **2:**278, 1965.
11. Alexander, S.P.: Dysrhythmia and oral surgery, Br. J. Anaesth. **43:**773, 1971.
12. Alexander, J.P., and others: Dysrhythmia and oral surgery II: Junctional rhythms, Br. J. Anaesth. **44:**1179, 1972.
13. Weiner, N.: Norepinephrine, epinephrine, and the sympathomimetic amines. In Gilman, A.G., Goodman, L.S., and Gilman, A., editors: The pharmaclogical basis of therapeutics, New York, 1980, MacMillan Publishing.
14. Katz, R.L., and Epstein, R.A.: The interaction of anesthetic agents and adrenergic drugs to produce cardiac arrhythmias, Anesthesiology **29:**763, 1968.
15. Katz, R.L.: Effects of alpha and beta adrenergic blocking agents on cyclopropane-catecholamine cardiac arrhythmias, Anesthesiology **26:**289, 1965.
16. Matteo, R.S., and others: The injection of epinephrine during general anesthesia with halogenated hydrocarbons and cyclopropane in man. 3. Cyclopropane, Anesthesiology **24:**327, 1963.
17. Price, H.L., and others: cyclopropane anesthesia. II. Epinephrine and norepinephrine in initiation of ventricular arrhythmias by carbon dioxide inhalation, Anesthesiology **19:**619, 1958.
18. Matteo, R.S., and others: The injection of epinephrine during general anesthesia with halogenated hydrocarbons and cyclopropane in man. 1. Trichloroethylene, Anesthesiology **23:**360, 1962.
19. Joas, T.A., and Stevens, W.C.: Comparison of the arrhythmic doses of epinephrine during forane, halothane, and fluroxene anesthesia in dogs, Anesthesiology **35:**48, 1971.
20. Wallbank, W.A.: Cardiac effects of halothane and adrenaline in hare-lip and cleft-palate surgery, Br. J. Anaesth. **42:**548, 1970.
21. Melgrave, A.P.: The use of epinephrine in the presence of halothane in children, Can. Anaesth. Soc. J. **17:**256, 1970.

Halothane–Phenytoin

3

Summary: Phenytoin may increase the likelihood of halothane-induced hepatotoxicity, and the hepatic dysfunction may reduce the clearance of phenytoin, resulting in phenytoin toxicity. One patient developed marked phenytoin toxicity 3 days after halothane anesthesia.[1]

Related Drugs: Phenytoin and phenobarbital have been implicated as contributing factors in a patient's fatal fluroxene-induced hepatotoxicity.[2] There is a lack of documentation concerning whether the hepatotoxic potential of other halogenated anesthetic agents (e.g., enflurane, isoflurane, methoxyflurane [see Appendix]) may be enhanced by phenytoin. However, the hepatotoxicity occurring with halothane is usually not seen with these agents, therefore a similar interaction would not be expected to occur. The other hydantoin anticonvulsants (ethotoin and mephenytoin) may interact with halothane similar to phenytoin based on pharmacologic similarity.

Mechanism: Hepatotoxicity following halothane anesthesia is not unexpected.[3] Whether concurrent administration of phenytoin actually increases the risk of halothane-induced hepatotoxicity has not been studied. Phenytoin metabolism is dependent on the liver microsomal system.[4,5] Injury to the microsomal system from any source would be expected to inhibit phenytoin metabolism.

Recommendations: Since it is not clear that phenytoin increases the likelihood of halothane-induced toxicity, no additional precautions are warranted. However, if patients receiving phenytoin show signs of hepatitis (fever, elevated transaminase levels, etc.) close monitoring of serum phenytoin concentrations and clinical signs of phenytoin toxicity (e.g., nystagmus, blurring of vision, ataxia) is indicated, and appropriate changes in doses should be made.

References

1. Karlin, J.M., and Kutt, H.: Acute diphenylhydantoin intoxication following halothane anesthesia, J. Pediatr. **76:**941, 1970.
2. Reynolds, E.S., and others: Massive hepatic necrosis after fluroxene anesthesia—a case of drug interaction?, N. Engl. J. Med. **286:**530, 1972.
3. Peters, R.L., and others: Hepatic necrosis associated with halothane anesthesia, Am. J. Med. **47:**748, 1969.
4. Kutt, H., and others: Inhibition of diphenylhydantoin metabolism in rats and in rat liver microsomes by antitubular drugs, Neurology **18:**706, 1968.
5. Butler, T.C.: The metabolic conversion of 5,5-diphenylhydantoin to 5-(p-hydroxyphenyl)-5-phenylhydantoin, J. Pharmacol. Exp. Ther. **119:**1, 1957.

Halothane–Rifampin

2

Summary: In a single case report, a patient who was started on rifampin and isoniazid immediately following halothane anesthesia developed serious hepatotoxicity.[1] In another patient, a nearly fatal hepatoxicity was reported when rifampin was administered following halothane anesthesia.[2] In both cases, a clear-cut cause and effect relationship could not be determined.

Related Drugs: There are no drugs related to rifampin. Documentation is lacking regarding a similar interaction between rifampin and the other halogenated inhalation anesthetics (enflurane, isoflurane, and methoxyflurane). However, the hepatotoxicity seen with halothane is usually not observed with these agents; therefore a similar interaction would not be expected to occur.

Mechanism: The mechanism is unknown. However, it has been suggested that the interaction is from the combined effects of the two agents on the liver, since halothane hepatotoxicity is well documented.

Recommendations: Although a cause and effect relationship was never clearly established, these agents should be used with caution and only when necessary.

References

1. Pessayne, D., and others: Isoniazid-rifampin fulminant hepatitis: a possible consequence of the enhancement of isoniazid hepatotoxicity by enzyme induction, Gastroenterology **72:**284, 1977.
2. Most, J.A., and Markle, G.B.: A nearly fatal hepatotoxic reaction to rifampin after halothane anesthesia. Am. J. Surg. **127:**593, 1974.

Ketamine–Diazepam

Summary: In a study involving 49 patients anesthetized with ketamine before abdominal surgery, the 10 patients who were pretreated with diazepam (10 mg) experienced significantly less initial tachycardia and hypertension after ketamine. They also required a significantly lower dose of ketamine during the initial 30 minutes of anesthesia, had a lower steady-state plasma concentration of ketamine, and the half-life of ketamine was significantly longer. Four patients who had received long-term diazepam had a shorter ketamine half-life than the pretreated patients or the control group.[1]

Related Drugs: Documentation is lacking regarding a similar interaction between ketamine and the other benzodiazepines (e.g., chlordiazepoxide, flurazepam, triazolam [see Appendix]). There are no drugs related to ketamine.

Mechanism: The mechanism of this interaction is unknown.

Recommendations: The clinician should be aware of this interaction, since a patient pretreated with diazepam may need a lower dose of ketamine.

Reference

1. Idvall, J., and others: Pharmacodynamic and pharmacokinetic interactions between ketamine and diazepam, Eur. J. Clin. Pharmacol. **24:**337, 1983.

Ketamine–Halothane

2

Summary: During halothane anesthesia, the concurrent use of ketamine caused a rapid increase in arteriolar peripheral resistance and a decrease in cardiac output, stroke volume, and systolic, diastolic, and mean arterial blood pressures in 3 studies.[1-3]

Related Drugs: Similar effects were seen when ketamine was used with enflurane, although the effects were less dramatic and developed slower than with halothane.[1] Documentation is lacking of an interaction with the other halogenated inhalation anesthetics (isoflurane and methoxyflurane), although a similar interaction may be expected to occur because of pharmacologic similarity.

Mechanism: Ketamine alone has cardiovascular stimulating properties including increased blood pressure and pulse rate.[1-3] Halothane, on the other hand, has been shown to induce cardiac depression.[1-3] It has been postulated that the autonomic stimulating properties of ketamine depend on an intact, nondepressed central nervous system. It is possible that halothane, acting as a sympatholytic, uncovers the direct negative inotropic effects of ketamine, resulting in significant hypotension.[2]

Recommendations: When halothane anesthesia is used, ketamine should be administered with caution.[1] The patient's blood pressure should be carefully monitored, because the hypotension has been severe enough in some reports to necessitate the use of a vasopressor.[2]

References

1. Bidwai, A.V., and others: Cardiovascular dynamics, Anesth. Analg. (Cleve.) **54**:588, 1975.
2. Stanley, T.H.: Blood-pressure and pulse-rate responses to ketamine during general anesthesia, Anesthesiology **36**:648, 1973.
3. Johnston, R.R., and others: The interaction of ketamine with d-tubocurarine, pancuronium, and succinylcholine in man, Anesth. Analg. (Cleve.) **53**:496, 1974.

Ketamine–Thyroid

3

Summary: In a study involving 2 patients receiving thyroid replacement therapy, the concurrent use of ketamine resulted in a marked hypertension and tachycardia.[1] The clinical significance of this interaction was not determined.

Related Drugs: There are no drugs related to ketamine. Documentation is lacking regarding an interaction between ketamine and the other thyroid drugs (e.g., levothyroxine, liothyronine, thyrotropin [see Appendix]), although because of pharmacologic similarity a similar interaction may be expected to occur.

Mechanism: The mechanism of this interaction is unknown. Ketamine alone has been shown to produce hypertension and tachycardia, although it is usually less severe than seen in this interaction. Therefore it is believed that the thyroid replacement was involved in these cases.[1]

Recommendations: Until further clinical studies are done, the concurrent use of these agents need not be avoided. However, if this interaction does occur, propranolol may be useful since it has been shown to control both the heart rate and the increase in blood pressure.[1]

Reference

1. Kaplan, J.A., and Cooperman, L.H.: Alarming reactions to ketamine in patients taking thyroid medication-treatment with propranolol, Anesthesiology **35:**229, 1971.

Methoxyflurane–Secobarbital

2

Summary: Of 13 patients studied for the effects of methoxyflurane on renal function, 1 patient who was receiving concurrent secobarbital developed nonoliguric renal insufficiency. This patient also had serum inorganic fluoride levels considerably higher than the other 12 patients.[1]

Related Drugs: A similar reaction has been described in a patient who had been receiving pentobarbital for several years until 3 days prior to anesthesia with methoxyflurane.[2] Methoxyflurane is metabolized by the liver to a greater extent than any other halogenated inhalation anesthetic agent (enflurane, halothane, and isoflurane). Therefore, a similar interaction between secobarbital and these other halogenated anesthetic agents would not be expected. Documentation is lacking of an interaction between methoxyflurane and the other barbiturates (e.g., amobarbital, butabarbital, phenobarbital [see Appendix]), although because of pharmacologic similarity a similar interaction may be expected to occur.

Mechanism: Patients who receive methoxyflurane have concentrations of toxic metabolites, mainly inorganic fluoride, as a result of liver biotransformation of the anesthetic, which directly damages the renal tubules. Barbiturates, which induce hepatic microsomal enzymes, lead to an increased production of methoxyflurane toxic metabolites, which increases the incidence of nephrotoxicity. This has been demonstrated in several animal studies.[2-7]

Recommendations: Methoxyflurane should be avoided in patients who are receiving barbiturates. If the use of methoxyflurane is necessary, the barbiturate should be discontinued well in advance of administering this anesthetic.

References

1. Churchill, D., and others: Toxic nephropathy after low-dose methoxyflurane anesthesia: drug interaction with secobarbital? Can. Med. Assoc. J. **114:**326, 1976.
2. Cousins, M.J., and Mazze, R.I.: Methoxyflurane nephrotoxicity: a study of dose response in man J.A.M.A. **225:**1611, 1973.
3. Mazze, R.I., and others: Effect of enzyme induction with phenobarbital on the in vivo and in vitro defluorination of isoflurane and methoxyflurane, J. Pharmacol. Exp. Ther. **190:**523, 1974.
4. Son, S.L., and others: The effect of phenobarbitone on the metabolism of methoxyflurane to oxalic acid in the rat, Br. J. Anesth. **44:**1224, 1972.
5. Cousins, M.J., and others: The etiology of methoxyflurane nephrotoxicity, J. Pharmacol. Exp. Ther. **190:**530, 1974.
6. Cook, T., and others: Renal effects and metabolism of methoxyflurane, Anesth. Analg. (Cleve.) **54:**829, 1975.
7. Brodeur, J., and others: Influence of phenobarbital pretreatment on methoxyflurane and sodium fluoride nephropathy in fischer 344 rats, Toxicol. Appl. Pharmacol. **37:**349, 1976.

Methoxyflurane–Tetracycline

Summary: Concurrent administration of tetracycline and methoxyflurane may result in severe nephrotoxicity.[1-3] Although based primarily on case reports, the interaction appears to be of sufficient importance to warrant avoiding concurrent use of these drugs.

Related Drugs: Other tetracyclines (e.g., methacycline, minocycline, oxytetracycline [see Appendix]) may exhibit the same pattern of toxicity and therefore would be expected to interact with methoxyflurane. There is a report that doxycycline may not exhibit a similar toxicity.[4]

Methoxyflurane is the only general anesthetic implicated as a causative agent of renal toxicity.

Mechanism: Prerenal azotemia caused by tetracyclines has been demonstrated in humans.[5] If renal function is impaired, elevated blood urea nitrogen occurs.[6] Methoxyflurane nephrotoxicity appears to be related[7] and is associated with an increase in serum inorganic fluoride[8] and renal oxalosis.[9] The nephrotoxic potential of methoxyflurane (administered in high doses) is well established.[10-11] Whether concurrent administration of tetracycline and methoxyflurane results in additive nephrotoxic effects or whether there is a synergistic basis for the toxicity is uncertain.[12]

Recommendations: Until more is known concerning the possible effects of concurrent tetracycline and methoxyflurane administration on renal function, these drugs should not be used together. When alternate therapy is not possible renal status should be carefully monitored. Concurrent administration of methoxyflurane and other antibiotics known to be nephrotoxic (e.g., aminoglycosides, polymyxin, etc.) should be avoided.

References

1. Kuzucu, E.Y.: Methoxyflurane, tetracycline, and renal failure, J.A.M.A. **211:**1162, 1970.
2. Proctor, E.A., and Barton, F.L.: Polyuric acute renal failure after methoxyflurane and tetracycline, Br. Med. J. **4:**661, 1971.
3. Albers, D.D., and others: Renal failure following prostatovesiculectomy related to methoxyflurane anesthesia and tetracycline—complicated by candida infection, J. Urol. **106:**348, 1971.
4. Little, P.J., and others: Tetracyclines and renal failure, N. Z. Med. J. **72:**183, 1970.
5. Shils, M.E.: Renal disease and the metabolic affects of tetracycline, Ann. Intern. Med. **58:**389, 1963.
6. Shils, M.E.: Some metabolic aspects of tetracyclines, Clin. Pharmacol. Ther. **3:**321, 1962.
7. Mazze, R.I., and others: Dose-related methoxyflurane nephrotoxicity in rats: a biochemical and pathologic correlation, Anesthesiology **36:**571, 1972.
8. Mazze, R.I., and others: Methoxyflurane metabolism and renal dysfunction: clinical correlation in man, Anesthesiology **35:**247, 1971.
9. Frascino, J.A., and others: Renal oxalosis and azotemia after methoxylfurane, N. Engl. J. Med. **283:**676, 1970.
10. Committee on Anesthesia, National Academy of Sciences-National Research Council: Statement regarding the role of methoxyflurane in the production of renal dysfunction, Anesthesiology **34:**505, 1971.
11. Mazze, R.I., and others: Renal dysfunction associated with methoxyflurane anesthesia: a randomized prospective clinical evaluation, J.A.M.A. **216:**278, 1971.
12. Stoelting, R.K., and Gibbs, P.S.: Effect of tetracycline therapy on renal function after methoxyflurane anesthesia, Anesth. Analog. (Cleve.) **52:**431, 1973.

Pancuronium–Aminophylline

2

Summary: The concurrent use of pancuronium and aminophylline has been reported to cause resistance to the neuromuscular blockade produced by pancuronium.[1] In a patient receiving aminophylline, supraventricular tachycardia was reported to occur after administration of pancuronium, although no cause and effect relationship was determined.[2]

Related Drugs: There is a lack of documentation regarding a similar interaction between pancuronium and the other theophylline derivatives (dyphylline, oxtriphylline, and theophylline). Documentation is also lacking regarding an interaction between the theophylline derivatives and the other neuromuscular blocking agents (depolarizing: succinylcholine; nondepolarizing: e.g., atracurium, metocurine, tubocurarine [see Appendix]).

Mechanism: The mechanism of this interaction is unknown.

Recommendations: Patients should be monitored during concurrent use of these agents, and the dose of the neuromuscular blocking agent may need to be increased.

References

1. Doll, D.C., and Rosenberg, H.: Antagonism of neuromuscular blockage by theophylline, Anesth. Analg. (Cleve.) **58:**139, 1979.
2. Belani, K.G., and others: Adverse drug interaction involving pancuronium and aminophylline, Anesth. Analg. (Cleve.) **61:**473, 1982.

Pancuronium–Azathioprine

3

Summary: In one patient, the administration of azathioprine antagonized the neuro-muscular blocking action of pancuronium. This was subsequently observed in 3 other patients who received either pancuronium or tubocurarine.[1]

Related Drugs: In an animal study, the use of azathioprine reversed the neuromuscular blockade produced by tubocurarine.[1] Similar results were observed when gallamine was used.[1] Documentation is lacking of an interaction with the other nondepolarizing neuromuscular blocking agents (atracurium and metocurine), although a similar interaction may be expected to occur because of pharmacologic similarity. In the same animal study, the effects of succinylcholine were potentiated by azathioprine.[1] Whether the other thiopurine antineoplastic agent (mercaptopurine) interacts similarly with pancuronium has not been documented.

Mechanism: It has been postulated that azathioprine inhibits the enzyme phosphodiesterase, which plays a key role in motor nerve terminal activity allowing cyclic AMP to accumulate. Increased concentrations of cyclic AMP prolong the time of depolarization causing generation of repetitive activity and also increasing transmitter release. This action of azathioprine has been shown to occur in vitro.[1]

Recommendations: Concurrent use or subsequent use of azathioprine following pancuronium administration should be avoided if neuromuscular blockade is desired. If concomitant use is necessary, the dose of pancuronium may need to be increased.

Reference

1. Dretchen, K.L., and others: Azathioprine: effects on neuromuscular transmission, Anesthesiology **45:**604, 1976.

Pancuronium–Clindamycin

2

Summary: Clindamycin, when administered intraoperatively, was reported to prolong the neuromuscular blockade produced by pancuronium in a case report. This blockade was unresponsive to calcium or anticholinesterase administration.[1]

Related Drugs: A similar interaction with clindamycin or lincomycin and two nondepolarizing neuromuscular blocking agents (pancuronium and tubocurarine) has been reported in several animal studies.[2,3] Lincomycin (600 mg IV) in 7 case studies has been reported to augment a partial pancuronium neuromuscular blockade. Neostigmine successfully reversed the blockade in several of these patients.[4] A similar interaction, although not documented, may be expected to occur with the other nondepolarizing neuromuscular blocking agents (atracurium, gallamine, and metocurine) based on pharmacologic similarity. The neuromuscular blockade of succinylcholine has also been reported to be enhanced by clindamycin.[5]

Mechanism: Clindamycin and lincomycin possess some inherent neuromuscular blockade alone and may have an additive or synergistic pharmacologic activity with the neuromuscular blocking agents.[2,3,6]

Recommendations: The concurrent use of these agents should be used with caution and only if concomitant use is necessary. It is important to be aware of prolonged neuromuscular blockade, and ventilatory assistance should be available if necessary.

References

1. Fogdall, R.P., and Miller, R.D.: Prolongation of a pancuronium-induced neuromuscular blockade by clindamycin, Anesthesiology **41**:407, 1974.
2. Becker, L.D., and Miller, R.D.: Clindamycin enhances a nondepolarizing neuromuscular blockade, Anesthesiology **45**:84, 1976.
3. Wright, J.M., and Collier, J.M.: Characterization of the neuromuscular block produced by clindamycin and lincomycin, Can. J. Physiol. Pharmacol. **54**:937, 1976.
4. Booij, L.H., and others: Neostigmine and 4-aminopyridine antagonism of lincomycin-pancuronium neuromuscular blockade in man, Anesth. Analg. (Cleve.) **57**:316, 1978.
5. Avery, D., and Finn, R.: Succinylcholine-prolonged apnea associated with clindamycin and abnormal liver function tests, Dis. Nerv. Syst. **38**:473, 1977.
6. Rubbo, J.T., and others: Comparative neuromuscular effects of lincomycin and clindamycin, Anesth. Analg. (Cleve.) **56**:329, 1977.

Pancuronium–Hydrocortisone

3

Summary: Following hydrocortisone administration during surgery in a hypophysectomized patient, partial recovery from the neuromuscular blockade produced by pancuronium was reported.[1]

Related Drugs: Prednisone (250 mg/day) was reported in one study to have decreased the neuromuscular blockade induced by pancuronium.[2] There is a lack of documentation regarding an interaction between pancuronium and the other corticosteroids (e.g., betamethasone, prednisolone, triamcinolone [see Appendix]) or between hydrocortisone and the other neuromuscular blocking agents (nondepolarizing: atracurium, metocurine, tubocurarine [see Appendix]; depolarizing: succinylcholine), although because of pharmacologic similarity a similar interaction may be expected to occur.

Mechanism: The mechanism of this interaction is unknown. However, it has been suggested that this interaction may involve competition at the myoneural junction, altered protein binding, or induction of hepatic biotransformation.[2]

Recommendations: If the patient is receiving corticosteroids, or if corticosteroids may be used during surgery, the dose of the neuromuscular blocking agent may need to be increased.

References

1. Meyers, E.F.: Partial recovery from pancuronium neuromuscular blockade following hydrocortisone administration, Anesthesiology **46:**148, 1977.
2. Laflin, M.J.: Interaction of pancuronium and corticosteroids, Anesthesiology **47:**471, 1977.

Pancuronium–Lithium Carbonate

3

Summary: One report involving a single patient described an enhanced or prolonged neuromuscular blockade following concurrent use of lithium carbonate and pancuronium.[1] This interaction has also been reported in several animal studies.[2-4] However, there is a conflicting report that did not find similar results.[5]

Related Drugs: There are no drugs related to lithium carbonate. In one report, a patient on long-term lithium therapy developed prolonged apnea following succinylcholine administration.[3] However, this has been disputed in a study involving 17 patients.[6] According to several studies, the effect of lithium on gallamine and tubocurarine is not clear; some investigators reported prolongation of the neuromuscular blockade[7] and others found no effect.[2,5] The neuromuscular blockade of succinylcholine and pancuronium was prolonged by lithium in animal studies.[2-4] Because of conflicting results it is difficult to determine whether an interaction would occur between lithium carbonate and the other nondepolarizing neuromuscular blocking agents (atracurium and metocurine).

Mechanism: Although the mechanism of this interaction is unknown, it has been suggested that it may be caused by the changes in electrolyte balance induced by lithium and the resultant reduction of acetylcholine release at the neuromuscular junction.[7] Regarding an interaction between lithium carbonate and the depolarizing neuromuscular blocking agent succinylcholine, one report indicated that lithium reversibly inhibits serum cholinesterase activity.[8] Since succinylcholine is inactivated by the cholinesterase enzyme, inhibition of this enzyme by lithium may be the mechanism responsible for prolonged apnea.

Recommendations: Pancuronium or other neuromuscular blocking agents should be used with caution in patients taking lithium carbonate. Patients should be closely monitored, and ventilatory assistance should be provided as necessary.

References

1. Borden, H., and others: The use of pancuronium bromide in patients receiving lithium carbonate, Can. Anaesth. Soc. J. **21:**79, 1974.
2. Hill, G.E., and others: Lithium carbonate and neuromuscular blocking agents, Anesthesiology **46:**122, 1977.
3. Hill, G.E., and others: Potentiation of succinylcholine neuromuscular blockade by lithium carbonate, Anesthesiology **44:**439, 1976.
4. Reimherr, F.W., and others: Prolongation of muscle relaxant effects by lithium carbonate, Am. J. Psychiatry **134:**205, 1977.
5. Waud, B.E., and others: Lithium and neuromuscular transmission, Anesth. Analg. (Cleve.) **61:**399, 1982.
6. Martin, B.A., and Kramer, P.M.: Clinical significance of the interaction between lithium and a neuromuscular blocker, Am. J. Psychiatry **10:**1326, 1982.
7. Basuray, B.N., and Harris, C.A.: Potentiation of d-tubocurarine (d-Tc) neuromuscular blockade in cats by lithium chloride, Eur. J. Pharmacol. **45:**79, 1977.
8. Choi, S.J., and Derman, R.M.: Lithium and cholinesterase, Prog. Neuropsychopharmacol. **4:**107, 1980.

Pancuronium–Nitroglycerin

3

Summary: Although not studied in humans, animal studies show that nitroglycerin, when used intravenously prior to pancuronium administration, increases the duration of the neuromuscular blockade produced by pancuronium. There is some evidence that nitroglycerin may also increase the depth of neuromuscular blockade.[1,2]

Related Drugs: In contrast to pancuronium, the neuromuscular blockade produced by tubocurarine,[1,2] succinylcholine,[1,2] and gallamine[2] was not prolonged by nitroglycerin. Because of conflicting reports and lack of documentation, it is difficult to determine whether an interaction would occur between nitroglycerin and the other nondepolarizing neuromuscular blocking agents (atracurium and metocurine) or between pancuronium and the other nitrates (e.g., amyl nitrite, isosorbide dinitrate, pentaerythritol tetranitrate [see Appendix]).

Mechanism: The mechanism of this interaction is unknown. However, it is known that this interaction is not caused by an altered plasma clearance of pancuronium, circulatory changes, or changes in the acid-base or electrolyte balance.[1,2]

Recommendations: Until further clinical studies are performed in humans, it is important to be aware of the possible prolongation of neuromuscular blockade. If nitroglycerin is to be used, it may be advisable to use a noninteracting neuromuscular blocking agent. Alternatively, neostigmine has been shown to rapidly and completely reverse muscle paralysis, even during the prolongation produced by nitroglycerin.[1,2]

References

1. Glisson, S.N., and others: Prolongation of pancuronium-induced neuromuscular blockade by intravenous infusion of nitroglycerin, Anesthesiology **51:**47, 1979.
2. Glisson, S.N., and others: Nitroglycerin and the neuromuscular blockade produced by gallamine, suuccinylcholine, d-tubocurarine, and pancuronium, Anesth. Analg. (Cleve.) **59:**117, 1980.

Pancuronium–Thiotepa (Triethylene-thiophosphoramide)

3

Summary: In one report, a myasthenic patient who received pancuronium and 90 minutes later an intraperitoneal thiotepa injection developed rapid and prolonged respiratory depression.[1]

Related Drugs: Documentation is lacking of a similar interaction between the other neuromuscular blocking agents (depolarizing: succinylcholine; nondepolarizing: e.g., atracurium, metocurine, tubocurarine [see Appendix]) and the other antineoplastic alkylating agents (nitrosoureas: e.g., busulfan, carmustine, uracil mustard [see Appendix]).

Mechanism: The mechanism of this interaction is unknown. In experimental animal preparations, thiotepa alone has not been shown to produce neuromuscular blockade,[2] therefore it does not appear to be an additive or synergistic effect with pancuronium.[1] It has been suggested that the presence of myasthenia gravis may have been the predisposing and critical factor in this interaction.[1] Also, since other drugs were also utilized in this patient (pyridostigmine for 6 months, and atropine and thiopental during surgery), a number of possibilities could have occurred, including a cholinergic crisis, a hexaflurenium type of blockade, or a carcinoma neuropathy.[1]

Recommendations: The concurrent use of these agents should be used with caution, and ventilatory assistance should be available.

References

1. Bennett, E.J., and others: Muscle relaxants, myasthenia, and mustards? Anesthesiology **46:**220, 1977.
2. Rylett, B.J., and Colhoun, E.H.: Effects of acetylcholine mustard aziridinium ion and its choline analogue on choline transport into synaptosomes, Can. J. Physiol. Pharmacol. **55:**769, 1977.

Succinylcholine–Cyclophosphamide

2

Summary: Cyclophosphamide may potentiate the neuromuscular blockade produced by succinylcholine by inhibiting its metabolism.[1-3] Prolonged respiratory depression may occur in patients receiving succinylcholine and cyclophosphamide concurrently.

Related Drugs: Since succinylcholine is the only neuromuscular blocking agent metabolized by pseudocholinesterase, the nondepolarizing neuromuscular blocking agents (e.g., atracurium, pancuronium, tubocurarine [see Appendix]) would not be expected to interact with cyclophosphamide. Other cytotoxic drugs that also inhibit pseudocholinesterase (e.g., triethylene-melamine, mechlorethamine, and triethylene-thiophosphoramide)[1,2] would be expected to interact in a similar manner with succinylcholine.

Mechanism: Studies in vitro and in vivo demonstrated that the intravenous administration of cyclophosphamide decreases pseudocholinesterase activity by 35% to 70%.[1,2] This effect may last for several days. Succinylcholine is hydrolyzed through the action of pseudocholinesterase. Therefore, a decrease in the amount of pseudocholinesterase may prolong the neuromuscular blockade produced by succinylcholine.

Recommendations: Although the information concerning the interaction between the two drugs is limited, it would be prudent to either determine pseudocholinesterase levels before administering these drugs concurrently in a patient on cyclophosphamide therapy, or avoid the concomitant use of these agents. Alternatively, choose another neuromuscular blocking agent other than succinylcholine to use with cyclophosphamide.

References

1. Mone, J.G., and Mathie, W.E.: Qualitative and quantitative defects of pseudocholinesterase activity, Anaesthesia **22:**55, 1967.
2. Zsigmond, E.K., and Robins, G.O.: The effect of a series of anti-cancer drugs on plasma cholinesterase activity, Can. Anaesth. Soc. J. **19:**75, 1972.
3. Wolff, H.: The inhibition of serum cholinesterase by cyclophosphamide, Klin. Wochenschr. **43:**819, 1965.

Succinylcholine–Dexpanthenol

Summary: A single case indicated that dexpanthenol prolonged the respiratory depression induced by succinylcholine.[1] A subsequent study failed to verify the effect.[2]

Related Drugs: There are no reports of this interaction occurring with the nondepolarizing neuromuscular blocking agents (e.g., atracurium, pancuronium, tubocurarine [see Appendix]), although because of a different metabolic fate than succinylcholine such a similar interaction would not be expected.

Mechanism: Succinylcholine is a skeletal muscle relaxant[3] with a duration of action dependent on the rate of hydrolysis by pseudocholinesterase.[4] Dexpanthenol is converted to pantothenic acid, which combines with a protein moiety to form coenzyme A, which then produces acetylcholine.[5] The excess acetylcholine may saturate its enzymatic metabolic pathway and then compete with succinylcholine for metabolism by pseudocholinesterase.

Recommendations: The possibility of an interaction between succinylcholine and dexpanthenol at usual doses appears to be unlikely. Therefore, no additional precautions are necessary when these compounds are used concurrently.

References

1. Stewart, P.: Case reports, J. Am. Assoc. Nurse Anesth. **28:**56, 1960.
2. Smith, R., and others: Succinylcholine-pantothenyl alcohol: a reappraisal, Anesth. Analg. (Cleve.) **48:**205, 1969.
3. Taylor, P.: Neuromuscular blocking agents. In Gilman, A.G., Goodman, L.S., and Gilman, A, editors: The pharmacologic basis of therapeutics, New York, 1980, Macmillan Publishing Co.
4. Gissen, A.J., and Nastuk, W.L.: Succinylcholine and decamethonium, Anesthesiology **33:**611, 1970.
5. Beckman, H.: Dilemmas in drug therapy, Philadelphia, 1967, W.B. Saunders Co.

Succinylcholine–Isoflurane

2

Summary: In a study involving 20 healthy patients scheduled for elective surgery, the use of isoflurane anesthesia potentiated the phase II (desensitizing) neuromuscular blockade produced by succinylcholine. The tachyphylaxis that occurs with prolonged succinylcholine administration is followed by a decrease in succinylcholine requirement during isoflurane anesthesia. The study indicated that isoflurane potentiates succinylcholine only when phase II block has developed.[1]

Related Drugs: Two studies demonstrated an acceleration of the onset of phase II block in the presence of enflurane but without a reduction in succinylcholine requirement.[2,3] Documentation is lacking of a similar interaction between succinylcholine and the other halogenated inhalation anesthetics (halothane and methoxyflurane). Because the features of the phase II block are also characteristic of the nondepolarizing neuromuscular blocking agents[4] (e.g., atracurium, pancuronium, tubocurarine [see Appendix]), a similar interaction may be expected to occur, although it is not possible to determine whether similar mechanisms are involved.[5]

Mechanism: The mechanism of this interaction is not fully known. However, in one study pseudocholinesterase levels were measured during isoflurane anesthesia, and no significant changes in enzyme activity were seen over time.[6] Therefore, decreased pseudocholinesterase (the enzyme that inactivates succinylcholine) levels cannot explain the reduced succinylcholine requirement. An increase in muscle blood flow induced by isoflurane has been suggested as an explanation for the increased effect of lower doses of succinylcholine, but this does not explain the difference observed with a continuous infusion. Differences in infusion rates were seen only after 2 hours, which suggests that muscle blood flow was not a factor.[1]

Recommendations: Patients should be closely observed during concurrent use of these agents because a decreased succinylcholine dose may be necessary.

References

1. Donati, F., and Bevan, D.R.: Potentiation of succinylcholine phase II block with isoflurane, Anesthesiology **58:**552, 1983.
2. Donati, F., and Bevan, D.R.: Effect of enflurane and fentanyl on the clinical characteristics of long-term succinylcholine infusion, Can. Anaesth. Soc. J. **29:**59, 1982.
3. Hilgenberg, S.C., and Stoelting, R.K.: Characteristics of succinylcholine-produced phase II neuromuscular block during influrane, halothane, and fentanyl anesthesia, Anesth. Analg. (Cleve.) **60:**192, 1981.
4. Lee, C., and Katz, R.L.: Neuromuscular pharmacology: a clinical update and commentary, Br. J. Anaesth. **52:**173, 1980.
5. Waud, B.E., and Ward, D.R.: The effects of diethyl ether, enflurane and isoflurane at the neuromuscular junction, Anesthesiology **42:**275, 1975.
6. Delisle, S., and others: Plasma cholinesterase activity and tachyphylaxis during prolonged succinylcholine infusion, Anesth. Analg. (Cleve.) **61:**941, 1982.

Succinylcholine–Lidocaine

2

Summary: Large doses of lidocaine (7.5 to 16.5 mg/kg/dose) administered intravenously may prolong and intensify the neuromuscular blocking effect and duration of apnea produced by succinylcholine.[1-5]

Concomitant use of succinylcholine and lidocaine more than doubled (179 seconds) and also tripled (219 seconds) the duration of apnea compared with succinylcholine alone (74 seconds).[1]

Related Drugs: Tubocurarine, a nondepolarizing neuromuscular blocking agent, interacts with lidocaine in a manner similar to succinylcholine.[6] Although documentation is not available, the other nondepolarizing neuromuscular blocking agents (e.g., atracurium, metocurine, pancuronium [see Appendix]) may interact with lidocaine because of similar pharmacologic action.

Local anesthetics such as bupivacaine, cocaine, etidocaine, mepivacaine, prilocaine, procaine and procaine methobromide have been reported to interact similarly with succinylcholine.[3,4] Although other local anesthetics (e.g., benzocaine, dibucaine, tetracaine [see Appendix]) have not been evaluated, they may also be expected to interact based on pharmacologic similarity.

Mechanism: The mechanism of this interaction has not been fully established. The greater than additive neuromuscular effect caused by the combination of lidocaine and succinylcholine has been explained by their different sites of action.[7,8] Studies report that lidocaine displaces succinylcholine from plasma protein and plasma pseudocholinesterase which results in a greater concentration of succinylcholine at the site of action.[1-3] Also, lidocaine may affect the motor end-plate directly, producing neuromuscular blockade, although this action is relatively weak.[9-11] In addition, lidocaine depresses respiration without depressing neuromuscular function in the absence of succinylcholine.[2,11] Therefore, the respiratory depression produced by lidocaine is probably through a central nervous system effect rather than through neuromuscular blockade.

Recommendations: Patients who receive lidocaine, especially in large intravenous doses concomitantly with succinylcholine, should be observed closely to determine the need for artificial ventilation.

References

1. Usubiaga, J.E., and others: Interaction of intravenously administered procaine, lidocaine and succinylcholine in anesthetized subjects, Anesth. Analg. (Cleve.) **46:**39, 1967.
2. Wikinski, J.A., and others: Mechanism of convulsions elicited by local anesthetic agents: I. Local anesthetic depression of electrically induced seizures in man, Anesth. Analg. (Cleve.) **49:**504, 1970.
3. Telivuo, L., and Katz, R.L.: The effects of modern intravenous local analgesics on respiration during partial neuromuscular blockade in man, Anaesthesia **25:**30, 1970.
4. Matsuo, S., and others: Interaction of muscle relaxants and local anesthetics at the neuromuscular junction, Anesth. Analg. (Cleve.) **57:**580, 1978.
5. De Kornfeld, T.J., and Steinhaus, J.E.: The effect of intravenously administered lidocaine and succinylcholine on the respiratory activity of dogs, Anesth. Analg. (Cleve.) **38:**173, 1959.

6. Bruckner, J., and others: Neuromuscular drug interactions of clinical importance, Anesth. Analg. (Cleve.) **59:**678, 1980.

7. Strichartz, G.: Inhibition of ionic current in myelinated nerves by quaternery derivatives of lidocaine. In Fink, B.R., editor: Molecular mechanisms of anesthesia, New York, 1975, Raven Press.

8. Maeno, T., and others: Difference in effects of endplate potentials between procaine and lidocaine as revealed by voltage-clamp experiments, J. Neurophysiol. **34:**32, 1971.

9. Maeno, T.: Analysis of sodium and potassium conductances in the procaine end-plate potential, J. Physiol. **183:**592, 1966.

10. Mathews, E.K., and Quilliam, J.P.: Effects of central depressant drugs upon acetylcholine release, Br. J. Pharmacol. **22:**415, 1964.

11. Katz, R.L., and Gissen, A.J.: Effects of intravenous and intraarterial procaine and lidocaine on neuromuscular transmission in man, Acta Anaesth. Scand. **36**(suppl.):103, 1969.

Succinylcholine–Neostigmine

Summary: Several studies reported that neostigmine may either antagonize or enhance the neuromuscular blocking effect of succinylcholine, depending on whether the blockade is in phase I (depolarizing) or phase II (desensitizing).[1-4] In a study involving 10 normal patients, neostigmine potentiated the block produced by succinylcholine whether it was of the depolarizing or desensitizing type. However, in 5 patients with atypical plasma cholinesterase, neostigmine potentiated the depolarizing phase while antagonizing the desensitizing phase.[1] Other studies in patients with atypical pseudocholinesterase found similar results.[2,3]

Related Drugs: In a study involving a patient with atypical pseudocholinesterase, edrophonium prolonged the neuromuscular blockade produced by succinylcholine, although it appeared to be administered in the depolarizing phase.[5] A patient with decreased pseudocholinesterase activity showed a prolonged duration of succinylcholine neuromuscular blockade after the use of pyridostigmine. When edrophonium was later used in the desensitizing phase, a persistent reversal of muscle weakness occurred.[6] A case study also reports the marked prolongation of succinylcholine after the use of physostigmine.[7] Documentation is lacking regarding an interaction between succinylcholine and the other anticholinesterases (ambenonium and demecarium), although because of related pharmacologic activity a similar interaction may be expected. The nondepolarizing neuromuscular blocking agents (e.g., atracurium, pancuronium, tubocurarine [see Appendix]) would not be expected to interact in a similar manner since they are not metabolized by pseudocholinesterase; however, documentation is lacking.

Mechanism: In patients with normal plasma cholinesterase activity, succinylcholine is rapidly hydrolyzed by plasma cholinesterase. Injection of neostigmine under such conditions will inhibit the cholinesterase and delay the hydrolysis of succinylcholine in phase I or II. In patients with atypical cholinesterase, the enzyme plays no part in the elimination of succinylcholine since there is virtually no hydrolysis of the drug. However, the action of neostigmine effectively increases the concentration of acetylcholine at the neuromuscular junction by decreasing its rate of hydrolysis. This will potentiate the depolarizing phase of succinylcholine and reverse its desensitizing phase.[1-4] Similar mechanisms were suggested for the other anticholinesterase drugs.[5-7]

Recommendations: The concurrent use of succinylcholine and an anticholinesterase agent should be avoided during the depolarizing phase of the neuromuscular blockade and should only be used with great caution if at all in the desensitizing phase. If concomitant use is necessary, closely monitor the patient and provide ventilatory assistance if necessary.

References

1. Baraka, A.: Suxamethonium-neostigmine interaction in patients with normal or atypical cholinesterase, Br. J. Anaesth. **49:**479, 1977.

2. Baraka, A.: Potentiation of suxamethonium blockade by neostigminé in patients with atypical cholinesterase, Br. J. Anaesth. **47:**416, 1975.
3. Miller, R.D., and Stevens, W.C.: Antagonism of succinylcholine paralysis in a patient with atypical pseudocholinesterase, Anesthesiology **36:**511, 1972.
4. Gissen, A.J., and others: Neuromuscular block in man during prolonged arterial infusion with succinylcholine, Anesthesiology **27:**242, 1966.
5. Vickers, M.D.A.: The mismanagement of suxamethonium apnoea, Br. J. Anaesth. **15:**260, 1963.
6. Bentz, E.W., and Stoelting, R.K.: Prolonged response to succinylcholine following pancuronium reversal with pyridostigmine, Anesthesiology **44:**258, 1976.
7. Kopman, A.F., and others: Prolonged response to succinylcholine following physostigmine, Anesthesiology **49:**142, 1978.

Succinylcholine–Procainamide

3

Summary: Studies have demonstrated that procainamide may prolong and intensify the neuromuscular blockade produced by succinylcholine in cats.[1] In humans, a smaller dose of succinylcholine may be required when it is administered concurrently with procainamide.[2]

Related Drugs: The same interaction with succinylcholine has been demonstrated in humans with procaine[3] and quinidine.[4-8] No documentation exists regarding an interaction between procainamide and the nondepolarizing neuromuscular blocking agents (e.g., atracurium, pancuronium, tubocurarine [see Appendix]). However, if the mechanism involves plasma cholinesterase, then these agents would not be expected to interact since they are not inactivated by plasma cholinesterase as is succinylcholine.

Mechanism: The mechanism through which procainamide exerts this effect may involve displacement of succinylcholine from the cholinesterase system or an inhibition of plasma cholinesterase activity. These actions would result in a greater concentration of succinylcholine at the site of action, thus enhancing the pharmacologic effect.

Recommendations: Patients receiving succinylcholine and procainamide concurrently should be observed for signs of neuromuscular blockade, especially prolonged apnea. Artificial ventilation may be required for a longer time in such patients.

References

1. Cuthbert, M.G.: The effect of quinidine and procainamide on the neuromuscular blocking action of suxamethonium, Br. J. Anaesth. **38:**775, 1966.
2. Valenti, F., and others: The interference of procainamide with the neuromuscular blockade of succinylcholine, Acta Anesth. (Padova) **18:**21, 1967.
3. Salgado, A.S.: Potentiation of succinylcholine by procaine, Anesthesiology **22:**897, 1961.
4. Grogono, A.W., and others: A guide to interaction in anesthetic practice, Drugs **19:**279, 1980.
5. Nugent, S.K.: Pharmacology and use of muscle relaxants in infants and children, J. Pediatr. **94:**481, 1979.
6. Harrah, M.D., and others: The interaction of d-tubocurarine with antiarrhythmic drugs, Anesthesiology **33:**406, 1970.
7. Mazin, E., and others: Interference by quinidine on the neuromuscular block caused by succinylcholine, Ann. Med. Psychol. (Paris) **103:**603, 1972.
8. Grogono, A.W.: Anesthesia for atrial fibrillation: effect of quinidine on muscular relaxation, Lancet **2:**193, 1963.

Succinylcholine–Promazine

2

Summary: The administration of promazine following a succinylcholine infusion resulted in total muscle relaxation and prolonged apnea in 1 patient. These reactions began within 3 minutes of promazine administration. The patient also became cyanotic and was unable to lift the head or move the extremities.[1]

Related Drugs: Although documentation is lacking, other phenothiazines (e.g., chlorpromazine, thioridazine, trifluoperazine [see Appendix]) may be expected to interact in a similar manner with succinylcholine because of pharmacologic similarity. Documentation is also lacking regarding an interaction between promazine and the nondepolarizing neuromuscular blocking agents (e.g., atracurium, pancuronium, tubocurarine [see Appendix]) However, because these agents are not inactivated by serum cholinesterase as is succinylcholine, a similar interaction would not be expected.

Mechanism: The mechanism is not fully known. However, it has been suggested that promazine may lower serum cholinesterase levels.[1] Because succinylcholine is inactivated by cholinesterase, the lower levels induced by promazine may result in succinylcholine remaining at the site of action for a prolonged period of time, thus resulting in prolonged apnea. The possibility of the existence of atypical plasma cholinesterase in this patient cannot be ruled out.[1]

Recommendations: Promazine should be used with caution in patients receiving succinylcholine, and ventilatory assistance should be made available. In this study, edrophonium successfully treated the prolonged apnea.[1]

Reference

1. Regan, A.G., and Aldrete, J.A.: Prolonged apnea after administration of promazine hydrochloride following succinylcholine infusion, Anesth. Analg. (Cleve.) **46:**315, 1967.

Succinylcholine–Trimethaphan

2

Summary: In one study, 10 patients were pretreated with trimethaphan and then given a succinylcholine injection; 9 showed an increased neuromuscular blocking effect as exhibited by prolonged apnea.[1] In a case report, a patient showed prolonged apnea after the concurrent use of succinylcholine and tubocurarine with trimethaphan (4500 mg over 90 minutes).[2] Another case report showed similar results.[3] There was variable response in an animal study, some of the animals showing a prolonged apnea whereas others did not.[4]

Related Drugs: Animal studies indicate the concurrent use of tubocurarine and trimethaphan may increase the neuromuscular blocking effect of tubocurarine.[5] Documentation is lacking regarding a similar interaction between trimethaphan and the other nondepolarizing neuromuscular blocking agents (e.g., atracurium, metocurine, pancuronium [see Appendix]). However, if the mechanism involves a direct neuromuscular blockade by trimethaphan, then these agents may also interact. There are no drugs related to trimethaphan.

Mechanism: It has been shown that trimethaphan can inhibit pseudocholinesterase in vitro.[1,4,6,8] The action of succinylcholine, which is metabolized by pseudocholinesterase, would be prolonged if trimethaphan does this in vivo as well. Rapid administration of trimethaphan has also caused respiratory paralysis,[7] and other reports suggest that trimethophan may have some direct neuromuscular blocking activity itself, possibly of the nondepolarizing type, which is not related to a cholinesterase inhibiting action.[5,7,8] This may explain the interaction with tubocurarine, which is not metabolized by pseudocholinesterase.

Recommendations: Trimethaphan and any neuromuscular blocking agent should be used concurrently with caution. If concomitant use is necessary, ventilatory assistance should be available.

References

1. Tewfik, G.I.: Trimethaphan, its effect on the pseudo-cholinesterase level of man, Anesthesia **12:**326, 1957.
2. Wilson, S.L., and others: Prolonged neuromuscular blockade associated with trimethaphan: a case report, Anesth. Analg. (Cleve.) **55:**353, 1976.
3. Poulton, T.J., and others: Prolonged apnea following trimethaphan and succinylcholine, Anesthesiology **50:**54, 1979.
4. Pearcy, W.C., and Wittenstein, E.S.: The interaction of trimethaphan (arfonad), suxamethonium and cholinesterase inhibition in the rat, Br. J. Anaesth. **32:**156, 1960.
5. Deacock, A.R., and Davies, T.D.: The influence of certain ganglionic blocking agents on neuromuscular transmission, Br. J. Anesth. **30:**217, 1958.
6. Sklar, G.S., and Lanks, K.W.: Effects of trimethaphan and sodium nitroprusside on hydrolysis of succinylcholine in vitro, Anesthesiology **47:**31, 1977.
7. Dale, R.C., and Schroeder, E.T.: Respiratory paralysis during treatment of hypertension with trimethaphan camsylate, Arch. Intern. Med. **136:**816, 1976.
8. Nakamura, K., and others: Prolonged neuromuscular blockade following trimethaphan infusion, Anesthesiology **35:**1202, 1980.

Thiopental–Morphine

2

Summary: The concurrent use of thiopental and morphine may lead to an increased respiratory depression greater than that seen with either agent alone. This was shown by a rise in end-expiratory carbon dioxide tensions and respiratory response to hypercapnia.[1]

Related Drugs: Similar results were seen with the concurrent use of thiopental and meperidine.[1] One study reported that small doses of thiopental antagonized the analgesia produced by 100 mg of meperidine, but respiratory depression was not discussed.[2] Although no documentation exists, a similar interaction may be expected between the other narcotics (e.g., codeine, hydromorphone, methadone [see Appendix]) and the other barbiturate anesthetics (methohexital and thiamylal), since they all produce a degree of respiratory depression alone.

Mechanism: Although the mechanism is not fully known, it has been suggested that because each agent produces respiratory depression on its own, an additive synergistic effect may be involved.

Recommendations: Patients should be closely monitored during concurrent use of these agents. If the dose of the narcotic cannot be lowered, it is important to be prepared for ventilatory assistance.

References

1. Eckenhoff, J.E., and Helrich, M.: The effect of narcotics, thiopental and nitrous oxide upon respiration and respiratory response to hypercapnia, Anesthesiology **19:**240, 1958.
2. Dundee, J.W.: Alterations in response to somatic pain associated with anaesthesia. II: The effect of thiopentone and pentobarbitone, Br. J. Anaesth. **32:**47, 1960.

Thiopental–Probenecid

3

Summary: Thiopental anesthesia was prolonged by 26% to 109% after probenecid administration in a double-blind controlled study involving 86 patients. The arterial blood pressure, heart rate, recovery time, tolerance to pain stimuli, and frequency of apnea were not altered by probenecid.[1]

Related Drugs: Documentation is lacking of an interaction between probenecid and the other barbiturate anesthetics (methohexital and thiamylal), although because they are related pharmacologically a similar interaction may occur. There is no documentation regarding a similar interaction between thiopental and the other uricosuric (sulfinpyrazone).

Mechanism: The mechanism of this interaction is unknown.

Recommendations: It is important to be aware of the possibility of prolonged anesthesia after concurrent use of thiopental and probenecid. Probenecid may need to be discontinued prior to the use of thiopental if this effect is not desired.

Reference

1. Kaukinen, S., and others: Prolongation of thiopentone anesthesia by probenecid, Br. J. Anaesth. **52:**603, 1980.

Thiopental–Reserpine

2

Summary: Reserpine may enhance the central nervous system (CNS) depression caused by thiopental prior to surgery, resulting in hypotension and bradycardia. In controlled studies, approximately 50% of both the control groups and the groups treated with reserpine developed bradycardia and hypotension after thiopental-induced anesthesia using various preoperative medications and gaseous anesthetics.[1,2] In a similar controlled study,[2] no difference in sleeping time or apnea were found between reserpine-treated patients and the control group. Other case reports of this interaction have been published.[3,4]

Related Drugs: Pentobarbital[5] and thiamylal[6] are reported to interact with reserpine in animals. There appears to be no documentation of interactions when other barbiturates (e.g., amobarbital, butabarbital, secobarbital [see Appendix]) are used with reserpine; however, they may be expected to interact similarly to pentobarbital because of pharmacologic similarity.

Because of similar pharmacologic action, all other rauwolfia alkaloids (alseroxylon, deserpidine, and rescinnamine) would probably have a potential for interacting with thiopental or other barbiturates.

Mechanism: The mechanism for this interaction is unknown. However, reserpine causes a depletion of catecholamines and serotonin in the central and peripheral nervous systems and cardiovascular tissue. Reserpine interferes with the binding of serotonin at the receptor sites, decreases the synthesis of norepinephrine and epinephrine by depleting their precursor dopamine, and competitively inhibits uptake of catecholamines into storage vesicles.[7] The action of barbiturates on the CNS is not fully understood, but they can produce hypnosis and anesthesia, anticonvulsant effects, and other actions such as autonomic nervous system depression and respiratory depression. Reserpine has been shown to prolong barbiturate-induced sleeping times[5,8] and respiratory depression[9] in animals.

Recommendations: Withdrawal of reserpine prior to surgery is not mandatory; however, it is important to be aware that the patient has been receiving rauwolfia alkaloids and that hypotension and bradycardia may occur. If reserpine is not withdrawn prior to surgery and if hypotension does occur, an exacerbated effect may be noticed since the endogenous catecholamines have already been chronically depleted by reserpine. Therefore, the use of an indirect-acting sympathomimetic agent would be ineffective, and a direct-acting sympathomimetic agent would be required to treat the hypotension.

References

1. Munson, W.M., and Jenicek, J.A.: Effect of anesthetic agents on patients receiving reserpine therapy, Anesthesiology **23:**741, 1962.
2. Tammisto, T., and others: The effect of reserpine, chlordiazepoxide and imipramine on the potency of thiopental in man, Ann. Chir. Gynaecol. **56:**323, 1967.

3. Coakley, C.S., and others: Circulatory responses during anesthesia of patients on rauwolfia therapy, J.A.M.A. **161:**1143, 1956.
4. Ziegler, C.H., and Lovette, J.B.: Operative complications after therapy with reserpine and reserpine compounds, J.A.M.A. **176:**916, 1961.
5. Garrattini, S., and others: Reserpine derivative with specific hypotensive or sedative activity, Nature **183:**1273, 1959.
6. Gray, W.D., and Rauh, C.E.: The anticonvulsant action of inhibitors of carbonic anhydrase: relation to endogenous amines in brain, J. Pharmacol. Exp. Ther. **155:**127, 1967.
7. Weiner, N.: Drugs that inhibit adrenergic nerves and block adrenergic receptors. In Gilman, A.G., Goodman, L.S., and Gilman, A., editors: The pahrmacologic basis of therapeutics, New York, 1980, Macmillan Publishing Co.
8. Brodie, B.B., and others: Potentiating action of chlorpromazine and reserpine, Nature **175:**1133, 1955.
9. Trapoid, J.H., and others: Cardiovascular and respiratory effects of serpasil, a new crystalline alkaloid from rauwolfia serpentina benth, in the dog, J. Pharmacol. Exp. Ther. **110:**205, 1954.

Thiopental–Sulfisoxazole

2

Summary: Intravenous sulfisoxazole reduces the amount of thiopental required for anesthesia and shortens the awakening time when administered immediately prior to the induction of anesthesia.[1,2]

Related Drugs: Information is not available regarding a similar interaction with other ultrashort-acting barbiturate anesthetics (thiamylal and methohexital); however, because of pharmacologic similarity, an interaction by be expected to occur. The effect of using longer-acting barbiturates (e.g., amobarbital, butabarbital, secobarbital [see Appendix]) with other sulfonamides (e.g., sulfamethizole, sulfamethoxazole, sulfasalazine [see Appendix]) is not known, but phenobarbital has been shown to produce little interaction with sulfisoxazole.[3]

Mechanism: It has been proposed that sulfisoxazole displaces thiopental from plasma protein binding sites, resulting in higher plasma concentrations of free thiopental.[4] More free thiopental is therefore available to exert an anesthetic effect, but it is also more rapidly metabolized.

Recommendations: When thiopental is used during long-term oral sulfisoxazole therapy, the thiopental dosage may have to be adjusted to provide smaller, more frequent doses in order to compensate for the effect of concomitant sulfisoxazole administration.

References

1. Cosgor, S.I., and Kerek, S.F.: Enhancement of thiopentone anesthesia by sulphafurazole, Br. J. Anaesth. **42:**988, 1970.
2. Cosgor, S.I., and others: Influence of sulfathiazole on thiopental and hexobarbital narcosis, Rev. Roum. Physiol. **8:**81, 1971.
3. Krauer, B.: Comparative investigations of elimination kinetics of two sulfonamides in children with and without phenobarbital administration, Schweiz. Med. Wochenschr. **101:**668, 1971.
4. Cosgor, S.I., and Papp, J.: Competition between sulphonamides and thiopental for binding sites of plasma proteins, Arzneimittelforsch. **20:**1925, 1970.

Tubocurarine–Chlorothiazide

3

Summary: Hypothetically an enhanced neuromuscular blockade can be predicted to arise from the combined action of a potassium-depleting diuretic such as chlorothiazide and the neuromuscular blocking agent d-tubocurarine.[1]

Related Drugs: Although documentation is lacking, the potential exists for an interaction between tubocurarine and other potassium-depleting diuretics such as the loop diuretics (bumetanide, ethacrynic acid, and furosemide), the mercurial diuretic (mersalyl), other thiazides (e.g., hydrochlorothiazide, methyclothiazide, polythiazide [see Appendix]) and thiazide related diuretics including chlorthalidone, metolazone, quinethazone, and indapamide. There are no reports of an interaction between chlorothiazide and other neuromuscular blocking agents (depolarizing: succinylcholine; nondepolarizing: atracurium, metocurine, pancuronium [see Appendix]), although based on the proposed mechanism a similar interaction may be expected to occur.

Mechanism: Clinical data are not available to verify the postulate that hypokalemia produced by chlorothiazide could enhance d-tubocurarine neuromuscular blockade. The potassium dependency of neuromuscular function has been demonstrated and this disruption of extracellular potassium levels by chlorothiazide could enhance actions of d-tubocurarine.[2]

Recommendations: Avoiding hypokalemia can reduce the potential risks of this interaction in a patient receiving diuretic therapy who will be given d-tubocurarine. The serum potassium level should be determined and corrected if necessary to avoid the possibility of prolonged neuromuscular blockade from a hypokalemic state.

References

1. Moyer, J.H., and others: Medical consideration in the hypertensive patient undergoing surgery, Am. J. Cardiol. **12:**286, 1963.
2. McLaughlin, A.P., and others: Hazards of gallamine administration in patients with renal failure, J. Urol. **108:**515, 1972.

Tubocurarine–Gentamicin

1

Summary: Aminoglycoside antibiotics produce a neuromuscular blockade that may prolong the respiratory depressant and muscle relaxant effects of tubocurarine and other neuromuscular depressant drugs.

Related Drugs: All aminoglycosides have been shown experimentally to produce neuromuscular blockade, with netilmicin and sisomicin being the most potent and tobramycin being the least potent.[1-7] Clinical potentiation of neuromuscular blocking agents has been reported with all currently available aminoglycosides (neomycin, streptomycin, gentamicin, kanamycin, tobramycin, and amikacin) as well as colistin.[3,8-23] Reports involving the recently released netilmicin will probably appear as the use of this agent increases. In addition to tubocurarine, clinical and experimental evidence indicates that the neuromuscular blockade produced by pancuronium, gallamine, vecuranium, succinylcholine, and atracurium may be potentiated by these antibiotics.[1,3-5,8,9,24,25]

Mechanism: The antibiotics produce neuromuscular blockade by inhibiting acetylcholine release presynaptically and by reducing the sensitivity of the postjunctional membrane.[2,26-28] The blockade, which is primarily caused by inhibition of presynaptic acetylcholine release, is similar to that produced by magnesium ions.[3] Alternatively, calcium ions antagonize the blockade, and it has been theorized that the antibiotics and calcium compete for a common receptor site on the presynaptic membrane.[3,27,28] Antibiotic-induced blockade is intensified by neuromuscular blocking agents, and vice versa, as well as by hypocalcemia.

Recommendations: Whenever possible, alternative antibiotics should be used perioperatively in patients who receive tubocurarine or other neuromuscular depressant drugs. Other antibiotics reported to prolong neuromuscular blockade include bacitracin, clindamycin, lincomycin, polymyxins, and tetracyclines.[3,24,29,30] Beta-lactams, chloramphenicol, erythromycin, and vancomycin seem to be free of the effect. When aminoglycosides or colistin must be used, the clinician should be aware of the potential dangers and exercise caution. Facilities for intubation and mechanical ventilation should be available both during and after surgery, and the patient should be continually observed for signs of respiratory depression.

    The interaction usually occurs when the antibiotic is given prior to or concurrently with the neuromuscular blocking drug, but it may also occur when given after, especially when depolarizing agents such as succinylcholine are involved.[8.9] The clinician should be aware that any antibiotic dose or route of administration including intravenous, intramuscular, oral, intraperitoneal, intrapleural, intraluminal, and irrigation can produce respiratory depression.[4-23]

    Clinically, the interaction is noted either intraoperatively as prolonged apnea or postoperatively as acute dyspnea progressing to prolonged apnea. Treatment centers around placing the patient on a respirator until respiratory function returns. Also, the blockade may be antagonized with calcium and neostigmine, since both have been used for this purpose. The efficacy of these agents in reversing neuromuscular blockade is variable and, as yet, unpredictable; however, calcium is usually more effective and should generally be tried first.[1,18,20,21,23,24,26,31] Neostigmine is not indicated in the treatment of neuromuscular blockade caused by depolarizing agents.[32]

References

1. Singh, Y.N., and others: Some effects of the aminoglycoside antibiotic amikacin on neuromuscular and autonomic transmissions, Br. J. Anesth. **50:**109, 1978.
2. Lee, C., and DeSilva, A.J.C.: Acute and subchronic neuromuscular blocking characteristics of streptomycin: a comparison with neomycin, Br. J. Anaesth. **58:**107, 1979.
3. Pittinger, C.B., and Adamson, R.: Antibiotic blockade of neuromuscular function, Ann. Rev. Pharmacol. **12:**169, 1972.
4. Warner, A.W., and Sanders, E.: Neuromuscular blockade associated with gentamicin therapy, J.A.M.A. **215:**1153, 1979.
5. Rutten, J.M.J., and others: The comparative neuromuscular blocking effects of some aminoglycoside antibiotics, Acta Anaesthesiol. Belg. **31:**293, 1980.
6. Albiero, L., and others: Comparison of neuromuscular effect and acute toxicity of some aminoglycoside antibiotic, Arch. Int. Pharmacodyn. Ther. **233:**343, 1978.
7. Poradelis, A.G., and others: Neuromuscular blocking activity of dibekacin, a new semisynthetic aminoglycoside antibiotic, Experimentia **36:**867, 1980.
8. Foldes, F.F., and others: Prolonged respiratory depression caused by drug combinations, muscle relaxants and intraperitoneal antibiotics as etiologic agents, J.A.M.A. **183:**672, 1963.
9. Benz, H.G., and others: "Recurarization" by intraperitoneal antibiotics, Br. Med. J. **2:**241, 1961.
10. Webber, B.W.: Respiratory arrest following intraperitoneal administration of neomycin, Arch. Surg. **75:**174, 1957.
11. Ferrera, B.E., and Phillips, R.D.: Respiratory arrest following intraperitoneal use of neomycin, Ann. Surg. **149:**546, 1959.
12. Doremus, W.P.: Respiratory arrest following intraperitoneal use of neomycin, Ann. Surg. **149:**546, 1959.
13. Stechishin, O., and others: Neuromuscular paralysis and respiratory arrest caused by intrapleural neomycin, Can. Med. Assoc. J. **81:**32, 1959.
14. Cooper, E.A., and Hanson, R. de G.: Oral neomycin and anaesthesia, Br. Med. J. **2:**1527, 1963.
15. Ream, C.R.: Respiratory and cardiac arrest after intravenous administration of kanamycin with reversal of toxic effects by neostigmine, Ann. Intern. Med. **59:**384, 1963.
16. Oriscello, R.G., and Depasqudle, N.P.: Neomycin wound irrigation: report of a case associated with massive absorption with nephro and neurotoxicity, Am. J. Ther. Clin. Rep. **1:**1, 1975.
17. Waterman, P.M., and Smith, R.B.: Tobramycin-curare interaction. Curr. Res. **56:**587, 1977.
18. Lilly, J.K.: Intraoperative aminoglycoside apnea, South. Med. J. **71:**979, 1978.
19. Hashimoto, Y., and others: A possible hazard of prolonged neuromuscular blockade by amikacin, Anesthesiology **49:**219, 1978.
20. Hashimoto, Y., and others: Neuromuscular blocking property of amikacin in man, Tohoku J. Exp. Med. **125:**11, 1978.
21. Giala, M.M., and Paradelis, A.G.: Two cases of prolonged respiratory depression due to interaction of pancuronium with colistin and streptomycin, J. Antimicrob. Chemother. **5:**234, 1979.
22. Regan, A.G., and Perumbetti, P.P.V.: Pancuronium and gentamicin interaction in patients with renal failure, Anesth. Analg. (Cleve.) **59:**393, 1980.
23. Giala, M., and others: Possible interaction of pancuronium and tubocurarine with oral neomycin, Anesthesiology **37:**776, 1982.
24. Burkett, L., and others: Mutual potentiation of the neuromuscular effects of antibiotics and relaxants, Anesth. Analg. (Cleve.) **58:**107, 1979.
25. Krieg, N., and others: Preliminary review of the interactions of ORG NC45 with anaesthetics and antibiotics in animals, Br. J. Anaeth. **52:**335, 1980.
26. Corrado, A.P., and others: Neuromuscular blockade by neomycin, potentiation by ether anesthesia and d-tubocurarine and antagonism by calcium and prostigmine, Arch. Int. Pharmacodyn. Ther. **121:**380, 1959.

27. Brazil, O.V., and Prado-Franceschi, J.: The nature of neuromuscular block produced by neomycin and gentamicin, Arch. Int. Pharmacodyn. Ther. **179:**78, 1969.
28. Farley, J.M., and others: Mechanism of neuromuscular block by streptomycin: a voltage clamp analysis, J. Pharmacol. Exp. Ther. **222:**488, 1982.
29. Fogdall, R.P., and Miller, R.D.: Prolongation of a pancuronium induced neuromuscular blockade by clindamycin, Anesthesiology **41:**407, 1974.
30. Small, G.A.: Respiratory paralysis after a large dose of intraperitoneal polymyxin B and bacitracin, Anesth. Analg. (Cleve.) **43:**137, 1964.
31. Jones, W.P.G.: Calcium treatment for ineffective respiration resulting from administration of neomycin, J.A.M.A. **170:**943, 1959.
32. Gilman, A.G., and others: The pharmacological basis of therapeutics, New York, 1980, Macmillan Publishing Co.

Tubocurarine–Ketamine

Summary: One human study[1] and 3 animal studies[2-4] have shown that a single intravenous dose of ketamine augments the neuromuscular blocking properties of tubocurarine.

Related Drugs: There are no drugs related to ketamine. The human study reports that neither succinylcholine nor pancuronium is affected by ketamine.[1] Conversely, 2 animal studies report that both succinylcholine and pancuronium are potentiated by ketamine.[2,3] Because of conflicting results, it is difficult to determine whether an interaction would occur between ketamine and the other nondepolarizing neuromuscular blocking agents (atracurium, gallamine, and metocurine).

Mechanism: Several mechanisms have been suggested. First, ketamine may decrease motor end-plate sensitivity and would therefore potentiate tubocurarine.[1-4] Also, ketamine may interfere with protein binding of tubocurarine, making more tubocurarine available to the neuromuscular junction. This effect would not be expected with succinylcholine or pancuronium since they do not significantly bind to protein.[4]

Recommendations: These agents should be used concurrently with caution. Patients should be closely monitored throughout anesthesia when ketamine and a neuromuscular blocking agent are used concurrently.

References

1. Johnston, R.R., and others: The interaction of ketamine with d-tubocurarine, pancuronium, and succinylcholine in man, Anesth. Analg. (Cleve.) **53:**496, 1974.
2. Amaki, Y., and others: Ketamine interaction with neuromuscular blocking agents in the phrenic nerve-hemidiaphragm preparation of the rat, Anesth. Analg. (Cleve.) **57:**238, 1978.
3. Kraunuk, P., and others: In vitro study of interaction between I.V. anaesthetics and neuromuscular blocking agents, Br. J. Anesth. **49:**768, 1977.
4. Cronnelly, R., and others: Ketamine: myoneural activity and interaction with neuromuscular blocking agents, Europ. J. Pharmacol. **22:**17, 1973.

Tubocurarine–Morphine

2

Summary: The intravenous or intramuscular administration of morphine augments the neuromuscular blockade produced by tubocurarine. Harmful effects from this interaction can be avoided by administering morphine only after the effects of tubocurarine have dissipated or by monitoring respiration and controlling it when necessary. Tubocurarine and morphine both reduce blood pressure and may produce hypotension if used concurrently.

Related Drugs: Documentation is lacking regarding an interaction between morphine and the other neuromuscular blocking agents (depolarizing: succinylcholine; nondepolarizing: e.g., atracurium, metocurine, pancuronium [see Appendix]), although because of similar pharmacologic action an interaction may occur. While there is also no documentation of an interaction between tubocurarine and other narcotics (e.g., codeine, hydromorphone, opium [see Appendix]), because they are related pharmacologically a similar interaction may be expected.

Mechanism: Morphine may augment the neuromuscular blockade of tubocurarine by a direct neuromuscular effect,[1,2] by causing central respiratory depression, or by elevating the partial pressure of carbon dioxide in the arterial blood.[3,4] Morphine also reduces neostigmine's ability to antagonize tubocurarine blockade.[5] The hypotensive effects of tubocurarine and morphine are thought to be caused in part to release of histamine.[6,7]

Recommendations: If morphine is given to a patient recovering from tubocurarine blockade or to one in whom the blockade has been antagonized recently by neostigmine, ventilation should be monitored and controlled so that the partial pressure of carbon dioxide in the arterial blood does not increase. If it does increase, tubocurarine blockade may reappear or recovery may be delayed.

Administration of morphine (5 mg/70 kg) and tubocurarine (9 mg/kg) in small intermittent doses rather than large bolus injections should minimize hypotension.

References

1. Fredickson, R.C., and Pinsky, C.: Morphine impairs acetylcholine release but facilitates acetylcholine action at skeletal neuromuscular junction, Nature New Biol. **231:**93, 1971.
2. Soteropoulos, G.C., and Standaert, F.G.: Neuromuscular effects of morphine and naloxone, J. Pharmacol. Exp. Ther. **184:**136, 1973.
3. Belville, J.W., and others: The interaction of morphine and d-tubocurarine on respiration and grip strength in man, Clin. Pharmacol. Ther. **5:**35, 1964.
4. Baraka, A.: The influence of carbon dioxide on the neuromuscular block caused by tubocurarine chloride in the human subject, Br. J. Anaesth. **36:**272, 1964.
5. Miller, R.D., and others: The effect of acid-base balance on neostigmine antagonism of a d-tubocurarine-induced neuromuscular blockade, Anesthesiology **42:**377, 1975.
6. Munger, W.L., and others: The dependence of d-tubocurarine-induced hypotension on alveolar concentration of halothane, Anesthesiology **40:**442, 1974.
7. Jaffe, J.H., and Martin, W.R.: Opioid analgesics and antagonists. In Gilman, A.G., Goodman, L.S., and Gilman, A., editors: The pharmacological basis of therapeutics, New York, 1980, Macmillan Publishing Co.

Tubocurarine–Propranolol

Summary: The neuromuscular blockade produced by tubocurarine was prolonged in 2 thyrotoxic patients receiving high doses (120 mg/day for 14 days) of propranolol.[1]

Related Drugs: The depolarizing neuromuscular blocking agent succinylcholine[2-4] has been shown to interact with propranolol in animals in a manner similar to tubocurarine. Although there is no documentation, the other nondepolarizing neuromuscular blocking agents (atracurium, gallamine, and pancuronium) might also interact with propranolol. However, no adverse effects were reported in 7 men who received metocurine, a nondepolarizing neuromuscular blocking analog of tubocurarine, 24 hours following the discontinuation of propranolol.[5]

Since the propranolol interaction with neuromuscular blocking agents may result from a number of mechanisms,[6] any of the other beta-blockers (e.g., atenolol, nadolol, timolol [see Appendix]) may potentially interact as well. However, one of the proposed mechanisms involves a local anesthetic or "quinidine-like" effect, involving depression of motor nerve terminal activity, of beta-blocking agents.[6] In this regard pindolol, which has less local anesthetic activity than propranolol, was less potent in causing neuromuscular blockade in frogs.[7]

Mechanism: Propranolol depresses post-tetanic repetitive activity that is thought to be localized at the motor nerve terminal and, therefore, may enhance the depression of motor nerve terminal activity of tubocurarine.[4,8] Propranolol may also render the postjunctional membrane insensitive to acetylcholine[4,9] and has been reported to induce symptoms of myasthenia gravis in 3 patients.[10] Propranolol may also enhance the duration of neuromuscular blockade through blocking the beta-adrenergic receptors.[6,11]

Theoretically, the hypotensive effect of tubocurarine may be augmented by blockade of the beta-adrenergic receptors in the heart by propranolol.[12-14]

Recommendations: Patients receiving propranolol or other beta-blocking agents should be observed closely for any unexpected prolongation of neuromuscular blockade (e.g., respiratory depression and apnea) or a hypotensive effect from tubocurarine or other neuromuscular blocking drugs. When neuromuscular blockade is prolonged, neostigmine (1 to 3 mg) with atropine (0.6 to 1.2 mg) may be given.[1,15] Although use of these agents may result in an excessive slowing of the heart rate in the presence of beta-blockers, this effect has not been consistently reported.[16]

References

1. Rosen, M.S., and Whan, F.: Prolonged curarization associated with propranolol, Med. J. Aust. **1:**467, 1972.
2. Wislicki, L., and Rosenblum, I.: Effects of propranolol on the action of neuromuscular blocking drugs, Br. J. Anaesth. **39:**939, 1967.
3. Wislicki, L., and Rosenblum, I.: The effects of propranolol on normal and denervated muscle, Arch. Int. Pharmacodyn. Ther. **170:**117, 1967.
4. Usubiga, J.E.: Neuromuscular effects of beta adrenergic blockers and their interaction with skeletal muscle relaxants, Anesthesiology **29:**484, 1968.

5. Zaidan, J., and others: Hemodynamic effects of metocurine in patients with coronary artery disease receiving propranolol, Anesth. Analg. (Cleve.) **56:**25, 1977.
6. Patel, V.K., and others: In vivo study of mechanism of propranolol-induced blockade of neuromuscular transmission, Indian J. Physiol. Pharmacol. **18:**126, 1974.
7. Nirmala, G., and Sastry, P.B.: Neuro-muscular depressant action of pindolol in comparison with propranolol and procaine, Arch. Int. Pharmacodyn. Ther. **238:**196, 1979.
8. Standaert, F.G., and Adams, J.E.: The actions of succinylcholine on the mammalian motor nerve terminal, J. Pharmacol. Exp. Ther. **149:**113, 1965.
9. Gill, E.W., and Vaughn-Williams, E.M.: Local anesthetic activity of beta receptor antagonist pronethalol, Nature **201:**199, 1964.
10. Herishanu, Y., and Rosenberg, P.: Beta-blockers and myasthenia gravis, Ann. Intern. Med. **83:**834, 1975.
11. Khetarpal, V.K., and Sharma, P.L.: Comparative effects of (+)- and (−)-isomers of propranolol and INPEA on (+) tubocararine and succinylcholine induced neuromuscular blockade, Eur. J. Pharmacol. **33:**325, 1975.
12. Stoelting, R.K.: Blood-pressure responses to d-tubocurarine and its preservatives in anesthetized patients, Anesthesiology **35:**325, 1975.
13. Smith, N.T., and Whitcher, C.E.: Hemodynamic effects of gallamine and tubocurarine administered during halothane anesthesia, J.A.M.A. **199:**704, 1967.
14. Munger, W.L., and others: The dependence of d-tubocurarine-induced hypotension on alveolar concentation of halothane, dose of d-tubocurarine and nitrous oxide, Anesthesiology **40:**442, 1974.
15. Taylor, P.: Neuromuscular blocking agents, In Gilman, A.G., Goodman, L.S., and Gilman, A., editors: The pharmacological basis of therapeutics, New York, 1980, Macmillan Publishing Co.
16. Wagner, D.L., and others: Administration of anticholinesterase drugs in the presence of beta-adrenergic blockade, Anesth. Analg. (Cleve.) **61:**153, 1982.

Tubocurarine–Quinidine

2

Summary: Quinidine, administered parenterally shortly after or simultaneously with tubocurarine, may enhance or cause recurrent neuromuscular effects of tubocurarine, resulting in prolonged or intensified respiratory depression and apnea. Although the evidence to support this drug interaction consists only of case reports,[1-4] potential hazards resulting from concurrent therapy require that the patient be observed closely for any unexpected increases in the intensity or duration of the neuromuscular blockade from tubocurarine.

Related Drugs: Gallamine triethiodide,[5] a nondepolarizing neuromuscular blocking agent similar to tubocurarine, has been shown to interact with quinidine in animals. Other nondepolarizing neuromuscular blocking agents (atracurium, metocurine, and pancuronium) may interact with quinidine in a similar manner because of pharmacologic similarity. The depolarizing neuromuscular blocking agent succinylcholine[1,5,6] has been reported to interact with quinidine in animals. In addition, succinylcholine has been reported to interact with quinidine in humans.[2] Although there is a lack of documentation regarding a similar interaction between tubocurarine and the other cinchona alkaloid (quinine), an interaction may be expected to occur based on similar pharmacologic activity.

Mechanism: Quinidine increases the refractory period of cardiac and skeletal muscle and reduces the responses to repetitive nerve stimulation and acetylcholine; it has been reported to precipitate symptoms of myasthenia gravis in a patient with Graves' disease.[7] The interaction with the neuromuscular blocking agent is therefore caused by a similarly additive pharmacologic effect of quinidine and the neuromuscular blocking agents on skeletal muscle.

Recommendations: Although the clinical documentation for this drug interaction is limited to case reports, the potential seriousness of the interaction requires that the patient be observed closely for any unexpected increases in the intensity or duration of respiratory depression when quinidine is given during or shortly following recovery from the effects of tubocurarine. If prolonged muscle paralysis causes respiratory depression, neostigmine (1 to 3 mg IV) administered with atropine sulfate (0.6 to 1.2 mg IV) may be used to antagonize the action of tubocurarine.[8] However, these drugs have been reported to be ineffective in 1 case[3] and are not recommended for treating toxic reactions of the depolarizing agents such as succinylcholine.[8]

References

1. Schmidt, J.L., and others: The effect of quinidine on the action of muscle relaxants, J.A.M.A. **183:**669, 1963.
2. Grogono, A.W.: Anaesthesia for atrial defibrillation, Lancet **2:**1039, 1963.
3. Way, W.L., and others: Recurarization with quinidine, J.A.M.A. **200;**163, 1967.
4. Boere, L.A.: Fehler und gefahren: Recurarisation nach chinindinsulfat, Der Anaesthesist. **13:**368, 1964.
5. Miller, R.D., and others: The potentiation of neuromuscular blocking agents by quinidine, Anesthesiology **28:**1036, 1967.

6. Cuthbert, M.F.: The effect of quinidine and procainamide on the neuromuscular blocking action of suxamethonium, Br. J. Anaesth. **38:**775, 1966.
7. Stoffer, S.S., and Chandler, J.H.: Quinidine-induced exacerbation of myasthenia gravis in patient with Graves' disease, Arch. Intern. Med. **140:**283, 1980.
8. Taylor, P.: Neuromuscular blocking agents. In Gilman A.G., Goodman, L.S., and Gilman, A., editors: The pharmacological basis of therapeutics, New York, 1980, MacMillan Publishing Co.

CHAPTER THREE

Antiarrhythmic Drug Interactions

TABLE 3. Antiarrhythmic Drug Interactions

Drug Interaction	Significance Code	Potential Effects	Recommendations	See Page
Disopyramide–Phenytoin	3	Phenytoin increases disopyramide's metabolism, which decreases plasma concentrations of disopyramide.	Since the metabolite of disopyramide has the same antiarrhythmic activity, the increased rate of metabolism cannot be equated with a shorter duration of response. Patients should be monitored for loss of antiarrhythmic effect.	114
Disopyramide–Quinidine	3	Concurrent use may lead to a small but significant increase in the disopyramide serum concentration and a small decrease in the quinidine serum concentration.	This may be of clinical significance in patients on high dose disopyramide therapy. Concurrent use need not be avoided. A longer interval between the last dose of disopyramide and the first dose of quinidine may be warranted.	115
Disopyramide–Rifampin	3	Rifampin may increase disopyramide metabolism.	The increased disopyramide metabolism cannot be equated with a shorter duration of response because the metabolite of disopyramide has some antiarrhythmic activity. Patients should be monitored for loss of antiarrhythmic effect.	116
Lidocaine–Cimetidine	1	Concurrent use of these agents results in reduced lidocaine clearance, prolonged half-life, and toxicity.	Monitor lidocaine plasma levels, reducing the dose if needed. Ranitidine may be a suitable alternative to cimetidine.	117
Lidocaine–Phenobarbital	3	Phenobarbital decreases plasma levels of lidocaine, probably by inducing lidocaine metabolism.	Monitor lidocaine levels. Because of pharmacologically active lidocaine metabolites, the implications of this interaction require further investigation.	118
Lidocaine–Propranolol	2	Beta-blocking agents may decrease the clearance of lidocaine, subsequently increasing lidocaine serum concentration, by decreasing cardiac output and hepatic blood flow.	Monitor lidocaine serum levels. Lidocaine dosage and infusion rate may need decreasing.	119
Procainamide–Alcohol, Ethyl	3	Alcohol may significantly reduce the half-life and increase the elimination half-life and total clearance of procainamide.	Monitor both procainamide and n-acetylprocainamide (a major metabolite) levels, and adjust the procainamide dosage if needed.	120

TABLE 3. Antiarrhythmic Drug Interactions—cont'd

Drug Interaction	Significance Code	Potential Effects	Recommendations	See Page
Quinidine– Aluminum Hydroxide	3	Combination antacids containing aluminum hydroxide may increase the urinary pH, thus decreasing the excretion of quinidine. Toxicity and an increased effect of quinidine may result.	Monitor for quinidine toxicity, reducing the quinidine dosage if needed.	121
Quinidine– Cimetidine	3	Cimetidine reduces quinidine clearance and increases its half-life and peak plasma concentration.	Monitor for quinidine toxicity especially in the initial stages of therapy.	122
Quinidine– Phenobarbital	2	Phenobarbital reduces the elimination half-life and area-under-curve of quinidine.	If loss of antiarrhythmic control is evident, the quinidine dosage may need increasing.	123
Quinidine– Phenytoin	2	Phenytoin may reduce serum levels of quinidine.	Monitor carefully and adjust the quinidine dosage if needed.	124
Quinidine– Reserpine	3	Reserpine may enhance the antiarrhythmic and cardiodepressant effects of quinidine.	Do not initiate treatment with these agents simultaneously. Reserpine should be started first. When quinidine is added, increase dosage cautiously and closely monitor cardiac function.	125
Quinidine– Rifampin	2	Rifampin may decrease the antiarrhythmic effects of quinidine.	Monitor carefully and adjust the quinidine dosage if needed.	126
Quinidine— Verapamil	2	Concurrent use of these agents in patients with hypertrophic cardiomyopathy may cause severe hypotension.	Use cautiously, since data are insufficient for determining which patients may be affected.	127
Verapamil– Calcium Gluconate	2	Calcium may antagonize the effects of verapamil and lead to reappearance of atrial fibrillation.	Monitor for change in response to verapamil if calcium is added to or withdrawn from therapy.	128
Verapamil– Propranolol	3	Serious hypotension, bradycardia, and rarely, ventricular asystole may result from concurrent use. Propranolol may also block the beta-adrenergic activity originally stimulated by verapamil.	Monitor blood pressure, heart rate, and clinical status, particularly during initial therapy.	129

Disopyramide–Phenytoin

3

Summary: Concomitant phenytoin therapy increased the metabolism of disopyramide twofold, which resulted in an approximate 30% decrease in disopyramide plasma concentrations.[1,2] Plasma concentrations of mono-N-dealkyldisopyramide (MND, a major metabolite) increased accordingly with concurrent phenytoin and MND has been reported to have some antiarrhythmic activity.[3] Disopyramide returned to pre-phenytoin levels within 2 weeks after phenytoin was discontinued.

Related Drugs: Documentation is lacking regarding an interaction between the other hydantoin anticonvulsants (ethotoin and mephenytoin) and disopyramide. However, a similar interaction may be expected since the action of ethotoin and mephenytoin on hepatic enzymes is similar.

Mechanism: The alterations in disopyramide disposition are consistent with the known hepatic enzyme induction properties of phenytoin.

Recommendations: Since phenytoin stimulates disopyramide metabolism, it is known that serum levels of disopyramide decrease.[4] However, because the metabolite of disopyramide has some antiarrhythmic activity, the increased rate of metabolism of disopyramide cannot be equated with a shorter duration of response. Therefore patients should be monitored for a loss of antiarrhythmic effect.

References

1. Aitio, M.L., and Vuorenmaa, T.: Enhanced metabolism and diminished efficacy of disopyramide by enzyme induction, Br. J. Clin. Pharmacol. **9:**149, 1980.
2. Aitio, M.L., and others: The effect of enzyme induction on the metabolism of disopyramide in man, Br. J. Clin. Pharmacol. **11:**279, 1981.
3. Aitio, M.L.: Plasma concentrations and protein binding of disopyramide and mono-N-dealkldisopyramide during chronic oral disopyramide therapy, Br. J. Clin. Pharmacol. **11:**369, 1981.
4. Kessler, J.M., and others: Disopyramide and phenytoin interaction, Clin. Pharm. **1:**263, 1982.

Disopyramide–Quinidine

Summary: In one study involving 16 healthy subjects, the concurrent use of disopyramide and quinidine led to a small but significant increase in disopyramide serum concentration and a small decrease in quinidine serum concentration. The elimination half-life was not significantly changed for either drug. The increased serum disopyramide may be of clinical significance in a patient on high dose disopyramide therapy since a small increase could lead to toxicity.[1]

Related Drugs: There are no drugs related to disopyramide. Documentation is lacking regarding a similar interaction between disopyramide and the other cinchona alkaloid (quinine).

Mechanism: The mechanism of this interaction is unknown.

Recommendations: The concurrent use of these agents need not be avoided. However, a longer interval between the last dose of disopyramide and the first dose of quinidine may be warranted.[1] Patients on high dose disopyramide therapy should be closely monitored.

Reference

1. Baker, B.J., and others: Concurrent use of quinidine and disopyramide: evaluation of serum concentration and electrocardiographic effects, Am. Heart J. **105:**12, 1983.

Disopyramide–Rifampin

3

Summary: Disopyramide metabolism is probably significantly increased with rifampin co-therapy. In 11 patients taking a combination of tuberculostatic drugs that included rifampin, disopyramide half-life was reduced by one-half. Disopyramide area-under-curve (AUC) was decreased to less than one-half whereas the area-under-curve for mono-N-dealkyldisopyramide (MND, a main metabolite) was almost doubled.[1] MND has been reported to have some antiarrhythmic activity. It is not certain if disopyramide will alter the disposition of rifampin.

Related Drugs: There are no drugs related to rifampin or disopyramide.

Mechanism: Rifampin accelerated disopyramide metabolism by enzyme induction, a well established action of rifampin.

Recommendations: Although the patients were taking other drugs that could have a role in this interaction, rifampin is still strongly suspected because of its known induction properties. Because the metabolite of disopyramide has some antiarrhythmic activity, the increased rate of metabolism of disopyramide cannot be equated with a shorter duration of response. Therefore patients should be monitored for a loss of antiarrhythmic effect.

Reference

1. Aitio, M.L., and others: The effects of enzyme induction on the metabolism of disopyramide in man, Br. J. Clin. Pharmacol. **11:**299, 1981.

Lidocaine–Cimetidine

1

Summary: Concomitant use of lidocaine and cimetidine has resulted in a reduction in lidocaine clearance, a prolongation of lidocaine half-life, and lidocaine toxicity.[1] Steady state serum lidocaine concentrations were increased 75% within 20 hours after initiation of cimetidine in patients hemodynamically stabilized on lidocaine.[2-4]

Related Drugs: Cimetidine has caused a similar increase in procainamide plasma concentrations and also decreased the renal clearance of n-acetylprocainamide, an active metabolite of procainamide.[5,6] Ranitidine has been shown not to interact with lidocaine.[7,8]

Mechanism: Several mechanisms have been suggested and more than one may be responsible for this interaction.[9] Proposed mechanisms are (1) cimetidine may inhibit the microsomal enzymes involved in the metabolism of lidocaine and (2) cimetidine induces a reduction in hepatic blood flow, which reduces the hepatic clearance of lidocaine.

Recommendations: Patients receiving cimetidine and lidocaine should be monitored for increasing plasma concentrations of lidocaine as well as possible toxicity. A reduction in the dosage of lidocaine may be necessary. An alternative would be to substitute ranitidine for cimetidine when using lidocaine.

References

1. Feely, J., and others: Increased toxicity and reduced clearance of lidocaine by cimetidine, Ann. Intern. Med. **96:**592, 1982.
2. Knapp, A.B.: Lidocaine-cimetidine interaction can be toxic, J.A.M.A. **247:**3174, 1982.
3. Knapp, A.B.: Toxic lidocaine/cimetidine interaction, Med. Sci. Bull. **5:**1, 1982.
4. Knapp, A.B., and others: The cimetidine-lidocaine interaction, Ann. Intern. Med. **98:**174, 1983.
5. Somogyi, A., and Heinzow, B.: Cimetidine reduces procainamide elimination, N. Engl. J. Med. **307:**1080, 1982.
6. Somogyi, A., and others: Cimetidine-procainamide pharmacokinetic interaction in man: evidence of competition for tubular secretion of basic drugs, Eur. J. Clin. Pharmacol. **25:**339, 1983.
7. Wood, J.R.: H₂ receptor antagonists: cimetidine and ranitidine, Br. Med. J. **286:**1440, 1983.
8. Feely, J., and Guy, E.: Lack of effect of ranitidine on the disposition of lidocaine, Br. J. Clin. Pharmacol. **15:**378, 1983.
9. Sorkin, E.M., and Darvey, D.L.: Review of cimetidine drug interactions, Drug Intell. Clin. Pharm. **17:**110, 1983.

Lidocaine–Phenobarbital

3

Summary: Studies in animals[1,2] and humans[3] indicate that plasma levels of lidocaine may be decreased during concurrent administration of phenobarbital. This could result in an increased dosage requirement of lidocaine for patients taking phenobarbital. It is unlikely that the interaction is of significance for patients who are having phenobarbital added to or removed from therapy since the time course of the induction of metabolism is likely to be substantially longer than the duration of lidocaine therapy.

Related Drugs: Documentation is lacking regarding whether other barbiturates (e.g. amobarbital, butabarbital, secobarbital [see Appendix]) may decrease lidocaine plasma levels. However a similar interaction may be expected to occur because of the similar pharmacologic action of the barbiturates.

Mechanism: It is likely that induction of lidocaine metabolism by phenobarbital is responsible for this interaction. A study in dogs revealed an increased removal of lidocaine by the liver after phenobarbital pretreatment at 18 mg/kg/day for 20 to 30 days.[1] Increased formation of lidocaine metabolites (monoethylglycylxylidine and glycine xylidide) was also observed. A recent study in dogs[2] showed a significant increase (75%) in lidocaine systemic clearance after 18 mg/kg/day for 10 to 12 days. Intrinsic clearance increased in a comparable manner.

Recommendations: It is recommended that lidocaine plasma levels be monitored to assure that they are in the therapeutic range. However, since induction of metabolism may result in increased levels of pharmacologically active metabolites,[4] the implications of the interaction for the clinical use of lidocaine require further investigation.

References

1. DiFazio, C.A., and Brown, R.E.: Lidocaine metabolism in normal and phenobarbital pretreated dogs, Anesthesiology **36:**238, 1972.
2. Esquivel, M., and others: Effect of phenobarbitone on the disposition of lignocaine and warfarin in the dog, J. Pharm. Pharmacol. **30:**804, 1978.
3. Heinonen, J.H., and others: Plasma lidocaine levels in patients treated with potential inducers of microsomal enzymes, Acta Anaesth. Scand. **14:**89, 1970.
4. Strong, J.M., and others: Pharmacological activity, metabolism, and pharmacokinetics of glycinexylidide, Clin. Pharmacol. Ther. **17:**184, 1975.

Lidocaine–Propranolol

2

Summary: The concurrent administration of propranolol and lidocaine significantly decreased the metabolic clearance of lidocaine.[1-5] When propranolol was given during lidocaine infusion, lidocaine clearance decreased approximately 25%, and the steady state serum levels of lidocaine increased 30% during concurrent administration.[1]

Related Drugs: When pindolol was used instead of propranolol in another study, no effect was noticed on lidocaine serum concentrations;[3] however, metoprolol was shown to reduce lidocaine clearance.[4] Because of conflicting data and lack of documentation, it is not known whether the other beta-adrenergic blocking agents (atenolol, nadolol, and timolol) would interact with lidocaine.

Mechanism: It is suggested that propranolol through its beta-blocking effect decreases the cardiac output and hepatic blood flow, thereby decreasing the metabolic clearance of lidocaine. It is also possible that propranolol influences hepatic drug metabolizing capacity.

Recommendations: Since lidocaine has a narrow therapeutic index, concurrent administration with a beta-blocking agent may require the dosage or infusion rate of lidocaine to be reduced. Lidocaine serum levels should be monitored with appropriate dosage adjustments.

References

1. Ochs, H.R. and others: Reduction in lidocaine clearance during continuous infusion and by coadministration of propranolol, N. Engl. J. Med. **303**:373, 1980.
2. Graham, C.F. and others: Lidocaine-propranolol interactions, N. Engl. J. Med. **304**:1301, 1981.
3. Svendsen, T.L. and others: Effects of propranolol and pindolol on plasma lidocaine clearance in man, Br. J. Clin. Pharmacol. **13**:223S, 1982.
4. Conrad, K.A. and others: Metoprolol reduces lidocaine elimination, Clin. Pharmacol. Ther. **31**:212, 1982.
5. Box, N.D.S., and others: Inhibition of drug metabolism by beta-adrenergic antagonists, Drugs **25** (suppl. 2): 121, 1983.

Procainamide–Alcohol, Ethyl

3

Summary: In a study involving 18 subjects, the concurrent ingestion of alcohol with procainamide resulted in a significant reduction in procainamide half-life and an increase in the elimination half-life and total clearance in both slow and fast acetylators, although total clearance was significantly higher in the slow acetylators. The volume of distribution and renal clearance were not affected by alcohol. The percentage of n-acetylprocainamide (a major metabolite) in the blood and urine increased to a greater extent in the presence of alcohol. In a second similar study, the procainamide area-under-curve was significantly reduced in the presence of alcohol, whereas that for n-acetylprocainamide was increased. Other parameters were similar to those found in the first report.[1] The clinical significance of this interaction was not determined.

Related Drugs: There are no drugs related to procainamide.

Mechanism: Acute alcohol ingestion leads to a decreased rate of hepatic microsomal enzyme metabolism, whereas chronic alcohol ingestion may cause the reverse effect. Procainamide is acetylated to n-acetylprocainamide in the liver; however, this takes place in the cystolic fraction of the hepatocytes, not in the microsomes. Therefore, considering the results of this study, it appears that alcohol may also affect the acetylation of drugs as seen with procainamide.[1] Further studies are needed.

Recommendations: Procainamide and n-acetylprocainamide levels should be monitored in patients concurrently ingesting alcohol while on procainamide therapy. The dosage of procainamide may need to be adjusted.

Reference

1. Olsen, H., and Morland, J.: Ethanol-induced increase in procainamide acetylation in man, Br. J. Clin. Pharmacol. **13**:203, 1982.

Quinidine–Aluminum Hydroxide

Summary: Although aluminum hydroxide may delay the gastrointestinal absorption of quinidine in animals,[1] it does not appear to decrease quinidine absorption in humans.[2] Because of the potential for aluminum containing combination antacids to increase urinary pH[3,4] and the potential for alkaline urine to decrease quinidine urinary excretion,[5] patients receiving both agents should be observed for signs and symptoms of quinidine toxicity.

Related Drugs: In rats, the presence of aluminum and magnesium hydroxides has been reported to delay the absorption of quinine, the stereoisomer of quinidine.[1] However, this interaction has not been documented in humans.

Although a suspension of aluminum hydroxide alone has been shown not to significantly increase urinary pH, the administration of antacids containing a combination of magnesium and aluminum hydroxides can significantly raise urine pH.[4] However, the effect of magnesium and aluminum hydroxide combination antacids on either quinidine absorption or elimination has not been clinically established.

Mechanism: Aluminum hydroxide gel may delay intestinal absorption of other drugs by physical adsorption onto the gel surface[3] or by causing a significant delay in gastric emptying.[6]

On the other hand, antacids, particularly the soluble (e.g. calcium carbonate, sodium bicarbonate), or combination magnesium and aluminum salt products, may alter the renal elimination of drugs by changing the urinary pH.[3,4] In the case of quinidine, an increase in urinary pH from less than 6.0 to greater than 7.5 has resulted in a 50% decrease in the average quinidine renal clearance and signs of increased quinidine effect.[5]

Recommendations: Aluminum hydroxide does not appear to significantly reduce single dose quinidine absorption.[2] However, considering its ability to slow gastric emptying,[6] the effect of larger aluminum hydroxide doses and long-term administration on quinidine absorption is not known. At this time it does not appear necessary to separate aluminum hydroxide and quinidine doses.

In addition, the potential exists for an increased urinary pH when aluminum hydroxide combination antacids are ingested,[4] with a resulting decrease in quinidine excretion, and possible toxicity development.[7] Therefore, patients receiving both agents should be monitored for the development of quinidine toxicity with urinary pH measurement, determination of serum quinidine concentration, and dosage reduction if necessary.

References

1. Hurwitz, A.: The effects of antacids on drug absorption in rats, J. Lab. Clin. Med. **76:**873, 1970.
2. Romankiewicz, J.A., and others: The noninterference of aluminum hydroxide gel with quinidine sulfate absorption: an approach to control quinidine-induced diarrhea, Am. Heart J. **96:**518, 1978.
3. Hurwitz, A.: Antacid therapy and drug kinetics, Clin. Pharmacokinet. **2:**269, 1977.
4. Gibaldi, M., and others: Effect of antacids on pH of urine, Clin. Pharmacol. Ther. **16:**520, 1974.
5. Gerhardt, R.E., and others: Quinidine excretion in aciduria and alkaluria, Ann. Intern. Med. **71:**927, 1969.
6. Hurwitz, A., and others: Effects of antacids on gastric emptying, Gastroenterology **71:**268, 1976.
7. Zinn, M.B.: Quinidine intoxication from alkali ingestion, Texas Med. J. **66:**64, 1970.

Quinidine–Cimetidine

3

Summary: Concurrent administration of cimetidine and quinidine resulted in reduced quinidine clearance, increased half-life, and increased peak plasma concentration in 6 normal volunteers. Plasma protein binding and urinary excretion of quinidine were unchanged.[1] Similar results were shown in another study[2] and a case report.[3]

Related Drugs: No documentation exists regarding a similar interaction between quinidine and the other H_2 receptor antagonist (ranitidine). However, if the mechanism involves hepatic enzyme inhibition by cimetidine, then ranitidine would not be expected to interact. There appear to be no reports involving the other cinchona alkaloid (quinine) with cimetidine, although because of pharmacologic similarity an interaction may be expected to occur.

Mechanism: Since quinidine is largely eliminated by hepatic biotransformation, it is potentially subject to interventions that alter liver metabolic activity. Cimetidine is known to affect the metabolism of drugs by the hepatic mixed function oxidase system. Therefore, the higher peak concentrations of quinidine and the delay in the time to achieve these peak concentrations with concurrent cimetidine may be related to hepatic enzyme inhibition, reduced liver blood flow, or both.[1-3] Also, it is suggested that an increase in quinidine absorption with concurrent cimetidine may explain the elevated quinidine plasma concentrations.[1]

Recommendations: Patients taking concurrent quinidine and cimetidine may require observation, especially in initial stages, for signs of quinidine toxicity (e.g., cinchonism, lethargy, tachyarrhythmias, vomiting). This may be done by monitoring quinidine levels, measuring electrocardiographic parameters, and making clinical assessments.

References

1. Hardy, B.G., and others: Effect of cimetidine on the pharmacokinetics and pharmacodynamics of quinidine, Am. J. Cardiol. **52:**172, 1983.
2. Fruncillo, R.J., and others: Effect of cimetidine on the pharmacokinetics of quinidine and lidocaine in the rat, J. Pharm. Sci. **72:**826, 1983.
3. Farringer, J.A., and others: Cimetidine-quinidine interaction, Clin. Pharm. **3:**81, 1984.

Quinidine–Phenobarbital

2

Summary: In a study of 4 normal subjects the concurrent administration of quinidine and phenobarbital resulted in reduction of the elimination half-life of quinidine by approximately 50% and the area-under-curve by approximately 60%.[1]

Related Drugs: Similar changes in quinidine levels after pentobarbital administration have been described in another report.[2] Although documentation is lacking, a similar interaction may be expected to occur between quinidine and the other barbiturates (e.g., amobarbital, butabarbital, secobarbital [see Appendix]) because of similar activity on hepatic enzymes. The half-life of the other cinchona alkaloid (quinine) was reported to be significantly decreased in epileptic patients receiving phenobarbital, primidone, or phenytoin either alone or in combination.[3]

Mechanism: Limited data suggest that phenobarbital, a known enzyme inducer, may increase the metabolism of quinidine.[1]

Recommendations: Quinidine plasma levels should be monitored during concurrent use of these agents. If a loss of arrhythmia control is evident, the dose of quinidine may need to be increased. Also, if a patient is stabilized on both agents, the dose of quinidine may have to be decreased upon withdrawal of the barbiturate.

References

1. Data, J.L., and others: Interaction of quinidine with anticonvulsant drugs, N. Engl. J. Med. **294:**699, 1976.
2. Chapron, D.J., and others: Apparent quinidine-induced digoxin toxicity after withdrawal of pentobarbital: a case of sequential drug interactions, Arch. Intern. Med. **139:**363, 1979.
3. Padgham, C. and Richens, A.: Quinine metabolism: a useful index of hepatic drug metabolizing capacity in man? Br. J. Clin. Pharmacol. **1:**352, 1974.

Quinidine–Phenytoin

2

Summary: Quinidine serum levels may be reduced by the concurrent use of phenytoin. Four weeks of concurrent phenytoin therapy decreased the half-life of quinidine an average of 50% and resulted in a 60% decrease in the quinidine area-under-curve.[1] Similar changes were seen within 3 weeks of initiating co-therapy in one patient.[2] Quinidine disposition had returned to pre-phenytoin controls within 2 to 3 weeks after phenytoin was discontinued.[1,2] Decreased quinidine serum levels and half-life were reported in one patient in another case study. However, this patient was on several other drugs concurrently.[3] In a case report involving a child, the dose of quinidine had to be increased (from 60 mg every 6 hours to 300 mg every 4 hours) to reach therapeutic levels in the presence of phenytoin.[4]

Related Drugs: Other hydantoin anticonvulsants (ethotoin and mephenytoin) may also interact with quinidine because of a similar activity on hepatic enzymes, but documentation is lacking. The half-life of quinine, also a cinchona alkaloid, was found to be significantly decreased in epileptic patients receiving phenobarbital, phenytoin, or primidone either alone or in combination.[5]

Mechanism: The decrease in quinidine half-life would be consistent with a mechanism that involved the induced metabolism of quinidine. Phenytoin has been shown to have enzyme induction properties, and quinidine is largely metabolized to hydroxylated metabolites by liver microsomal enzymes.[1,3] The metabolite levels of 3-hydroxyquinidine were elevated after concurrent phenytoin,[2] a finding that lends support to the proposed mechanism of enzyme induction.

Recommendations: Combination therapy of quinidine and phenytoin will probably require an alteration in quinidine dosage to maintain therapeutic quinidine serum levels. Careful monitoring and possible readjustment of quinidine levels will be required when phenytoin therapy is begun or discontinued, as seen in one patient where decreasing the phenytoin dosage resulted in an increased quinidine level.[6]

References

1. Data, J.L., and others: Interaction of quinidine with anticonvulsant drugs, N. Engl. J. Med. **294:**699, 1976.
2. Pershing, L.K., and others: An HPLC method for the quantitation of quinidine and its metabolites in plasma and application to a quinidine-phenytoin drug interaction study, J. Anal. Toxicol. **6:**153, 1982.
3. Kroboth, F.J., and others: Phenytoin-quinidine interaction, N. Engl. J. Med. **308:**725, 1983.
4. Rodgers, G.C., and Blackman, M.S.: Quinidine interaction with anticonvulsants, Drug Intell. Clin. Pharm. **17:**24, 1983.
5. Padgham, C., and Richens, A.: Quinine metabolism: a useful index of hepatic drug metabolizing capacity in man? Br. J. Clin. Pharmacol. **1:**352, 1974.
6. Urbano, A.M.: Phenytoin-quinidine interaction in a patient with recurrent ventricular tachyarrhythmias, N. Engl. J. Med. **308:**225 1983.

Quinidine–Reserpine

3

Summary: Clinical and experimental studies show that the antiarrhythmic and cardio-depressant effects of quinidine may be enhanced by the administration of reserpine, although the data about the drug interaction are limited and unreliable.

Related Drugs: Quinidine is available as the sulfate, gluconate, and polygalacturonate salts; all salts may have a similar interaction with reserpine. There is no documentation regarding an interaction with the other cinchona alkaloid, quinine. In addition to reserpine, the other rauwolfia alkaloids (e.g. alseroxylon, deserpidine, rescinnamine [see Appendix]) may be expected to exhibit a similar activity with quinidine because of pharmacologic similarity.

Mechanism: Reserpine depletes myocardial tissue of 80% to 95% of its catecholamine stores[1-3] by causing the intraneural release of norepinephrine and by blocking the uptake of the neurotransmitter into the storage granules of the sympathetic nerve ending.[4] This catecholamine depletion causes a decrease in the electrical automaticity and excitability of the myocardial tissue, which results in decreased atrial and ventricular rates.[1] This effect may enhance quinidine's direct myocardial tissue depressant activity[4] and may result in the heart becoming less excitable. These combined effects could result in quinidine toxicity, manifested as cardiac asystole or excessive bradycardia.[4]

Recommendations: To minimize the possible toxic effects resulting from concurrent administration of quinidine and reserpine, treatment with these agents should not be initiated simultaneously. Treatment with reserpine should be initiated first and an interval of at least 24 hours should be allowed before introducing quinidine. When quinidine is added to the regimen of a reserpine-treated patient, the dose should be increased cautiously and cardiac function should be monitored closely.

References

1. Roberts, J., and others: Some aspects of the cardiac actions of reserpine and pronethalol, Fed. Proc. **24:**1421, 1965.
2. Lee, W.C., and Shideman, F.E.: The role of myocardial catecholamines in cardiac contractility, Science **129:**967, 1959.
3. Pasonen, M.K., and Krayer, C.: The release of norepinephrine from the mammalian heart by reserpine, J. Pharmacol. Exp. Ther. **123:**153, 1958.
4. Weiner, N.: Drugs that inhibit adrenergic nerves and block adrenergic receptors: In Gilman, A.G., Goodman, L.S., and Gilman, A., editors: The pharmacological basis of therapeutics, New York, 1980, MacMillan Publishing.

Quinidine–Rifampin

Summary: The antiarrhythmic effect of quinidine was diminished within 1 week in a patient who received rifampin concurrently with quinidine.[1] When isoniazid was substituted for rifampin, plasma quinidine concentrations returned to therapeutic levels.

Related Drugs: Although no documentation exists of rifampin altering the disposition of quinine, another cinchona alkaloid, an interaction may occur because of pharmacologic similarity. There are no drugs related to rifampin.

Mechanism: Rifampin is a known inducer of microsomal enzymes responsible for the metabolism of many drugs. In 2 reports, it was demonstrated that rifampin induced the enzymes that metabolize antipyrine and simultaneously reduced quinidine plasma concentrations, area-under-curve, and half-life.[2,3]

Recommendations: When using rifampin concurrently with quinidine, the response to quinidine should be closely monitored, and a dosage increase made if necessary.

References

1. Ahmad, D., and others: Rifampicin-quinidine interaction, Br. J. Dis. Chest. **73:**409, 1979.
2. Twum-Barima, Y., and Carruthers, S.G.: Evaluation of rifampin-quinidine interaction, Clin. Pharmacol. Ther. **27:**290, 1980.
3. Twum-Barima, Y., and Carruthers, S.G.: Quinidine-rifampin interaction, N. Engl. J. Med. **304:**1466, 1981.

Quinidine–Verapamil

2

Summary: In a small number of patients with hypertrophic cardiomyopathy, concomitant use of verapamil and quinidine resulted in significant hypotension.[1] The onset of hypotension occurred in 3 patients within 4 days of beginning co-therapy. Two of the 3 patients developed acute pulmonary edema coincident with the hypotension.

Related Drugs: In a case study the concurrent use of nifedipine and quinidine in a diabetic patient without hypertrophic cardiomyopathy resulted in decreased quinidine serum levels which led to inadequate control of the patient's dysrhythmia. When nifedipine was discontinued, the quinidine levels increased.[2] No documentation is available regarding an interaction between quinidine and the other calcium channel blocker (diltiazem), although because of pharmacologic similarity an interaction may be expected to occur. No documentation is available regarding any interaction between the calcium channel blockers and the other cinchona alkaloid (quinine).

Mechanism: The exact mechanism of the interaction is not known. However, verapamil, in addition to its main mechanism of action, also prolongs A-V nodal refractoriness and slows A-V conduction,[3] and quinidine depresses conduction velocity and prolongs the refractory period.[4] Therefore, the concomitant use of these agents may result in a hypotension related to both a peripheral vascular and a myocardial component, which are affected by both agents.

Recommendations: One factor predisposing patients with hypertrophic cardiomyopathy to such an interaction is their sensitivity to hypotension with the obstructive form of the disease. Not enough evidence exists to determine which patients will be affected. Therefore, until definitive studies are available, the concomitant use of these agents should be undertaken only with extreme caution.

References

1. Epstein, S.E., and Rosing, D.R.: Verapamil—its potential for causing serious complications in patients with hypertrophic cardiomyopathy, Circulation **64:**437, 1981.
2. Green, J.A., and others: Nifedipine-quinidine interaction, Clin. Pharm. **2:**461, 1983.
3. Mitchell, L.B., and others: Comparative clinical electrophysiologic effects of diltiazem, verapamil and nifedipine: a review, Am. J. Cardiol. **46:**629, 1982.
4. Bigger, J.T. Jr., and Hoffman, B.F.: Antiarrhythmic drugs. In Gilman, A.G., Goodman, L.S., and Gilman, A., editors: The pharmacological basis of therapeutics, New York, 1980, MacMillan Publishing.

Verapamil–Calcium Gluconate

Summary: A 70-year-old patient receiving verapamil for atrial fibrillation was treated with calcium and calciferol for osteoporosis. Within one week the atrial fibrillation reappeared, and the serum calcium also increased. Subsequent doses of furosemide and verapamil were successful in reversing the fibrillation.[1] Since calcium has also been used to treat verapamil overdose,[2-4] it appears that calcium and calciferol were responsible for this interaction.

Related Drugs: Documentation is lacking regarding an interaction between calcium gluconate and the other calcium channel blockers (diltiazem and nifedipine), although because of pharmacologic similarity a similar interaction may be expected to occur. The other salts of calcium (e.g., carbonate, chloride, lactate) may be expected to interact similarly to calcium gluconate.

Mechanism: Calcium has successfully been used to treat verapamil overdose,[2-4] and verapamil also reversed the calcium-induced fibrillation.[1] Therefore, it appears this interaction results from an antagonistic effect between the 2 agents.

Recommendations: Patients should be monitored for a change in their response to verapamil if calcium is added to or withdrawn from their therapy.

References

1. David, B.O., and Yoel, G.: Calcium and calciferol antagonize effect of verapamil in atrial fibrillation, Br. Med. J. **282**:1585, 1981.
2. Perkins, C.M.: Serious verapamil poisoning: treatment with intravenous calcium gluconate, Br. Med. J. **4**:1127, 1978.
3. Woie, L., and Storestein, L.: Successful treatment of suicidal verapamil poisoning with calcium gluconate, Eur. Heart J. **2**:239, 1981.
4. Chimienti, M., and others: Acute verapamil: successful treatment with epinephrine, Clin. Cardiol. **5**:219, 1982.

Verapamil–Propranolol

3

Summary: Concurrent use of verapamil and propranolol may result in serious hypotension, bradycardia, and rarely, ventricular asystole in both children and adults.[1-9] The onset of the adverse effects occurs within 48 hours after concurrent therapy begins. The effects are generally transient and subside within 1 to 7 days.

A number of predisposing factors have been observed in patients who developed adverse effects. These include left ventricular function impairment, cardiac arrhythmia, aortic stenosis during large doses, and intravenous administration of one or both agents.

Related Drugs: Similar effects have been seen in patients receiving pindolol or metoprolol and verapamil.[6,8,10] There appear to be no reports regarding the effects of concurrent verapamil with the other beta-blockers (atenolol, timolol, or nadolol) although because of pharmacologic similarity, a similar interaction may occur.

Concurrent use of nifedipine and propranolol or atenolol has led to hypotension or heart failure in a few patients.[11-16] Although adverse reactions with beta-adrenergic blocking agents and the other calcium channel blocker, diltiazem, have not been reported, they may be expected to occur since diltiazem possesses many of the pharmacologic properties of verapamil.

Mechanism: The mechanism involved in the interaction is complex. Verapamil exerts potent negative inotropic and chronotropic effects as a result of its ability to inhibit calcium and sodium transport across cell membranes in cardiac muscle. Beta-blockade produces similar hemodynamic effects. Therefore, an additive cardiodepressive response may be seen with concomitant use of these agents. Verapamil also has peripheral vasodilator properties because of inhibition of slow-channel activity in vascular smooth muscle. The resultant decrease in systemic vascular resistance and blood pressure stimulates beta-adrenergic activity, which serves to increase heart rate and contractility and offset the depressant effects of verapamil. Therefore, concurrent administration of propranolol may block the beta-adrenergic activity originally stimulated by verapamil.[6]

Recommendations: In view of studies indicating the concurrent use of these drugs as a superior therapy for angina pectoris, such patients need to be carefully selected since several predisposing factors appear to increase the risk of an interaction.[6-8,17-21] During treatment patients should be monitored closely for blood pressure, heart rate, and clinical status, especially during the first few days of initiating concomitant therapy.[10] One report indicates that this interaction may be avoided by withdrawal of the beta-blocking agent for 24 hours before verapamil administration.[8]

References

1. Singh, B.N., and others: Verapamil: a review of its pharmacological properties and therapeutic use, Drugs **15**:169, 1981.
2. Frishman, W.H., and Subramanian, V.B.: Calcium blockers for heart disease: two approved, more to come, J.A.M.A. **247**:1911, 1982.

3. Kieval, J., and others: The effects of intravenous verapamil on hemodynamic status of patients with coronary artery disease receiving propranolol, Circulation **65:**653, 1982.
4. Shahar, E., and others: Verapamil in the treatment of paroxysmal supraventricular tachycardia in infants and children, J. Pediatr. **98:**323, 1981.
5. Opie, L.H.: Drugs and the heart. III. Calcium antagonists, Lancet **1:**806, 1980.
6. Packer, M., and others: Hemodynamic consequences of combined beta-adrenergic and slow calcium channel blockade in man, Circulation **65:**660, 1982.
7. Subramanian, B., and others: Combined therapy with verapamil and propranolol in chronic stable angina, Am. J. Cardiol. **49:**125, 1982.
8. Packer, M., and others: Hemodynamic consequences of combined beta-adrenergic and slow calcium channel blockade in man, Circulation **65:**660, 1982.
9. Leon, M.B., and others: Clinical efficacy of verapamil alone and combined with propranolol in treating patients with chronic stable angina pectoris, Am. J. Cardiol. **48:**131, 1981.
10. Wayne, V.S., and others: Adverse interaction between beta-adrenergic blocking drugs and verapamil: report of three cases, Aust. N. Z. J. Med. **12:**285, 1982.
11. Anastassiades, C.J.: Nifedipine and beta-blocker drugs, Br. Med. J. **281:**1251, 1980.
12. Opie, L.H., and White, D.A.: Adverse interaction between nifedipine and beta-blockade, Br. Med. J. **281:**1462, 1980.
13. Staffurth, J.S., and Emery, P.: Adverse interaction between nifedipine and beta-blockade, Br. Med. J. **282:**225, 1981.
14. Robson, R.H., and Vishwanath, M.C.: Nifedipine and beta-blockade as a cause of cardiac failure, Br. Med. J. **284:**104, 1982.
15. Anastassiades, C.J.: Nifedipine and beta-blockade as a cause of cardiac failure, Br. Med. J. **284:**506, 1982.
16. Dargie, H.J., and others: Nifedipine and propranolol: a beneficial drug interaction, Am. J. Med. **71:**676, 1981.
17. Mueller, H.S., and others: Nifedipine therapy for angina pectoris, Pharmacother. **1:**78, 1981.
18. Tweddel, A.C., and others: The combination of nifedipine and propranolol in the management of patients with angina pectoris, Br. J. Clin. Pharmacol. **12:**229, 1981.
19. Ekelund, L.G., and Oro, L.: Antianginal efficiency of nifedipine with and without a beta-blocker, studied with exercise test: a double-blind, randomized subacute study, Clin. Cardiol. **2:**203, 1979.
20. DePonti, C., and others: Effects of nifedipine, acebutolol, and their association on exercise tolerance in patients with effort angina, Cardiol. **68**(suppl. 2):195, 1981.
21. Eggersten, R., and Hansson, L.: Effects of treatment with nifedipine and metoprolol in essential hypertension, Eur. J. Clin. Pharmacol. **21:**389, 1982.

CHAPTER FOUR

Anticoagulant Drug Interactions

*Not available in the U.S.

TABLE 4. Anticoagulant Drug Interactions

Drug Interaction	Significance Code	Potential Effects	Recommendations	See Page
Dicumarol–Allopurinol	1	Allopurinol may significantly prolong the half-life of dicumarol.	Monitor closely for increased anticoagulant response. The dicumarol dose may need decreasing.	140
Dicumarol–Chloramphenicol	2	Chloramphenicol inhibits dicumarol metabolism, thus enhancing the anticoagulant action.	The concurrent use of these agents should be avoided. Monitor prothrombin levels frequently if concomitant use is necessary.	141
Dicumarol–Corticotropin	2	Corticosteroids both increase and decrease the activity of dicumarol and other anticoagulants and may increase blood coagulability or lower the vascular integrity.	Monitor carefully and adjust the dosage of anticoagulant as needed.	142
Dicumarol–Methylphenidate	3	Methylphenidate may increase dicumarol's half-life, although 1 study is conflicting and reports no effect.	Concurrent use need not be avoided, although it is important to be aware of a possible interaction.	143
Dicumarol–Oral Contraceptive Agents	2	Concurrent use results in a diminished anticoagulant response, although a conflicting report shows increased anticoagulation with acenocoumarol.*	Adjustment in the anticoagulant dosage may be necessary.	144
Dicumarol–Phenytoin	2	Dicumarol may increase serum levels and half-life of phenytoin, however phenytoin may decrease serum levels and anticoagulant action of dicumarol.	Monitor levels of both agents and adjust dosages if needed.	145
Heparin–Aspirin	1	Both agents prolong bleeding time, and concurrent use may result in serious bleeding complications.	Although both may be used concurrently in low doses for postoperative thromboembolism, observe patients for hemorrhagic complications throughout therapy.	147
Heparin–Carbenicillin	2	The penicillins prolong bleeding time and may theoretically increase the effects of heparin. This interaction may also occur with oral anticoagulants.	Monitor coagulation frequently; if bleeding occurs, protamine will correct excessive anticoagulation. Low doses of carbenicillin may avoid this interaction.	149
Heparin–Dextran	2	Concurrent use of heparin and dextran 70 or 75 is associated with a statistically higher incidence of bleeding than either agent alone.	Use concurrently only when close monitoring is possible. Dextran 40 has been used without untoward effects.	150

*Not available in the U.S.

Abbreviations: GI, gastrointestinal; NSAIA, nonsteroidal antiinflammatory agent.

TABLE 4. Anticoagulant Drug Interactions—cont'd

Drug Interaction	Significance Code	Potential Effects	Recommendations	See Page
Phenindione– Haloperidol	3	Haloperidol may reduce the anticoagulant effect of phenindione.	Concomitant use need not be avoided. If inadequate anticoagulation occurs, decrease the haloperidol dose or increase the phenindione dose.	152
Warfarin– Acetaminophen	3	In therapeutic doses, concurrent use results in only a slight, if any, effect on the hypoprothrombinemic response to the anticoagulant.	Monitor the prothrombin time, even though the interaction appears minor.	153
Warfarin– Alcohol, Ethyl	3	Moderate, occasional ingestion of alcohol appears to have little effect on oral anticoagulant control. Patients consuming large amounts, who have long histories of ingestion, or who have liver dysfunction may have a shortened serum half-life of the oral anticoagulants with antagonism of drug activity.	Moderate to heavy alcohol consumption should be avoided, especially over long periods. Sudden changes in amount ingested may require alterations in the oral anticoagulant dosage.	154
Warfarin– Ascorbic Acid	4	High doses of ascorbic acid are associated with a decreased total warfarin plasma concentration, although no alterations in warfarin action were noted.	Concurrent use need not be avoided. However, if the patient's dose requirements of warfarin are increasing, ascorbic acid should be eliminated as a causative factor.	155
Warfarin– Aspirin	1	High doses of aspirin (>3 g/day) may potentiate the anticoagulant action of warfarin, increase the risk of bleeding, or both. This interaction appears to be dose-related.	Avoid concurrent use when possible. Acetaminophen or a noninteracting NSAIA should be substituted for aspirin, depending on the indication.	156
Warfarin– Chloral Hydrate	2	Chloral hydrate may transiently increase warfarin anticoagulation.	Monitor during initial concurrent administration. Dosage adjustment of warfarin is usually not necessary.	158
Warfarin– Chlordiazepoxide	4	Warfarin pharmacokinetics or anticoagulant action are not significantly affected by concurrent use.	Concurrent use need not be avoided. Monitor warfarin routinely.	159
Warfarin– Cholestyramine	2	Cholestyramine decreases the half-life and increases the total body clearance of warfarin; it is unknown if this results in a decreased warfarin effect. Cholestyramine-induced vitamin K deficiency and hemorrhagic episodes have been reported.	Avoid concomitant use when possible, but if unavoidable cholestyramine may be given 3-6 hours after warfarin.	160

TABLE 4. Anticoagulant Drug Interactions—cont'd

Drug Interaction	Significance Code	Potential Effects	Recommendations	See Page
Warfarin– Cimetidine	1	Cimetidine prolongs the hypoprothrombinemic response of warfarin. Ranitidine may not affect warfarin concentration.	The hypoprothrombinemic response to warfarin should be closely monitored when cimetidine is added or discontinued.	162
Warfarin– Clofibrate	1	Clofibrate may enhance the anticoagulant action of warfarin, increasing the risk of excessive anticoagulation and hemorrhage.	Prothrombin time should be frequently monitored and a warfarin dosage reduction should be expected.	164
Warfarin– Diphenhydramine	4	No significant effect on anticoagulation occurs with concurrent use of these agents.	Concurrent use of these agents need not be avoided.	165
Warfarin– Disopyramide	3	Disopyramide may enhance the hypoprothrombinemic response to warfarin.	Monitor warfarin activity when disopyramide is added to or withdrawn from therapy.	166
Warfarin– Disulfiram	1	Disulfiram may elevate serum warfarin levels and enhance the hypoprothrombinemic response.	Concurrent use should be avoided. When concomitant use is necessary a decrease of warfarin dosage may be required.	167
Warfarin– Erythromycin	2	Erythromycin may increase the hypoprothrombinemic action of warfarin.	Monitor patients during concurrent use. Adjustment of the warfarin dosage may be necessary.	168
Warfarin– Ethacrynic Acid	2	Ethacrynic acid markedly increases prothrombin time. Furosemide and bumetanide reportedly have no effect on warfarin.	Monitor prothrombin time when ethacrynic acid is added to warfarin therapy.	169
Warfarin– Ethchlorvynol	2	Ethchlorvynol may significantly decrease the anticoagulant activity of warfarin.	A benzodiazepine, which does not significantly affect warfarin, may be substituted for ethchlorvynol.	170
Warfarin– Glucagon	1	Glucagon may increase the hypoprothrombinemic effect of warfarin, possibly in a dose-dependent manner.	If more than 25 mg/day of glucagon is given, reduce the warfarin dosage.	171
Warfarin– Glutethimide	1	Glutethimide stimulates warfarin metabolism, thus reducing its anticoagulant effect.	If used concurrently, warfarin dosages may need to be increased. Glutethimide withdrawal may cause severe bleeding unless warfarin dosage is decreased.	172
Warfarin– Griseofulvin	2	Griseofulvin may decrease the hypoprothrombinemic action of warfarin in some, but not all, patients.	Monitor prothrombin times frequently. Warfarin dosage may need to be increased during initial concurrent therapy and decreased on withdrawal of griseofulvin.	173

TABLE 4. Anticoagulant Drug Interactions—cont'd

Drug Interaction	Significance Code	Potential Effects	Recommendations	See Page
Warfarin–Ibuprofen	3	Although ibuprofen may cause some displacement of warfarin from plasma binding sites and may decrease platelet aggregation, anticoagulation is not significantly affected. Increased GI bleeding associated with ibuprofen may be complicated by warfarin.	Carefully monitor coagulation at beginning of concurrent use and monitor for GI bleeding.	174
Warfarin–Indomethacin	2	Indomethacin can cause gastric ulceration and bleeding and inhibit platelet aggregation. It may also decrease the albumin binding of warfarin, although hypoprothrombinemic effects are not significantly enhanced.	Use cautiously, monitor prothrombin times, and observe for signs of increased anticoagulation such as easy bruising or bleeding.	176
Warfarin–Influenza Virus Vaccine	1	Patients stabilized on warfarin may experience massive upper GI hemorrhage, increased prothrombin time, and diffuse gastric bleeding after an influenza vaccination.	Monitor closely after vaccination and lower the warfarin dosage if necessary.	178
Warfarin–Isoniazid	3	Isoniazid may cause bleeding and increased prothrombin time with concurrent warfarin, possibly in a dose-related manner.	Monitor for increased anticoagulation and decrease the warfarin dosage if needed.	179
Warfarin–Magnesium Hydroxide	4	Concurrent use of antacids containing aluminum or magnesium ions has no significant effect on warfarin.	Concurrent use need not be avoided. However, as a routine practice simultaneous administration should not be encouraged.	180
Warfarin–Mefenamic Acid	3	Mefenamic acid may increase the hypoprothrombinemic response to warfarin.	Monitor prothrombin times and decrease the warfarin dosage if necessary.	181
Warfarin–Meprobamate	3	Meprobamate may antagonize the anticoagulant activity of warfarin; however, during concurrent use prothrombin times are unchanged.	Concurrent use need not be avoided, although prothrombin times should be checked routinely.	182
Warfarin–Mercaptopurine	3	Mercaptopurine decreases the anticoagulant effect of warfarin.	Monitor the anticoagulant effect of warfarin if mercaptopurine is added to or withdrawn from therapy.	183

TABLE 4. Anticoagulant Drug Interactions—cont'd

Drug Interaction	Significance Code	Potential Effects	Recommendations	See Page
Warfarin–Methaqualone*	4	No significant effect on warfarin activity occurs with concurrent use.	Concurrent use need not be avoided because of the relatively minor effect on warfarin metabolism.	184
Warfarin–Methyltestosterone	1	Methyltestosterone may increase the hypoprothrombinemic action of warfarin.	Monitor prothrombin times and decrease the warfarin dosage if needed.	185
Warfarin–Metronidazole	1	Metronidazole significantly enhances the hypoprothrombinemic action of warfarin.	Monitor prothrombin levels and decrease the warfarin dosage if needed.	187
Warfarin–Miconazole	2	Miconazole can increase the anticoagulant effect of warfarin and this effect is manifested within 12 days.	Warfarin dosage may need to be decreased initially, then gradually increased as concurrent therapy proceeds.	188
Warfarin–Nalidixic Acid	1	Nalidixic acid may potentiate the action of warfarin, resulting in purpuric rash and bruising.	Monitor patients and decrease the warfarin dosage if necessary.	189
Warfarin–Neomycin	3	Neomycin may slightly increase the hypoprothrombinemic effect of warfarin; this may only be significant in those who have a dietary deficiency of vitamin K and/or who are receiving large doses of neomycin.	Monitoring of prothrombin activity is warranted when the 2 drugs are administered concurrently especially in those patients with a vitamin K deficiency or those receiving large doses of neomycin.	190
Warfarin–Nortriptyline	4	Concurrent use apparently does not affect warfarin. Nortriptyline inhibits dicumarol metabolism and may slow GI motility allowing greater absorption of dicumarol.	The concurrent use of warfarin and nortriptyline need not be avoided; however, patients should be monitored for changes in the anticoagulant response.	191
Warfarin–Phenobarbital	1	Phenobarbital may decrease the anticoagulant effect of warfarin. Barbiturates also increase the synthesis of clotting factors.	Avoid concurrent use of these agents if possible. When phenobarbital is initiated, an increase in the warfarin dose may be anticipated. Also, the dose of warfarin may need to be decreased when phenobarbital is discontinued.	192
Warfarin–Phenylbutazone	1	Phenylbutazone enhances the hypoprothrombinemic effect of warfarin and can cause serious bleeding episodes. Phenylbutazone alone may cause gastric ulceration and decrease platelet aggregation.	Avoid concurrent therapy, using alternatives to phenylbutazone whenever possible. Phytonadione (vitamin K) can be used to treat excessive hypoprothrombinemia.	194

TABLE 4. Anticoagulant Drug Interactions—cont'd

Drug Interaction	Significance Code	Potential Effects	Recommendations	See Page
Warfarin– Phytonadione	1	Warfarin inhibits vitamin K–dependent synthesis of clotting factors II, VII, IX, and X. Vitamin K antagonizes the inhibitory effect of warfarin, and in excess of normal dietary consumption the vitamin may impair anticoagulation.	Monitor prothrombin time during concurrent therapy and after withdrawing vitamin K since the effects of vitamin K may last for several days after intake is stopped. Also, vitamin K is an effective antidote for warfarin overdose.	196
Warfarin– Propoxyphene	2	Concurrent use of these agents may lead to decreased prothrombin levels and bleeding episodes.	Monitor prothrombin times closely. Decreased warfarin dosage, discontinuing propoxyphene, or substituting a noninteracting analgesic may be considered.	198
Warfarin– Quinidine	2	Quinidine may enhance the hypoprothrombinemic activity of warfarin. The cinchona alkaloids can depress vitamin K–dependent clotting factor production.	Monitor prothrombin times frequently and monitor for clinical symptoms of warfarin overdose. The use of a noninteracting antiarrhythmic agent may be preferable (e.g., procainamide).	199
Warfarin– Rifampin	1	Rifampin may decrease the pharmacologic effects of warfarin during long-term (21 day) therapy.	Monitor prothrombin times closely. The dose of warfarin may need to be increased and readjusted downward after rifampin discontinuation.	200
Warfarin– Spironolactone	3	Spironolactone may decrease the hypoprothrombinemic effect of warfarin.	Adjustment of warfarin dosage may be indicated, although the clinical significance of long-term co-therapy has not been determined.	201
Warfarin– Sucralfate	3	A patient given sucralfate and magaldrate had a delayed response in prothrombin time elevation after warfarin administration. When sucralfate was withdrawn, serum warfarin concentration and prothrombin time gradually rose.	Monitor prothrombin times closely and adjust the warfarin dosage if needed.	202
Warfarin– Sulfamethoxazole	1	Sulfamethoxazole augments the hypoprothrombinemic effect of warfarin. Serum warfarin levels may or may not be increased.	Appropriate precautions should be taken to prevent excessive hypoprothrombinemia and bleeding.	203

TABLE 4. Anticoagulant Drug Interactions—cont'd

Drug Interaction	Significance Code	Potential Effects	Recommendations	See Page
Warfarin–Sulfinpyrazone	1	Sulfinpyrazone enhances the anticoagulant effect of warfarin, sometimes within 48 hours of initiating co-therapy.	Monitor the prothrombin time carefully and reduce the warfarin dosage if needed. Some practitioners have used one-half the usual warfarin dosage.	205
Warfarin–Sulindac	2	Sulindac may enhance the anticoagulant effect of warfarin, although studies are conflicting.	Monitor for increased anticoagulant activity since a decrease in the warfarin dosage may be necessary.	206
Warfarin–Tetracycline	3	Tetracycline may potentiate the hypoprothrombinemic effect of warfarin, although there is limited clinical evidence to substantiate a drug interaction.	Monitor the prothrombin time closely during concurrent use and when either drug is withdrawn from the regimen.	207
Warfarin–Thyroid	1	Thyroid compounds increase the hypoprothrombinemic effect of warfarin. Hypothyroidism may reduce serum albumin as well as its actual protein binding capacity, or it may enhance degradation of vitamin K–dependent clotting factor.	Either agent should be initiated in small doses. Monitor thyroid levels and prothrombin time closely throughout therapy.	208
Warfarin–Vitamin E	2	Vitamin E may enhance the hypoprothrombinemic effect of warfarin. One study indicated this effect is apparent only in vitamin K deficiency.	Until further studies are done, concurrent use need not be avoided. However, monitor and reduce the warfarin dosage if needed.	210

Dicumarol—Allopurinol

1

Summary: The concurrent use of dicumarol and allopurinol in 6 healthy subjects resulted in a significantly prolonged dicumarol half-life.[1] In another study involving 3 subjects, only one showed an increased dicumarol half-life after allopurinol administration.[2]

Related Drugs: Two patients receiving phenprocoumon had bleeding episodes after allopurinol treatment was started.[3] A single case report showed an enhanced warfarin activity with a sharp increase in prothrombin time when allopurinol was added to the drug regimen.[4] However, 2 other controlled studies showed no change in warfarin activity in 5 of 6 patients[5] or in 2 patients[2] after concurrent allopurinol. Because results conflict, it is difficult to determine whether a similar interaction would occur with the indandione derivatives (anisindione and phenindione). There are no drugs related to allopurinol.

Mechanism: It has been postulated that allopurinol inhibits the hepatic metabolism of dicumarol, thereby prolonging its half-life.[1,5] However, there appears to be wide individual variability with respect to this interaction.[2]

Recommendations: Patients should be closely monitored for an increased anticoagulant response during concurrent use of dicumarol and allopurinol. If necessary, the dose of the anticoagulant may need to be decreased.

References

1. Vesell, E.S., and others: Impairment of drug metabolism in man by allopurinol and nortriptyline, N. Engl. J. Med. **283:**1484, 1970.
2. Pond, S.M., and others: The effects of allopurinol and clofibrate on the elimination of coumarin anticoagulants in man, Aust. N.Z. J. Med. **5:**324, 1975.
3. Jahnchen, E., and others: Interaction of allopurinol with phenprocoumon in man, Klin. Wochenschr. **55:**759, 1977.
4. Self, T.H., and others: Drug enhancement of warfarin activity, Lancet **2:**557, 1975.
5. Rawlins, M.D., and Smith, S.E.: Influence of allopurinol on drug metabolism in man, Br. J. Pharmacol. **48:**693, 1973.

Dicumarol–Chloramphenicol

2

Summary: The anticoagulant activity of dicumarol may be enhanced by the concurrent administration of chloramphenicol.[1] Chloramphenicol increased the average dicumarol half-life approximately 3-fold in 4 patients.[2]

Related Drugs: Although no documentation exists, a similar interaction may be expected to occur with the other coumarin anticoagulants (phenprocoumon and warfarin) and the indandione derivatives (anisindione and phenindione) because of pharmacologic similarity. There are no drugs related to chloramphenicol.

Mechanism: Chloramphenicol is capable of inhibiting microsomal enzymes,[3] which may be involved in the hydroxylation and subsequent glucuronide conjugation of the anticoagulants.[4] It has also been proposed that chloramphenicol may enhance the anticoagulant activity by reducing the availability of vitamin K.[1,5-7] However, one of these studies suggests that changes in the absorption of vitamin K from bacterial sources during antibiotic therapy are relatively unimportant compared with diet and have little influence on prothrombin-complex synthesis even in anticoagulated patients.[7] It has also been proposed that chloramphenicol interferes with the production of prothrombin at the hepatic cellular level.[1]

Recommendations: The concurrent use of dicumarol and chloramphenicol should be avoided. If concomitant use is necessary, frequent monitoring of prothrombin levels is required, and patients should be observed for clinical signs of dicumarol overdosage (e.g., hematuria, melena, bruising).

References

1. Klippel, A.P., and Pitsinger, B.: Hypoprothrombinemia secondary to antibiotic therapy and manifested by massive gastrointestinal hemorrhage: report of three cases, Arch. Surg. **96:**266, 1968.
2. Christensen, L.K., and Stousted, L.: Inhibition of drug metabolism by chloramphenicol, Lancet **2:**1397, 1969.
3. Dixon, R.L., and Fouts, J.R.: Inhibition of microsomal drug metabolic pathways by chloramphenicol, Biochem. Pharmacol. **11:**715, 1962.
4. O'Reilly, R.A.: The pharmacodynamics of the oral anticoagulant drugs, Prog. Hemost. Thromb. **2:**175, 1974.
5. Koch-Weser, J., and Sellers, E.M.: Drug interactions with coumarin anticoagulants, N. Engl. J. Med. **285:**487, 1971.
6. O'Reilly, R.A., and Aggeler, P.M.: Determinants of the response to oral anticoagulant drugs in man, Pharmacol. Rev. **22:**35, 1970.
7. Udall, J.A.: Human sources and absorption of vitamin K in relation to anticoagulation stability, J.A.M.A. **194:**107, 1965.

Dicumarol–Corticotropin

2

Summary: Corticotropin and corticosteroids have been shown to both increase[1-4] and decrease[5-7] the hypoprothrombinemic effect of dicumarol and other oral anticoagulants. Hemorrhagic episodes have been associated with concurrent use of these medications.[1,2]

Related Drugs: The activity of the indandione anticoagulant phenindione is enhanced by corticotropin.[1,3] Likewise, increased sensitivity to the coumarin anticoagulant warfarin was noted in a patient receiving prednisone.[8] Although not documented, the other coumarin anticoagulant (phenprocoumon) and the other indandione derivative (anisindione) may also interact with corticotropin or corticosteroids because of pharmacologic similarity.

There is evidence that cortisone[7] and prednisone[4] interact with dicumarol. Although there is no documentation, other corticosteroids (e.g., betamethasone, hydrocortisone, triamcinolone [see Appendix]) would be expected to interact with dicumarol in a similar manner.

Mechanism: The exact mechanisms by which corticotropin may affect the response to oral anticoagulants are not known. Corticosteroids have been shown to increase the coagulability of the blood, which may explain the reduction of anticoagulant effect seen.[7,9] Alternatively, corticotropin and corticosteroids may lower vascular integrity, which could increase the risk of hemorrhage.[1,10]

Recommendations: Clotting time tests and clinical signs of hemorrhage should be monitored closely during concurrent administration of dicumarol and corticotropin or corticosteroids. The dosage of the anticoagulant may need to be either increased or decreased based on the results of such monitoring.

References

1. Van Cuwenberge, H., and Jacques, L.B.: Hemorrhagic effect of ACTH with anticoagulants, Can. Med. Assoc. J. **79:**536, 1958.
2. O'Connell, T.X., and Aston, S.J.: Acute adrenal hemorrhage complicating anticoagulant therapy, Surg. Gynecol. Obstet. **139:**355, 1974.
3. Hellem, A.J., and Solem, J.H.: Influence of ACTH on prothrombin-proconvertin values in blood during treatment with dicumarol and phenylindanedione, Acta Med. Scand. **150:**389, 1954.
4. Sievers, J., and others: The corticosteroid treatment of acute myocardial infarction, Cardiologia **45:**65, 1964.
5. Chatterjea, J.B., and Solomon, L.: Antagonistic effect of ACTH and cortisone on the anticoagulant activity of ethyl biscoumacetate, Br. Med. J. **2:**790, 1954.
6. Menczel, J., and Dreyfuss, F.: Effect of prednisone on blood coagulation time in patients on dicumarol therapy, J. Lab. Clin. Med. **56:**14, 1960.
7. Cosgriff, S.W., and others: Hypercoagulability of the blood associated with ACTH and cortisone therapy, Am. J. Med. **9:**752, 1950.
8. Brozovic, M., and Curd, L.J.: Prothrombin during warfarin treatment, Br. J. Haematol. **24:**579, 1973.
9. Ozsoylu, S., and others: Effects of corticosteroids on coagulation of the blood, Nature **195:**1214, 1962.
10. Hamblin, T.J.: Interaction between warfarin and phenformin, Lancet **2:**1323, 1971.

Dicumarol–Methylphenidate

3

Summary: In one study involving 4 normal subjects given dicumarol, after 3 to 5 days of concurrent methylphenidate, the half-life of dicumarol was approximately doubled.[1] However, a double-blind study with 12 healthy volunteers failed to show any effect of methylphenidate on either the half-life or hypoprothrombinemic action of dicumarol.[2]

Related Drugs: Because results are conflicting and documentation is lacking, it is difficult to determine whether a similar interaction would occur between methylphenidate and the other coumarin anticoagulants (phenprocoumon and warfarin) or the indandione derivatives (anisindione and phenindione), as well as an interaction between dicumarol and the other indirect-acting sympathomimetic agents (e.g., amphetamine, mephentermine, phendimetrazine [see Appendix]).

Mechanism: It has been suggested that methylphenidate may inhibit the hepatic metabolism of dicumarol.[1]

Recommendations: The concurrent use of these agents need not be avoided. However, it is prudent to be aware of a possible interaction, and prothrombin levels should be frequently monitored.

References

1. Garrettson, L.K., and others: Methylphenidate interaction with both anticonvulsants and ethyl biscoumacetate, J.A.M.A. **207:**2053, 1969.
2. Hague, D.E., and others: The effect of methylphenidate and prolintane on the metabolism of ethyl biscoumacetate, Clin. Pharmacol. Ther. **12:**259, 1971.

Dicumarol–Oral Contraceptive Agents

2

Summary: The concurrent administration of oral contraceptive agents and dicumarol resulted in a diminished anticoagulant response in 75% of the subjects tested. The plasma half-life of dicumarol was the same in these women before and after treatment.[1]

Related Drugs: Conflicting results have been reported in other studies where the degree of anticoagulation was increased in 12 female patients who were concurrently receiving oral contraceptive agents and acenocoumarol.[*,2,3] Because of conflicting results and a lack of information, it is difficult to determine whether a similar interaction would occur with the other coumarin anticoagulants (phenprocoumon and warfarin) or the indandione derivatives (anisindione and phenindione).

Mechanism: Although oral contraceptive steroids are known to cause an increase in the plasma concentrations of certain blood clotting factors,[4] how these changes might account for the conflicting results is not understood. It has been suggested that the estrogenic component of the oral contraceptive agent is responsible for the alterations in blood coagulation.[5]

Recommendations: The evidence is limited, but does indicate that the blood coagulation response of some oral anticoagulant agents may be changed with concurrent oral contraceptive agents. Some adjustment in the anticoagulant dosage may be necessary.

References

1. Schrogie, J.J., and others: Effect of oral contraceptives on vitamin K-dependent clotting activity, Clin. Pharmacol. Ther. **8:**670, 1967.
2. DeTeresa, E., and others: Interaction between anticoagulants and contraceptives: an unsuspected finding, Br. Med. J. **2:**1260, 1979.
3. Pangrazzi, J., and others: Oral contraceptives and the prothrombin time, Br. Med. J. **280:**332, 1980.
4. Breckenridge, A.M., and others: Interactions between oral contraceptives and other drugs, Pharmacol. Ther. **7:**617, 1979.
5. Poller, L., and others: Progesterone oral contraception and blood coagulation, Br. Med. J. **1:**554, 1969.

* Not available in the U.S.

Dicumarol–Phenytoin

2

Summary: Concurrent administration of dicumarol and phenytoin may result in a significant increase in the half-life and serum level of phenytoin.[1-3] Phenytoin may decrease serum dicumarol levels and decrease its anticoagulant effect.[4] However, the effect of phenytoin on the pharmacologic action of the anticoagulant is variable and dependent on the anticoagulant used.

Related Drugs: Warfarin has been reported to cause phenytoin toxicity in 2 cases[5,6] and to have no effect in another study,[2] whereas phenytoin has been reported to enhance the anticoagulant effect of warfarin.[7-9] One case report describes an interaction in which the addition of phenytoin appeared to alter the effect of warfarin in a biphasic manner. For the first 6 days of co-therapy the patient's sensitivity to warfarin increased but then declined to a level lower than that observed before phenytoin therapy.[10] Phenprocoumon has been reported to impair phenytoin metabolism,[2] whereas phenindione had no effect.[2] Phenytoin[11] causes no uniform change in the serum level of phenprocoumon or its anticoagulant effect; some patients experience decreased and others increased prothrombin times. Because of conflicting results, it is difficult to determine whether an interaction would occur with the other indandione derivative (anisindione).

Although not documented, other hydantoin anticonvulsants (ethotoin and mephenytoin) may be expected to interact with dicumarol because of pharmacologic similarity. Carbamazepine[5,12-15] reduces the anticoagulant effect of warfarin through enhanced hepatic warfarin metabolism.

Mechanism: Dicumarol may impair the hepatic p-hydroxylation of phenytoin causing a subsequent increase in phenytoin half-life, accumulation, and intoxication.[1,2] Phenytoin may induce the hepatic enzyme systems responsible for dicumarol metabolism and impair those for warfarin, thereby decreasing serum dicumarol levels and its anticoagulant effect[3] and increasing serum warfarin levels and its anticoagulant effect.[8] Phenytoin alone may prolong the prothrombin time in some patients.[16,17] Similarly, carbamazepine may induce the hepatic enzyme systems responsible for warfarin.[5] Being highly protein bound, both dicumarol (and warfarin) and phenytoin have the potential to compete with one another for protein binding sites, with displacement resulting in increased free phenytoin or anticoagulant concentrations in the plasma. However, the clinical significance of this effect has not been demonstrated.

Recommendations: If dicumarol, warfarin, or phenprocoumon and phenytoin are co-administered, an increase in phenytoin half-life, serum levels, or side effects should occur within the first 4 weeks of therapy, particularly when the anticoagulant is added to the drug regimen of a patient previously stabilized on phenytoin. If signs and symptoms of phenytoin toxicity develop (e.g., nystagmus, gait ataxia, poor muscle tone, or lethargy), serum phenytoin levels should be determined and doses of phenytoin reduced to establish therapeutic levels. Similarly, prothrombin times should be monitored closely. Caution should be exercised when establishing anticoagulant doses after discontinuation of phenytoin or carbamazepine because of the possibility of a subsequent increase in anticoagulant effect, which takes approximately 3 weeks to develop.[3]

References

1. Hansen, J.M., and others: Dicumarol-induced diphenylhydantoin intoxication, Lancet **2:**265, 1966.
2. Skovsted, L., and others: The effect of different oral anticoagulants on diphenylhydantoin and tolbutamide metabolism, Acta Med. Scand. **199:**513, 1976.
3. Frantzen, E., and others: Phenytoin (dilantin) intoxication, Acta Neurol. Scand. **43:**440, 1967.
4. Hansen, J.M., and others: Effect of diphenylhydantoin on the metabolism of dicumarol in man, Acta Med. Scand. **189:**15, 1971.
5. Hansen, J.M., and others: Carbamazepine-induced acceleration of diphenylhydantoin and warfarin metabolism in man, Clin. Pharmacol. Ther. **12:**539, 1971.
6. Rothermick, N.O.: Diphenylhydantoin intoxication, Lancet **2:**640, 1966.
7. Koch-Weser, J.: Hemorrhagic reactions and drug interactions in 500 warfarin-treated patients, Clin. Pharmacol. Ther. **14:**139, 1973.
8. Nappi, J.M.: Warfarin and phenytoin interaction, Ann. Intern. Med. **90:**852, 1979.
9. Taylor, J.W., and others: Oral anticoagulant-phenytoin interactions, Drug Intell. Clin. Pharm. **14:**669, 1980.
10. Levine, M., and Sheppard, I.: Biphasic interaction of phenytoin with warfarin, Clin. Pharm. **3:**200, 1984.
11. Chrishe, H.W., and others: Effect of phenytoin on the metabolism of phenprocoumon, Eur. J. Clin. Invest. **4:**331, 1974.
12. Kendall, A.G., and Boivin, M.: Warfarin-carbamazepine interaction, Ann. Intern. Med. **94:**280, 1981.
13. Massey, E.W.: Effect of carbamazepine on coumadin metabolism, Ann. Neurol. **13:**691, 1983.
14. Penry, J.K., and Newmark, M.E.: The use of antiepileptic drugs, Ann. Intern. Med. **90:**207, 1979.
15. Ross, J.R.Y., and Beeley, L.: Interaction between carbamazepine and warfarin, Br. Med. J. **1:**1415, 1980.
16. Andreason, P.B., and others: Abnormalities in liver function tests during long-term diphenylhydantoin therapy in epileptic outpatients, Acta Med. Scand. **194:**261, 1973.
17. Solomon, G.E., and others: Coagulation defects caused by diphenylhydantoin, Neurology **22:**1165, 1972.

Heparin–Aspirin

Summary: The combined use of heparin and aspirin may result in serious bleeding complications.[1-3] The risk of developing these complications while on the combination may be 1.5 to 2.4 times greater than with heparin therapy alone.[4] These observations have been confirmed by careful epidemiologic study[4] and controlled clinical trials.[5-7] Although some studies have reported no increased complication rate,[8] the preponderance of data would suggest a significant risk for bleeding complications from the concurrent use of heparin and aspirin.

Aspirin also prevents heparin-induced platelet aggregation and has been used to clinical advantage for this effect in several circumstances.[9,10]

Related Drugs: No available drugs are related to heparin and there are no reports of heparin interactions with other salicylates (e.g., choline salicylate, salicylamide, sodium salicylate [see Appendix]) other than aspirin. However, since it is believed that the acetyl group accounts for the altered platelet function, the other salicylates that do not contain this moiety would not be expected to interact in a similar manner.[11]

Mechanism: Both heparin[12,13] and aspirin[14] prolong bleeding time, and heparin potentiates aspirin-induced prolongation of the bleeding time.[13] Aspirin may cause gastrointestinal bleeding and decrease platelet aggregation.[14] Inhibition of platelet aggregation removes a hemostatic mechanism for protection against heparin-induced bleeding.

Recommendations: Since the combination of low dose heparin and aspirin is effective prophylaxis for postoperative thromboembolism,[5] this combination will continue to be used. Patients should be closely observed for hemorrhagic complications; however, these may not always be predicted by laboratory monitoring of coagulation status.[15] Heparinized patients requiring antipyresis or analgesia should receive acetaminophen rather than aspirin.

References

1. Yett, H.S., and others: The hazards of aspirin plus heparin, N. Engl. J. Med. **298:**1092, 1978.
2. Rubenstein, J.J.: Aspirin, heparin and hemorrhage, N. Engl. J. Med. **294:**1122, 1976.
3. Davis, G.L., and Mutnick, A.H.: Case study: complications associated with anticoagulant therapy, Am. J. Med. Technol. **47:**179, 1981.
4. Walker, A.M., and Jick, H.: Predictors of bleeding during heparin therapy, J.A.M.A. **244:**1209, 1980.
5. Vinazzer, H., and others: Prophylaxis of postoperative thromboembolism by low dose heparin and by acetylsalicylic acid given simultaneously: a double blind study, Thromb. Res. **17:**177, 1980.
6. Loew, D., and others: Acetylsalicylic acid, low dose heparin, and a combination of both substances in the prevention of postoperative thromboembolism: a double blind study. Thromb. Res. **11:**81, 1974.
7. Flicoteaux, H., and others: Comparison of low dose heparin and low dose heparin combined with aspirin in prevention of deep vein thrombosis after total hip replacement, Pathol. Biol. (Paris) **25**(suppl.):55, 1977.

8. Schondorf, T.H., and Hey, D.: Combined administration of low dose heparin and aspirin as prophylaxis of deep vein thrombosis after hip joint surgery, Haemostasis **5:**250, 1976.

9. Janson, P.A., and others: Aspirin prevents heparin-induced platelet aggregation in vivo, Br. J. Haematol. **53:**166, 1983.

10. Flye, M.W., and others: Successful creation of arteriovenous fistulas in nonuremic patients with heparin and aspirin therapy, Am. J. Surg. **142:**759, 1981.

11. O'Reilly, R.A.: Anticoagulant antithromboic and thrombolytic drugs, In Gilman, A.G., Goodman, L.S., and Gilman, A., editors: The pharmacological basis of therapeutics. New York, 1980, MacMillan Publishing.

12. Heiden, D., and others: Heparin bleeding, platelet dysfunction and aspirin, J.A.M.A. **246:**330, 1981.

13. Kelton, J.G., and Hirsh, J.: Bleeding associated with antithrombotic therapy, Semin. Hematol. **17:**259, 1980.

14. Rothschild, B.M.: Hematologic perturbations associated with salicylate, Clin. Pharmacol. Ther. **26:**145, 1979.

15. Coon, W.W., and others: Hemorrhagic complications of anticoagulant therapy, Arch. Intern. Med. **133:**386, 1976.

Heparin–Carbenicillin

Summary: Carbenicillin and other penicillins have been shown to prolong bleeding time[1-7] and may therefore theoretically increase the effects of heparin when used concurrently. Although this specific interaction has not been studied, the clinical implications must be considered in uremic patients who already have abnormal platelet function, where heparin treatment is required for hemodialysis, and where heparin's action may be enhanced by the heparin-like activity of carbenicillin.[1] The effects of carbenicillin and other penicillins may be dose related.

Related Drugs: Similar effects on bleeding have been reported with penicillin G,[2] ticarcillin,[3] ampicillin,[4] and methicillin.[4] Since all penicillins (e.g., azlocillin, mezlocillin, oxacillin [see Appendix]) share the same basic structure, they may all be able to alter platelet function[4] and may theoretically interact with heparin. There are no drugs related to heparin. Although specific documentation is lacking, a similar interaction between carbenicillin and the coumarin anticoagulants (dicumarol, phenprocoumon, and warfarin) and the indandione derivatives (anisindione and phenindione) may also theoretically occur.

Mechanism: The coagulation disorder seen with the penicillins is the composite result of platelet dysfunction, disturbed conversion of fibrinogen to fibrin, and increased antithrombin-III activity.[1-7] The inhibition of factor-Xa activity seen with carbenicillin corresponds to that seen after low-dose heparin prophylaxis.[5] It has been suggested that this mechanism, along with the mechanism of action of heparin, may result in an additive pharmacologic activity when these agents are used concurrently.

Recommendations: Since the effect of the penicillins on bleeding function appears to occur only at high doses, it is suggested that lower doses be used if heparin is to be administered concurrently or if carbenicillin is to be given to uremic patients. One report suggests that in cases where creatinine clearance is lower than 10 ml/min, the dose of carbenicillin should not exceed 3 to 4 g/day.[1] Coagulation must always be frequently monitored if bleeding occurs. Also, protamine may be used if bleeding arises since one study shows the anticoagulant action of carbenicillin may be corrected without impairing its bactericidal activity.[1]

References

1. Tabernero Romo, J.M., and others: Effects of carbenicillin on blood coagulation: a study in patients with chronic renal failure, Clin. Nephrol. **11:**31, 1979.
2. Cazenave, J.P., and others: Effects of penicillin G on platelet aggregation, release, and adherence to collagen, Proc. Soc. Exp. Biol. Med. **142:**159, 1973.
3. Brown, C.H., and others: Study of the effects of ticarcillin on blood coagulation and platelet function, Antimicrob. Agents Chemother. **7:**652, 1975.
4. Brown, C.H., and others: Defective platelet function following the administration of penicillin compounds, Blood **47:**949, 1976.
5. Andrassy, K., and others: Penicillin-induced coagulation disorder, Lancet **2:**1039, 1976.
6. Andrassy, K., and others: Bleeding in uremic patients after carbenicillin, Thromb. Haemost. **36:**115, 1976.
7. Brown, C.H., and others: The hemostatic defect produced by carbenicillin, N. Engl. J. Med. **291:**265, 1974.

Summary: Limited information from 2 studies in humans suggests that the use of dextran 70[1] or dextran 75[2] in combination with heparin is associated with a statistically significant higher incidence of bleeding than the use of either agent alone. However, dextran 40 has been administered concomitantly with heparin without untoward effects.[3-7]

Related Drugs: There are no commercially available drugs chemically related to either dextran or heparin.

Mechanism: Heparin and dextran have been proved in humans to possess independent and synergistic effects to prolong coagulation time and reduce clot strength.[2] Heparin functions as an anticoagulant by accelerating the rate at which antithrombin III normally inactivates thrombin, factor Xa, and other factors.[8] Dextran has various effects on hemostasis including reduced viscosity, hemodilution, altered suspension stability of cells, prevention of erythrocyte agglutination, impairment of bleeding time and platelet function, and alteration of the sol-gel transformation from fibrinogen to fibrin.[2,9-11] Dextran 40 has been shown to retard rouleau formation and sludging of red blood cells whereas dextran 70 has not been shown to possess these properties.[12] Both heparin and dextran sulfate competitively inhibit prostaglandin E (PGE), sensitize adenylate cyclase activity in human platelets, and antagonize the antiaggregating action of PGE, in vitro.

Recommendations: Data pertaining to the concurrent use of dextran 40 and heparin suggest baseline studies (thrombin time, activated prothrombin time, or the Lee White clotting time) should be performed before and intermittently during therapy until anticoagulation is achieved.

Although sufficient data to formulate a conclusive recommendation for the concomitant use of dextran 70 or 75 and heparin are lacking, the two should only be used in combination when patients can be closely monitored. Limited data suggest dextran 70 or 75 may cause a greater incidence of adverse reactions and have less effect on the sludging of red blood cells than the use of dextran 40; however, a firm recommendation as to the preferred agent cannot be offered.

References

1. Morrison, N.D., and others: Deep vein thrombosis after femoropopliteal bypass grafting with observations on the incidence of complications following the use of dextran 70, N. Z. Med. J. **84:**233, 1976.
2. Bloom, W.L., and Brewer, S.S.: The independent yet synergistic effects of heparin and dextran, Acta Chir. Scand. **387**(suppl.):53, 1968.
3. Schondorf, T.H., and Weber, V.: Prevention of deep venous thrombosis in orthopedic surgery with the combination of low dose heparin plus either dihydroergotamine or dextran, Scand. J. Haematol. **36**(suppl.):126, 1980.
4. Evarts, C-M: Diagnosis and treatment of fat embolism, J.A.M.A. **194:**899, 1965.
5. Serjeant, J.C.B.: Mesenteric embolus treated with low-molecular-weight dextran, Lancet **1:**139, 1965.

6. Gregory, R.J.: The rapid lowering of hematocrit by exchange transfusion of rheomacrodex dextran 40, Acta. Med. Scand. **189:**551, 1971.
7. Munster, A.M.: Low molecular weight dextran in the treatment of phlegmasia caerulea dolens, Med. J. Aust. **1:**851, 1965.
8. Jaques, L.B.: Heparins-anionic polyelectrolyte drugs, Pharmacol. Rev. **31:**99, 1979.
9. O'Reilly, R.A.: Anticoagulant, antithrombotic, and thrombolytic drugs. In Gilman, A.G., Goodman, L.S., and Gilman, A., editors: The pharmacological basis of therapeutics, ed. 6, New York, 1980, Macmillan Publishing Co.
10. Kluge, T.H., and others: Thrombosis propyhlaxis with dextran and warfarin in vascular operations, Surg. Gynecol. Obstet. **135:**941, 1972.
11. Davies, W.T.: Dextran or heparin? Lancet **2:**732, 1978.
12. Moore, F.D.: Tris buffer, mannitol and low viscous dextran, Surg. Clin. North Am. **43:**577, 1963.

Phenindione–Haloperidol

3

Summary: The concurrent use of phenindione and haloperidol may lead to a reduction in the anticoagulant effect of phenindione. A single case report showed that a patient maintained on phenindione needed an increased dosage when haloperidol was added to his therapy. Not until the haloperidol was withdrawn was it possible to return to the original phenindione dose.[1]

Related Drugs: There is no documentation regarding an interaction between haloperidol and the coumarin anticoagulants (dicumarol, phenprocoumon, and warfarin) or the other indandione derivative (anisindione). Documentation is lacking regarding an interaction between phenindione and the other antipsychotic agents including the phenothiazines (e.g., chlorpromazine, thioridazine, triflupromazine [see Appendix]), thioxanthenes (chlorprothixene and thiothixene), as well as the dihydroindolone (molindone) and dibenzoxazepine (loxapine).

Mechanism: The mechanism of this interaction is unknown.

Recommendations: Until further clinical studies are performed, the concurrent use of these agents need not be avoided. However, it is important to be aware of a possible interaction, and if inadequate anticoagulation occurs a decrease in the haloperidol dose or an increase in the phenindione dose may be necessary.

Reference

1. Oakley, D.P., and Lautch, H.: Haloperidol and anticoagulant treatment, Lancet **2:**1231, 1963.

Warfarin–Acetaminophen

3

Summary: In therapeutic dosages, coadministration of acetaminophen with warfarin resulted in only a slight, if any, effect on the hypoprothrombinemic response to the anticoagulant.[1-4] However, one study reported that high daily doses of acetaminophen (four 500 mg tablets, 4 times a day) significantly prolonged prothrombin times in patients on coumarin derivatives.[5]

Related Drugs: Dicumarol and phenprocoumon[2] have also been reported to interact with acetaminophen in a dosage of 2600 mg/day and to cause a slight elevation of the prothrombin time. While no evidence of this interaction has appeared in the biomedical literature, the indandione derivatives (anisindione and phenindione) may also be expected to interact with acetaminophen in a similar manner since they are pharmacologically related.

Mechanism: The mechanism of this interaction is unknown.

Recommendations: Enhancement of warfarin's hypoprothrombinemic effect by acetaminophen appears to be controversial. The use of therapeutic dosages of acetaminophen would thus be preferable to aspirin as an antipyretic or analgesic in the patient requiring oral anticoagulants. However, the use of high doses of acetaminophen may result in an increased prothrombin time. Therefore, the need for monitoring prothrombin time is still necessary for individual patient response to acetaminophen-anticoagulant coadministration.

References

1. Antlitz, A.M., and Awalt, L.F.: A double-blind study of acetaminophen used in conjunction with oral anticoagulant therapy, Curr. Ther. Res. **11:**360, 1969.
2. Antlitz, A.M., and others: Potentiation of oral anticoagulant therapy by acetaminophen, Curr. Ther. Res. **10:**501, 1968.
3. Udall, J.A.: Drug interference with warfarin therapy, Clin. Med. **77:**20, 1970.
4. Orme, M., and others: Warfarin and distalgesic interaction, Br. Med. J. **1:**200, 1976.
5. Boeijinga, J.J., and others: Interactions between paracetamol and coumarin anticoagulants, Lancet **1:**506, 1982.

Warfarin–Alcohol, Ethyl

3

Summary: The use of small or moderate amounts of alcohol (<120 ml of 100 proof whiskey) by patients receiving warfarin is unlikely to produce any significant effect on warfarin pharmacokinetics or pharmacodynamics.[1] However, continuous heavy alcohol consumption, particularly in patients with hepatic dysfunction, may significantly alter warfarin metabolism and patient response.

Related Drugs: Alcohol may be expected to interact with the other coumarin anticoagulants (dicumarol and phenprocoumon) and the indandione derivatives (anisindione and phenindione) in a manner similar to that with warfarin because of pharmacologic similarity.

Mechanism: Ingestion of moderate to substantial quantities of alcohol has little effect on warfarin action,[2] although acute ingestion in individual cases may transiently impair warfarin metabolism.[3] Regular use of moderate quantities of alcohol produces no significant effect on warfarin anticoagulant response, although more substantial use may be associated with an increased rate of warfarin metabolism.[4] Chronic alcohol abuse resulting in hepatic dysfunction may result in exaggerated response to warfarin.[5] This may reflect impaired hepatic synthesis of clotting factor (i.e., II, VII, IX, X) precursors or impaired hepatic drug metabolism capacity.

Recommendations: No special precautions are necessary when administering warfarin to patients reporting minimal to moderate alcohol consumption as long as routine prothrombin time determinations are regularly obtained. Administration of warfarin to patients who chronically abuse alcohol may require frequent laboratory evaluation to prevent excessive warfarin anticoagulation.

References

1. O'Reilly, R.A.: Lack of effect of mealtime wine on the hypoprothrombinemia of oral anticoagulants, Am. J. Med. Sci. **277**:189, 1979.
2. Waris, E.: Effect of ethyl alcohol on some coagulation factors in man during anticoagulant therapy, Ann. Med. Int. Fenn. **41**:45, 1963.
3. Breckenridge, A., and Orme, M.: Clinical implications of enzyme induction, Ann. N.Y. Acad. Sci. **179**:421, 1971.
4. Kater, R.M.H., and others: Increased rate of clearance of drugs from the circulation of alcoholics, Am. J. Med. Sci. **258**:35, 1969.
5. Udall, J.A.: Drug interference with warfarin therapy, Clin. Med. **77**(8):20, 1970.

Warfarin–Ascorbic Acid

4

Summary: No clinically significant alteration of warfarin anticoagulant action by concurrently administered ascorbic acid has been demonstrated in controlled clinical studies.[1,2] Of 2 cases reported to demonstrate antagonism of warfarin effect by ascorbic acid,[3,4] only one showed a reasonable temporal relationship between altered anticoagulant action and ascorbic acid administration, and other possible contributing factors were not evaluated. Although high doses of concurrently administered ascorbic acid have been associated with decreases of 2% to 40% in total warfarin plasma concentration,[1] no alterations in warfarin action were noted.

Related Drugs: There are no reports demonstrating a similar interaction between ascorbic acid and the other coumarin anticoagulants (dicumarol and phenprocoumon) and the indandione derivatives (anisindione and phenindione). There are no drugs related to ascorbic acid.

Mechanism: The observed decrease in plasma warfarin concentration during concurrent administration of ascorbic acid (3 to 10 g/day) is thought to result from diarrhea occurring in a number of subjects, particularly at higher doses.

Recommendations: No routine adjustment of warfarin dose needs to be made during concurrent ascorbic acid therapy. However, in patients exhibiting changing (increasing) dosage requirements of warfarin during maintenance anticoagulant therapy, possible concurrent ascorbic acid ingestion should be eliminated as a causative factor.

References

1. Feetam, C.L., and others: Lack of a clinically important interaction between warfarin and ascorbic acid, Toxicol. Appl. Pharmacol. **31:**544, 1975.
2. Smith, E.C., and others: Interaction of ascorbic acid and warfarin, J.A.M.A. **219:**1479, 1972.
3. Rosenthal, G.: Interaction of ascorbic acid and warfarin, J.A.M.A. **215:**671, 1971.
4. Hume, R., and others: Interaction of ascorbic acid and warfarin, J.A.M.A. **219:**479, 1972.

Warfarin–Aspirin

1

Summary: Concurrent administration of moderate to large doses of aspirin (>3 g/day) and warfarin may potentiate the anticoagulant action of warfarin, increase the risk of warfarin-induced bleeding, or both. Although the effects of lower doses of aspirin on warfarin hypoprothrombinemic action may be less substantial, concurrent administration of aspirin and warfarin should be avoided.

The effects of aspirin on warfarin action appear to be dose-related. Lower doses of aspirin (1.95 g/day) in patients or healthy volunteers do not alter warfarin effects on prothrombin time, whereas larger doses (3.9 g/day) may be associated with substantial prothrombin time prolongation.[1-3] However, some patients receiving warfarin may exhibit an initial rise in prothrombin time following the initiation of aspirin therapy in a dose of 1 g/day.[4] This transient effect may disappear within 4 to 5 days of therapy. After discontinuing salicylates, warfarin effect declines substantially and there may be a lag time before it returns to pre-salicylate levels.

Related Drugs: One study has shown that dicumarol and phenindione do not interact with low doses of aspirin.[5] Dicumarol and phenindione as well as the other coumarin anticoagulant (phenprocoumon) and indandione derivative (anisindione) may interact with higher doses of aspirin in a manner similar to warfarin, although documentation is lacking.

Sodium salicylate and diflunisal are analogs of aspirin and have also been shown to interact with anticoagulants.[6] The newer salicylic acid derivative, diflunisal, has been shown to significantly influence warfarin pharmacokinetics and anticoagulant effect.[6] Administration of diflunisal (1 g/day) for 2 weeks significantly increased plasma free warfarin fraction while decreasing total warfarin concentration. The possible interaction between other salicylates (e.g., choline salicylate, salicylamide, salsalate [see Appendix]) with warfarin has not been documented, but because of their effect on gastric mucosa and the potential binding sites, they may be expected to interact similarly to diflunisal and sodium salicylate.

Mechanism: Aspirin may augment the action of anticoagulants such as warfarin through several mechanisms. Aspirin and related compounds, including sodium salicylate and diflunisal, will displace warfarin from plasma protein binding sites, causing a transient increase in anticoagulant effect (elevated prothrombin time) and a corresponding decrease in total plasma warfarin concentrations.[6] At the same time, aspirin but not nonacetylated salicylates will directly decrease platelet aggregation and prolong bleeding time, and oral salicylate administration may have a direct toxic effect on gastric mucosa and cause gastrointestinal bleeding.

Recommendations: Concurrent administration of warfarin and salicylate compounds, including aspirin, sodium salicylate, and diflunisal, should be avoided whenever possible. Either acetaminophen or another nonsteroidal anti-inflammatory agent that does not interact with warfarin should be substituted for aspirin according to the indication present. If warfarin and aspirin in moderate to large dosages are administered together, frequent prothrombin time determinations should be performed initially to monitor the transient increase in warfarin effect which is likely to occur.

References

1. O'Reilly, R.A., and Aggeler, P.M.: Determinants of the response to oral anticoagulant drugs in man, Pharmacol. Rev. **22:**35, 1970.
2. O'Reilly, R.A.: Impact of aspirin and chlorthalidone on the pharmacodynamics of oral anticoagulant drugs in man, Ann. N. Y. Acad. Sci. **179:**173, 1971.
3. Udall, J.A.: Drug interference with warfarin therapy, Clin. Med. **77**(8):20, 1970.
4. Donaldson, D.R., and others: Assessment of the interaction of warfarin with aspirin and dipyridamole, Thromb. Haemost. **47:**77, 1982.
5. Jarnum, S.: Cinchophen and acetylsalicylic acid in anticoagulant treatment, Scand. J. Lab. Clin. Invest. **6:**91, 1954.
6. Serlin, M.J., and others: Interaction between diflunisal and warfarin, Clin. Pharmacol. Ther. **28:**493, 1980.

Warfarin–Chloral Hydrate

Summary: Concurrent administration of chloral hydrate and warfarin may be associated with a transient increase in warfarin anticoagulant action.[1,2] Alterations in warfarin pharmacokinetics, specifically decreased warfarin plasma protein binding, and increased systemic drug clearance are induced by chloral hydrate administration. However, during long-term therapy these effects do not significantly alter the hypoprothrombinemic response to warfarin.[1-3]

Related Drugs: Chloral betaine* and triclofos, which undergo enteral hydrolysis to chloral hydrate, produce similar effects on warfarin metabolism and pharmacodynamics.[4,5] Dicumarol has been shown to interact with chloral hydrate in a manner similar to warfarin.[6] Studies of the effect of chloral hydrate on the other coumarin anticoagulant (phenprocoumon) and the indandione derivatives (anisindione and phenindione) have not been reported, although a similar interaction may be expected to occur since they are pharmacologically related.

Mechanism: The major metabolite of chloral hydrate, trichloroacetic acid, displaces warfarin from plasma protein (albumin) binding sites,[1] increasing the warfarin free fraction in plasma. Although this elevated free drug concentration is associated with an increased hypoprothrombinemic effect, it also promotes increased systemic drug clearance. The increased hypoprothrombinemic response to warfarin administration after initiation of chloral hydrate therapy parallels changes in plasma concentration of trichloroacetic acid.[1] During continuous concurrent administration, the prothrombin time returns to pre-chloral hydrate values, although the associated total plasma warfarin concentration may be lower.[2] Similarly, continued administration of chloral betaine does not substantially alter warfarin response.[3]

Recommendations: During initial concurrent administration of warfarin and chloral hydrate, frequent prothrombin time determinations should be made to monitor possible increases in warfarin anticoagulant action. Although temporary warfarin dosage adjustments are not generally necessary, changes in warfarin therapy should be determined on an individual patient basis. For long-term sedative hypnotic therapy, a benzodiazepine is a choice preferable to chloral hydrate (see Warfarin-Chlordiazepoxide, p. 159).

References

1. Sellers, E.M., and Koch-Weser, J.: Kinetics and clinical importance of displacement of warfarin from albumin by acidic drugs, Ann. N. Y. Acad. Sci. **179:**213, 1971.
2. Weiner, M.: Species differences in the effect of chloral hydrate on coumarin anticoagulants, Ann. N. Y. Acad. Sci. **179:**226, 1971.
3. Griner, P.F., and others: Chloral hydrate and warfarin interaction: clinical significance, Ann. Intern. Med. **74:**540, 1971.
4. McDonald, M.G., and others: The effects of phenobarbital, chloral betaine and glutethimide administration on warfarin plasma levels and hypoprothrombinemic responses in man, Clin. Pharmacol. Ther. **10:**80, 1969.
5. Seller, E.M., and Koch-Weser, J.: Enhancement of warfarin-induced hypoprothrombinemia by triclofos, Clin. Pharmacol. Ther. **13:**911, 1972.
6. Cucinell, S.A., and others: The effect of chloral hydrate on bishydroxycoumarin metabolism, J.A.M.A. **197:**366, 1966.

*Not available in the U.S.

Warfarin–Chlordiazepoxide

4

Summary: Concurrent administration of chlordiazepoxide and warfarin produces no clinically significant effect on warfarin pharmacokinetics or anticoagulant action.[1-3]

Related Drugs: The majority of other studies regarding the effects of benzodiazepines on warfarin have involved diazepam[3-6] or nitrazepam[*3,5,7] in addition to chlordiazepoxide.[1-3] These studies have not demonstrated any interaction with warfarin.[1-6] Although documentation is lacking, other benzodiazepines (e.g., clonazepam, flurazepam, triazolam [see Appendix]) may also be expected not to interact. The coumarin anticoagulant, phenprocoumon, has been demonstrated not to interact with nitrazepam.[7] One case report of an enhanced dicumarol effect during diazepam administration has been described.[8] No data describing the indandione derivatives (anisindione and phenindione) have been presented, and because results are conflicting it is not possible to determine whether an interaction would occur with chlordiazepoxide.

Mechanism: The benzodiazepines may induce hepatic microsomal enzymes; however, documentation is lacking in regard to the significance of this effect at usual therapeutic dosages.[1,2,4-7]

Recommendations: Warfarin therapy during concurrent chlordiazepoxide administration should be monitored in a routine fashion. Therefore, no special precautions are necessary when these drugs are given concurrently.

References

1. Lackner, H., and Hunt, V.E.: The effect of librium on hemostasis, Am. J. Med. Sci. **256:**368, 1968.
2. Robinson, D.S., and Sylvester, D.: Interactions of commonly prescribed drugs and warfarin, Ann. Intern. Med. **72:**853, 1970.
3. Solomon, H.M., and others: Mechanisms of drug interactions, J.A.M.A. **216:**1997, 1971.
4. Orme, M., and others: Interactions of benzodiazepines with warfarin, Br. Med. J. **3:**611, 1972.
5. Ristola, P., and Pyorala, K.: Determinants of response to coumarin anticoagulants in patients with acute myocardial infarction, Acta Med. Scand. **192:**183, 1972.
6. Whitfield, J.B., and others: Change in plasma gamma-glutamyl transpeptidase activity and altered drug metabolism in man, Br. Med. J. **1:**316, 1973.
7. Beiger, R., and others: Influence of nitrazepam on oral anticoagulation with phenprocoumon, Clin. Pharmacol. Ther. **13:**361, 1972.
8. Taylor, P.J.: Hemorrhage while on anticoagulant therapy precipitated by drug interaction, Ariz. Med. **24:**697, 1967.

*Not available in the U.S.

Warfarin–Cholestyramine

Summary: Concurrent administration of oral cholestyramine and oral or parenteral warfarin may result in a significant alteration of warfarin anticoagulant action.[1-3] Cholestyramine has been demonstrated to decrease warfarin half-life and increase warfarin total body clearance after oral and parenteral warfarin administration.[1,2] Although studies in normal subjects and case reports in patients suggest that this interaction will result in decreased warfarin effect, the magnitude of the interaction cannot be predicted.

Related Drugs: Cholestyramine-induced enhancement of phenprocoumon elimination, and consequent decrease in anticoagulant effect, is similar to that observed with warfarin.[4,5] A similar interaction may be expected to occur between cholestyramine and the other coumarin anticoagulant (dicumarol) and the indandione derivatives (anisindione and phenindione) because of pharmacologic similarity. Colestipol, another anion exchange resin, has been reported not to interact with phenprocoumon.[6] Whether warfarin and the other coumarin and indandione anticoagulants would also fail to interact with colestipol has not been documented.

Mechanism: Cholestyramine is an insoluble chloride salt of a basic ion-exchange resin that binds to anionic substances in a pH-dependent fashion. In vitro experiments have demonstrated that cholestyramine also binds warfarin in a pH-dependent fashion, suggesting possible direct interaction of the 2 drugs in the gut.[2] Additional studies with intravenous warfarin have demonstrated that cholestyramine may inhibit the entrohepatic recycling of warfarin and thereby increase systemic drug clearance and decrease anticoagulant effect.

At the same time, cholestyramine-induced vitamin K deficiency and hemorrhagic episodes have also been reported. The clinical influence of this effect in patients receiving oral anticoagulants has not been identified, however.[7]

Recommendations: Concurrent administration of warfarin and cholestyramine should be avoided whenever possible. If the 2 drugs must be used concurrently, a portion of the cholestyramine effect may be minimized by delaying administration of cholestyramine for 3 to 6 hours after oral warfarin administration. During concurrent therapy, prothrombin time should be closely monitored to ensure adequate therapeutic anticoagulation.

References

1. Janchen, E., and others: Enhanced elimination of warfarin during treatment with cholestyramine, Br. J. Clin. Pharmacol. **5:**437, 1978.
2. Robinson, D.S., and others: Interaction of warfarin and nonsystemic gastrointestinal drugs, Clin. Pharmacol. Ther. **12:**491, 1971.
3. Levy, R.I., and others: Dietary and drug treatment of primary hyperlipoproteinemia, Ann. Intern. Med. **77:**267, 1972.
4. Meinertz, T., and others: Intoxication with phenprocoumon (Marcumar): cholestyramine enhances the elimination of the drug from the body, Br. Med. J. **2:**439, 1977.

5. Meinertz, T., and others: Interruption by cholestyramine of the enterohepatic circulation of phenprocoumon, Clin. Pharmacol. Ther. **21:**731, 1977.
6. Harvengt, C., and Desager, G.P.: Effect of colestipol a bile acid sequester on the absorption of phenprocoumon in man, Eur. J. Clin. Pharmacol. **4:**142, 1972.
7. Gross, L., and Brotman, M.: Hypoprothrombinemia and hemorrhage associated with cholestyramine therapy, Ann. Intern. Med. **72:**95, 1970.

Warfarin–Cimetidine

1

Summary: The hypoprothrombinemic response of warfarin is prolonged when cimetidine is given concurrently.[1-9] The addition of cimetidine results in a gradual increase in hypoprothrombinemia over a 1 or 2 week period. When cimetidine is discontinued, the prothrombin time returns to pre-cimetidine values in approximately 1 week.

Related Drugs: Cimetidine caused prolonged prothrombin times in patients receiving the indandione derivative phenindione.[9] However, the anticoagulant effects of the coumarin anticoagulant phenprocoumon were not altered with concurrent cimetidine.[10,11] There is no documentation regarding an interaction with the other coumarin anticoagulant (dicumarol) or the other indandione derivative (anisindione), and because of conflicting results it is not possible to determine whether an interaction would occur. Ranitidine, another histamine H_2-receptor antagonist, did not affect prothrombin time or plasma warfarin concentration in 5 subjects.[12]

Mechanism: When cimetidine is added to warfarin therapy, warfarin plasma levels increase and the clearance significantly decreases.[4,8,9] Cimetidine inhibited the hydroxylation of coumarin and the 0-deethylation of 7-ethoxycoumarin in human liver, as demonstrated in biopsies.[13] It is therefore thought that cimetidine inhibits warfarin metabolism.[14,15] It has been suggested that phenprocoumon is metabolized by glucuronidation, which appears to be unaffected by cimetidine.[16]

Recommendations: The hypoprothrombinemic response to warfarin should be closely monitored when cimetidine is added or discontinued. In those patients receiving cimetidine in whom warfarin therapy is begun, the possibility exists of an increased sensitivity to the hypoprothrombinemic warfarin effect.

References

1. Silver, B.A., and Bell, W.R.: Cimetidine potentiation of the hypoprothrombinemic effect of warfarin, Ann. Intern. Med. **90:**348, 1979.
2. Wallin, B.A., and others: Cimetidine and effect of warfarin, Ann. Intern. Med. **90:**993, 1979.
3. Flind, A.C.: Cimetidine and oral anticoagulants, Br. Med. J. **2:**1367, 1978.
4. Hetzel, D., and others: Cimetidine interaction with warfarin, Lancet **2:**639, 1979.
5. Flind, A.C.: Cimetidine and oral anticoagulants, Lancet **2:**1054, 1978.
6. Kerley, B., and Ali, M.: Cimetidine potentiation of warfarin action, Can. Med. Assoc. J. **126:**116, 1982.
7. Devanesen, S.: Prolongation of prothrombin time with cimetidine, Med. J. Aust. **1:**537, 1981.
8. Breckenridge, A.M., and others: Cimetidine increases the action of warfarin in man, Br. J. Clin. Pharmacol. **8:**393, 1979.
9. Serlin, J.J., and others: Cimetidine: interaction with oral anticoagulants in man, Lancet **2:**317, 1979.
10. Harenberg, J., and others: Influence of cimetidine on the pharmacodynamics of phenprocoumon, Clin. Pharmacol. Ther. **31:**233, 1982.
11. Harenberg, J., and others: Lack of effect of cimetidine on action of phenprocoumon, Eur. J. Clin. Pharmacol. **23:**365, 1982.

12. Serlin, M.J., and others: Lack of effect of ranitidine on warfarin action, Br. J. Clin. Pharmacol. **12:**791, 1981.
13. Puurunen, J., and others: Effect of cimetidine on microsomal drug metabolism in man, Eur. J. Clin. Pharmacol. **18:**185, 1980.
14. Sorkin, E.M., and Darvey, D.L.: Review of cimetidine drug interactions, Drug Intell. Clin. Pharm. **17:**110, 1983.
15. Mangini, R.J.: Clinically important cimetidine drug interactions, Clin. Pharm. **1:**433, 1982.
16. Harenberg, J., and others: Cimetidine does not increase the anticoagulant effect of phenprocoumon, Br. J. Clin. Pharmacol. **14:**292, 1982.

Warfarin–Clofibrate

Summary: Concurrent administration of oral clofibrate and warfarin may substantially enhance warfarin's anticoagulant action, predisposing patients to significant risk of excessive anticoagulation and hemorrhage.[1-5]

Related Drugs: Phenindione and dicumarol[6,7] have been reported to interact with clofibrate in a fashion similar to warfarin. The other coumarin anticoagulant (phenprocoumon) and indandione derivative (anisindione) may also interact with clofibrate because of pharmacologic similarity, although no documentation of an interaction exists.

Mechanism: Clofibrate displaces warfarin from plasma protein binding sites in both a competitive and noncompetitive fashion.[4,5] This effect occurs with both the R(−) and S(−) warfarin isomers, although the effect on the S(−) isomer may be greater.[4] However, these changes do not necessarily result in significant alterations in free plasma warfarin fraction[5] or in changes in warfarin elimination half-life or clearance.[8] The lack of correlation between clofibrate-induced alterations in warfarin pharmacokinetics and the observed enhancement of anticoagulant effect suggests the possibility of a direct receptor-site interaction. However, clofibrate does not appear to enhance warfarin inhibition of vitamin K epoxide reductase.[9]

It has also been suggested that the enhancement of warfarin effect in patients may be directly associated with clofibrate's hypolipidemic action. These proposed mechanisms have not been proved in clinical investigations, however, and the precise mechanism of clofibrate enhancement of warfarin action remains to be determined.

Recommendations: Because the concurrent use of clofibrate and warfarin may lead to excessive warfarin-induced anticoagulation and clinically significant hemorrhagic side effects, frequent prothrombin time determinations should be made during concurrent therapy. A reduction in warfarin dosage requirements should be expected,[1,7] although the magnitude of clofibrate effect will vary among individual patients.[3] Warfarin dosage in patients concurrently receiving clofibrate should be individually titrated using appropriate laboratory evaluation.

References

1. Roberts, S.D., and Pantridge, J.F.: Effects of Atromid on requirements of warfarin, J. Atherosclerosis Res. **3**:655, 1963.
2. O'Reilly, R.A., and others: Studies on the interaction of warfarin and clofibrate in man, Thromb. Haemost. **27**:309, 1972.
3. Udall, J.A.: Drug interference with warfarin therapy, Clin. Med. **77**(8):20, 1970.
4. Bjornsson, T.D., and others: Interaction of clofibrate with warfarin. 1. Effect of clofibrate on the disposition of the optical enantiomorphs of warfarin, J. Pharmacokinet. Biopharm. **5**:495, 1977.
5. Bjornsson, T.D., and others: Clofibrate displaced warfarin from plasma proteins in man: an example of a pure displacement interaction, J. Pharmacol. Exp. Ther. **210**:316, 1979.
6. Williams, G.E., and others: Atromid and anticoagulant therapy, J. Atherosclerosis Res. **3**:655, 1963.
7. Rogen, A.S., and Ferguson, J.C.: Clinical observations on patients treated with Atromid and anticoagulants, J. Atherosclerosis Res. **3**:671, 1963.
8. Pond, S.M., and others: The effects of allopurinol and clofibrate on the elimination of coumarin anticoagulants in man, Aust. N. Z. J. Med. **5**:324, 1975.
9. Bjornsson, T.D., and others: Effects of clofibrate and warfarin alone and in combination on the disposition of vitamin K, J. Pharmacol. Exp. Ther. **210**:322, 1979.

Warfarin–Diphenhydramine

4

Summary: Concurrent administration of oral diphenhydramine and warfarin produces no clinically significant effect on warfarin pharmacodynamics or anticoagulant action. Although reviews of warfarin drug interactions have suggested possible interactions between antihistamines and warfarin,[1,2] no clinical documentation through case reports or controlled clinical studies has been presented.

Related Drugs: No documentation exists regarding an interaction between diphenhydramine and the other coumarin anticoagulants (dicumarol and phenprocoumon) and the indandione derivatives (anisindione and phenindione). However, a similar lack of an interaction may be expected. There is also a lack of documentation of this interaction with the other antihistamines (e.g., brompheniramine, chlorpheniramine, tripelennamine [see Appendix]), although because they are pharmacologically related a similar lack of an interaction with warfarin may be expected.

Mechanism: A number of antihistamines, including diphenhydramine, have been shown to induce hepatic microsomal enzymes in animal studies.[3,4] Although this effect may cause increased metabolism of selected sedative-hypnotic compounds by in vitro rat hepatic microsomal preparations, no effect on oral anticoagulants has been demonstrated.

Recommendations: No specific precautions need be taken during concurrent administration of diphenhydramine and warfarin.

References

1. Hartshorn, E.A.: Drug interactions. III. Classes of drugs and their interactions, Drug Intell. Clin. Pharm. **2:**198, 1968.
2. Formiller, N., and Cohon, M.S.: Coumarin and indandione anticoagulants: potentiators and antagonists, Am. J. Hosp. Pharm. **26:**574, 1969.
3. Kato, R., and others: Further studies on the inhibition and stimulation of microsomal drug-metabolizing enzymes of rat liver by various compounds, Biochem. Pharmacol. **13:**69, 1964.
4. Conney, A.H., and others: Adaptive increases in drug-metabolizing enzymes induced by phenobarbital and other drugs, J. Pharmacol. Exp. Ther. **130:**1, 1960.

Warfarin–Disopyramide

3

Summary: Disopyramide may enhance the hypoprothrombinemic response to warfarin. A patient receiving warfarin, disopyramide, and other medications developed general malaise and was found to be hypotensive.[1] Disopyramide was discontinued, and the previously stable prothrombin time fell, necessitating incremental doses of warfarin. More recent studies have failed to confirm this relationship.[2,3]

Related Drugs: Documentation is lacking regarding an interaction between disopyramide and the other coumarin anticoagulants (dicumarol and phenprocoumon) and the indandione derivatives (anisindione and phenindione), although such an interaction may be possible if the mechanism involves competition for the same metabolic pathways. There are no drugs related to disopyramide.

Mechanism: The mechanism of interaction is not known. One suggested mechanism is that disopyramide and warfarin compete for the same hepatic metabolic pathways.

Recommendations: The pharmacologic activity of warfarin may need to be monitored when disopyramide is added to or deleted from therapy.

References

1. Haworth, E., and Burroughs, A.K.: Disopyramide and warfarin interaction, Br. Med. J. **4:**866, 1977.
2. Ryll, C., and others: Warfarin-disopyramide interaction? Drug Intell. Clin. Pharm. **13:**260, 1979.
3. Sybren, C., and Anderson, P.: Evidence that disopyramide does not interact with warfarin, Br. Med. J. **286:**1181, 1983.

Warfarin–Disulfiram

1

Summary: Concurrent administration of warfarin and disulfiram may result in elevated serum warfarin levels and an enhanced hypoprothrombinemic response.[1-3]

Related Drugs: Although interactions have not been documented, disulfiram may interact with other coumarin anticoagulants (dicumarol and phenprocoumon) and the indandione derivatives (anisindione and phenindione) because of pharmacologic similarity. No drugs are related to disulfiram.

Mechanism: Because hydroxylation is the primary pathway in the metabolism of warfarin, it has been proposed that inhibition of this hepatic enzyme system by disulfiram results in increased warfarin levels and an enhanced hypoprothrombinemic effect.[4-8] However, it has been shown that the interaction of disulfiram with the separated enantiomorphs of warfarin is stereoselective. Since disulfiram did not change the plasma concentration of either enantiomorph, the interaction is not the result of disulfiram's effect on the metabolic disposition of warfarin enantiomorphs. Therefore, it is suggested that disulfiram augments the anticoagulant effect of racemic warfarin by directly affecting the hepatic mechanism responsible for the hypoprothrombinemia.[9]

Recommendations: The concurrent use of warfarin and disulfiram should be avoided. When these drugs must be administered concurrently, a decrease of usual dosages of warfarin may be necessary. Patient education and careful monitoring of prothrombin activity are recommended.

References

1. Rothstein, E.: Warfarin effect enhanced by disulfiram, J.A.M.A. **206:**1574, 1968.
2. Rothstein, E.: Warfarin effect enhanced by disulfiram (Antabuse), J.A.M.A. **221:**1052, 1972.
3. O'Reilly, R.A.: Interaction of sodium warfarin and disulfiram in man, Ann. Intern. Med. **78:**73, 1973.
4. Kjeldgaard, N.O.: Inhibition of aldehyde oxidase from the liver by tetraethylthiuramidisulphide (Antabuse), Acta Pharmacol. Toxicol. **5:**397, 1949.
5. Goldstein, M., and others: Inhibition of dopamine-beta-hydroxylase by disulfiram, Life Sci. **3:**763, 1964.
6. Stripp, B., and others: Disulfiram impairment of drug metabolism by rat liver microsomes, J. Pharmacol. Exp. Ther. **170:**347, 1969.
7. Vessel, E.S., and others: Impairment of drug metabolism by disulfiram in man, Clin. Pharmacol. Ther. **12:**785, 1971.
8. O'Reilly, R.A.: The pharmacodynamics of the oral anticoagulant drugs, Prog. Hemost. Thromb. **2:**175, 1974.
9. O'Reilly, R.A.: Dynamic interaction between disulfiram and separated enantiomorphs of racemic warfarin, Clin. Pharmacol. Ther. **29:**332, 1981.

Warfarin–Erythromycin

2

Summary: Two case reports indicate that the hypoprothrombinemic action of warfarin may be increased by concurrent administration of erythromycin.[1,2] One patient developed bruising, hematuria, and an increase in prothrombin time when erythromycin stearate was added to the drug regimen,[1] whereas the other patient who developed similar adverse effects received erythromycin ethyl succinate.[2] Both patients were on multiple drug therapy and the first patient improved and prothrombin time returned to normal on withdrawal of erythromycin.[1] In another case report a patient on erythromycin stearate and warfarin also had increased prothrombin times. When erythromycin was discontinued, his prothrombin time decreased.[3]

Related Drugs: The other erythromycin salts (estolate and lactobionate as well as the free base) may be expected to interact with warfarin in a similar manner. There is no documentation regarding an interaction with the other macrolide antibiotics (oleandomycin and troleandomycin); however, because of similar pharmacologic activity an interaction may be expected to occur.

Documentation is lacking regarding an interaction between erythromycin and the other coumarin anticoagulants (dicumarol and phenprocoumon) and the indandione derivatives (anisindione and phenindione), although a pharmacologically similar interaction may be expected.

Mechanism: The mechanism is unknown. The multiple drug therapy of the 2 patients makes it difficult to determine the exact mechanism of this interaction until further clinical studies are done. However, several mechanisms have been postulated, such as antibiotic induced reduction of vitamin K–producing bacterial flora in the intestine, inhibition of warfarin metabolism, and enhanced responsiveness to warfarin as a result of altered ribosomal function.[2] However, one study suggests that changes in the absorption of vitamin K from bacterial sources during antibiotic therapy are relatively unimportant compared with diet and have little influence on the prothrombin complex synthesis even in anticoagulated patients.[4]

Recommendations: Because of lack of clinical evidence, it is prudent to monitor prothrombin levels in patients receiving erythromycin and warfarin concurrently, with an adjustment of warfarin dosage if necessary.

References

1. Bartle, W.R.: Possible warfarin-erythromycin interaction, Arch. Intern. Med. **140:**985, 1980.
2. Schwartz, J. and others: Interaction between warfarin and erythromycin, South. Med. J. **76:**91, 1983.
3. Husserl, F.E.: Erythromycin-warfarin interaction, Arch. Intern. Med. **143:**1831, 1983.
4. Serlin, M.J., and Breckenridge, A.M.: Drug interaction with warfarin, Drugs **25:**610, 1983.

Warfarin–Ethacrynic Acid

2

Summary: Ethacrynic acid, when added to the drug regimen of a patient previously stabilized on warfarin, resulted in a marked increase in prothrombin time.[1]

Related Drugs: The other coumarin anticoagulants (dicumarol and phenprocoumon) and the indandione derivatives (anisindione and phenindione) may also have the potential for interacting with ethacrynic acid, if the mechanism involves displacement of the anticoagulant from albumin, but there have been no such reports. Other loop diuretics (bumetanide and furosemide) have been reported in some studies[2-4] to have no effect on warfarin.

Mechanism: Ethacrynic acid has been shown to displace warfarin from human albumin in vitro[5] and enhance warfarin–induced hypoprothrombinemia in rats.[6]

Recommendations: Patients stabilized on warfarin should be monitored for prothrombin activity whenever ethacrynic acid is added to or withdrawn from the regimen. Furosemide or bumetanide may be suitable alternatives since some studies[2-4] have reported that warfarin is unaffected by their concurrent use. Since intravenously administered ethacrynic acid has been associated with gastrointestinal bleeding,[7] patients should also be monitored for possible hemorrhage.

References

1. Petrick, R.J., and others: Interactions between warfarin and ethacrynic acid, J.A.M.A. **231:**843, 1975.
2. Nilsson, C.M., and others: The effect of furosemide and bumetanide on warfarin metabolism and anticoagulant response, J. Clin. Pharmacol. **18:**91, 1978.
3. Foged, I., and others: Protein binding of phenprocoumon in the absence and presence of furosemide, Acta Pharmacol. Toxicol. **39:**312, 1976.
4. Nipper, H., and others: The effect of bumetanide on the serum disappearance of warfarin sodium, J. Clin. Pharmacol. **21:**654, 1981.
5. Sellers, E.M., and Koch-Weser, J.: Displacement of warfarin from human albumin by diazoxide and ethacrynic, mefenamic and nalidixic acids, Clin. Pharmacol. Ther. **11:**524, 1970.
6. Buu-Hoi, N.P.: Effects de deux duretiques, 1-hydrochlorothiazide et 1-acide ethacrynique sur la coagulation sanguine chez le rat normal et chez rat recevant des antivitamines K, C. R. Acad. Sci. **265:**2165, 1967.
7. Sloan, D., and others: Intravenously given ethacrynic acid and gastrointestinal bleeding: a finding resulting from comprehensive drug surveillance, J.A.M.A. **209:**1668, 1969.

Warfarin–Ethchlorvynol

Summary: Ethchlorvynol may significantly decrease the anticoagulant activity of warfarin when these drugs are administered concurrently.[1,2]

Related Drugs: Dicumarol has also been shown to interact with ethchlorvynol.[1] The other coumarin anticoagulant (phenprocoumon) and the indandione derivatives (anisindione and phenindione) may interact in a similar manner, if the mechanism involves induction of hepatic enzymes by ethchlorvynol, but there are no reports of such interactions.

Mechanism: The mechanism of the interaction is unknown, although it has been suggested that ethchlorvynol increases warfarin metabolism by induction of hepatic microsomal enzymes.[2] However, another study suggests that ethchlorvynol neither induces nor inhibits the liver enyzmes that metabolize drugs.[3]

Recommendations: Patients stabilized on dicumarol or warfarin should be monitored for prothrombin activity whenever ethchlorvynol is added to or withdrawn from the drug regimen. The substitution of benzodiazepine compounds as an alternative to ethchlorvynol should be considered since benzodiazepines do not significantly affect the activity of oral anticoagulants[4] (see Warfarin-Chlordiazepoxide, p. 159).

References

1. Johansson, S.A.: Apparent resistance to oral anticoagulant therapy and influence of hypnotics on some coagulation factors, Acta Med. Scand. **184:**297, 1968.
2. Cullen, S.I., and Catalano, P.M.: Griseofulvin-warfarin antagonism, J.A.M.A. **199:**582, 1967.
3. Martin, Y.C.: The effect of ethchlorvynol on the drug-metabolizing enzymes of rats and dogs, Biochem. Pharmacol. **16:**2041, 1967.
4. Robinson, D.S., and Amidon, E.L.: Interaction of benzodiazepines with warfarin in man. In Garattini, S., and others, editors: The benzodiazepines. New York, 1973, Raven Press.

Warfarin–Glucagon

1

Summary: The hypoprothrombinemic effect of warfarin was shown to increase in 8 of 9 patients who received glucagon for 2 or more days, with the total dose of glucagon exceeding 50 mg/day. Three of these patients had bleeding episodes. Eleven patients received a total glucagon dose of 30 mg over 1 to 2 days and failed to show an increased anticoagulant response.[1] This interaction appears to be dependent on the glucagon dose administered.

Related Drugs: Documentation is lacking regarding an interaction between glucagon and the other coumarin anticoagulants (dicumarol and phenprocoumon) or the indandione derivatives (anisindione and phenindione), although because of pharmacologic similarity a similar interaction may be expected to occur. No drugs are related to glucagon.

Mechanism: The mechanism of this interaction is unknown. However, it has been suggested that glucagon may potentiate the hypoprothrombinemic action of warfarin by acting synergistically to depress hepatic synthesis of vitamin K–sensitive clotting proteins or by increasing the affinity of warfarin for its receptor site.[1]

Recommendations: It has been suggested that if more than 25 mg of glucagon per day is to be given for longer than 1 to 2 days, the dosage of warfarin should be reduced and prothrombin time should be monitored closely.[1]

Reference

1. Koch-Weser, J.: Potentiation by glucagon of the hypoprothrombinemic action of warfarin, Ann. Intern. Med. **72**:331, 1970.

Warfarin–Glutethimide

1

Summary: Glutethimide stimulates the metabolism of warfarin, thereby reducing its anticoagulant effect. A decrease of approximately 15% in the hypoprothrombinemic response[1] and decreases in the warfarin half-life of approximately 33% to 50% have been reported.[1,2]

Related Drugs: Although results of the concurrent use of the other piperidine derivative (methyprylon) with oral anticoagulants have not been reported, a similar interaction may be expected to occur because methyprylon also induces hepatic enzymes. Pretreatment with glutethimide in rats for 14, 21, and 28 days resulted in a significant decrease in dicumarol plasma levels.[3] The other coumarin anticoagulant (phenprocoumon) as well as the indandione derivatives (anisindione and phenindione) may interact similarly to warfarin if the mechanism involves induction of hepatic enzymes by glutethimide.

Mechanism: Glutethimide is capable of increasing the activity of the hepatic microsomal enzymes involved in drug metabolism.[1,3,4] This effect can appear from several days to 1 week after initiation of glutethimide and may continue for several weeks after its withdrawal.[1] When administered to dogs for 12 days, glutethimide (80 mg/kg/day) reduced the serum warfarin half-life by approximately 50%.[5]

Recommendations: If glutethimide is administered to patients receiving oral anticoagulants, they should be carefully monitored and the dosage adjusted upward as needed. Conversely, the withdrawal of glutethimide from the drug regimen could lead to severe bleeding unless the patient is monitored and the anticoagulant dosage adjusted downward as needed. After the discontinuation of glutethimide, it may take up to 4 weeks for the prothrombin time to return to pretreatment levels.[6] In patients requiring a hypnotic agent, a benzodiazepine can be used as an alternative to glutethimide since these compounds do not significantly affect the prothrombin time achieved with anticoagulants (see Warfarin-Chlordiazepoxide, p. 159).

References

1. MacDonald, M.G., and others: The effects of phenobarbital, chloral betaine, and glutethimide administration on warfarin plasma levels and hypoprothrombinemic responses in man, Clin. Pharmacol. Ther. **10:**80, 1969.
2. Corn, M.: Effect of phenobarbital and glutethimide on biological half-life of warfarin, Thromb. Diath. Haeorrh. **16:**606, 1966.
3. Zaroslinski, J., and others: Effect of subacute administration of methaqualone, phenobarbital and glutethimide on plasma levels of bishydroxycoumarin, Arch. Int. Pharmacodyn. Ther. **195:**185, 1972.
4. Conney, A.H.: Pharmacological implications of microsomal enzyme induction, Pharmacol. Rev. **19:**317, 1967.
5. Hunninghake, D.B., and Azarnoff, D.L.: Drug interactions with warfarin, Arch. Intern. Med. **121:**349, 1968.
6. Udall, J.A.: Clinical implications of warfarin interactions with five sedatives, Am. J. Cardiol. **35:**67, 1975.

Warfarin–Griseofulvin

2

Summary: Griseofulvin (1 g/day orally) may decrease the hypoprothrombinemic effects of warfarin in some,[1] but not all,[2] patients receiving these drugs concurrently.

Related Drugs: The other coumarin anticoagulants (dicumarol and phenprocoumon) and the indandione derivatives (anisindione and phenindione) might be expected to interact with griseofulvin in a manner similar to warfarin because of pharmacologic similarity, although no interactions have been reported.

Mechanism: Griseofulvin may decrease the hypoprothrombinemic effect of warfarin by inducing liver microsomal enzymes[1] and increasing the metabolic biotransformation of warfarin. It also has been suggested that griseofulvin may interfere with the absorption of warfarin.[3]

Recommendations: Although only reported in 2 patients, a decrease in the anticoagulant effect of warfarin should be considered when warfarin and griseofulvin are administered concurrently.[1] Prothrombin times should be determined 2 or 3 times weekly until a stable level is attained. In some patients receiving griseofulvin the warfarin dosage may need to be increased to attain therapeutic anticoagulant effect. On discontinuing griseofulvin, the anticoagulant dosage may need to be reduced and the prothrombin time should be monitored to prevent potential hemorrhage. Many patients may require no adjustment of anticoagulant dosage, as a controlled study of 10 patients indicated.[2]

References

1. Cullen, S.I., and Catalano, P.M.: Griseofulvin-warfarin antagonism, J.A.M.A. **199:**582, 1967.
2. Udall, J.A.: Drug interference with warfarin therapy, Clin. Med. **77:**20, 1970.
3. Koch-Weser, J., and Sellers, E.M.: Drug interactions with coumarin anticoagulants, N. Engl. J. Med. **285:**487, 1971.

Warfarin–Ibuprofen

Summary: Concurrent administration of recommended therapeutic doses of oral ibuprofen (1600 to 2400 mg/day) and warfarin should not significantly affect warfarin's anticoagulant action.[1,2] Ibuprofen may cause some displacement of warfarin from plasma binding sites[3,4] and may individually decrease platelet aggregation and theoretically contribute to prolonged bleeding times.[5,6] However, the clinical significance of these effects is unclear. Because ibuprofen and related drugs may cause gastritis and possibly gastric ulcer as a result of inhibition of prostaglandin synthesis,[5,6] the potential for adverse hemorrhagic reactions to warfarin administration may be increased.

Related Drugs: Fenoprofen in high concentrations displaces warfarin from protein binding in vitro,[7] has caused gastrointestinal bleeding, and may inhibit platelet function. Tolmetin in doses of 800 to 1200 mg/day does not appear to affect the hypoprothrombinemic response to oral anticoagulants.[8,9] Naproxen does not enhance the hypoprothrombinemic effect of warfarin,[10,11] however it does affect platelet function and causes gastric irritation.[12] Piroxicam has been reported to cause a slight increase in the hypoprothrombinemic response to acenocoumarol.*[13] Whether this also occurs with warfarin is not known. Documentation is lacking regarding an interaction between warfarin and meclofenamate, although meclofenamate (as well as piroxicam) may inhibit platelet function and cause gastric irritation as do the other nonsteroidal anti-inflammatory agents. The effects of other nonsteroidal anti-inflammatory agents on warfarin metabolism and clinical symptoms appear to be drug-specific and are discussed in individual monographs. Data describing the effect of ibuprofen and another coumarin anticoagulant (phenprocoumon) have been presented, and a similar lack of effect by ibuprofen was noted.[14-16] There appears to be no documentation regarding an interaction between ibuprofen and the other coumarin anticoagulant (dicumarol) and the indandione derivatives (anisindione and phenindione) although a similar interaction may be expected because of pharmacologic similarity.

Mechanism: Studies in rats have demonstrated that ibuprofen may significantly affect warfarin plasma protein binding and consequently, the biological half-life and total body clearance of warfarin.[4] It may also alter the relationship between warfarin-induced anticoagulant effects and total warfarin plasma concentrations, as a result of displacement of warfarin from binding sites. However, these effects have been noted at ibuprofen plasma concentrations higher than those encountered during routine clinical use of this drug in humans. In in vitro studies using human plasma, the presence of ibuprofen in clinically expected concentrations (30 to 40 μg/ml) will slightly increase the warfarin free fraction.[3]

Ibuprofen may decrease platelet aggregation and prolong bleeding time in a manner similar to that observed with other nonsteroidal anti-inflammatory

*Not available in the U.S.

agents.[5,6] This prolonged bleeding time has not been specifically demonstrated to produce adverse effects.

Recommendations: No specific adjustments of warfarin maintenance dosage need to be made during concurrent administration of ibuprofen and warfarin. However, because initial administration of ibuprofen during maintenance warfarin therapy may displace warfarin from protein binding sites and transiently increase its anticoagulation action, coagulation studies should be carefully monitored at the beginning of ibuprofen therapy. In addition, because of the possibility of increased risk of gastrointestinal bleeding associated with ibuprofen and complicated by warfarin administration, patients should be carefully monitored for this complication.

References

1. Concalves, L: Influence of ibuprofen on hemostasis in patients on anticoagulant therapy, J. Int. Med. Res. **1:**180, 1973.
2. Penner, J.A., and Abbrecht, P.H.: Lack of interaction between ibuprofen and warfarin, Curr. Ther. Res. **18:**862, 1975.
3. Slattery, J.T., and Levy, G.: Effect of ibuprofen on protein binding of warfarin in human serum, J. Pharm. Sci. **66:**1060, 1977.
4. Slattery, J.T., and others: Comparative pharmacokinetics of warfarin induced anticoagulants XXV: warfarin-ibuprofen interaction in rats, J. Pharm. Sci. **66:**943, 1977.
5. Davies, E.F., and Avery, G.S.: Ibuprofen: a review of its pharmacologic properties and therapeutic efficacy in rheumatic disorders, Drugs **2:**416, 1971.
6. Lewis, J.R.: Evaluation of ibuprofen (Motrin), J.A.M.A. **233:**364, 1975.
7. Rubin, A. and others: A profile of the physiological disposition of fenoprofen in man, Pharmacol. Exp. Ther. **183:**449, 1972.
8. Ascione, F.J.: Oral anticoagulants with aspirin alternatives, Drug Ther. **3:**63, 1978.
9. Pullar, T.: Interaction between oral anticoagulant drugs and nonsteroidal anti-inflammatory agents: a review, Scott. Med. J. **28:**42, 1983.
10. Slattery, J.T., and others: Effect of naproxen on the kinetics of elimination and anticoagulant activity of a single dose of warfarin, Clin. Pharmacol. Ther. **25:**51, 1979.
11. Jain, A., and others: Effect of naproxen on the steady-state serum concentration and anticoagulant activity of warfarin, Clin. Pharmacol. Ther. **25:**61, 1979.
12. Cuthbert, M.F.: Adverse reactions to non-steroidal antirheumatic drugs, Curr. Med. Res. Opin. **2:**600, 1974.
13. Dahl, S.L., and Ward, J.R.: Pharmacology, clinical efficacy, and adverse effects of piroxicam, a new nonsteroidal anti-inflammatory agent, Pharmacother. **2:**80, 1982.
14. Thilo, D., and Nyman, D.: A study of the effects of the antirheumatic drug ibuprofen (Brufen) on patients being treated with the oral anticoagulant phenprocoumon (Marcoumar), J. Int. Med. Res. **2:**276, 1974.
15. Boekhout-Mussert, M.J., and Loeliger, E.A.: Influence of ibuprofen on oral anticoagulation with phenprocoumon, J. Int. Med. Res. **2:**274, 1974.
16. Duckert, F.: The absence of effect of the antirheumatic drug ibuprofen on oral anticoagulation with phenprocoumon, Curr. Med. Res. Opin. **3:**556, 1975.

Warfarin–Indomethacin

Summary: Although 2 case reports[1,2] have suggested an interaction between indomethacin and warfarin, other reports[3-8] and 2 double-blind controlled studies[9] indicate that indomethacin does not significantly enhance the hypoprothrombinemic effect of warfarin or other anticoagulants during concurrent administration of both drugs. However, indomethacin can cause gastric ulceration and hemorrhage, and it inhibits platelet aggregation. Therefore, indomethacin should still be used cautiously in patients receiving oral anticoagulants.[10]

Related Drugs: Sulindac, which is structurally and pharmacologically related to indomethacin, has been reported to increase the hypoprothrombinemic effect of warfarin in case reports (see Warfarin-Sulindac, p. 206).[11-13] However, a double-blind placebo controlled study of normal volunteers indicated that sulindac did not significantly affect the hypoprothrombinemic response to warfarin or warfarin plasma concentrations.[13] Other nonsteroidal anti-inflammatory agents are discussed in other monographs. The other coumarin anticoagulants (dicumarol[14] and phenprocoumon[4,15]) and the indandione derivatives (anisindione and phenindione) do not appear to interact with indomethacin since documented evidence is lacking.

Mechanism: Although the mechanism is unknown, the interaction may be related to indomethacin decreasing the albumin binding of warfarin.[5,14]

Recommendations: Although available data indicate that indomethacin generally causes no significant enhancement of oral anticoagulant activity,[3-9] it can cause gastric ulceration and may inhibit platelet aggregation.[16] A similar situation appears to exist with the structurally related drug, sulindac, which may also cause thrombocytopenia.[17] Thus, both drugs should be used cautiously in patients receiving oral anticoagulants. Prothrombin times should be monitored routinely in patients receiving indomethacin and warfarin, and patients should be observed for signs of increased anticoagulant effect, such as easy bruising or bleeding.

References

1. Self, T.H., and others: Drug enhancement of warfarin activity, Lancet **2:**557, 1975.
2. Self, T.H., and others: Possible interaction of indomethacin and warfarin, Drug Intell. Clin. Pharm. **12:**580, 1978.
3. Gaspardy, G., and others: Effect of combination of indomethacin and Syncumar (acenocoumarol) on the prothrombin level in the blood plasma, Z. Rheumaforsch. **26:**332, 1967.
4. Muller, K.H., and Herman, K.: Is a simultaneous treatment with anticoagulants and indomethacin compatible, Med. Welt. **29:**1553, 1966.
5. Solomon, H.M., and others: The displacement of phenylbutazone-C^{14} and warfarin-C^{14} from human albumin by various drugs and fatty acids, Biochem. Pharmacol. **17:**143, 1968.
6. Muller, G., and Zollinger, W.: Indomethacin influence on blood clotting with particular respect to the interference of anticoagulants, Praxis **55:**1462, 1966.
7. Hoffbrand, B.I., and Kininmonth, D.A.: Potentiation of anticoagulants, Br. Med. J. **2:**838, 1967.
8. Wanwimolruk, S., and others: Protein binding of some non-steroidal anti-inflammatory drugs in rheumatoid arthritis, Clin. Pharmacokinet. **7:**85, 1982.

9. Vesell, E.S., and others: Failure of indomethacin and warfarin to interact in normal human volunteers, J. Clin. Pharmacol. **15:**486, 1975.
10. Pullar, T., and Capell, H.A.: Interaction of indomethacin and warfarin, Br. Med. J. **284:**198, 1982.
11. Ross, J.R.Y., and Beeley, L.: Sulindac, prothrombin time, and anticoagulants, Lancet **2:**1075, 1979.
12. Carter, S.A.: Potential effect of sulindac on response of prothrombin time to oral anticoagulants, Lancet **2:**698, 1979.
13. Loftin, J.P., and Vesell, E.S.: Interaction between sulindac and warfarin: different results in normal subjects and in an unusual patient with a potassium-losing renal tubular defect, J. Clin. Pharmacol. **19:**733, 1979.
14. Koch-Weser, J., and Sellers, E.M.: Drug interactions with coumarin anticoagulants, N. Engl. J. Med. **285:**547, 1971.
15. Frost, H., and Hess, H.J.: Concomitant administration of indomethacin and anticoagulants, In Heister, R. and Hofmann, H.F., editors: International Symposium on Inflammation, Friedburg in Breisgau, Germany, May 4-6, 1966. Munich, Germany, 1966, Urban and Schwarzenberg.
16. O'Brien, J.R., and others: A comparison of an effect of different anti-inflammatory drugs on human platelets, J. Clin. Pathol. **23:**522, 1970.
17. Rosenbaum, J.T., and O'Connor, M.: Thrombocytopenia associated with sulindac, Arthritis Rheum. **24:**753, 1981.

Warfarin–Influenza Virus Vaccine

1

Summary: In a case report, a patient stabilized on warfarin for 12 years received an influenza vaccination. Ten days later, the patient developed massive upper gastrointestinal hemorrhage, an increased prothrombin time, and diffuse gastric bleeding without gastritis or ulceration.[1] In another patient stabilized on warfarin, a serious bleeding episode developed after the administration of influenza vaccine.[2]

Related Drugs: Documentation is lacking regarding a similar interaction between influenza virus vaccine and the other coumarin anticoagulants (dicumarol and phenprocoumon) or the indandione derivatives (anisindione and phenindione). However, if the mechanism involves decreased metabolism of warfarin as a result of the influenza vaccine, then these agents may be expected to interact in a similar manner.

Mechanism: Influenza vaccine decreases the metabolism of aminopyrine, a drug that undergoes N-demethylation. Since no other potential cause for the augmented anticoagulation could be identified, it was concluded that the metabolism of warfarin was reduced by the influenza vaccination, suggesting that warfarin is partially eliminated by N-demethylation.[1]

Recommendations: After the administration of influenza vaccine, patients should be closely monitored since a reduction in the warfarin dose may be necessary.

References

1. Kramer, P., and McClain, C.J.: Depression of aminopyrine metabolism by influenza vaccination, N. Engl. J. Med. **305:**1262, 1981.
2. Sumner, H.W., and others: Drug-induced liver disease, Geriatrics **36:**83, 1981.

Warfarin–Isoniazid

3

Summary: In a single case report, a patient on warfarin (10 mg) received concurrent isoniazid (300 mg). When the patient inadvertently doubled the isoniazid dosage (to 600 mg), he developed bleeding gums, hematuria, and an increased prothrombin time. This patient was then stabilized on 7.5 mg of warfarin and 300 mg of isoniazid with no further bleeding episodes.[1] Conversely, in an animal study, no effect on warfarin kinetics or hypoprothrombinemic action could be demonstrated with concurrent isoniazid.[2]

Related Drugs: There are no drugs related to isoniazid. In another animal study using dicumarol, the prothrombin time and blood levels were both increased after administration of isoniazid.[3] There is no documentation of an interaction with the other coumarin anticoagulant (phenprocoumon) or the indandione derivatives (anisindione and phenindione). However, if the mechanism of the interaction is related to inhibition of hepatic metabolism by isoniazid, then a similar interaction may be expected with these agents.

Mechanism: The mechanism is unknown. However, it has been suggested that isoniazid may inhibit the hepatic microsomal enzymes responsible for the metabolism of the anticoagulant.[3] Also, this interaction might be dependent on the dose of isoniazid as indicated by the case report.[1]

Recommendations: Until further clinical studies are available, patients should be monitored for an increased anticoagulant action after isoniazid is added to warfarin therapy. The dosage of warfarin may need to be decreased.

References

1. Rosenthal, A.R., and others: Interaction of isoniazid and warfarin, J.A.M.A. **238:**2177, 1977.
2. Kiblawi, S.S., and others: Influence of isoniazid on the anticoagulant effect of warfarin, Clin. Ther. **2:**235, 1979.
3. Eade, N.R., and others: Potentiation of bishydroxycoumarin in dogs by isoniazid and p-aminosalicylic acid, Am. Rev. Resp. Dis. **103:**792, 1971.

Warfarin–Magnesium Hydroxide

4

Summary: Concurrent administration of warfarin with antacids containing aluminum or magnesium hydroxide, or both, does not produce any significant effect on warfarin pharmacokinetics or pharmacodynamics.

Related Drugs: The interaction of dicumarol with magnesium hydroxide has been shown to differ from that with warfarin. It has been reported that the absorption of dicumarol is slightly enhanced by the simultaneous administration of magnesium hydroxide suspension, although little effect on resulting anticoagulation could be demonstrated.[1] No effect of concurrently administered aluminum hydroxide gel on dicumarol absorption or action was observed. The effects of aluminum or magnesium hydroxide products on the other coumarin anticoagulant (phenprocoumon) or the indandione derivatives (anisindione and phenindione) have not been evaluated.

Mechanism: Theoretical effects of antacid-induced increases in intestinal pH thus decreasing the absorption of warfarin, a weak acid, have been proposed. However, they have not been verified in clinical studies in normal subjects.[1-3]

Recommendations: No special precautions are necessary when antacids containing aluminum or magnesium hydroxide are concurrently administered with warfarin. As a routine practice, however, simultaneous administration of antacids with warfarin should not necessarily be encouraged.

References

1. Ambre, J.J., and Fisher, L.J.: The effect of coadministration of aluminum and magnesium hydroxides on absorption of anticoagulants in man, Clin. Pharmacol. Ther. **14:**231, 1973.
2. Robinson, D.S., and others: Interaction of warfarin and nonsystemic gastrointestinal drugs, Clin. Pharmacol. Ther. **12:**491, 1971.
3. McElnay, J.C., and others: Interaction of warfarin with antacid constituents, Br. Med. J. **2:**1166, 1978.

Warfarin–Mefenamic Acid

3

Summary: Concurrent administration of warfarin and mefenamic acid has been reported to result in an increased hypothrombinemic response of warfarin.[1] Several review articles[2-6] confirm this interaction and refer to it as clinically significant. However, they either cite the previously mentioned studies[7-9] or offer no documentation at all. Hemorrhagic complications resulting from concurrent use of these drugs have not been reported, suggesting that the interaction may be of minor importance.

Related Drugs: Other coumarin anticoagulants (dicumarol and phenprocoumon) and the indandione derivatives (anisindione and phenindione) may undergo a similar interaction with mefenamic acid, if the mechanism involves displacement of the anticoagulant from albumin binding sites, but documentation is lacking. Other nonsteroidal anti-inflammatory agents are discussed in other monographs.

Mechanism: Mefenamic acid is an acidic drug that is highly bound to human albumin.[7] Several in vitro studies have shown that mefenamic acid displaces warfarin from human albumin binding sites[7,10,11] and may double the free warfarin level in vivo.[7,9]

Recommendations: Although the lack of a significant interaction has yet to be firmly established, the possibility of an increase in warfarin anticoagulant effect must be kept in mind if mefenamic acid is used concurrently. Prothrombin levels should be monitored with an appropriate decrease in warfarin dosage if necessary.

References

1. Holmes, E.L.: Pharmacology of the fenamates: IV toleration by normal human subjects, Ann. Phys. Med. **9**(suppl.):36, 1966.
2. Reiss, B.S.: Interactions of drugs and laboratory tests, J. Clin. Pharmacol. **15**:74, 1975.
3. Bernstein, D.L., and Thompson, G.A.: Drug-altered warfarin anticoagulation, Drug Therapy **5**:95, 1975.
4. Koch-Weser, J., and Sellers, S.M.: Binding of drugs to serum albumin, N. Engl. J. Med. **294**:526, 1976.
5. Sher, P.P.: Drug interference with laboratory tests, Drug Therapy **6**:149, 1976.
6. Wormser, H.C.: Pharmacology of anticoagulant, antithrombotic, and thrombolytic drugs, Hosp. Form. **13**:438, 1978.
7. Sellers, E.M., and Koch-Weser, J.: Displacement of warfarin from human albumin by diazoxide and ethacrynic, mefenamic, and nalidixic acids, Clin. Pharmacol. Ther. **11**:524, 1970.
8. Koch-Weser, J., and Sellers, E.M.: Drug interactions with coumarin anticoagulants, N. Engl. J. Med. **285**:487, 1971.
9. Koch-Weser, J., and Sellers, E.M.: Drug interactions with coumarin anticoagulants, N. Engl. J. Med. **285**:547, 1971.
10. Sellers, E.M., and Koch-Weser, J.: Kinetics and clinical importance of displacement of warfarin from albumin by acidic drugs, Ann. N.Y. Acad. Sci. **179**:213, 1971.
11. McElnay, J.C., and D'Arcy, P.F.D.: Displacement of albumin-bound warfarin by anti-inflammatory agent in vitro, J. Pharm. Pharmacol. **32**:709, 1980.

Warfarin–Meprobamate

3

Summary: Meprobamate has been reported to induce the hepatic microsomal enzymes that metabolize warfarin in animals.[1,2] However, a clinically significant interaction between meprobamate and warfarin leading to increased anticoagulant activity has not been consistently reported in humans.[3-5] Meprobamate has been reported to have no consistent effect on the prothrombin time in patients stabilized on warfarin, with the mean prothrombin times remaining unchanged.[4]

Related Drugs: There is a lack of documentation of a similar interaction with the propanediol derivatives, which are structurally related to meprobamate (e.g., carisoprodol, chlorphenesin, methocarbamol [see Appendix]). However, an interaction may be expected if these agents also induce hepatic enzymes.

Interactions between meprobamate and the other coumarin anticoagulants (dicumarol and phenprocoumon) or the indandione derivatives (anisindione and phenindione) have not been documented. However, if the mechanism involves hepatic microsomal enzyme induction, a similar interaction may occur.

Mechanism: Meprobamate is capable of inducing the hepatic microsomal enzymes involved in drug metabolism in animals.[1] Therefore, it may accelerate the metabolic inactivation of drugs metabolized by a similar enzyme system in humans. Meprobamate was reported to have accelerated its own metabolism in humans when given for prolonged periods[1] and reduced the serum warfarin half-life in dogs when administered in a dosage of approximately 100 mg/kg for 12 days.[2]

Recommendations: Since there may be a significant decrease in the prothrombin time only in a rare patient receiving meprobamate and warfarin,[5] it is prudent to routinely check weekly prothrombin times for the first 4 weeks after initiating meprobamate in warfarin stabilized patients. The use of another antianxiety agent such as a benzodiazepine may be a satisfactory alternative.

References

1. Conney, A.H.: Pharmacological implications of microsomal enzyme induction, Pharmacol. Rev. **19:**317, 1967.
2. Hunninghake, D.B., and Azarnoff, D.L.: Drug interactions with warfarin, Arch. Intern. Med. **121:**349, 1968.
3. DeCarolis, P.P., and Gelfand, M.L.: Effect of tranquilizers on prothrombin time response to coumarin, J. Clin. Pharmacol. **19:**557, 1975.
4. Udall, J.A.: Warfarin therapy not influenced by meprobamate: a controlled study in nine men, Curr. Ther. Res. **12:**724, 1970.
5. Gould, L., and others: Prothrombin levels maintained with meprobamate and warfarin, J.A.M.A. **220:**1460, 1972.

Warfarin–Mercaptopurine

Summary: A single case report described a reduction in the anticoagulant effect of warfarin during concurrent treatment with mercaptopurine, a thiopurine antineoplastic agent, in a patient on long-term anticoagulation therapy.[1] The hypoprothrombinemic response was reduced on each of 2 occasions and returned to normal when mercaptopurine was withdrawn.

Related Drugs: There have been no reports of an interaction between mercaptopurine and the other coumarin anticoagulants (dicumarol and phenprocoumon) or the indandione derivatives (anisindione and phenindione), although because of pharmacologic similarity an interaction may be expected.

   The hypoprothrombinemic response of warfarin was not altered when the patient received other antineoplastic agents (e.g., melphalan, busulfan, cyclophosphamide, or cytarabine). However, another case report stated that cyclophosphamide reduced the anticoagulant effect of warfarin.[2] No documentation demonstrates that azathioprine, another thiopurine, interacts with warfarin; however, an interaction may be expected if azathioprine also induces hepatic enzymes.

Mechanism: Although the exact mechanism is unknown, mercaptopurine might induce the hepatic microsomal enzymes responsible for warfarin metabolism, but a decreased gastrointestinal absorption of warfarin cannot be disregarded. Animal experiments have suggested that synthesis or inactivation of the prothrombin complex may also be involved.[3]

Recommendations: On the basis of the limited reports, it appears that mercaptopurine and warfarin may be used concurrently. It would be advisable to monitor the anticoagulant effect of warfarin if mercaptopurine is added to or withdrawn from therapy.

References

1. Spiers, A.S.D., and Mibasham, R.S.: Increased warfarin requirement during mercaptopurine therapy: a new drug interaction, Lancet **2:**221, 1974.
2. Tashima, C.K.: Cyclophosphamide effect on courmarin anticoagulation, South. Med. J. **72:**633, 1979.
3. Martini, A., and Jahnchen, E.: Studies in rats on the mechanism by which 6-mercaptopurine inhibits the anticoagulant effect of warfarin, J. Pharmacol. Exp. Ther. **201:**547, 1977.

Warfarin–Methaqualone*

Summary: Oral administration of methaqualone produces no significant pharmacologic or pharmacokinetic effects on warfarin.[1,2]

Related Drugs: There appears to be no documentation regarding an interaction between methaqualone and the other coumarin anticoagulants (dicumarol and phenprocoumon) and the indandione derivatives (anisindione and phenindione), although no interaction may be expected with methaqualone because of pharmacologic similarity. No drugs are related to methaqualone.

Mechanism: Studies in humans[1] have demonstrated that methaqualone is a relatively weak inducer of microsomal enzymes. Although methaqualone may induce the formation of certain hepatic microsomal enzymes,[3] the resulting effects on warfarin metabolism are clinically insignificant.[1]

Recommendations: Because of the relatively minor effect of methaqualone on warfarin metabolism, no specific precautions are necessary when methaqualone and warfarin are concurrently administered.

References

1. Whitfield, J.B., and others: Changes in plasma gamma-glutamyl transpeptidase associated with alterations in drug metabolism in man, Br. Med. J. **1**:316, 1973.
2. Udall, J.A.: Clinical implications of warfarin interactions with five sedatives, Am. J. Cardiol. **35**:67, 1975.
3. Nayak, R.K., and others: Methaqualone pharmacokinetics after single and multiple dose administration in man, J. Pharmacokinet. Biopharm. **2**:107, 1974.

*Not available in the U.S.

Warfarin–Methyltestosterone

1

Summary: Concurrent administration of warfarin and methyltestosterone in therapeutic doses can significantly increase the hypoprothrombinemic actions of warfarin.[1-11]

Related Drugs: Clinical evidence has demonstrated that oxymetholone[2] and danazol[12,13] increase the hypoprothrombinemic action of warfarin and the other similar anticoagulants dicumarol[1] and phenindione.[4] Although no documentation exists, a similar interaction may be expected with the other coumarin anticoagulant (phenprocoumon) and the other indandione derivative (anisindione) because of pharmacologic similarity.

   Other C-17-alkylated androgen derivatives (e.g., methandriol, fluoxymesterone, stanozolol [see Appendix]) may be expected to interact similarly. Limited data suggest that non-C-17-alkylated androgens (e.g., nandrolone, dromostanolone, testosterone [see Appendix]) may not cause a similar effect.[8]

Mechanism: The precise mechanism for this interaction is unknown. The mode of action may be a possible increase in the rate of decay of clotting proteins or a decrease in the availability of vitamin K to receptor sites in the liver.[1] Another suggestion[1] was the enhancement of the anticoagulant effect by an increase in the affinity of receptor sites for warfarin. Because these drugs are known to produce minor changes in liver function, there is a possibility that the hepatic synthesizing capacity for vitamin K–sensitive clotting factors is altered. None of the C-17-alkylated androgens cause an alteration in the metabolism of warfarin.[1-6]

Recommendations: If methyltestosterone or other C-17-alkylated androgens are administered concomitantly with oral anticoagulants, the anticoagulant dosage may need to be decreased based on changes in prothrombin time.

References

1. Schrogie, J.J., and Solomon, H.M.: The anticoagulant response to bishydroxycoumarin. II. The effect of D-thyroxine, clofibrate, and norethandrolone, Clin. Pharmacol. Ther. **8:**70, 1967.
2. Robinson, B.H.B., and others: Anticoagulant tolerance with oxymetholone, Lancet, **1:**1356, 1971.
3. De Oya, J.C., and others: Decreased anticoagulant tolerance with oxymetholone in paroxysmal nocturnal haemoglobinuria, Lancet **2:**259, 1971.
4. Longridge, K., and others: Decreased anticoagulant tolerance with oxymetholone, Lancet **2:**90, 1971.
5. Pyorala, K., and Kekki, M.: Decreased anticoagulant tolerance during methandrostenolone therapy, Scand. J. Clin. Lab. Invest. **15:**367, 1963.
6. Koch-Weser, J., and Sellers, E.M.: Drug interactions with coumarin anticoagulants, N. Engl. J. Med. **285:**547, 1971.
7. McLaughlin, G.E., and others: Hemarthrosis complicating anticoagulant therapy: report of three cases, J.A.M.A. **196:**1020, 1966.
8. Edwards, M.S., and Curtis, J.R.: Decreased anticoagulant tolerance with oxymetholone, Lancet **2:**221, 1971.
9. Dresdale, F.C., and Hayes, J.C.: Potential dangers in the combined use of methandrostenolone and sodium warfarin, J. Med. Soc. N.S. **64:**609, 1967.

10. Murakami, M., and others: Effects of anabolic steroids on anticoagulant requirements, Jpn. Circ. J. **29:**243, 1965.
11. Husted, S., and others: Increased sensitivity to phenprocoumon during methyltestosterone therapy, Eur. J. Clin. Pharmacol. **10:**209, 1976.
12. Goulbourne, I.A., and Macleod, D.A.: An interaction between danazol and warfarin, Br. J. Obstet. Gynecol. **88:**950, 1981.
13. Small, S., and others: Danazol and oral anticoagulants, Scott. Med. J. **27:**331, 1982.

Warfarin–Metronidazole

1

Summary: In 2 studies metronidazole significantly enhanced the hypoprothrombinemic effect of warfarin.[1,2] The onset of the interaction occurred with 4[1] to 10 days[2] and appeared as excessive bruising of the legs.

Related Drugs: Since the mechanism appears to involve a specific warfarin racemate, it is not known if a similar interaction would occur between metronidazole and the other coumarin anticoagulants (dicumarol and phenprocoumon) and the indandione derivatives (anisindione and phenindione). However, phenprocoumon is a racemic mixture, as is warfarin, and may be expected to interact similarly. No drugs are related to metronidazole.

Mechanism: In 8 normal subjects, metronidazole significantly increased the half-life of racemic and S(−) warfarin.[3] R(+) warfarin, which is metabolized primarily by the reduction of side chains, was unaffected by metronidazole. Therefore, it was suggested that metronidazole inhibits only the enzymatic pathway responsible for the ring hydroxylation of S(−) warfarin. This indicates that the S(−) racemate, which is the more potent, is retained in the body whereas the R(+) racemate is unaffected.[3]

Recommendations: The racemic mixture is the usual commercially available warfarin given, and therefore it can be anticipated that excessive hypoprothrombinemia and bleeding will occur in patients receiving concurrent metronidazole. Appropriate precautions and monitoring of prothrombin levels should be undertaken if these agents are to be used concomitantly, with a decrease in the warfarin dosage if necessary.

References

1. Dean, R.P., and Talbert, R.L.: Bleeding associated with concurrent warfarin and metronidazole therapy, Drug Intell. Clin. Pharm. **14:**864, 1980.
2. Kazmier, F.J.: A significant interaction between metronidazole and warfarin, Mayo Clin. Proc. **51:**782, 1976.
3. O'Reilly, R.A.: The stereoselective interaction of warfarin and metronidazole in man, N. Engl. J. Med. **295:**354, 1976.

Warfarin–Miconazole

2

Summary: Miconazole is capable of increasing the anticoagulant effect of warfarin.[1,2] The interaction is manifested within 12 days and first appears as bruising, prolonged prothrombin times, or both.[1]

Related Drugs: Although no documentation exists, if the mechanism involves displacement from protein binding sites the other coumarin anticoagulants (dicumarol and phenprocoumon) and the indandione derivatives (anisindione and phenindione) may also interact similarly with miconazole. No information is available regarding an interaction between the other antifungal, ketoconazole, and warfarin.

Mechanism: The mechanism is currently not known. It has been suggested that miconazole displaces warfarin from plasma protein binding sites. However, such an interaction generally produces transient increases in the free fraction of warfarin, which disappear within a week.[3] This is not consistent with the time that the manifestations of the interaction appeared.

Recommendations: Patients receiving these agents concomitantly should be monitored for changes in the anticoagulant effect of warfarin. The dosage of warfarin may need to be initially decreased and then gradually increased as co-therapy proceeds.

References

1. Watson, P.G., and others: Drug interaction with coumarin derivative anticoagulants, Br. Med. J. **285:**1045, 1982.
2. Goenen, M., and others: A case of Candida albicans endocarditis 3 years after an aortic valve replacement, J. Cardiovasc. Surg. **18:**391, 1977.
3. Kelly, J.G., and O'Malley, K.: Clinical pharmacokinetics of oral anticoagulants, Clin. Pharmacokinet. **4:**1, 1979.

Warfarin–Nalidixic Acid

Summary: In a single case report, a patient maintained on warfarin developed a purpuric rash on the abdomen and bruising on the left leg and back within 6 days of starting concurrent nalidixic acid. This patient's prothrombin time was also increased but returned to normal after nalidixic acid was withdrawn.[1]

Related Drugs: A similar interaction was reported involving nicoumalone (a warfarin derivative not available in the United States) and nalidixic acid in another case study.[2] Documentation is lacking regarding a similar interaction between warfarin and cinoxacin, a synthetic organic acid urinary antiinfective chemically related to nalidixic acid. Documentation is also lacking of an interaction between nalidixic acid and the other coumarin anticoagulants (dicumarol and phenprocoumon) and the indandione derivatives (anisindione and phenindione). However, if the mechanism involves displacement from protein binding sites, then a similar interaction may be expected.

Mechanism: Nalidixic acid can displace warfarin from its binding sites on plasma albumin in vitro.[2,3] Whether this is also the mechanism in vivo remains to be determined.

Recommendations: It is important to monitor patients for an increased anticoagulant response when these agents are used concurrently. The dosage of warfarin may need to be decreased.

References

1. Hoffbrand, B.I.: Interaction of naldixic acid and warfarin, Br. Med. J. **2:**666, 1974.
2. Sellers, E.M., and Koch-Weser, J.: Displacement of warfarin from human albumin by diazoxide and ethacrynic, mefanamic, and naldixic acids, Clin. Pharmacol. Ther. **11:**524, 1970.
3. Sellers, E.M., and Koch-Weser, J.: Kinetics and clinical importance of displacement of warfarin from albumin by acidic drugs, Ann. N.Y. Acad. Sci. **179:**213, 1971.

Warfarin–Neomycin

3

Summary: Concurrent administration of warfarin and oral neomycin may result in a slight increase in the hypoprothrombinemic effect of warfarin.[1,2] This may be significant only in certain patients who may have a dietary deficiency of vitamin K, are receiving large doses of neomycin, or both.

Related Drugs: Although this has not been documented, the other oral aminoglycosides (kanamycin and paromomycin) may also interact with warfarin.

Documentation is lacking of an interaction between neomycin and the other coumarin anticoagulants (dicumarol and phenprocoumon) and the indandione derivatives (anisindione and phenindione), although a similar interaction may be expected because of pharmacologic similarity.

Mechanism: Neomycin may enhance the hypoprothrombinemic response to oral anticoagulants by decreasing vitamin K availability. This decrease may result from suppression of intestinal bacteria that produce vitamin K or from a decreased absorption of vitamin K.[1,3] However, one study reports that although intestinal bacteria may produce vitamin K_2, there is no convincing evidence that these compounds are available for absorption, and it is possible that the main or only source of vitamin K for humans is the diet.[4] Therefore, neomycin would not produce vitamin K deficiency. A previously mentioned study suggests that changes in the absorption of vitamin K from bacterial sources during antibiotic therapy are relatively unimportant compared with diet and have little influence on prothrombin complex synthesis, even in anticoagulated patients.[1] Impaired renal function with decreased antibiotic clearance may exacerbate the severity and increase the susceptibility to this drug interaction.

Recommendations: The possibility of a clinically significant enhancement of warfarin activity by the oral aminoglycosides may occur only in certain patients who have a dietary deficiency of vitamin K and are receiving large doses of the aminoglycoside. Nevertheless, monitoring of prothrombin activity is warranted when the 2 drugs are administered concurrently, as it is whenever any drug is added to or deleted from the regimen of a patient receiving an oral anticoagulant.

References

1. Udall, J.A.: Human sources and absorption of vitamin K in relation to anticoagulation stability, J.A.M.A. **194:**127, 1965.
2. Udall, J.A.: Drug interference with warfarin therapy, Clin. Med. **77:**20, 1970.
3. Faloon, W.W., and others: Effect of neomycin and kanamycin upon intestinal absorption, Ann. N.Y. Acad. Sci. **132:**879, 1966.
4. Barkham, P., and Shearer, M.J.: Metabolism of vitamin K (phylloquinone) in man, Proc. R. Soc. Med. **70:**93, 1977.

Warfarin–Nortriptyline

4

Summary: Nortriptyline has been reported not to interfere with warfarin half-life, metabolism, or elimination.[1] The possibility of this interaction occurring seems remote.

Related Drugs: The half-life of dicumarol was reported to be significantly increased (up to 3 times longer) in 6 patients after nortriptyline treatment[2]; however, hypoprothrombinemic effects were not reported in this single dose study. A subsequent controlled study of 12 patients demonstrated no significant effect of amitriptyline or nortriptyline on the half-life of dicumarol or warfarin.[1] In another report, concurrent administration of amitriptyline to warfarin-treated patients may have contributed to hemorrhagic complications; however, a causal relationship could not be established from the data presented.[3] In animal studies, a dose-dependent effect of nortriptyline and amitriptyline on anticoagulant response to warfarin was demonstrated in rats, suggesting competitive inhibition of warfarin metabolism.[4] On the other hand, high-dose desipramine had no effect on the hypoprothrombinemic response to dicumarol in guinea pigs.[5]

Because of conflicting reports, it is difficult to determine whether an interaction would occur between the other coumarin anticoagulant (phenprocoumon) or the indandione derivatives (anisindione and phenindione) with nortriptyline, or between warfarin and the other tricyclic antidepressants (e.g., doxepin, protriptyline, trimipramine [see Appendix]) or the tetracyclic antidepressant maprotiline.

Mechanism: It has been suggested that nortriptyline inhibits the metabolism of dicumarol, thereby prolonging its half-life.[2] Another proposed mechanism is that tricyclic antidepressants, by virtue of their anticholinergic properties, slow gastrointestinal motility and allow for greater absorption of dicumarol.[1] It has been shown that warfarin is not affected by nortriptyline.[1]

Recommendations: Avoidance of concurrent administration of these 2 agents does not appear necessary. However, patients should be monitored for changes in anticoagulant response when antidepressants are added to an oral anticoagulant regimen.

References

1. Pond, S.M., and others: Effects of tricyclic antidepressants on drug metabolism, Clin. Pharmacol. Ther. **18:**191, 1975.
2. Vesell, E.S., and others: Impairment of drug metabolism in man by allopurinol and nortriptyline, N. Engl. J. Med. **283:**1484, 1970.
3. Koch-Weser, J.: Hemorrhagic reactions and drug interactions in 500 warfarin treated patients, Clin. Pharmacol. Ther. **14:**139, 1973.
4. Loomis, C.W., and Racz, W.J.: Drug interactions of amitriptyline and nortriptyline with warfarin in the rat, Res. Commun. Chem. Pathol. Pharmacol. **30:**41, 1980.
5. Weiner, M.: Effect of centrally active drugs on the actions of coumarin anticoagulants, Nature **212:**1599, 1966.

Warfarin–Phenobarbital

1

Summary: The anticoagulant effect of warfarin can be decreased by concurrent administration of phenobarbital. It may be necessary to increase the dosage of warfarin to maintain adequate anticoagulation. However, if the phenobarbital is then discontinued, the warfarin dose must be decreased to avoid overanticoagulation.

Related Drugs: Amobarbital,[1-3] aprobarbital,[4] barbital,[5,6] butabarbital,[7] pentobarbital,[8] and secobarbital,[1-3,9-11] also interact with coumarin anticoagulants. All other barbiturates (e.g., mephobarbital, metharbital, tolbutal [see Appendix]) may act in a manner similar to that of phenobarbital, although there are no specific reports.

Although most reports of barbiturate-anticoagulant interactions involved the use of phenobarbital with warfarin[12-15] or dicumarol,[16-20] the other commercially available coumarin anticoagulant (phenprocoumon)[8] is influenced similarly. Similar caution is also indicated with the indandione derivatives (anisindione and phenindione) because of a similar metabolic fate; however, no interactions have been reported.

Mechanisms: Phenobarbital increases the activity of the hepatic microsomal enzymes responsible for metabolizing warfarin,[12,21-26] resulting in a decreased anticoagulant response.[16,19,27-29] Barbiturates have also been shown to increase the synthesis of clotting factors,[8,12,29] and decrease the absorption of dicumarol from the gastrointestinal tract, although the absorption of warfarin is unaffected.[13,16,17]

Recommendations: If possible, it is best to avoid the concurrent use of warfarin and phenobarbital. If phenobarbital therapy is initiated in a patient stabilized on a particular dosage of warfarin, it is likely that an increase in the dosage of warfarin will be required. If phenobarbital is discontinued, the therapy should be monitored closely and the need for reducing the anticoagulant dosage must be carefully considered.

References

1. Breckenridge, A., and Orme, M. Clinical implications of enzyme induction, Ann. N.Y. Acad. Sci. **179:**421, 1971.
2. Robinson, D.S., and Sylwester, D.: Interaction of commonly prescribed drugs and warfarin, Ann. Intern. Med. **72:**853, 1970.
3. Hunninghake, D.B., and Azarnoff, D.L.: Drug interactions with warfarin, Arch. Intern. Med. **121:**349, 1968.
4. Johansson, S.: Apparent resistance to oral anticoagulant therapy and influence of hypnotics on some coagulation factors, Acta Med. Scand. **184:**297, 1968.
5. Welch, R.M., and others: An experimental model in dogs for studying interactions of drugs with bishydroxycoumarin, Clin. Pharmacol. Ther. **10:**817, 1969.
6. Weiner, M.: Effect of centrally active drugs on the action of coumarin anticoagulants, Nature **212:**1599, 1966.
7. Antlitz, A.M., and others: Effect of butabarbital on orally administered anticoagulants, Curr. Ther. Res. **10:**70, 1968.

8. Lucas, O.N.: Study of the interaction of barbiturates and dicumarol and their effect on prothrombin activity, hemorrhage, and sleeping time in rats, Can. J. Physiol. Pharmacol. **45:**905, 1967.

9. Cucinell, S.A., and others: The effect of choral hydrate on bishydroxycoumarin metabolism: a fatal outcome, J.A.M.A. **197:**366, 1967.

10. Breckenridge, A., and others: Dose-dependent enzyme induction, Clin. Pharmacol. Ther.**14:**514, 1973.

11. O'Reilly, R.A., and others: Interaction of secobarbital with warfarin pseudoracemates, Clin. Pharmol. Ther. **28:**187, 1980.

12. Levy, G., and others: Pharmacokinetic analysis of the effect of barbiturate on the anticoagulant action of warfarin in man, Clin. Pharmacol. Ther. **11:**372, 1970.

13. Dayton, P.G., and others: The influence if barbiturates on coumarin plasma levels and prothrombin response, J. Clin. Invest. **40:**1797, 1961.

14. Corn, M.: Effect of phenobarbital and glutethimide on biological half-life of warfarin, Thromb. Diath. Haemorrh. **16:**606, 1966.

15. MacDonald, M.G., and others: The effects of phenobarbital, chloral betaine, and glutethimide administration on warfarin plasma levels and hypoprothrombinemic responses in man, Clin. Pharmacol. Ther. **10:**80, 1969.

16. O'Reilly, R.A., and Aggeler, P.M.: Effect of barbiturates on oral anticoagulants in man, Clin. Res. **17:**153, 1969.

17. Aggeler, P.M., and O'Reilly, R.A.: Effect of heptabarbital on the response to bishydroxycoumarin in man, J. Lab. Clin. Med. **74:**229, 1969.

18. Cucinell, S.A., and others: Drug interactions in man. I. Lowering effect of phenobarbital on plasma levels of bishydroxycoumarin (dicumarol) and diphenylhydantoin (dilantin), Clin. Pharmacol. Ther. **6:**420, 1965.

19. Goss, J.E., and Dickhaus, D.W.: Increased bishydroxycoumarin requirements in patients receiving phenobarbital, N. Engl. J. Med. **273:**1094, 1965.

20. Zaroslinski, J., and others: Effect of subacute administration of methaqualone, phenobarbital and glutethimide on plasma levels of bishydroxycoumarin, Arch. Int. Pharmacodyn. Ther. **195:**185, 1972.

21. Koch-Weser, J., and Seller, E.M.: Drug interactions with coumarin anticoagulants, N. Engl. J. Med. **285:**547, 1971.

22. Yacobi, A,. and others: Comparative pharmacokinetics of coumarin anticoagulants. XLVI. Effect of treatment with phenobarbital on pharmacokinetics of (S)-(--)-warfarin in rats, J. Pharm. Sci. **69:**634, 1980.

23. Yacobi, I., and Levy, G.: Comparative pharmacokinetics of coumarin anticoagulants: relationship between protein binding distribution, and elimination kinetics of warfarin in rats, J. Pharm. Sci. **64:**1660, 1975.

24. Ikeda, M., and others: Stimulatory effect of phenobarbital and insecticides on warfarin metabolism in the rat, J. Pharmacol. Exp. Ther. **162:**338, 1968.

25. Fasco, M.J., and Cashin, M.J.: Effects on induction on R- and S- warfarin and metabolite concentrations in rat plasma, Toxicol. Appl. Pharmacol. **56:**101, 1980.

26. Breckenridge, A., and others: Increased rates of drug oxidation in man. In Morselli, P.L., and Garattini, S. editors: Drug interaction. New York, 1974, Raven Press.

27. Robinson, D.S., and MacDonald, M.G.: The effect of phenobarbital administration on the control of coagulation achieved during warfarin therapy, Hosp. Form. Management **2:**43, 1967.

28. MacDonald, M.G., and Robinson, D.S.: Clinical observations of possible barbiturate interference with anticoagulation, J.A.M.A. **204:**97, 1968.

29. Yacobi, A., and others: Procoagulant effect of phenobarbital in rats, Life Sci. **26:**1379, 1980.

Warfarin–Phenylbutazone

1

Summary: Phenylbutazone enhances the hypoprothrombinemic effect of warfarin and can cause serious bleeding episodes. Concurrent use of these drugs should be avoided.

Related Drugs: The coumarin anticoagulant phenprocoumon[1,2] has also been reported to interact with phenylbutazone or its analogs.

Enhanced anticoagulant effect of the indandione derivative phenindione has been attributed to phenylbutazone in 2 patients.[3] However, in vitro studies using human plasma indicate that phenylbutazone does not alter the plasma binding of phenindione.[4] An interaction between the other coumarin anticoagulant (dicumarol) and the other indandione derivative (anisindione) and phenylbutazone has not been reported, but these anticoagulants would probably interact with phenylbutazone in a similar manner because of pharmacologic similarity.

Oxyphenbutazone, a metabolite of phenylbutazone, also interacts with the coumarin anticoagulants.[5-7]

Mechanism: There are several postulated mechanisms responsible for this interaction. Phenylbutazone increases the plasma concentration of unbound warfarin by displacing warfarin from protein binding sites.[8,9] It also inhibits the metabolism of the $S(-)$ isomer of warfarin, which is the more potent of the 2 isomers.[10-13] Phenylbutazone alone may cause gastric ulceration and decrease platelet aggregation.[14,15]

Recommendations: Concurrent warfarin and phenylbutazone therapy threatens all patients with the potential for serious hemorrhage and should be avoided. If the combination must be used, close observation for bleeding is mandatory, and alternatives to phenylbutazone should be administered whenever possible. These alternatives (e.g., acetaminophen, other nonsteroidal anti-inflammatory agents) are discussed in other monographs.

Excessive hypoprothrombinemia can be treated with phytonadione (vitamin K, 5 to 10 mg) given subcutaneously or orally and by discontinuing the anticoagulant until prothrombin levels return to the proper range. Larger doses of vitamin K do not hasten response and will make the patient resistant to subsequent warfarin therapy. Evidence of hemorrhage requires immediate return of prothrombin levels to normal ranges, attention to blood volume restoration, and other medical and surgical treatments as indicated. If hemorrhage is severe, fresh frozen plasma may be given to supply clotting factors.[16,17]

References

1. Seiler, K., and Duckert, F.: Properties of 3-(1-phenyl-propyl)-4- oxycoumarin (Marcoumar) in plasma when tested in normal cases and under the influence of drugs, Thromb. Diath. Haemorrh. **19:**89, 1968.
2. O'Reilly, R.A.: Phenylbutazone and sulfinpyrazone interaction with oral anticoagulant phenprocoumon, Arch. Intern. Med. **142:**1634, 1982.
3. Kindermann, A.: Vascular allergies due to butalidon and hazards of its combined use with athrombon (phenylindandione), Dermatol. Wochenschr. **143:**172, 1961.

4. Tillement, J.P., and others: Effect of phenylbutazone on the binding of vitamin K antagonists to albumin, Eur. J. Clin. Pharmacol. **6:**15, 1973.

5. Hobbs, C.B., and others: Potentiation of anticoagulant therapy by oxyphenylbutazone: a probable case, Postgrad. Med. J. **41:**563, 1965.

6. Fox, S: Potentiation of anticoagulants caused by pyrazole compounds, J.A.M.A. **188:**320, 1964.

7. Kaplinsky, N., and others: Transient pulmonary infiltrates associated with warfarin, J.A.M.A. **243:**513, 1980.

8. O'Reilly, R.A., and Levy, G.: Pharmacokinetic analysis of potentiating effect of phenylbutazone on anticoagulant action of warfarin in man, J. Pharm. Sci. **59:**1258, 1970.

9. Aggeler, P.M., and others: Potentiations of anticoagulant effect on warfarin by phenylbutazone, N. Engl. J. Med. **276:**496, 1967.

10. O'Reilly, R.A., and others: Stereoselective interaction of phenylbutazone with $^{12}C/^{13}C$ warfarin pseudoracemates in man, J. Clin. Invest. **65:**746, 1980.

11. Lewis, R.J., and others: Warfarin, stereochemical aspects of its metabolism and the interaction with phenylbutazone, J. Clin. Invest. **537:**1607, 1974.

12. O'Reilly, R.A., and Aggeler, P.M.: Phenylbutazone potentiation of anticoagulant effects: fluorometric assay of warfarin, Soc. Exp. Biol. Med. **128:**1080, 1968.

13. Schary, W.L., and others: Warfarin-phenylbutazone interaction in man: a long term multiple dose study, Res. Commun. Chem. Pathol. Pharmacol. **10**(4):663, 1975.

14. Koch-Weser, J., and Seller, E.M.: Drug interaction with coumarin anticoagulants, N. Engl. J. Med. **285:**487,547, 1971.

15. O'Reilly, R.A., and Aggeler, P.M.: Determinants of the response to oral anticoagulant drugs in man, Pharmacol. Rev. **22:**35, 1970.

16. Bruno, J.J., and others: Effects of naproxen on bleeding time and platelet function in normal subjects, Clin. Pharmacol. Ther. **27:**247, 1980.

17. Coon, W.W., and Willis, P.W.: Some aspects of the pharmacology of oral anticoagulants, Clin. Pharmacol. Ther. **11:**312, 1970.

Warfarin–Phytonadione

1

Summary: The interaction between warfarin and phytonadione is well documented. Warfarin inhibits the vitamin K–dependent synthesis of clotting factors II, VII, IX, and X, and vitamin K antagonizes the inhibitory effect of warfarin. In cases of excessive hypoprothrombinemia caused by warfarin, phytonadione (vitamin K_1) is the preparation of choice.[1,2] However, excessive intake of this vitamin, particularly from foods such as green leafy vegetables, should be avoided in patients stabilized on oral anticoagulants.[3,4]

Related Drugs: The coumarin anticoagulants (dicumarol and phenprocoumon) and the indandione derivatives (anisindione and phenindione) all have essentially the same action as warfarin within the body, their differences being mainly quantitative rather than qualitative.[5] Therefore, vitamin K would be expected to affect all of these agents in a similar manner. Available drugs with vitamin K activity include menadione (vitamin K_3), its watersoluble derivative menadione sodium diphosphate, and phytonadione. Even with relatively small doses, these compounds can help normalize decreased prothrombin activity resulting from warfarin therapy.[6] In addition, vitamin K can be found in green leafy vegetables and in many oral nutritional supplements. If these substances are taken in large amounts, the warfarin response may be affected.[3,4,7]

Mechanism: Compounds with vitamin K activity are essential for the hepatic synthesis and release of the clotting factors II, VII, IX, and X, collectively called the vitamin K–dependent clotting factors. Coumarin anticoagulants inhibit the vitamin K–dependent synthesis of these factors. Although the exact mechanism of coumarin interference with the action of vitamin K remains unclear,[8] warfarin may act by inhibiting the cyclic regeneration of vitamin K_1 from its inactive epoxide, which is formed during synthesis of the vitamin K–dependent clotting factors.[9,10] Since the amount of vitamin K available at the site of synthesis influences the rate of clotting factor synthesis,[11] vitamin K intake in excess of normal dietary consumption and intestinal bacterial production may reverse or impair the anticoagulant effect of warfarin.

Recommendations: Cases of warfarin resistance and increased warfarin dosage requirements have been reported in patients receiving a variety of enteral nutrition supplements, apparently resulting from the relatively high vitamin K content in these products.[12-17] Although these products have since been reformulated to provide amounts of vitamin K more consistent with the normal dietary intake of 300 to 500 mg/day,[7,17] 1 report suggests that these products may still affect the warfarin dosage required.[7] As a result, it is prudent to monitor the prothrombin time of patients stabilized on warfarin when large quantities of tube feedings are initiated or stopped. Excessive intake of foods containing vitamin K, such as green leafy vegetables, should also be avoided in patients stabilized on warfarin.[4,18] The effects of vitamin K ingestion may persist for several days after intake is stopped.[6,14] On the other hand, the effectiveness of vitamin K as an antidote for warfarin overdose is well documented,[5,11] with phytonadione reported to be more effective than menadione and the drug of choice for this condition.[1,2]

References

1. Finkel, M.J.: Vitamin K and the vitamin K analogues, Clin. Pharmacol. Ther. **2:**794, 1961.
2. Griminger, P.: Biological activity of the various vitamin K forms, Vitam. Horm. **24:**605, 1966.
3. Anon.: Leafy vegetables in diet alter prothrombin time in patients taking anticoagulant drugs, J.A.M.A. **187:**27 1964.
4. Fletcher, D.C.: Do clotting factors in vitamin K–rich vegetables hinder anticoagulant therapy? J.A.M.A. **237:**1871, 1977.
5. O'Reilly, R.A., and Aggeler, P.M.: Determinants of the response to oral anticoagulant drugs in man, Pharmacol. Rev. **22:**35, 1970.
6. Andersen, P., and Godal, H.C.: Predictable reduction in anticoagulant activity of warfarin by small amounts of vitamin K, Acta Med. Scand. **198:**269, 1975.
7. Parr, M.D., and others: Effect of enteral nutrition on warfarin therapy, Clin. Pharm. **1:**274, 1982.
8. Deykin, D.: Warfarin therapy, N. Engl. J. Med. **283:**691, 801, 1970.
9. Carlisle, D.M., and Blaschke, T.F.: Vitamin K_1, vitamin K_1 epoxide and warfarin interrelationships in the dog, Biochem. Pharmacol. **30:**2931, 1981.
10. Shearer, M.J., and Barkhan, P.: Vitamin K_1 and therapy of massive warfarin overdose, Lancet **1:**266, 1979.
11. Koch-Weser, J., and Sellers, E.M.: Drug interactions with coumarin anticoagulants, N. Engl. J. Med. **285:**487, 1971.
12. Westfall, J.K.: An unrecognized cause of warfarin resistance, Drug Intell. Clin. Pharm. **15:**131, 1981.
13. Zallman, J.A., and others: Liquid nutrition as a cause of warfarin resistance, Am. J. Hosp. Pharm. **38:**1174, 1981.
14. Michaelson, R., and others: Inhibition of the hypoprothrombinemic effect of warfarin (coumadin) by Ensure Plus, a dietary supplement, Clin. Bull. **10:**171, 1980.
15. Lader, E., and others: Warfarin dosage and vitamin K in osmolite, Ann. Intern. Med. **93:**373, 1980.
16. O'Reilly, R.A., and Rytand, D.A.: "Resistance" to warfarin due to unrecognized vitamin K supplementation, N. Engl. J. Med. **303:**160, 1980.
17. Lee, M., and others: Warfarin resistance and vitamin K, Ann. Intern. Med. **94:**140, 1981.
18. Kempin, S.J.: Warfarin resistance caused by broccoli, N. Engl. J. Med. **308:**1229, 1983.

Warfarin–Propoxyphene

Summary: The concurrent use of warfarin and propoxyphene may lead to decreased prothrombin levels and bleeding episodes. One patient showed marked hematuria and another had increased prothrombin times when taking warfarin concomitantly with a propoxyphene-acetaminophen combination.[1] This interaction was also observed in another patient.[2]

Related Drugs: Since the exact mechanism is not known, it is unknown whether an interaction would occur between warfarin and the other narcotic analgesics (e.g., codeine, meperidine, morphine [see Appendix]) although because of pharmacologic similarity an interaction may be expected. Documentation is also lacking regarding a similar interaction between propoxyphene and the other coumarin anticoagulants (dicumarol and phenprocoumon) and the indandione derivatives (anisindione and phenindione). However, based on pharmacologic similarity and the proposed mechanism, the other oral anticoagulants may be expected to interact similarly.

Mechanism: Although the specific drug component that may have caused the interaction was not identified (acetaminophen or propoxyphene), it seems unlikely that the interaction results from acetaminophen since it has been shown in low doses to have little if any effect on warfarin (see Warfarin-Acetaminophen, p. 153). The specific mechanism is not known, but in vitro experiments have shown that this is not a displacement interaction.[3] It has been suggested that propoxyphene, which is metabolized by the same hepatic microsomal enzymes that hydroxylate warfarin, competes for metabolism.[1]

Recommendations: Patients' prothrombin times should be monitored closely during concurrent use of these agents. The dose of warfarin may need to be decreased, the propoxyphene may need to be discontinued, or the use of a noninteracting analgesic may be considered.

References

1. Orme, M., and Breckenridge, A.: Warfarin and distalgesic interaction, Br. Med. J. **1:**200, 1976.
2. Jones, R.V.: Warfarin and distalgesic interaction, Br. Med. J. **1:**460, 1976.
3. Toribara, T.Y., and others: The ultrafilterable calcium of human serum. I. Ultrafiltration methods and normal values, J. Clin. Invest. **36:**738, 1957.

Warfarin–Quinidine

2

Summary: Concurrent administration of quinidine and warfarin may result in enhanced hypoprothrombinemic activity.[1-4] Quinidine can also inhibit the production of the vitamin K–dependent clotting factors and may result in synergism. However, other reports are conflicting. One study found a decreased anticoagulant effect when warfarin was combined with quinidine.[5] In a study involving 8 patients, neither the administration nor the withdrawal of quinidine were associated with major changes in prothrombin complex activity.[6]

Related Drugs: Quinine may also exert a direct hypoprothrombinemic effect.[3] Dicumarol and the indandione anticoagulant phenindione have been reported to enhance hypoprothrombinemic activity when used with quinidine.[2] However, dicumarol has also been reported to decrease the anticoagulant effect when used concurrently with quinidine.[5] Because of pharmacologic similarity, the other coumarin anticoagulant (phenprocoumon) and the other indandione derivative (anisindione) may interact with quinidine, although no documentation exists.

Mechanism: Quinidine alone will probably not cause a problem in all patients, but it may be clinically significant in patients whose synthesis of the vitamin K–dependent clotting factors (factors II, VII, IX, and X) has been depressed by warfarin.[3] The additive effect shown by quinidine is presumed to be related to the ability of the cinchona alkaloids to also depress the vitamin K–dependent clotting factor production by a direct effect on the enzyme system.[1-3] Regarding the decreased anticoagulant effect of warfarin, it has been suggested that in the conversion of atrial fibrillation to regular sinus rhythm by quinidine, regular atrial contractions might contribute to increased cardiac output and increased liver blood flow. Therefore, this may result in an enhanced production of prothrombin and other coagulation factors.[5]

Recommendations: Concurrent administration of warfarin and quinidine is not recommended, but if necessary there should be frequent monitoring of prothrombin times as well as monitoring for clinical symptoms of warfarin overdose. Use of an alternative antiarrhythmic agent that does not interact with the anticoagulant may be preferable to the use of quinidine.

References

1. Pirk, L.A., and Engelberg, R.: Hypoprothrombinemic action of quinidine sulfate, J.A.M.A. **128**:1093, 1945.
2. Jarnum, S.: Cinchophen and acetylsalicylic acid in anticoagulant treatment, Scand. J. Clin. Lab. Invest. **6**:91, 1954.
3. Koch-Weser, J.: Quinidine-induced hypoprothrombinemic hemorrhage in patients on chronic warfarin therapy, Ann. Intern. Med. **68**:511, 1968.
4. Gazzaniga, A.B., and Stewart, D.R.: Possible quinidine-induced hemorrhage in a patient on warfarin sodium, N. Engl. J. Med., **280**:711, 1969.
5. Sylven, C., and Anderson, P.: Evidence that disopyramide does not interact with warfarin, Br. Med. J., **286**:1181, 1983.
6. Jones, F.L.: More on quinidine-induced hypoprothrombinemia (letter), Ann. Intern. Med. **69**:1074, 1968.

Warfarin–Rifampin

1

Summary: The pharmacologic effect of warfarin can be decreased as a result of an enhancement of its metabolism when used concurrently with rifampin during long-term (21 days) therapy.[1-6]

Related Drugs: The coumarin anticoagulant phenprocoumon[7] has also been reported to interact with rifampin. Although not documented, because of pharmacologic similarity the other coumarin anticoagulant (dicumarol) and indandione derivatives (anisindione and phenindione) may have their hypoprothrombinemic effect changed by rifampin as well.

Mechanism: Rifampin is known to be a potent inducer of hepatic microsomes responsible for drug metabolism.[8,9] Warfarin is known to be metabolized in the liver via hydroxylation and to be affected by enzyme inducers such as rifampin.[9,10]

Recommendations: Close monitoring of the prothrombin time is needed when these 2 drugs are used together. Concurrent administration of warfarin and rifampin may require an increase in warfarin dosage to achieve the clinical anticoagulant effect. Conversely, when rifampin is discontinued from the patient's drug regimen, the warfarin dosage may have to be readjusted downward to avoid excessive anticoagulation.

References

1. O'Reilly, R.A.: Interaction of sodium warfarin and rifampin: studies in man, Ann. Intern. Med. **81:**337, 1974.
2. O'Reilly, R.A.: Interaction of chronic daily warfarin therapy and rifampin, Ann. Intern. Med. **83:**506, 1975.
3. Romankiewicz, J.A., and Ehrman, M.: Rifampin and warfarin: a drug interaction, Ann. Intern. Med. **82:**224, 1975.
4. Self, T.H., and Mann, R.B.: Interaction of rifampin and warfarin, Chest **67:**490, 1975.
5. O'Reilly, R.A.: Interaction of rifampin and warfarin in man, Clin. Res. **21:**207, 1973.
6. Felty, P.: Warfarin-rifampin interaction, Med. J. Aust. **62:**60, 1982.
7. Boekhout-Mussert, R.J., and others: Inhibition by rifampin of the anticoagulant effect of phenprocoumon, J.A.M.A. **229:**1903, 1974.
8. Fouts, J.R.: Factors influencing metabolism of drugs by liver microsomes, Ann. N.Y. Acad. Sci. **104:**875, 1964.
9. Conney, A.H.: Pharmacological implications of microsomal enzyme induction, Pharmacol. Rev. **19:**317, 1967.
10. Ikeda, M., and others: Stimulatory effect of phenobarbital and insecticides on warfarin metabolism in the rat, J. Pharmacol. Exp. Ther. **162:**338, 1968.

Warfarin–Spironolactone

3

Summary: Concurrent administration of spironolactone for 7 days decreased the hypoprothrombinemic effect of warfarin approximately 25% as determined by prothrombin time in 9 normal subjects.[1]

Related Drugs: Although documentation is lacking, based on pharmacologic similarity an interaction may be expected between spironolactone and other coumarin anticoagulants (dicumarol and phenprocoumon) and the indandione derivatives (anisindione and phenindione).

Although no documentation exists that other potassium sparing diuretics (amiloride and triamterene) will interact similarly with warfarin, pharmacologically such an interaction may be expected.

Mechanism: It has been suggested but not documented that spironolactone-induced diuresis concentrated the blood clotting factors as a result of plasma water loss and may have led to the reduced anticoagulant effect.[1]

Recommendations: The clinical significance of long-term co-therapy has not been determined. If a reduction in the hypoprothrombinemic effect should occur with long-term administration, suitable dosage adjustments of warfarin may be indicated.

Reference

1. O'Reilly, R.A.: Spironolactone and warfarin interaction, Clin. Pharmacol. Ther. **27:**198, 1980.

Warfarin–Sucralfate

3

Summary: A patient who was administered sucralfate and magaldrate showed a delayed response in prothrombin time elevation after warfarin administration. When sucralfate was withdrawn, the serum warfarin concentration gradually rose as well as the prothrombin time.[1]

Related Drugs: There are no drugs related to sucralfate. No documentation exists concerning whether a similar interaction would occur between sucralfate and the other coumarin anticoagulants (dicumarol and phenprocoumon) and the indandione derivatives (anisindione and phenindione).

Mechanism: The mechanism of this interaction is unknown.

Recommendations: Until further clinical studies are done, the concurrent use of these agents should be approached cautiously. Prothrombin times should be closely monitored as the dosage of warfarin may need adjustment.

Reference

1. Mungall, D., and others: Sucralfate and warfarin, Ann. Intern. Med. **98:**557, 1983.

Warfarin–Sulfamethoxazole

Summary: Concurrent administration of sulfamethoxazole and trimethoprim, as co-trimoxazole, has augmented the hypoprothrombinemic effect of warfarin within 2 to 6 days.[1-9] The interaction usually occurs without any change in serum warfarin concentrations, but some reports indicate that warfarin levels are significantly increased.[10,11]

Related Drugs: The hypoprothrombinemic activity of warfarin has also been increased with concomitant sulfisoxazole.[12] Warfarin half-life was significantly increased in two patients also receiving sulfamethazole.[13] There appear to be no reports of warfarin interacting with the other currently available sulfonamides (e.g., sulfadiazine, sulfasalazine, sulfapyridine [see Appendix]), although based on pharmacologic similarity an interaction may be expected.

One report states that phenindione did not interact with co-trimoxazole.[14] No documentation demonstrates that the other coumarin anticoagulants (dicumarol and phenprocoumon) or the other indandione derivative (anisindione) interact similarly with sulfonamides.

Mechanism: The mechanism, though not clearly established, may involve several processes. It has been shown that sulfonamides displace plasma protein bound warfarin.[15-17] Further, antibiotics may enhance anticoagulant activity by reducing vitamin K synthesis by gut flora.[10] However, one study suggests that changes in absorption of vitamin K from bacterial sources during antibiotic therapy is relatively unimportant as compared to diet and have little influence on prothrombin complex synthesis even in anticoagulated patients.[18] Third, the sulfonamides may inhibit warfarin metabolism stereoselectively.[5]

Recommendations: Patients receiving sulfamethoxazole, either alone or as co-trimoxazole, and warfarin would be expected to display enhanced anticoagulant effects. Appropriate precautions should be taken to prevent excessive hypoprothrombinemia and bleeding.

References

1. O'Reilly, R.A., and Motley, C.H.: Racemic warfarin and trimethoprim-sulfamethoxazole interaction in humans, Ann. Intern. Med. **91:**34, 1979.
2. Greenlaw, C.W.: Drug interaction between co-trimoxazole and warfarin, Am. J. Hosp. Pharm. **36:**1155, 1979.
3. Keys, P.W.: Drug interaction between co-trimoxazole and warfarin, Am. J. Hosp. Pharm. **36:**1155, 1979.
4. Hassall, C., and others: Potentiation of warfarin by co-trimoxazole, Lancet **2:**1155, 1975.
5. O'Reilly, R.A.: Stereoselective interaction of trimethoprim-sulfamethoxazole with the separated enantiomorphs of racemic warfarin in man, N. Engl. J. Med. **302:**33, 1980.
6. Tilstone, W.J., and others: Interaction between warfarin and sulphamethoxazole, Postgrad. Med. J. **53:**388, 1977.
7. Perkash, A.: Experience with the management of deep vein thrombosis in patients with spinal cord injury. II. A critical evaluation of the anticoagulant therapy, Paraplegia **18:**2, 1980.

8. Brooks, B.J., and Mocklin, K.E.: Retropharyngeal hematoma as a complication of warfarin therapy, J. La. State Med. Soc. **133:**156, 1981.
9. Hansen, J.M., and others: Potentiation of warfarin by co-trimoxazole, Br. Med. J. **2:**684, 1975.
10. Serlin, M.J.: Antimicrobial drug interactions with oral anticoagulants, J. Antimicrob. Chemother. **5:**628, 1979.
11. Barnett, D.B., and Hancock, B.W.: Anticoagulant resistance: an unusual case, Br. Med. J. **1:**608, 1975.
12. Sioris, L.J., and others: Potentiation of warfarin anticoagulation by sulfisoxazole, Arch. Intern. Med. **140:**546, 1980.
13. Lumholtz, B., and others: Sulfamethizole-induced inhibition of diphenylhydantoin, tolbutamide, and warfarin metabolism, Clin. Pharmacol. Ther. **17:**731, 1975.
14. De Swiet, J.: Potentiation of warfarin by co-trimoxazole, Br. Med. J. **3:**491, 1975.
15. Deykin, D.: Warfarin therapy, N. Engl. J. Med. **283:**801, 1970.
16. Koch-Weser, J., and Sellers, E.M.: Drug interactions with coumarin anticoagulants, N. Engl. J. Med. **285:**487, 1971.
17. Koch-Wesser, J., and Sellers, E.M.: Drug interactions with coumarin anticoagulants, N. Engl. J. Med. **285:**547, 1971.
18. Serlin, M.J., and Breckenridge, A.M.: Drug interaction with warfarin, Drugs **25:**610, 1983.

Warfarin–Sulfinpyrazone

1

Summary: The anticoagulant effect of warfarin has been enhanced with concomitant sulfinpyrazone therapy, in some cases within 48 hours.[1-10] In many of these episodes associated bleeding was observed. One report indicated a return to warfarin pretreatment levels and a reversal of the original interaction when co-therapy was discontinued.[6]

Related Drugs: In one study sulfinpyrazone did not interact with phenprocoumon.[11] Because the mechanism appears to involve a specific warfarin racemate, it is not known if an interaction would occur between sulfinpyrazone and the other coumarin anticoagulant (dicumarol) or the indandione derivatives (anisindione and phenindione).

Mechanism: Sulfinpyrazone is highly plasma protein bound and has been thought to displace warfarin[12] from such binding sites. Sulfinpyrazone did displace phenprocoumon from plasma proteins in vitro.[13] However, it was found that warfarin was not displaced,[8] but rather that sulfinpyrazone stereoselectively inhibited the metabolism of S(−) warfarin,[14] which is more potent than R(+) warfarin. Warfarin is commercially available as a racemic mixture of both of these forms.

Recommendations: When these agents are used concurrently, prothrombin time should be carefully monitored, with a reduction in warfarin dosage if necessary. Some practitioners have used one-half the usual warfarin dosage,[10,15] but patients will have to be individually monitored.

References

1. Barley, R.R., and Reddy, J.: Potentiation of warfarin action by sulphinpyrazone, Lancet **1:**254, 1978.
2. Gallus, A., and Birkett, D.: Sulphinpyrazone and warfarin: a probable drug interaction, Lancet **1:**609, 1979.
3. Weiss, M.: Potentiation of coumarin effect by sulfinpyrazone, Lancet **1:**609, 1979.
4. Mattingly, D., and others: Hazards of sulphinpyrazone, Br. Med. J. **2:**1786, 1978.
5. Jamel, A., and others: Interaction between sulphinpyrazone and warfarin, Chest, **79:**375, 1981.
6. Nence, G.G., and others: Biphasic sulphinpyrazone-warfarin interaction, Br. Med. J. **282:**1361, 1981.
7. Thompson, P.L., and Serjeant, C.: Potentially serious interaction of warfarin with sulphinpyrazone, Med. J. Aust. **1:**41, 1981.
8. Miners, J.O., and others: Interaction of sulphinpyrazone with warfarin, Eur. J. Clin. Pharmacol. **22:**327, 1982.
9. Daves, J.W., and Johns, L.E.: Possible interaction of sulfinpyrazone with coumarins, N. Engl. J. Med. **299:**955, 1978.
10. Stockley, I.H.: Drug interactions with sulphinpyrazone, Pharmacol. J. **230:**163, 1983.
11. O'Reilly, R.A.: Phenylbutazone and sulfinpyrazone interaction with oral anticoagulant phenprocoumon, Arch. Intern. Med. **142:**1634, 1982.
12. Ahmad, S.: Drug interactions with oral anticoagulants, Postgrad. Med. **67:**47, 1980.
13. Seiler, K., and Duckert, F.: Properties of 3-(1-phenyl-propyl) 4-oxycoumarin (Marcoumar) in the plasma when tested in normal cases and under the influence of drugs, Throm. Diathesis. Haemorrh. **19:**389, 1968.
14. O'Reilly, R.A.: Sulfinpyrazone-racemic warfarin: a stereoselective interaction in man, Clin. Res. **29:**276A, 1981.
15. Tulloch, J.A., and Marr, T.C.K.: Sulphinpyrazone and warfarin after myocardial infarction, Br. Med. J. **2:**133, 1979.

Warfarin–Sulindac

2

Summary: Four patients have shown a marked enhancement of the anticoagulant effect of warfarin within 4 to 7 days after initiating concurrent sulindac therapy.[1-3] However, 7 days of sulindac treatment did not significantly affect warfarin-induced hypoprothrombinemia in normal subjects.[1] Sulindac has also been implicated as a cause of thrombocytopenia.[4]

Related Drugs: No other documentation appears to be available regarding a similar interaction with the other coumarin anticoagulants (dicumarol and phenprocoumon) and indandione derivatives (anisindione and phenindione). The interactions between warfarin and other nonsteroidal anti-inflamatory agents are discussed in separate monographs.

Mechanism: The mechanism of this interaction is not known.

Recommendations: Patients should be monitored for increased anticoagulant activity. Such increased anticoagulant activity may necessitate a reduction in warfarin dosage, which may enable the successful coadministration of these agents.[2]

References

1. Loftin, J.P., and Vesell, E.S.: Interaction between sulindac and warfarin: different results in normal subjects and in an unusual patient with a potassium-losing renal tubular defect, J. Clin. Pharmacol. **19:**733, 1979.
2. Carter, S.A.: Potential effect of sulindac on response of prothrombin-time to oral anticoagulants, Lancet **2:**698, 1979.
3. Ross, J.R.Y., and Beeley, L.: Sulindac, prothrombin time, and anticoagulants, Lancet **2:**1075, 1979.
4. Rosenbaum, J.T., and O'Connor, M.: Thrombocytopenia associated with sulindac, Arthritis Rheum. **24:**753, 1981.

Warfarin–Tetracycline

3

Summary: Although limited clinical evidence is available to substantiate a drug inter-action, broad spectrum antibiotics such as tetracycline that significantly inhibit gut flora with a subsequent decrease in vitamin K production can theoretically potenti-ate the hypoprothrombinemic effect of warfarin. On the other hand, a vitamin K deficient coagulopathy has been described in patients receiving antibiotics alone. This condition has usually occurred in severely ill, hospitalized patients with dietary deficits and renal dysfunction who are receiving parenteral drug therapy. In these patients administration of exogenous vitamin K is warranted if the prothrombin time is prolonged.[1]

Related Drugs: Various tetracycline analogs (e.g., chlortetracycline, minocycline, oxy-tetracycline [see Appendix]) may interact in a similar manner, although no docu-mentation exists. A recent case report has implicated oral doxycycline as the cause of an increased hypothrombinemic effect of warfarin.[2] The other coumarin anticoag-ulants (dicumarol and phenprocoumon) and the indandione derivatives (anisin-dione and phenindione) may interact similarly, because they are related pharmaco-logically, although no documentation exists.

Mechanism: In humans, the mechanism of this interaction has often been considered to be inhibition of bacterial synthesis of vitamin K by the antibiotic, resulting in an increased hypoprothrombinemic effect.[3] However, although broad spectrum antibi-otics such as tetracycline do block the synthesis of vitamin K by intestinal microflora, present evidence suggests that changes in the absorption of vitamin K from bacterial sources during antibiotic therapy are relatively unimportant compared with diet and have little influence on prothrombin complex synthesis even in anticoagulated patients.[3,4]

Impaired renal function with decreased antibiotics clearance may exacerbate the severity and increase the susceptibility to this drug interaction.

Recommendations: The possibility of enhanced warfarin activity caused by tetracy-cline or its analogs appears to be slight when dietary intake of vitamin K is main-tained at adequate levels and antibiotic clearance is normal. Nevertheless, close monitoring of prothrombin activity is warranted when the 2 drugs are administered concurrently or when one or the other is deleted from the regimen.

References

1. Pineo, G.F., and others: Unexpected vitamin K deficiency in hospitalized patients, Can. Med. Assoc. J. **109**:880, 1973.
2. Westfall, L.K., and others: Potentiation of warfarin by tetracycline, Am. J. Hosp. Pharm. **37**:1620, 1980.
3. Koch-Wesser, J., and Sellers, E.M.: Drug interactions with coumarin anticoagulants: part 2. N. Engl. J. Med. **285**:547, 1971.
4. Serlin, M.J., and Breckenridge, A.M.: Drug interaction with warfarin, Drugs **25**:610, 1983.

Warfarin–Thyroid

Summary: Thyroid compounds increase the hypoprothrombinemic effect of warfarin and other anticoagulants.[1-7] Conversely, a reduction in the effects of warfarin may be expected in hypothyroid patients or those who are receiving antithyroid drugs (methimazole and propylthiouracil), although this has not been specifically documented.[8-10]

Related Drugs: A case study reports a patient who developed prolonged prothrombin time and partial thromboplastin time after the concurrent administration of warfarin and levothyroxine. When warfarin was discontinued and vitamin K administered, the prothrombin time returned to normal within 4 to 5 hours.[11] Of the anticoagulants currently commercially available, the coumarin anticoagulant dicumarol[1] and the indandione derivative phenindione[2] have been shown to interact with thyroid derivatives. Although documentation is lacking, the other coumarin anticoagulant (phenprocoumon) and the other indandione derivative (anisindione) may be expected to interact in a similar manner with thyroid compounds. Also, since all thyroid compounds (e.g., liothyronine, liotrix, thyroglobulin [see Appendix]) are similar structurally and therapeutically, all should be expected to interact with anticoagulants in the same manner.

Mechanism: A number of possible explanations for the enhanced effect of thyroid compounds and hyperthyroidism on the anticoagulant response to warfarin have been postulated. Hyperthyroidism may significantly reduce serum albumin, the major plasma protein responsible for warfarin binding,[3] as well as reducing its actual protein binding capacity.[4]

An alternative explanation is that of enhanced degradation of vitamin K–dependent factors, particularly factor II, as a result of hyperthyroidism itself.[5]

Propylthiouracil, in the absence of an oral anticoagulant, has occasionally been reported to cause hypoprothrombinemia and bleeding, which would increase rather than decrease warfarin's effect.[10]

Recommendations: Initiation of thyroid replacement therapy in patients stabilized on warfarin carries a significant risk of excessive prothrombin response and hemorrhage. Conversely, warfarin therapy should be started in small doses in hyperthyroid patients, and any change of thyroid status in patients already receiving warfarin may necessitate a change in warfarin dosage requirement. A decrease in the dosage of warfarin required for anticoagulation usually becomes necessary within 1 to 4 weeks after starting therapy with thyroid compounds.[6] Since hyperthyroidism may increase patient sensitivity to warfarin, individuals undergoing unexplained changes in warfarin requirements should have an evaluation of thyroid function.[7] Patients' prothrombin times should be closely monitored while they are on antithyroid therapy, since a dosage increase or discontinuation of the antithyroid drug may necessitate an increase or a decrease, respectively, of the warfarin dosage.

References

1. Schrogie, J.J., and Solomon, H.M.: The anticoagulant response to bishydroxycoumarin. II. The effect of D-thyroxin, clofibrate and norethandrolone, Clin. Pharmacol. Ther. **8:**70, 1967.
2. Walters, M.B.: The relationship between thyroid function and anticoagulant therapy, Am. J. Cardiol. **11:**112, 1969.
3. Kimberg, D.V.: Liver. In Werner, S.C., and Ingbar, S.H., editors: The thyroid, New York, 1971, Harper & Row, Publishers, p. 569.
4. Feeley, J., and others: Altered plasma protein binding of drugs in thyroid disease, Clin. Pharmacokinet. **6:**298, 1981.
5. Weintraub, M., and others: The effects of dextrothyroxine on the kinetics of prothrombin activity: proposed mechanism of the potentiation of warfarin by D-thyroxine, J. Lab. Clin. Med. **81:**273, 1973.
6. Owens, J.C., and others: Effect of sodium dextrothyroxine in patients receiving anticoagulants, N. Engl. J. Med. **266:**76, 1962.
7. Self, T., and others: Warfarin-induced hypoprothrombinemia: potentiation by hyperthyroidism, J.A.M.A. **231:**1165, 1975.
8. Rice, A.J., and others: Decreased sensitivity to warfarin in patients with myxedema, Am. J. Med. Sci. **262:**211, 1971.
9. Vagenakis, A.G.: Enhancement of warfarin-induced hypoprothrombinemia by thyrotoxicosis, Johns Hopkins Med. J. **131:**69, 1972.
10. Gotta, A.W., and others: Prolonged intraoperative bleeding caused by propylthiouracil-induced hypoprothrombinemia, Anesthesiology **37:**562, 1972.
11. Costigan, D.C., and others: Potentiation of oral anticoagulant effect of L-thyroxine, Clin. Pediatr. **23:**172, 1984.

Warfarin–Vitamin E

2

Summary: The concurrent use of vitamin E may enhance the hypoprothombinemic effect of warfarin. In one report, a patient developed ecchymosis and hematuria after ingestion of up to 1200 IU/day of vitamin E over the previous 2 months while receiving warfarin. A further test study in this patient indicated that concurrent vitamin E (800 IU/day) could reduce the plasma levels of vitamin K-dependent clotting factors II, VII, IX, and X, and demonstrated that bleeding could be induced. The clotting factors returned to baseline levels and bleeding stopped after vitamin E was discontinued.[1]

Related Drugs: One study involving 3 healthy volunteers showed a mild increase in the hypoprothrombinemic response to dicumarol after ingesting 42 IU of vitamin E for 30 days.[2] There is a lack of documentation regarding an interaction between vitamin E and the other coumarin anticoagulant (phenprocoumon) and the indandione derivatives (anisindione and phenindione), although based on pharmacologic similarity an interaction may be expected to occur. No drugs are related to vitamin E.

Mechanism: The mechanism is unknown. Studies in humans report that large doses of vitamin E (2 to 4 mg) alone does not affect the coagulation mechanism;[3] however, animal studies show that vitamin E enhances the anticoagulant response to warfarin.[2] One study reports that the effect of vitamin E is apparent only in the vitamin K–deficient state, and the effect is not clinically obvious with doses of 400 IU/day or less. It has been suggested that vitamin E, an antioxidant, interferes with the oxidation of the reduced form of vitamin K.[4]

Recommendations: Until further clinical studies are reported, the concurrent use of these agents need not be avoided. However, it is prudent to monitor patients during concomitant administration, and a lower dose of warfarin may be necessary. It should be noted that the vitamin E effect can be overcome by either stopping the vitamin E or administering vitamin K.[1,4]

References

1. Corrigan, J.J., and Marcus, F.I.: Coagulopathy associated with vitamin E ingestion, J.A.M.A. **230:**1300, 1974.
2. Schrogie, J.J.: Coagulopathy and fat-soluble vitamins, J.A.M.A. **232:**19, 1975.
3. Hillman, R.W.: Tocopherol excess in man: creatinuria associated with prolonged ingestion, Am. J. Clin. Nutr. **5:**597, 1957.
4. Corrigan, J.J., and Ulfers, L.L.: Effect of vitamin E on prothrombin levels in warfarin-induced vitamin K deficiency, Am. J. Clin. Nutr. **34:**1701, 1981.

CHAPTER FIVE

Anticonvulsant Drug Interactions

TABLE 5. Anticonvulsant Drug Interactions

Drug Interaction	Significance Code	Potential Effects	Recommendations	See Page
Carbamazepine–Charcoal	2	Charcoal, when given 5 minutes after carbamazine, may reduce the drug's absorption by 95%; when given 1 hour later, absorption is reduced by 59%. Carbamazepine elimination may be increased 2-fold after multiple doses of charcoal.	Give charcoal immediately after carbamazeine overdose. For other uses, these agents should be given as far apart as possible.	219
Carbamazepine–Cimetidine	3	Cimetidine may decrease the clearance of carbamazepine, resulting in an increased carbamazepine plasma concentration.	Monitor for alterations in plasma levels of carbamazepine and adjust the dosage if needed.	220
Carbamazepine–Erythromycin	2	Erythromycin increases the plasma concentration of carbamazepine, and these changes occur within 1 day of co-therapy and subside within 2 to 3 days after erythromycin is discontinued.	Monitor plasma levels of carbamazepine and adjust the dosage if needed or select another antibiotic.	221
Carbamazepine–Isoniazid	2	Concurrent use may cause neurologic changes from elevated carbamazepine levels. Isoniazid hepatotoxicity may also be induced by carbamazepine.	Monitor carbamazepine levels. A reduction in the dose has been shown to reverse toxicity.	222
Carbamazepine–Phenobarbital	3	Phenobarbital decreases the half-life and plasma concentration of carbamazepine.	Monitor carefully to ensure maintenance of adequate levels of carbamazepine.	223
Carbamazepine–Propoxyphene	2	Propoxyphene may increase carbamazepine concentrations, and this has been associated with toxic symptoms.	Monitor carbamazepine levels and adjust the dosage as needed. An alternate analgesic may be necessary.	224
Clonazepam–Carbamazepine	3	Carbamazepine decreases the half-life and plasma concentrations of clonazepam. These drugs may have an additive anticonvulsant action, so the effect on seizure control has not been established.	Monitor clonazepam levels when carbamazepine is added or discontinued due to the possibility of subtherapeutic or toxic levels. Seizure control may not be affected.	225
Clonazepam–Primidone	4	Reports are conflicting: increased primidone concentrations, lack of effect, and decreased half-life and increased clearance of clonazepam have all been reported. These agents may have an additive anticonvulsant action, so the effect on seizure control has not been established.	The clinical significance is difficult to predict since clonazepam exhibits therapeutic effects over a wide range of plasma concentrations.	226

TABLE 5. Anticonvulsant Drug Interactions

Drug Interaction	Significance Code	Potential Effects	Recommendations	See Page
Phenobarbital–Valproic Acid	2	Concurrent use increases phenobarbital concentrations, which can lead to sedation and in some cases phenobarbital toxicity. Decreased valproic acid concentration may also occur.	Reduced phenobarbital dosage may be required. The significance of decreased valproic acid levels is not clear.	227
Phenytoin–Acetazolamide	4	One report suggested concurrent use may accelerate the osteomalacia induced by anticonvulsant therapy, although it is impossible to conclude a direct cause and effect relationship.	The concurrent use of these agents need not be avoided. However, monitor for early signs of osteomalacia in patients receiving the combination.	229
Phenytoin–Alcohol, Ethyl	2	Previous reports state that chronic alcohol ingestion increased the metabolism and clearance of phenytoin. However, recently it has been postulated that long-term alcohol ingestion may inhibit phenytoin metabolism, and alcohol withdrawal increases clearance and decreases levels of phenytoin. Small amounts of alcohol may not produce these effets.	Monitor patients closely and adjust the phenytoin dosage as needed, depending on chronic use of alcohol or the discontinuation of alcohol.	230
Phenytoin–Allopurinol	2	One report found increased phenytoin serum concentration with concurrent use of allopurinol, necessitating a phenytoin dosage reduction.	Monitor closely and decrease the phenytoin dosage if phenytoin toxicity appears.	231
Phenytoin–Aspirin	4	Aspirin may transiently increase phenytoin plasma levels. Metabolic phenytoin clearance may also increase, resulting in lower total phenytoin plasma levels.	Since increased effects of phenytoin have not been clinically established, concurrent use of these agents need not be avoided.	232
Phenytoin–Carbamazepine	3	Decreased phenytoin serum concentrations and half-life have been reported, as have decreased carbamazepine concentration.	Monitor levels of both agents when either drug is added to or withdrawn from therapy.	233
Phenytoin–Carmustine, Methotrexate, Vinblastine	3	A high incidence of partial seizures has been reported in a patient maintained on phenytoin after concurrent chemotherapy including these agents.	Monitor phenytoin levels both during and between chemotherapy cycles.	235

TABLE 5. Anticonvulsant Drug Interactions—cont'd

Drug Interaction	Significance Code	Potential Effects	Recommendations	See Page
Phenytoin–Charcoal	2	Phenytoin absorption is reduced as much as 98% when charcoal is given within 5 minutes after phenytoin. When charcoal is given 1 hour after phenytoin, absorption is reduced by 80%.	Activated charcoal can be given for phenytoin overdose. If charcoal is not used in this situation, give these agents as far apart as possible.	236
Phenytoin–Chloramphenicol	2	Concurrent use may inhibit phenytoin metabolism, decrease the serum chloramphenicol concentration, or increase the peak serum chloramphenicol concentration.	Obtain frequent phenytoin levels after chloramphenicol is initiated and monitor chloramphenicol levels as well.	237
Phenytoin–Chlorpheniramine	2	Two cases of phenytoin toxicity have been reported with concurrent chlorpheniramine.	Monitor patients frequently. If toxicity occurs, decrease the phenytoin dosage or withdraw chlorpheniramine.	239
Phenytoin–Chlorpromazine	3	Chlorpromazine may increase the half-life and serum levels of phenytoin. Chlorpromazine itself may also produce seizure activity.	Monitor for an increase in seizure frequency and for phenytoin toxicity. Reduce the phenytoin dosage if needed.	240
Phenytoin–Cimetidine	2	Cimetidine decreases phenytoin clearance and increases serum levels, possibly resulting in toxicity. One case of severe neutropenia has also been reported.	A lower cimetidine dosage or substituting ranitidine, which does not interact with phenytoin, may be indicated.	242
Phenytoin–Cyclosporine	3	Reduced cyclosporine area-under-curve may result from concurrent use; the clinical significance has not been determined.	Monitor for decreased cyclosporine bioavailability and increase the cyclosporine dosage if needed.	243
Phenytoin–Dexamethasone	2	Phenytoin impairs the response to dexamethasone in the dexamethasone suppression test and may decrease the therapeutic response. Half-life and serum levels of phenytoin may also be increased.	A higher dose of dexamethasone may be necessary and/or a decrease in phenytoin dosage may also be required.	244
Phenytoin–Diazepam	3	Conflicting reports on concurrent use include increased and decreased phenytoin concentrations and enhanced diazepam elimination.	Clinical effects cannot be predicted; however, monitor and adjust dosages as needed.	244

TABLE 5. Anticonvulsant Drug Interactions—cont'd

Drug Interaction	Significance Code	Potential Effects	Recommendations	See Page
Phenytoin–Diazoxide	2	Oral diazoxide may reduce phenytoin serum levels to subtherapeutic concentrations. The effects of diazoxide (oral or IV) may also be reduced.	Monitor phenytoin plasma levels and increase the dosage if needed.	248
Phenytoin–Disulfiram	1	Addition of disulfiram to a stable phenytoin regimen decreases the metabolism and increases the levels of phenytoin.	Monitor phenytoin levels frequently especially during initial co-therapy. Decreased phenytoin dosage may be sufficient, but withdrawal of disulfiram may be necessary.	249
Phenytoin–Dopamine	1	Severe hypotension occurred when IV phenytoin was given to 5 patients receiving dopamine infusions to support blood pressure. This interaction was thought to be the cause of death in 2 of the patients.	Phenytoin should be used with greatest caution or not at all in patients receiving dopamine to support blood pressure.	250
Phenytoin–Ethosuximide	3	Increased phenytoin concentrations may result from concurrent use, although some studies report no interaction.	Monitor for increased phenytoin levels.	251
Phenytoin–Folic Acid	2	High doses (≥ 5 mg) of folic acid to patients stabilized on phenytoin has been associated with increased seizure frequency and lowered phenytoin concentrations. Long-term phenytoin therapy may cuase low serum folate concentration, which may result in congenital malformations, though a causal relationship has not been established.	Observe for symptoms of folic acid deficiency. Large doses of folic acid should be avoided. Monitor the serum phenytoin concentration.	252
Phenytoin–Ibuprofen	3	Ibuprofen may increase phenytoin plasma levels and result in phenytoin toxicity.	Phenytoin dosage may need adjusting, especially when ibuprofen is given in a high dosage range.	254
Phenytoin–Imipramine	3	Imipramine may increase phenytoin levels by inhibiting phenytoin's metabolism.	Monitor for signs of phenytoin toxicity and adjust the dose accordingly.	255
Phenytoin–Isoniazid	2	Isoniazid may increase phenytoin serum concentrations in a dose-dependent manner. This interaction may be more significant in slow acetylators.	In slow acetylators, reduce the phenytoin dosage when isoniazid is added to regimen. Monitor other patients periodically.	257

TABLE 5. Anticonvulsant Drug Interactions

Drug Interaction	Significance Code	Potential Effects	Recommendations	See Page
Phenytoin– Levodopa	3	Phenytoin may inhibit therapeutic effects of levodopa. Symptoms of parkinsonism may worsen, and a reduction of levodopa-dependent dyskinesias may occur.	Higher levodopa doses may be required if concomitant use is necessary.	258
Phenytoin– Methylphenidate	3	Methylphenidate may raise serum phenytoin concentrations in some children. This has not been observed in adults.	Monitor phenytoin serum levels and adjust the dose if necessary.	259
Phenytoin– Nitrofurantoin	3	Nitrofurantoin may reduce plasma phenytoin levels, possibly resulting in seizures.	Concurrent use need not be avoided. However, monitor patients and increase the phenytoin dosage if needed.	260
Phenytoin– Oral Contraceptive Agents	3	The concurrent use of these agents may cause breakthrough bleeding, spotting, and in some cases pregnancy. However, a clear-cut cause and effect relationship has not been determined. Concomitant use may lead to loss of seizure control.	An alternate form of contraception may be necessary, as well as an increased phenytoin dosage.	261
Phenytoin– Phenobarbital	3	Phenobarbital may increase, decrease, or cause no change in phenytoin concentrations. Increased phenobarbital levels have also been reported.	Concurrent use need not be avoided, but monitor the serum levels of both drugs frequently.	262
Phenytoin– Phenylbutazone	2	Phenylbutazone may increase the half-life, free fraction, and serum level of phenytoin.	Monitor phenytoin serum levels and adjust the dosage as needed.	264
Phenytoin– Pyridoxine	3	Large doses (200 mg/day) of pyridoxine may cause marked reduction in phenytoin serum levels. The effect of smaller doses is unknown.	Concurrent use need not be avoided. However, monitor patients for loss of seizure control and monitor serum phenytoin concentrations.	266
Phenytoin– Sulfamethizole	2	Concurrent use of these agents may increase phenytoin half-life and serum levels.	Monitor phenytoin and reduce the dosage if necessary.	267
Phenytoin– Trimethoprim	2	Trimethoprim may increase phenytoin elimination half-life and reduce its metabolic clearance rate.	Monitor and decrease the phenytoin dosage if needed.	268

TABLE 5. Anticonvulsant Drug Interactions

Drug Interaction	Significance Code	Potential Effects	Recommendations	See Page
Phenytoin– Valproic Acid	3	Valproic acid decreases total plasma phenytoin concentrations while the percentage of free phenytoin increases, although phenytoin levels usually return to pre–valproic acid levels as combined therapy continues. The overall result depends on the combination of the two opposing trends.	Measurement of free phenytoin levels should provide a better therapeutic guide than total serum concentrations.	269
Primidone– Acetazolamide	3	Acetazolamide decreases or delays absorption of primidone.	Monitor patients for lack of seizure control.	271
Primidone– Phenytoin	2	Phenytoin increases plasma concentrations of phenobarbital (derived from primidone metabolism) but only slightly decreases primidone plasma concentrations.	Concurrent use need not be avoided, but monitor for phenobarbital toxicity and to ensure effective seizure control.	272
Valproic Acid– Aluminum Hydroxide, Magnesium Hydroxide	3	Concurrent use of these agents may significantly increase the bioavailability of valproic acid. Since none of valproic acid's side effects are serum level dependent, whether the increase is clinically significant at steady state levels remains to be determined.	Monitor for valproic acid toxicity.	274
Valproic Acid– Aspirin	3	Aspirin may increase the half-life and serum valproic acid free fraction and decrease the renal clearance. This may result in increased therapeutic and toxic effects.	Monitor for valproic acid toxicity and decrease the dosage as needed.	275
Valproic Acid– Carbamazepine	2	Carbamazepine decreases serum valproic acid concentrations. Valproic acid may increase serum carbamazepine concentrations, but some studies report no effect.	Adjust the valproic acid dosage as needed.	276
Valproic Acid– Clonazepam	3	Concurrent use does not appear to alter concentrations of either drug; however, absence seizures in some patients and drowsiness in others have been reported.	The incidence of this interaction is expected to be low. Clonazepam dosage may need to be reduced if drowsiness occurs.	277

Carbamazepine–Charcoal

2

Summary: In a crossover study involving 5 subjects, 50 g of activated charcoal was administered 5 minutes after carbamazepine ingestion. The absorption of carbamazepine was reduced by more than 95%. When activated charcoal was administered 1 hour after carbamazepine, the absorption was reduced only 59% compared to control values. After multiple doses of activated charcoal, the elimination of carbamazepine was increased about 2-fold.[1]

Related Drugs: There are no drugs related to carbamazepine or charcoal.

Mechanism: Charcoal adsorbs carbamazepine and prevents its absorption. It was suggested that activated charcoal prevents enterohepatic recycling of carbamazepine, thus increasing its elimination.[1]

Recommendations: It has been recommended that activated charcoal be administered as soon as possible after an acute carbamazepine overdose. Also, activated charcoal may significantly increase the elimination of carbamazepine if given in multiple doses thereafter. If charcoal is not used for carbamazepine overdose, it may be advisable to separate the administration of these agents by as much time as possible.

Reference

1. Neuvonen, P.J., and Elonen, E.: Effect of activated charcoal on absorption and elimination of phenobarbitone, carbamazepine, and phenylbutazone in man, Eur. J. Clin. Pharmacol. **17**:51, 1980.

Carbamazepine–Cimetidine

3

Summary: Cimetidine may decrease the clearance of concurrent carbamazepine, resulting in increased carbamazepine plasma concentrations. In a single case study, a patient developed somnolence, nystagmus, dizziness, and involuntary twitching after the concomitant use of these agents. After cimetidine was discontinued, carbamazepine concentrations declined and the patient's clinical condition improved.[1] However, in a study involving 7 epileptic patients receiving carbamazepine, the addition of cimetidine (200 mg 3 times a day and 400 mg at night for 7 days) did not result in any neurologic side effects or other adverse effects. Also, no significant alteration of the steady-state level of carbamazepine or its metabolite was noted.[2]

Related Drugs: There are no drugs related to carbamazepine. If the mechanism involves inhibition of hepatic metabolism by cimetidine, then ranitidine, which is not involved in inhibition of hepatic enzymes, would not be expected to interact with carbamazepine.

Mechanism: It has been suggested that cimetidine inhibits the metabolism of carbamazepine.[1] This has been supported by animal studies.[3]

Recommendations: Because of conflicting results, the concurrent use of carbamazepine and cimetidine need not be avoided but should be approached with caution. If cimetidine is added to or withdrawn from concomitant carbamazepine, the patient should be monitored for alterations in plasma carbamazepine concentrations. The dose of carbamazepine may need to be adjusted accordingly.

References

1. Telerman-Toppet, N., and others: Cimetidine interaction with carbamazepine, Ann. Intern. Med. **94:**544, 1981.
2. Sonne, J., and others: Lack of interaction between cimetidine and carbamazepine, Acta Neurol. Scand. **68:**253, 1983.
3. Grasela, D.M., and others: Inhibition of carbamazepine metabolism by cimetidine, Clin. Pharmacol. Ther. **33:**252, 1983.

Carbamazepine–Erythromycin

2

Summary: Concurrent use of erythromycin and carbamazepine has resulted in increased plasma concentrations of carbamazepine and symptoms of nausea, nystagmus, vomiting, dizziness, ataxia, and drowsiness.[1-5] These changes occur within 1 day of the beginning of co-therapy and subside within 2 to 3 days after erythromycin is discontinued. In one study 4 children developed carbamazepine toxicity after erythromycin administration, and symptoms disappeared when erythromycin was discontinued. Serum carbamazepine levels were measured before, during, and after the toxic episodes, and in all cases carbamazepine levels increased sharply after erythromycin therapy and rapidly decreased on discontinuing erythromycin.[4]

Related Drugs: Concurrent administration of troleandomycin produced a similar interaction in epileptic patients.[2,6] There are no reports that oleandomycin, another macrolide antibiotic, has produced such an interaction with carbamazepine, although one may be expected to occur.

Although the specific erythromycin salt form was not reported,[1-4] it is expected that carbamazepine will interact with erythromycin estolate, stearate, ethylsuccinate, and the free base. There are no drugs related to carbamazepine.

Mechanism: Although the mechanism is undocumented, it may involve erythromycin inhibiting the metabolism of carbamazepine in the liver.[2]

Recommendations: Patients receiving erythromycin and carbamazepine concurrently should be monitored closely, and adjustment of carbamazepine dosage or selection of an alternate antibiotic may be necessary.

References

1. Straughan, J.: Erythromycin-carbamazepine interaction? South Afr. Med. J. **61:**420, 1982.
2. Mesdjian, E., and others: Carbamazepine intoxication due to triacetyloleandomycin administration in epileptic patients, Epilepsia **21:**489, 1980.
3. Wong, Y.Y., and others: Effect of erythromycin on carbamazepine kinetics, Clin. Pharmacol. Ther. **33:**460, 1983.
4. Hedrick, R., and others: Carbamazepine-erythromycin interaction leading to carbamazepine toxicity in four epileptic children, Ther. Drug Monit. **5:**405, 1983.
5. Vajda, F.J.E., and Bladin, P.F.: Carbamazepine-erythromycin-base interaction, Med. J. Aust. **140:**81, 1984.
6. Dravet, C., and others: Interaction between carbamazepine and triacetyleandomycin, Lancet **1:**810, 1977.

Carbamazepine–Isoniazid

2

Summary: Concurrent administration of carbamazepine and isoniazid may lead to neurologic changes (e.g., ataxia, lethargy, nystagmus, somnolence) as a result of elevated carbamazepine levels. Several studies reported toxic carbamazepine levels after initiation of isoniazid,[1-3] and in one study[1] these toxic symptoms disappeared when the carbamazepine dose was lowered. One study also reported isoniazid hepatotoxicity induced by carbamazepine.[3]

Related Drugs: There are no drugs related to carbamazepine or isoniazid.

Mechanism: Isoniazid is known to inhibit the metabolism of several drugs, and it has been postulated that isoniazid inhibits the hepatic metabolism of carbamazepine as well.[1-3] A mechanism for the carbamazepine-induced hepatotoxicity has been suggested. Isoniazid-induced hepatotoxicity has been attributed to the microsomal metabolism of acetylhydrazine, a major metabolite, to a reactive intermediate that results in cell death. Carbamazepine, a known inducing agent, may increase the formation of the reactive intermediate and thereby contribute to the toxicity.[3]

Recommendations: It is important to monitor carbamazepine levels during concurrent use of these agents. It may be necessary to reduce the dose of carbamazepine if toxic symptoms appear since this has been shown to reverse toxicity.

References

1. Valsalan, V.C., and others: Carbamazepine intoxication caused by interaction with isoniazid, Br. Med. J. **285**:261, 1982.
2. Block, S.H.: Carbamazepine-isoniazid interaction, Pediatrics **69**:494, 1982.
3. Wright, J.M., and others: Isoniazid-induced carbamazepine toxicity and vice versa, N. Engl. J. Med. **307**:1325, 1982.

Carbamazepine–Phenobarbital

3

Summary: Phenobarbital has been shown to decrease serum carbamazepine half-life and plasma concentration levels when given in combination.[1-4] Significant changes in carbamazepine serum concentrations were seen within 5 days after the addition of phenobarbital to the therapeutic regimen.[2] Conversely, carbamazepine appears to have no effect on serum phenobarbital levels.[2]

Related Drugs: Carbamazepine has been reported to lower serum concentrations of primidone, but the decrease does not appear to be clinically significant.[5] Other barbiturates (e.g., amobarbital, butabarbital, secobarbital [see Appendix]) may interact in a manner similar to phenobarbital because of pharmacologic similarity, but no documentation substantiates this. There are no drugs related to carbamazepine.

Mechanism: Phenobarbital is thought to induce the metabolism of carbamazepine to its epoxide metabolite.[3] Accordingly, after phenobarbital administration, decreased serum carbamazepine concentrations were accompanied by increased epoxide levels.[6]

Recommendations: Careful monitoring should be done on patients receiving both phenobarbital and carbamazepine to assure that adequate therapeutic carbamazepine concentrations are maintained. The possibility of shortened carbamazepine half-life should be taken into consideration when establishing dosage frequency to prevent large fluctuations in plasma concentration. One report[4] suggests giving carbamazepine 3 times a day—morning, evening, and bedtime—to keep carbamazepine plasma levels fairly constant during the day and to counteract subtherapeutic levels in the morning.

References

1. Christiansen, J., and Dam, M.: Influence of phenobarbital and diphenylhydantoin on plasma carbamazepine levels in patients with epilepsy, Acta Neurol. Scand. **49:**543, 1973.
2. Cereghino, J.J., and others: The efficacy of carbamazepine combinations in epilepsy, Clin. Pharmacol. Ther. **18:**733, 1975.
3. Rane, A., and others: Kinetic of carbamazepine and its 10,11-epoxide metabolite in children, Clin. Pharmacol. Ther. **19:**276, 1976.
4. Dam, M.: Recent advances in the treatment of epilepsy, Acta Neurol. Scand. suppl. **78:**88, 1980.
5. Windorfer, A., and Sauer, W.: Drug interactions during anticonvulsant therapy in childhood: diphenylhydantoin, primidone, phenobarbitone, clonazepam, nitrazepam, carbamazepine and dipropylacetate, Neuropadiatrie **8:**29, 1977.
6. Dam, M., and others: Plasma level and effect of carbamazepine in grand mal and psychomotor epilepsy, Acta Neurol. Scand. suppl. **60:**33, 1975.

Carbamazepine–Propoxyphene

Summary: Concurrent propoxyphene in epileptic patients receiving carbamazepine resulted in a 66% increase in carbamazepine serum concentrations within 1 week.[1] The decreased carbamazepine clearance has been associated with toxic symptoms such as headache, dizziness, ataxia, nausea, and tiredness.[2] During concurrent therapy, propoxyphene serum concentrations declined.[1]

Related Drugs: There are no reports of an interaction between carbamazepine and the other narcotic analgesics (e.g., codeine, meperidine, morphine [see Appendix]). There are no drugs related to carbamazepine.

Mechanism: The mechanism is not clearly understood. It has been proposed that this interaction results from propoxyphene-induced reduction in hepatic carbamazepine metabolism.[3]

Recommendations: Patients receiving both agents should be monitored for increasing carbamazepine serum concentrations, and dosage adjustments made as necessary. Selection of an alternate analgesic may be necessary.

References

1. Hansen, B.S., and others: Influence of dextropropoxyphene on steady-state serum levels and protein binding of three antiepileptic drugs in man, Acta Neurol. Scand. **61:**357, 1980.
2. Dam, M., and Christiansen, J.: Interaction of propoxyphene with carbamazepine, Lancet **2:**509, 1977.
3. Kabacha, R.T., and Ferrante, J.A.: Carbamazepine-propoxyphene interaction, Clin. Pharm. **2:**104, 1983.

Clonazepam–Carbamazepine

3

Summary: Concurrent carbamazepine reduced steady-state plasma clonazepam concentrations 19% to 37% over a 5 to 15 day period.[1] The half-life of clonazepam was significantly reduced from an average of 32 hours to 22 hours. Another report indicated a reduction in carbamazepine half-life by clonazepam in 1 patient.[2] The effect this interaction may have on seizure control is difficult to assess since these agents may have an additive anticonvulsant action during concomitant use.

Related Drugs: The other benzodiazepines that are metabolized by phase I (N-dealkylation or hydroxylation) reactions (e.g., chlordiazepoxide, diazepam, triazolam [see Appendix]) as is clonazepam may be expected to similarly interact with carbamazepine if the mechanism involves induction of hepatic enzymes by carbamazpine; however, documentation is lacking. It has not been determined if the benzodiazepines that are dependent on phase II (glucuronidation) metabolism (lorazepam, oxazepam, and temazepam), would interact in a similar manner. There are no drugs related to carbamazepine.

Mechanism: Carbamazepine is known to induce hepatic enzymes, which is thought to be responsible for the reduced clonazepam levels.[1] D-Glucaric acid excretion, a commonly used index of enzyme induction, was increased when these agents were used concomitantly. No mechanism has been postulated for the manner by which clonazepam reduces carbamazepine's half-life.

Recommendations: The addition or removal of carbamazepine may necessitate serum clonazepam monitoring to avoid subtherapeutic or toxic levels, respectively. There is insufficient evidence to predict the clinical effect of reduced clonazepam levels, since seizure control may not be affected. This may result from possible additive anticonvulsant action when carbamazepine is added to the regimen.

References

1. Lai, A.A., and others: Time course of interaction between carbamazepine and clonazepam in normal man, Clin. Pharmacol. Ther. **24:**316, 1978.
2. Eichelbaum, M., and others: Kinetics and metabolism of carbamazepine during combined antiepileptic drug therapy, Clin. Pharmacol. Ther. **26:**366, 1979.

Clonazepam–Primidone

4

Summary: Reports concerning an interaction between primidone and clonazepam are contradictory. Two reports state that concurrent use of these agents can lead to an increase in primidone serum concentrations.[1,2] Two other studies report a lack of effect between primidone and clonazepam.[3,4] Another report stated that phenobarbital (an active metabolite of primidone) can result in a decrease in the half-life and a corresponding increase in the clearance of clonazepam.[5] The effect this interaction may have on seizure control is difficult to assess since these agents may have an additive anticonvulsant action during concomitant use.

Related Drugs: Nitrazepam* also has been reported to decrease the primidone serum concentration.[2] Clorazepate, another benzodiazepine, given with primidone resulted in personality changes (aggression, irritability, and depression).[6] There is no other documentation of other benzodiazepines (e.g., chlordiazepoxide, flurazepam, triazolam [see Appendix]) interacting with primidone or of other barbiturates (e.g., amobarbital, butabarbital, secobarbital [see Appendix]) interacting with clonazepam. However, because of pharmacologic similarities an interaction may be expected to occur.

Mechanism: The mechanism is unknown. One proposed mechanism is that phenobarbital, a known inducer of microsomal enzymes, can cause an increased clearance of drugs that undergo hepatic elimination. However, this does not account for the increase in primidone levels noted in 2 studies.[1,2]

Recommendations: The clinical significance of this interaction is difficult to assess. Clonazepam has exhibited therapeutic effects over a wide range of plasma concentrations, and the possible change in primidone levels may offset any decreased levels of clonazepam.

References

1. Windorfer, P.: Drug interaction during anticonvulsant therapy, Int. J. Clin. Pharmacol. Biopharm. **14**:236, 1976.
2. Windorfer, A., and Sauer, W.: Drug interactions during anticonvulsant therapy in childhood: diphenylhydantoin, primidone, phenobarbitone, clonazepam, nitrazepam, carbamazepine and dipropylacetate, Neuropadiatrie **8**:29, 1977.
3. Johannessen, S.I., and others: Lack of effect of clonazepam on serum levels of diphenylhydantoin, phenobarbital and carbamazepine, Acta Neurol. Scand. **55**:506, 1977.
4. Huang, C.Y., and others: Clonazepam in the treatment of epilepsy, Med. J. Aust. **2**:5, 1974.
5. Khoo, K.C., and others: Influence of phenytoin and phenobarbital on the disposition of a single oral dose of clonazepam, Clin. Pharmacol. Ther. **28**:368, 1980.
6. Feldman, R.G.: Chlorazepate in temporal lobe epilepsy, J.A.M.A. **236**:2603, 1976.

*Not available in the U.S.

Phenobarbital–Valproic Acid

2

Summary: Coadministration of valproic acid and phenobarbital will result in increased serum phenobarbital concentrations, which can lead to sedation and in some cases phenobarbital intoxication.[1-9] The concurrent use of these agents may result in decreased serum valproic acid concentrations compared with valproic acid alone.[2,8-10]

Related Drugs: Serum primidone concentrations increased in a group of children when valproic acid was added, necessitating a reduction in primidone dosage.[8,11] The primidone dose subsequently was increased since serum levels continued to decline. Reports have stated that valproic acid increases, decreases,[9,10] or does not alter primidone levels in adults,[10,12] whereas primidone causes valproic acid levels to fall.[2,9] Phenobarbital, as a major metabolite of primidone, may slightly increase[5,8] or not change[12] with concurrent valproic acid. Mephobarbital significantly reduced serum valproic acid concentrations in one adult patient.[10] Other barbiturates (e.g., amobarbital, butabarbital, secobarbital [see Appendix]) may be expected to interact in a similar manner because they also induce hepatic enzymes, although this has not been documented. Although there are no drugs related to valproic acid, its sodium salt, sodium valproate, and divalproex sodium, a stable coordination compound containing equal proportions of valproic acid and sodium valproate, would be expected to interact similarly.

Mechanism: Valproic acid alters many pharmacokinetic parameters of phenobarbital. The half-life is prolonged,[13,14] the plasma clearance[13-15] and metabolic clearance[8,14] are decreased, and an increased fraction of the dose is excreted unchanged.[13,14,16] These changes are consistent with an inhibition of phenobarbital metabolism by valproic acid. Valproic acid has no enzyme induction properties of its own but is thought to bind to hepatic microsomes, thus blocking phenobarbital metabolism.[3] Phenobarbital is capable of inducing the metabolism of valproic acid, leading to the increased valproate clearance and subsequent decline in serum concentrations.[2,3,8]

Recommendations: A reduction in phenobarbital dosage will be required when valproic acid is added to therapy. Reductions of 30% to 75% of the phenobarbital dosage have been suggested.[1,3,5,7,17] Because of the long biologic half-life of phenobarbital, 15 to 20 days will be required to reach new steady-state levels.[2,4,8] The significance of decreased valproic acid levels is not clear, but serum valproic acid monitoring may be useful in adjusting valproic acid dosage.

References

1. Bruni, J., and Wilder, B.J.: Valproic acid: review of a new antiepileptic drug, Arch. Neurol. **36:**393, 1979.
2. Gugler, R., and von Unruh, G.E.: Clinical pharmacokinetics of valproic acid, Clin. Pharmacokinet. **5:**67, 1980.
3. Pinder, R.M., and others: Sodium valproate: a review of its pharmacological properties and therapeutic efficacy in epilepsy, Drugs **13:**81, 1977.

4. Simon, D., and Penry, J.K.: Sodium di-n-propylacetate (DPA) in the treatment of epilepsy, Epilepsia **16**:549, 1975.
5. Wilder, B.J., and others: Valproic acid: interaction with other anticonvulsant drugs, Neurology **28**:892, 1978.
6. Schobben, F., and others: Pharmacokinetics of di-n-propylacetate in epileptic patients, Eur. J. Clin. Pharmacol. **8**:97, 1975.
7. Keys, P.A.: Valproic acid: interactions with phenytoin and phenobarbital, Drug Intell. Clin. Pharm. **16**:737, 1982.
8. Levy, R.H., and Koch, K.M.: Drug interactions with valproic acid, Drugs **24**:543, 1982.
9. Perucca, E.: Pharmacokinetic interactions with antiepileptic drugs, Clin. Pharmacokinet. **7**:57, 1982.
10. Sackellares, J.C., and others: Reduction of steady-state valproic levels by other antiepileptic drugs, Epilepsia **22**:437, 1981.
11. Windorfer, A., and others: Elevation of diphenylhydantoin and primidone serum concentration by addition of dipropylacetate, a new anticonvulsant drug, Acta Paediatr. Scand. **64**:771, 1975.
12. Bruni, J.: Valproic acid and plasma levels of primidone and derived phenobarbital, Can. J. Neurol. Sci. **8**:91, 1981.
13. Kapetanovic, I.M., and others: Mechanism of valproate-phenobarbital interaction in epileptic patients, Clin. Pharmacol. Ther. **29**:480, 1981.
14. Patel, I.H., and others: Phenobarbital-valproic acid interaction, Clin. Pharmacol. Ther. **27**:515, 1980.
15. Baruzzi, A., and others: Plasma levels of di-n-propylacetate and clonozepam in epileptic patients, Int. J. Clin. Pharmacol. Biopharm. **15**:403, 1977.
16. Bruni, J., and others: Valproic acid and plasma levels of phenobarbital, Neurology **30**:94, 1980.
17. Gram, L. and others: Valproate sodium: a controlled clinical trial including monitoring of drug levels, Epilepsia **18**:141, 1977.

Phenytoin–Acetazolamide

4

Summary: One report has suggested that concurrent use of phenytoin and acetazolamide can accelerate the osteomalacia induced by anticonvulsant therapy.[1] However, the patients in these reports were taking other drugs, making it impossible to conclude a direct cause and effect relationship.

Related Drugs: An interaction between acetazolamide and other hydantoin anticonvulsants (ethotoin and mephenytoin) has not been documented. Also, no reports are available regarding an interaction between hydantoins and the other carbonic anhydrase inhibitors (dichlorphenamide, ethoxzolamide, and methazolamide).

Mechanism: Several pharmacologic actions of acetazolamide could accelerate the development of osteomalacia.[2] Acetazolamide enhances urinary calcium excretion, urinary phosphate excretion, and causes systemic acidosis, which retards the conversion of 25-hydroxycholecalciferol to 1,25-dihydroxycholecalciferol. The exact manner in which one or more of these actions leads to osteomalacia is not clearly understood.

Recommendations: The concurrent use of these agents need not be avoided. However, special attention to the early detection of osteomalacia should be given to patients receiving this combination of agents.

References

1. Mallette, L.E.: Anticonvulsants, acetazolamide and osteomalacia, N. Engl. J. Med. **293:**668, 1975.
2. Mallette, L.E.: Acetazolamide-accelerated anticonvulsant osteomalacia, Arch. Intern. Med. **137:**1013, 1977.

Phenytoin–Alcohol, Ethyl

2

Summary: The effect of chronic alcohol ingestion on phenytoin metabolism appears complex. Previously it had been reported that long-term alcohol ingestion may increase the metabolism and thereby increase the clearance of phenytoin.[1-3] However, recently it has been postulated that long-term alcohol ingestion can inhibit phenytoin metabolism causing levels of phenytoin to increase and that during alcohol withdrawal phenytoin clearance seems to increase, thereby resulting in a decrease in serum phenytoin levels.[4] The use of small amounts of alcohol does not produce these effects.[3]

Related Drugs: The other hydantoin derivatives (ethotoin and mephenytoin) may interact with alcohol in a similar manner because they are pharacologically related, but documentation is lacking.

Mechanism: Although the mechanism is unclear, a recent hypothesis states that increased phenytoin clearance during alcohol withdrawal results from the increased metabolic rate of the drug secondary to enzyme induction by alcohol, which becomes unmasked on cessation of alcohol consumption.[4]

Recommendations: If phenytoin is administered to patients who ingest alcohol chronically, the serum phenytoin level should be monitored to assure that they are in the therapeutic range. Conversely, in alcoholic patients whose phenytoin dose has been titrated to therapeutic levels, a decrease in serum phenytoin levels may occur when alcohol is discontinued, necessitating an increase in the phenytoin dose.

References

1. Birkett, D.S., and others: Multiple drug interaction with phenytoin, Med. J. Aust. **2:**467, 1977.
2. Kater, R.M.H., and others: Increased rate of clearance of drugs from the circulation of alcoholics, Am. J. Med. Sci. **258:**35, 1969.
3. Schmidt, D.: Effect of ethanol intake on phenytoin metabolism in volunteers, Experimentia **31:**1313, 1975.
4. Sandor, D.S., and others: Effect of short and long-term alcohol use on phenytoin kinetics in chronic alcoholics, Clin. Pharmacol. Ther. **30:**390, 1981.

Phenytoin–Allopurinol

2

Summary: In one study involving a child with Lesch-Nyhan syndrome who was taking multiple anticonvulsant agents (phenytoin, phenobarbital, clonzaepam, and valproic acid), concurrent allopurinol resulted in an increase in phenytoin serum concentration. This necessitated a reduction in the dose of phenytoin by 22.8% and 35.4% when allopurinol was given in 150 and 200 mg/day doses, respectively. The other anticonvulsant drugs may have affected this interaction, but they were held constant throughout the study peroid.[1]

Related Drugs: Documentation is lacking regarding an interaction between allopurinol and the other hydantoin anticonvulsants (ethotoin and mephenytoin), although because of pharmacologic similarity, a similar interaction may be expected to occur. There are no drugs related to allopurinol.

Mechanism: Allopurinol appears to be an inhibitor not only for xanthine oxidase but also for mixed-function oxidase systems. Since phenytoin is almost totally metabolized by the hepatic microsomal mono-oxygenase system, the results of this study suggest that allopurinol inhibits the oxidative metabolism of phenytoin in the liver, resulting in the increase in serum concentration.[1]

Recommendations: Close patient attention is necessary during the concurrent administration of phenytoin and allopurinol. If phenytoin toxicity appears, the dosage may need to be adjusted downward.

Reference

1. Yokochi, K., and others: Phenytoin-allopurinol interaction: Michaelis-Menten kinetic parameters of phenytoin with and without allopurinol in a child with Lesch-Nyhan syndrome, Ther. Drug Monit. **4:**353, 1982.

Phenytoin–Aspirin

4

Summary: Several studies have indicated that aspirin and other salicylates may cause a transient increase in phenytoin plasma levels.[1-8] However, whether the effects of phenytoin also increase has never been clinically established, and further studies are needed to determine the significance of this interaction.

Related Drugs: There is no documentation regarding a similar interaction between the other hydantoin anticonvulsants (ethotoin and mephenytoin) and the other salicylates (e.g., choline salicylate, salicylamide, sodium salicylate [see Appendix]). However, because of pharmacologic similarity an interaction may be expected.

Mechanism: In vitro and in vivo studies have demonstrated that salicylates displace phenytoin from plasma protein binding sites.[1-8] However, it has been suggested that the metabolic clearance of phenytoin increases as well, which may result in a lower total phenytoin plasma level.

Recommendations: Although the patient's phenytoin levels (free and total) should be monitored closely during concurrent salicylate therapy, these agents need not be avoided.

References

1. Lunde, P.K.M., and others: Plasma protein binding of diphenylhydantoin in man: interaction with other drugs and the effect of temperature and plasma dilution, Clin. Pharmacol. Ther. **11:**846, 1970.
2. Odar-Cederlof, I., and Borga, O.: Impaired plasma protein binding of phenytoin in uremia and displacement effect of salicylic acid, Clin. Pharmacol. Ther. **20:**36, 1976.
3. Ehrnebo, M., and Odar-Cederof, I.: Distribution of phenobarbital and diphenylhydantoin between plasma and cells in blood: effect of salicylic acid temperature and total drug concentration, Eur.J. Clin. Pharmacol. **11:**37, 1977.
4. Fraser, D.G., and others: Displacement of phenytoin from plasma binding sites by salicylate, Clin. Pharmacol. Ther. **27:**165, 1980.
5. Paxton, J.W.: Effects of aspirin on salivary and serum phenytoin kinetics in healthy subjects, Clin. Pharmacol. Ther. **27:**170, 1980.
6. Leonard, R.F., and others: Phenytoin-salicylate interaction, Clin. Pharmacol. Ther. **29:**56, 1981.
7. Olanow, C.W., and others: The effects of salicylate on the pharmacokinetics of phenytoin, Neurology **31:**341, 1981.
8. Inoui, F., and Walsh, R.J.: Folate supplements and phenytoin salicylate interaction, Neurology **33:**115, 1983.

Phenytoin–Carbamazepine

3

Summary: A dual interaction has been observed when carbamazepine and phenytoin are administered simultaneously. In several studies, phenytoin's half-life and/or serum concentrations were found to decrease when carbamazepine therapy was instituted.[1-5] In other studies, carbamazepine serum concentrations were reduced by concurrent phenytoin.[3,5-11] The phenytoin half-life decreased from 10.6 to 6.4 hours after at least 9 days of combined therapy,[1] while significant changes in the serum carbamazepine concentrations were detected in 24 hours.[8]

Related Drugs: Ethosuximide plasma concentrations were similarly reduced by carbamazepine.[5] In one study involving 6 healthy subjects, the steady-state levels of ethosuximide decreased by 17% and its clearance increased by 20% with concomitant carbamazepine. The half-life of ethosuximide was reduced approximately 20%.[12] Ethosuximide and phensuximide have been reported to induce the metabolism of carbamazepine, resulting in decreased carbamazepine levels.[13] There is no documentation regarding an interaction between carbamazepine and other hydantoin anticonvulsants (ethotoin and mephenytoin), although based on the mechanism of the interaction, a similar effect may be expected. There are no drugs related to carbamazepine.

Mechanism: Induction of hepatic metabolism is the proposed mechanism for both cases of this interaction.[1,6-9,14] Carbamazepine serum concentrations decrease while the epoxide metabolite concentrations increase when phenytoin is administered concurrently.[7,15] However, 1 study found a decrease in carbamazepine levels, but unaltered epoxide levels, suggesting that phenytoin may increase the drug's biotransformation to a metabolite other than the epoxide.[14] An interaction at the absorption site might be an explanation for the rapid effect seen on carbamazepine serum concentration when phenytoin is given acutely.[8]

Recommendations: If patients are to be treated with both phenytoin and carbamazepine, serum concentrations should be monitored after combination therapy is instituted to assure that adequate blood levels of both agents are maintained. To maintain adequate seizure control, patients previously stabilized on either agent should be monitored closely when the second drug is added. The shortened half-lives should be taken into consideration when determining dosage frequency to prevent great fluctuation in plasma levels.

References

1. Hansen, J.M., and others: Carbamazepine-induced acceleration of diphenylhydantoin and warfarin metabolism in man, Clin. Pharmacol. Ther. **12:**539, 1971.
2. Windorfer, P.: Drug interaction during anticonvulsant therapy, Int. J. Clin. Pharmacol. Biopharm. **14:**236, 1976.
3. Hooper, W.D., and others: Preliminary observations on the clinical pharmacology of carbamazepine ('Tegretol'), Proc. Aust. Assoc. Neurol. **11:**189, 1974.
4. Windorfer, A., and Sauer, W.: Drug interactions during anticonvulsant therapy in childhood: diphenyl-

hydantoin, primidone, phenobarbitone, clonazepam, nitrazepam, carbamazepine and dipropyl-acetate, Neuropadiatrie **8:**29, 1977.

5. Dam, M.: Recent advances in the treatment of epilepsy, Acta Neurol. Scand. suppl. **78:**88, 1980.
6. Christiansen, J., and Dam, M.: Influence of phenobarbital and diphenylhydantoin on plasma carba-mazepine levels in patients with epilepsy, Acta Neurol. Scand. **49:**543, 1973.
7. Eichelbaum, M., and others: Kinetics and metabolism of carbamazepine during combined antiepi-leptic drug therapy, Clin. Pharmacol. Ther. **26:**366, 1979.
8. Perucca, E., and Richens, A.: Reversal by phenytoin of carbamazepine-induced water intoxication: a pharmacokinetic interaction, J. Neurol. Neurosurg. Psychiatry **43:**540, 1980.
9. Lander, C.M., and others: Interactions between anticonvulsants, Proc. Aust. Assoc. Neurol. **12:**111, 1975.
10. Lander, C.M., and others: Factors influencing plasma carbamazepine concentrations, Clin. Exp. Neurol. **14:**184, 1977.
11. Cereghino, J.J., and others: The efficacy of carbamazepine combinations in epilepsy, Clin. Pharmacol. Ther. **18:**733, 1975.
12. Warren, J.W., and others: Kinetics of a carbamazepine-ethosuximide interaction, Clin. Pharmacol. Ther. **28:**646, 1980.
13. Sillampaa, M.: Carbamazepine: pharmacology and clinical uses, Acta Neurol. Scand. suppl. **64:**1, 1981.
14. McKauge, L., and others: Factors influencing simultaneous concentrations of carbamazepine and its epoxide in plasma, Ther. Drug Monit. **3:**63, 1981.
15. Dam, M., and others: Plasma level and effect of carbamazepine in grand mal and psychomotor epilepsy, Acta Neurol. Scand. suppl. **60:**33, 1975.

Phenytoin–Carmustine, Methotrexate, Vinblastine

3

Summary: A high incidence of partial seizures was noted in a patient maintained on phenytoin and phenobarbital after concurrent chemotherapy of carmustine, methotrexate, and vinblastine. Plasma levels of phenytoin fell by almost 4 μg/ml in a 24 hour period after initiation of chemotherapy. Phenytoin concentrations returned to the previous level 2 weeks after the completion of chemotherapy.[1]

Related Drugs: In a study involving an epileptic patient maintained on phenytoin, the dosage had to be doubled to maintain therapeutic levels after initiation of combination chemotherapy with bleomycin, cisplatin, and vinblastine. The phenytoin dosage had to be reduced between chemotherapy cycles to prevent toxicity.[2] There is a lack of documentation regarding a similar interaction with the other hydantoin anticonvulsants (ethotoin and mephenytoin). However, because of pharmacologic similarity an interaction may be expected.

Mechanism: Although the mechanism is unknown, it may involve decreased gastrointestinal absorption of phenytoin resulting from the antineoplastic agents.

Recommendations: It is difficult to determine whether this interaction was caused by the combination of the antineoplastic agents or if an individual agent is responsible. In any case, it is important to monitor phenytoin levels both during and between chemotherapy cycles and adjust the dosage if necessary.

References

1. Bollini, P., and others: Decreased phenytoin level during antineoplastic therapy: a case report, Epilepsia **24:**75, 1983.
2. Fincham, R.W., and Schottelius, D.D.: Decreased phenytoin levels in antineoplastic therapy, Ther. Drug. Monit. **1:**277, 1979.

Phenytoin–Charcoal

Summary: In a cross-over study involving 6 healthy subjects, 50 g of activated charcoal was administered within 5 minutes of phenytoin ingestion. Plasma phenytoin levels revealed a 98% reduction in the absorption of phenytoin. When activated charcoal was administered 1 hour after phenytoin ingestion, the phenytoin absorption was reduced by 80%.[1]

Related Drugs: The other hydantoin anticonvulsants (ethotoin and mephenytoin) may also interact with charcoal because of pharmacologic similarity. However, documentation is lacking.

Mechanism: Charcoal adsorbs phenytoin, thereby limiting its absorption. It has also been shown that phenytoin delays the gastric emptying time, and it has been suggested that this delay results in an increase in the phenytoin adsorbed by the charcoal.[1]

Recommendations: It has been recommended that activated charcoal (50 to 100 g) be given for acute phenytoin overdose to limit phenytoin absorption. If charcoal is not used to treat phenytoin toxicity, it is advisable to administer charcoal as far apart from phenytoin administration as possible.

Reference

1. Neuvonen, P.J., and others: Reduction of absorption of digoxin, phenytoin, and aspirin by activated charcoal in man, Eur. J. Clin. Pharmacol. **13:**213, 1978.

Phenytoin–Chloramphenicol

2

Summary: When administered concurrently, it has been shown that chloramphenicol has a direct inhibitory effect on the metabolism of phenytoin, thus decreasing the metabolic clearance and increasing the serum concentration of the latter.[1-8] Two other studies have offered conflicting findings on the effect of phenytoin on chloramphenicol disposition, one indicating a lowered serum chloramphenicol concentration,[9] the other an elevated peak serum concentration.[10]

Related Drugs: Although documentation is lacking, other hydantoin anticonvulsants (ethotoin and mephenytoin) may be expected to interact with chloramphenicol in an analogous manner based on a similar metabolic fate. There are no drugs related to chloramphenicol.

Mechanism: The most important pathway for chloramphenicol metabolism is glucuronide conjugation,[11] whereas the rate-limiting pathway for phenytoin is hydroxylation by the mixed function oxidase system.[12] Since both routes involve cytochrome P-450,[1] concurrent administration of chloramphenicol might inhibit phenytoin metabolism causing elevated serum levels. No mechanism was proposed for the phenytoin enhancement of chloramphenicol metabolism.[9] However, competition for hepatic enzyme binding sites was postulated as the most probable explanation for the inhibition of chloramphenicol metabolism by phenytoin.[10]

Recommendations: In view of the increases in serum phenytoin concentration that have been observed after a single dose of chloramphenicol, it is recommended that frequent phenytoin levels be obtained after the initiation of chloramphenicol therapy, and that careful observation of the patient for signs and symptoms of phenytoin toxicity (e.g., ataxia, nystagmus) be undertaken with subsequent proper phenytoin dosage adjustments if needed. With regard to potential chloramphenicol toxicity, it has been recommended that a dosage of chloramphenicol no greater than 75 mg/kg/day be considered in patients receiving phenytoin concomitantly.[10]

References

1. Christensen, L.K., and Skovsted, L.: Inhibition of drug metabolism by chloramphenicol, Lancet **2:**1397, 1969.
2. Bullek, R.E., and others: Inhibition of diphenylhydantoin metabolism by chloramphenicol, Lancet **1:**150, 1973.
3. Houghton, G.W., and Richens, A.: Inhibition of phenytoin metabolism by other drugs used in epilepsy, Int. J. Clin. Pharmacol. Biopharm. **12:**210, 1975.
4. Rose, J.Q., and others: Intoxication caused by interaction of chloramphenicol and phenytoin, J.A.M.A. **237:**2630, 1977.
5. Vincent, F.M., and others: Chloramphenicol-induced phenytoin intoxication, Ann. Neurol. **3:**469, 1978.
6. Harper, J.M., and others: Phenytoin-chloramphenicol interaction: a retrospective study, Drug Intell. Clin. Pharm. **13:**425, 1979.
7. Greenlaw, C.W.: Chloramphenicol-phenytoin drug interaction, Drug Intell. Clin. Pharm. **13:**609, 1979.

8. Saltiel, M., and Stephen, N.M.: Phenytoin-chloramphenicol interaction, Drug Intell. Clin. Pharm. **14:**221, 1980.
9. Powell, D.A., and others: Interactions among chloramphenicol, phenytoin and phenobarbital in a pediatric patient, J. Pediatr. **98:**1001, 1981.
10. Krasinski, K., and others: Pharmacologic interactions among chloramphenicol, phenytoin and phenobarbital, Pediatr. Infect. Dis. **1:**232, 1982.
11. Richens, A.: Interactions with antiepileptic drugs, Drugs **13:**266, 1977.
12. Powell, D.A., and Nahata, M. C.: Chloramphenicol: new perspectives on an old drug, Drug Intell. Clin. Pharm. **16:**295, 1982.

Phenytoin–Chlorpheniramine

Summary: Two isolated cases of phenytoin toxicity have been reported after concurrent administration of chlorpheniramine.[1,2] An epileptic woman on phenytoin and phenobarbital had serum phenytoin levels of 65 μg/ml after a week of chlorpheniramine (4 mg 3 times a day). When the chlorpheniramine was discontinued, the toxic symptom disappeared and phenytoin levels decreased.[1] The other case involved an epileptic woman who developed facial and jaw movements (without ataxia or nystagmus) 12 days after concurrent therapy was initiated, and phenytoin levels were 30 μg/ml. When chlorpheniramine was discontinued, the movements disappeared and phenytoin levels fell to 16 μg/ml.[2]

Related Drugs: There is no documentation concerning whether an interaction will occur between phenytoin and the other antihistamines (e.g., brompheniramine, diphenhydramine, tripelennamine [see Appendix]), however based on pharmacologic similarity an interaction may be expected to occur. Also, because of similar pharmacologic action, an interaction between chlorpheniramine and the other hydantoin anticonvulsants (ethotoin and mephenytoin) may be expected, although documentation is lacking.

Mechanism: The mechanism is unknown; however, it has been postulated that chlorpheniramine may inhibit the liver microsomal enzymes responsible for phenytoin metabolism.

Recommendations: Although this interaction is based on isolated case reports, it is necessary to monitor phenytoin levels during concurrent use of these agents. If toxicity does occur, the dose of phenytoin may need to be decreased or chlorpheniramine may need to be discontinued.

References

1. Pugh, R. N. H., and others: Interaction of phenytoin with chlorpheniramine, Br. J. Clin. Pharmacol. **2:**173, 1975.
2. Ahmad, S., and others: Involuntary movements caused by phenytoin intoxication in epileptic patients, J. Neurol. Neurosurg. Psychiatry **38:**225, 1975.

Phenytoin–Chlorpromazine

Summary: Concurrent administration of chlorpromazine and phenytoin may result in an increase in the half-life and serum level of phenytoin in some patients.[1-3] Chlorpromazine may affect the action of phenytoin indirectly by producing seizure activity in both epileptic and nonepileptic patients.[4-6] This interaction is uncommon and subject to large individual variability.

Related Drugs: Prochlorperazine[7] and thioridazine[8] have been reported to impair phenytoin metabolism, but not consistently, since 4 patients receiving thioridazine had depressed levels of phenytoin. Other phenothiazines, especially propylamino or aliphatic derivatives like promazine and triflupromazine, share similar biotransformation pathways and would be expected to interact with phenytoin in a similar manner.

Other antipsychotic drugs, including other phenothiazines (e.g., fluphenazine, mesoridazine, trifluoperazine [see Appendix]), the thioxanthenes (chlorprothixene and thiothixene), as well as the butyrophenone (haloperidol), dihydroinidolone (molindone), and dibenzoxazepine (loxapine) based on pharmacologic similarity, may affect the action of phenytoin indirectly, although possibly to a lesser degree. These agents may lower the seizure threshold and produce seizure activity in both epileptic and nonepileptic patients.[4-6]

One study showed the elimination of mianserin* is enhanced when given concurrently with phenytoin (in combination with phenobarbital or carbamazepine). Peak plasma levels, elimination half-life, and area-under-curve of mianserin were significantly higher in healthy volunteers not receiving an anticonvulsant.[9]

Other hydantoin anticonvulsants (ethotoin and mephenytoin) may interact with chlorpromazine and other phenothiazines in a similar manner, although this has not been documented.

Mechanism: Chlorpromazine, other phenothiazines, and phenytoin probably compete for the limited metabolic capacity of the microsomal hydroxylation enzymes in the liver.[10] Since phenytoin metabolism is saturable within the normal therapeutic range,[11] phenytoin p-hydroxylation is impaired with subsequent phenytoin accumulation and intoxication. This mechanism is subject to large individual variability.

Most antipsychotic drugs induce discharge patterns in the electroencephalogram similar to those associated with epileptic seizure disorders and can also lower the seizure threshold.[4-6] The degree of this effect varies greatly with drug class, drug, dose, and route of administration (highest with parenteral administration).[4]

Recommendations: Epileptic patients should be monitored closely for a possible increase in seizure frequency whenever an antipsychotic drug is administered. If chlorpromazine and phenytoin are coadministered, an increase in phenytoin half-life, serum levels, or side effects may occur within the first 4 weeks of therapy. If signs and symptoms of phenytoin toxicity develop (e.g., nystagmus, gait ataxia, poor

*Not available in the U.S.

muscle tone, or lethargy), serum phenytoin levels should be determined and doses of phenytoin reduced to establish therapeutic levels.

Antipsychotic drugs that are least likely to lower the seizure threshold (e.g., thioxanthenes, piperidine phenothiazines, and molindone) may be selected for psychotic patients with seizure disorders.[4-6]

References

1. Kutt, H., and McDowell, F.: Management of epilepsy with diphenylhydantoin, J.A.M.A. **203:**969, 1968.
2. Houghton, G.W., and Richens, A.: Inhibition of phenytoin metabolism by other drugs used in epilepsy, Int. J. Clin. Pharmacol. Biopharm. **12:**210, 1975.
3. Kutt, H.: Interactions of antiepileptic drugs, Epilepsia **16:**394, 1975.
4. Sriwatanakul, K.: Minimizing the risk of antipsychotic-associated seizures, Drug Ther. **13:**207, 1983.
5. Logothetis, J.: Spontaneous epileptic seizures and electroencephalographic changes in the course of phenothiazine therapy, Neurology **17:**869, 1967.
6. Itil, T.M.: Effects of psychotropic drugs in human EEG. In Clark, W.G., and Del Guidice, J., editors: Principles of psychopharmacology, second edition. New York, 1978, Academic Press.
7. Siris, J.H., and others: Anticonvulsant drug-serum levels in psychiatric patients with seizure disorders: effects of certain psychotropic drugs, N.Y. State J. Med. **74:**1554, 1974.
8. Vincent, F.M.: Phenothiazine-induced phenytoin intoxication, Ann. Intern. Med. **93:**56, 1980.
9. Nawishy, S., and Dawling, S.: Antidepressant drugs, convulsions and epilepsy, Br. J. Clin. Pharmacol. **13:**612, 1982.
10. Glazko, A.J.: Antiepileptic drugs: biotransformation, metabolism, and serum half-life, Epilepsia, **16:**367, 1975.
11. Bochner, F., and others: Effects of dosage increments on blood phenytoin concentration, J. Neurol. Neurosurg. Psychiatry **35:**874, 1972.

Phenytoin–Cimetidine

2

Summary: The concurrent use of phenytoin and cimetidine results in decreased phenytoin clearance and increased phenytoin serum levels with toxicity occurring in some patients.[1-6] One study reported a case of severe neutropenia when both agents were used in high doses.[7,8]

Related Drugs: Documentation is lacking regarding an interaction between cimetidine and the other hydantoin anticonvulsants (ethotoin and mephenytoin), although because of pharmacologic similarity an interaction may be expected. Ranitidine, another H_2 receptor antagonist, does not appear to interact similarly with phenytoin.[9]

Mechanism: Cimetidine inhibits hepatic microsomal enzymes and impairs the metabolism of phenytoin, resulting in increased serum phenytoin levels.[1-4,6,7,9] Also, since both drugs are known to depress bone marrow activity in some patients, a synergistic action may account for the neutropenia described in one report.[7]

Recommendations: Patients should be monitored for increased phenytoin levels, and a decrease in phenytoin dosage may be necessary if toxicity appears (e.g., nystagmus, ataxia). Conversely, since this interaction may be dependent on the dose of cimetidine, a reduction in cimetidine dosage may be indicated or the use of ranitidine may avoid the interaction.

References

1. Hetzel, D.J., and others: Cimetidine interaction with phenytoin, Br. Med. J. **282**:1512, 1981.
2. Algozzine, G.J., and others: Decreased clearance of phenytoin with cimetidine, Ann. Intern. Med. **95**:244, 1981.
3. Neuvonan, P.J., and others: Cimetidine-phenytoin interaction: effect on serum phenytoin concentration and antipyrine test, Eur. J. Clin. Pharmacol. **21**:215, 1981.
4. Bartle, W.R., and others: Dose-dependent effect of cimetidine on phenytoin kinetics, Clin. Pharmacol. Ther. **33**:649, 1983.
5. Salem, R.B., and others: The effect of cimetidine on phenytoin clearance, Epilepsia **24**:284, 1983.
6. Iteogu, M.O., and others: Effect of cimetidine on single-dose phenytoin kinetics, Clin. Pharm. **2**:302, 1983.
7. Sazie, E., and Jaffe, J.P.: Severe granulocytopenia with cimetidine and phenytoin, Ann. Intern. Med. **93**:151, 1980.
8. Al-Kawas, F.H., and others: Cimetidine and agranulocytosis, Ann. Intern. Med. **90**:991, 1979.
9. Watts, R.W., and others: Lack of interaction between ranitidine and phenytoin Br. J. Clin. Pharmacol. **15**:499, 1983.

Phenytoin–Cyclosporine

Summary: In 5 renal transplant patients, the concurrent administration of cyclosporine and phenytoin resulted in a reduction in the cyclosporine area-under-curve. The interaction disappeared within 72 hours after discontinuing phenytoin.[1] The clinical significance of this interaction was not determined in this uncontrolled study.

Related Drugs: Documentation is lacking regarding a similar interaction between cyclosporine and the other hydantoin anitconvulsants (ethotoin and mephenytoin). There are no drugs related to cyclosporine.

Mechanism: The mechanism of this interaction is unknown.

Recommendations: Patients should be monitored for a decrease in cyclosporine bioavailability during concomitant use of phenytoin. An increase cyclosporine dosage may be necessary.

Reference

1. Keown, P.A., and others: The effects and side effects cyclosporine: relationship to drug pharmacokinetics, Transplant Proc. **14:**659, 1982.

Phenytoin–Dexamethasone

2

Summary: Phenytoin impairs the response to dexamethasone in the dexamethasone suppression test.[1-4] The concurrent administration of phenytoin may result in a decrease in the therapeutic response to dexamethasone as well.[5,6] Concurrent administration of dexamethasone may result in a significant increase in the half-life and serum level of phenytoin.[7]

Related Drugs: Phenytoin has been reported to increase the metabolism of hydrocortisone (cortisol),[8-10] methylprednisolone,[11,12] prednisolone,[13] and prednisone.[14] Although not documented, other corticosteroids (e.g., betamethasone, cortisone, triamcinolone [see Appendix]) may interact with phenytoin in a like manner because of a similar metabolic fate.

Primidone has increased the metabolism of dexamethasone and reduced its clinical effectiveness.[15] Although not documented, the other hydantoin anticonvulsants (ethotoin and mephenytoin) and other anticonvulsants that cause enzyme induction (e.g., carbamazepine) may interact with dexamethasone and other corticosteroids in a similar manner.

Mechanism: Phenytoin affects corticosteroid metabolism, most notably dexamethasone, by stimulating hepatic microsomal hydroxylating enzymes responsible for corticosteroid metabolism.[4] Phenytoin and dexamethasone probably compete for the limited metabolic capacity of these microsomal hydroxylating enzymes as well. Since phenytoin metabolism is saturable within the normal therapeutic range,[16] phenytoin p-hydroxylation is impaired, which results in phenytoin accumulation and intoxication.

Recommendations: If the dexamethasone suppression test is used in patients who have been receiving phenytoin long-term, the test should be interpreted with caution and a higher dose of dexamethasone may be necessary.

Patients receiving both drugs concurrently should be observed for possible diminution of the therapeutic effect of dexamethasone or other corticosteroids and/or signs and symptoms of phenytoin toxicity (e.g., nystagmus, gait ataxia, poor muscle tone, or lethargy). These effects may require an increase in corticosteroid dosage, a decrease in phenytoin dose, or both, to establish therapeutic levels.

References

1. Werk, E.E., and others: Interference in the effect of dexamathasone by diphenylhydantoin, N. Engl. J. Med. **281**:32, 1969.
2. Jubiz, W., and others: Effect of diphenylhydantoin on the metabolism of dexamethasone: mechanism of the abnormal dexamethasone suppression in humans, N. Engl. J. Med. **283**:11, 1970.
3. Jubiz, W., and others: Failure of dexamethasone suppression in patients on chronic diphenylhydantoin therapy, Clin. Res. **17**:106, 1969.
4. Haque, N., and others: Studies on dexamethasone metabolism in man: effect of diphenylhydantoin, J. Clin. Endocrinol. Metab. **34**:44, 1972.
5. McLelland, J., and Jack, W.: Phenytoin-dexamethasone interaction: a clinical problem, Lancet **1**:1096, 1978.

6. Boylan, J.J., and others: Phenytoin interference with dexamethasone, J.A.M.A. **235:**803, 1976.
7. Lawson, L.A., and others: Phenytoin-dexamethasone interaction: a previously unreported observation, Surg. Neurol. **16:**23, 1981.
8. Werk, E.E., and others: Cortisol production in epileptic patients treated with diphenylhydantoin, Clin. Pharmacol. Ther. **12:**698, 1971.
9. Werk, E.E., and others: Effect of diphenylhydantoin on cortisol metabolism in man, J. Clin. Invest. **43:**1824, 1964.
10. Choi, Y., and others: Effect of diphenylhydantoin on cortisol kinetics in humans, J. Pharmacol. Exp. Ther. **176:**27, 1971.
11. Stjernholm, M.J., and Katz, F.H.: Effect of diphenylhydantoin, phenobarbital, and diazepam on the metabolism of methylprednisolone and its sodium succinate, J. Clin. Endocrinol. Metab. **41:**887, 1975.
12. Sells, R.A., and others: Methylprednisolone blood levels in cadaveric renal allograft recipients, Transplant. Proc. **10;**651, 1978.
13. Petereit, L.B., and Meikle, A.W.: Effectiveness of prednisolone during phenytoin therapy, Clin. Pharmacol. Ther. **22:**912, 1977.
14. Wassner, S.J., and others: The adverse effect of anticonvulsant therapy on renal allograft survival, J. Pediatr. **88:**134, 1976.
15. Hancock, K.W., and Levell, M.J.: Primidone-dexamethasone interaction, Lancet **2:**97, 1978.
16. Bochner, F. and others: Effects of dosage increments on blood phenytoin concentration, J. Neurol. Neurosurg. Psychiatry **35:**874, 1972.

Summary: There are conflicting reports regarding the effect of diazepam on phenytoin serum concentrations. Increased phenytoin serum concentrations have been reported in numerous studies.[1-3] However, concurrent diazepam has also decreased phenytoin levels.[4] Other reports have suggested that diazepam alters phenytoin concentrations, but poor study design prevents definitive conclusions.[5,6] One report indicates that diazepam elimination is enhanced with concurrent phenytoin.[7]

Related Drugs: Phenytoin serum levels have been shown to be increased during administration of the following benzodiazepines: chlordiazepoxide,[1,8] clonazepam,[9-13] and an insignificant increase with nitrazepam.[*9] Phenytoin levels have been shown to be decreased with chlordiazepoxide[4] and clonazepam.[12-16] Other benzodiazepines (e.g., flurazepam, halazepam, triazolam [see Appendix]) have not been reported to alter phenytoin levels. Because of conflicting results, it is difficult to determine whether a similar interaction would occur between diazepam and the other hydantoin anticonvulsants (ethotoin and mephenytoin).

Mechanism: The inconsistency of the effect of these 2 agents is not understood. Possible mechanisms include a benzodiazepine microsomal enzyme induction or inhibition of phenytoin metabolism.[4,13,14] The apparent volume of distribution of phenytoin may also be affected by benzodiazepines.

Recommendations: The effect of concomitant use of these 2 agents cannot be predicted. However, the inconsistent changes in phenytoin levels require that patients be monitored closely during concurrent benzodiazepine therapy. Phenytoin dosage may need to be adjusted depending on the individual patient's response to these agents.

References

1. Vajda, F.J.E., and others: Interaction between phenytoin and the benzodiazepines, Br. Med. J. **1:**346, 1971.
2. Rogers, H.J., and others: Diphenylhydantoin-diazepam interactions; a pharmacokinetic analysis, Pediatr. Res. **9:**286, 1975.
3. Rogers, H.J., and others: Phenytoin intoxication during concurrent diazepam therapy, J. Neurol. Neurolsurg. Psychiatry **40:**890, 1977.
4. Houghton, G.W., and Richens, A.: The effect of benzodiazepines and pheneturide on phenytoin metabolism in man, Br. J. Clin. Pharmacol. **1:**344P, 1974.
5. Kariks, J., and others: Serum folic acid and phenytoin levels in permanently hospitalized epileptic patients receiving anticonvulsant drug therapy, Med. J. Aust. **2:**368, 1971.
6. Shuttleworth, E., and others: Choreoathetosis and diphenylhydantoin intoxication, J.A.M.A. **230:**1170, 1974.
7. Hepner, G.W., and others: Disposition of aminopyrine, antipyrine, diazepam, and indocyanine green in patients with liver disease or an anticonvulsant drug therapy: diazepam breath test and correlations in drug eliminations, J. Lab. Clin. Med. **90:**440, 1977.
8. Kutt, H., and McDowell, F.: Management of epilepsy with diphenylhydantoin sodium, J.A.M.A. **203:**167, 1968.

*Not available in the U.S.

9. Windorfer, A., and Sauer, W.: Drug interactions during anticonvulsant therapy in childhood: diphenylhydantoin, primidone, phenobarbitone, clonazepam, nitrazepam, carbamazepine and dipropylacetate, Neuropadiatrie **8:**29, 1977.
10. Windorfer, P.: Drug interaction during anticonvulsive therapy, Int. J. Clin. Pharmacol. **14:**231, 1976.
11. Eeg-Olofsson, O.: Experiences with Rivotril in treatment of epilepsy—particularly minor motor epilepsy—in mentally retarded children, Acta Neurol. Scand. suppl. 53 **49:**29, 1973.
12. Huang, C.Y., and others: Clonazepam in the treatment of epilepsy, Proc. Aust. Assoc. Neurol. **10:**67, 1973.
13. Huang, C.Y., and others: Clonazepam in the treatment of epilepsy, Med. J. Aust. **2:**5, 1974.
14. Edwards, V.E., and Eadie, M.J.: Clonazepam—a clinical study of its effectiveness as an anticonvulsant, Proc. Aust. Assoc. Neurol. **10:**61, 1973.
15. Sjo, O., and others: Pharmacokinetics and side-effects of clonazepam and its 7-amino-metabolite in man, Eur. J. Clin. Pharmacol. **8:**249, 1975.
16. Khoo, K., and others: Influence of phenytoin and phenobarbital on the disposition of a single oral dose of clonazepam, Clin. Pharmacol. Ther. **28:**368, 1980.

Phenytoin–Diazoxide

2

Summary: Phenytoin serum levels may be decreased to subtherapeutic levels by concurrent oral diazoxide.[1,2] In one study, when diazoxide was withdrawn the phenytoin levels returned to therapeutic levels, but when diazoxide was again started phenytoin concentration fell to undetectable levels and seizures occurred.[1] The effects of diazoxide (oral and intravenous) were also reduced during concurrent use as demonstrated by the appearance of symptomatic hypoglycomia in several case reports.[2,3]

Related Drugs: Although documentation is lacking, a similar interaction may be expected to occur between diazoxide and the other hydantoin anticonvulsants (ethotoin and mephenytoin) because of pharmacologic similarity. There are no drugs related to diazoxide.

Mechanism: Diazoxide may increase the hepatic metabolism of phenytoin and increase its clearance as well.[1-2] It has been suggested that displacement from plasma protein binding sites also plays a role.[1] The reduced effects of diazoxide may be the result of induction of diazoxide's metabolism by phenytoin.[2,3]

Recommendations: Phenytoin plasma levels should be monitored, and an increased phenytoin dosage may be necessary if loss of seizure control occurs. Also, when diazoxide is discontinued, phenytoin dosage may need to be decreased to avoid toxicity.

References

1. Roe, T.F., and others: Drug interaction: diazoxide and diphenylhydantoin, J. Pediatr. **87**:480, 1975.
2. Petro, D.J., and others: Diazoxide-diphenylhydantoin interaction, J. Pediatr. **89**:331, 1975.
3. Pruitt, A.W., and others: Disposition of diazoxide in children, Clin. Pharmacol. Ther. **14**:73, 1973.

Phenytoin–Disulfiram

Summary: Addition of disulfiram to a stable phenytoin regimen will result in decreased phenytoin metabolism and increased phenytoin levels that may lead to toxicity.[1-8]

Related Drugs: The other hydantoin anticonvulsants (ethotoin and mephenytoin) have not been reported to interact with disulfiram. However, because their chemical structure and metabolism are similar to that of phenytoin, they may be expected to interact with disulfiram in a similar manner.

Mechanism: Increased phenytoin levels result from disulfiram inhibition of the major route of metabolism of phenytoin.[1-3] Pharmacokinetic analysis suggests that this inhibition of hepatic microsomal enzymes is noncompetitive.[4]

Recommendations: If a patient must be treated with both drugs, a baseline phenytoin level should be drawn before disulfiram is added to the regimen. The levels should be measured again in 2 to 4 days, and once or twice weekly until a new steady-state is established. In most cases, the plateau will be reached 2 to 3 weeks after the last dosage adjustment.[6] The patient should also be monitored clinically for signs of phenytoin toxicity (e.g., ataxia, nystagmus) since symptom severity and height of serum level usually are parallel. Both parameters may be used as guides for adjusting the phenytoin dose if necessary.

In most cases, decreasing the phenytoin dose will be sufficient to avoid toxicity, but some patients may require withdrawal of the disulfiram.[3]

References

1. Notten, W.R., and others: Effect of disulfiram on the urinary d-glucuric acid excretion and activity of some enzymes involved in drug metabolism in guinea-pig, Arch. Int. Pharmacodyn. Ther. **205:**199, 1973.
2. Kutt, H., and others: Metabolism of phenytoin by rat liver microsomes, Biochem. Pharmacol. **19:**675, 1970.
3. Svendsen, T.L.: Influence of disulfiram on half-life and metabolic clearance of phenytoin and tolbutamide in man, Eur. J. Clin. Pharmacol. **9:**439, 1976.
4. Taylor, J.W., and others: Mathematical analysis of a phenytoin-disulfiram interaction, Am. J. Hosp. Pharm. **38:**93, 1981.
5. Olesen, O.V.: The influence of disulfiram and calcium carbimide on the serum diphenylhydantoin excretion of HPPH in the urine, Arch. Neurol. **16:**642, 1967.
6. Olesen, O.V.: Disulfiram (Antabuse) as inhibitor of phenytoin metabolism, Acta Pharmacol. Toxicol. **24:**317, 1966.
7. Kiorboe, E.: Phenytoin intoxication during treatment with Antabuse (disulfiram), Epilepsia **7:**246, 1966.
8. Loiseau, P., and others: Poisoning during disulfiram therapy, Nouv. Presse. Med. **4:**504, 1975.

Phenytoin–Dopamine

1

Summary: Five patients in shock who were given a dopamine infusion to support their blood pressure had a rapid decline in blood pressure when intravenous phenytoin was begun. Death of 2 patients was attributed to the concurrent use of these agents.[1] The hypothesis that dopamine and phenytoin produced the dramatic hypotension has been verified by animal studies.

Related Drugs: There is no documentation concerning the interaction of dopamine with the other hydantoin anticonvulsants (ethotoin and mephenytoin). No reports are available regarding an interaction between phenytoin and other agents used to treat shock (e.g., dobutamine, epinephrine, isoproterenol, [see Appendix]). Therefore, because of the lack of available information it cannot be determined at this time if an interaction exists between other anticonvulsants and other sympathomimetics used in the treatment of shock.

Mechanism: The mechanism is unknown. However, one possible explanation is related to the fact that dopamine is known to prevent uptake at sympathetic storage sites and increase the synthesis of norepinephrine, whereas phenytoin exerts a greater myocardial depressant effect in the presence of catecholamine depletion. This may be the mechanism of hypotension, although many other effects of the 2 drugs could explain the observations.[1]

Recommendations: Although this precaution is based on one report, phenytoin should be used with the greatest care, or not at all, in patients receiving dopamine to support blood pressure. If hypotension occurs, discontinue phenytoin.

Reference

1. Bivins, B.A., and others: Dopamine-phenytoin interaction, Arch. Surg. **113:**245, 1978.

Phenytoin–Ethosuximide

3

Summary: Increased serum phentoin concentrations with concurrent administration of ethosuximide have been reported in a few patients receiving only these 2 agents.[1,2] In one case report the patient was receiving several other drugs when ethosuximide was added and toxicity developed.[3] There have also been reports that no interaction occurs with these agents.[4,5]

Related Drugs: Increased serum phenytoin concentrations have been seen with concurrent methsuximide.[6] There is no documentation regarding an interaction between ethosuximide and the other hydantoin anticonvulsants (ethotoin and mephenytoin) or between phenytoin and the other succinimide (phensuximide), although a similar interaction may be expected to occur because of a similar metabolic fate.

Mechanism: The exact mechanism is unknown. However, ethosuximide induced inhibition of phenytoin metabolism is a suggested mechanism for this interaction.

Recommendations: Patients receiving phenytoin should be closely monitored for increased serum phenytoin concentrations or signs of toxicity (e.g., ataxia, nystagmus) when ethosuximide is coadministered. Patients stabilized on both drugs should also be monitored for subtherapeutic phenytoin levels if ethosuximide is discontinued.

References

1. Lander, C.M., and others: Interactions between anticonvulsants, Proc. Aust. Assoc. Neurol. **12:**111, 1975.
2. Frantzen, E., and others: Phenytoin (dilantin) intoxication, Acta Neurol. Scand. **43:**440, 1967.
3. Dawson, G.W., and others: Serum phenytoin and ethosuximide, Ann. Neurol. **4:**583, 1978.
4. Perucca, E.: Pharmacokinetic interactions with antiepileptic drugs, Clin. Pharmacokinet. **7:**57, 1982.
5. Smith, G.A., and others: Factors influencing plasma concentrations of ethosuximide, Clin. Pharmacokinet. **4:**38, 1979.
6. Rambeck, B.: Pharmacological interactions of methsuximide with phenobarbital and phenytoin in hospitalized epileptic patients, Epilepsia **20:**147, 1979.

Phenytoin–Folic Acid

2

Summary: Folic acid administration of 5 mg or more to patients previously stabilized on phenytoin has been associated with increased seizure frequency[1-5] and lowered serum phenytoin concentrations.[1,3,4,6-8] Long-term administration of phenytoin may cause low serum folate concentrations in some patients and may precipitate symptoms of folic acid deficiency (e.g., mental dysfunction, neuropathy, psychiatric disorders and, rarely, megaloblastic anemia).[9-13] Phenytoin-induced folate deficiency may be responsible for congenital malformations, but a causal relationship has not been established.[13-16]

Related Drugs: Phenobarbital and primidone have also been associated with decreased serum folate concentrations.[2,10,14,17] The other hydantoin anticonvulsants (ethotoin and mephenytoin) may also interact with folic acid in a manner similar to phenytoin because they are pharmacologically related, but this has not been documented. There are no drugs related to folic acid.

Mechanism: The mechanism of the phenytoin-induced folate deficiency is unclear. An early theory that phenytoin inhibited the intestinal absorption of folic acid has been disputed.[18-20] A second theory is that the phenytoin-induced increase in hepatic metabolizing enzymes causes an increased demand for folate.[7] A third possibility is that phenytoin interferes with the conversion of folate to a form that is transported into the brain and cerebrospinal fluid, which results in higher serum folate and lower cerebrospinal fluid folate concentrations.[4,11]

Folic acid, when administered is doses of 5 mg or more, enhances the para-hydroxylation of phenytoin[1] perhaps by an unknown pathway.[21,22] Other investigators have failed to find a change in the phenytoin half-life after folic acid administration.[23] Folic acid alone has caused seizures in animals,[11] and the anticonvulsant properties of phenytoin have been attributed to the antifolate acitivty.[10]

Recommendations: Many studies of patients receiving phenytoin and folic acid showed no significant interaction[22,24-26] although shortcomings of these trials have also been reported.[8,27-30] Patients receiving phenytoin should be observed closely for symptoms of folic acid deficiency. If these symptoms are observed serum folate concentrations should be obtained and, if necessary, folic acid (0.1 to 1 mg/day orally) may be added as supplemental therapy.[31] Larger doses of folic acid are no more effective in correcting folate deficiency[31] and should be avoided because of the possible detrimental effect on seizure control.[1-3] Pregnant patients have a greater folate requirement than others. However, although some recommend adding folic acid as a prophylactic measure,[14] others believe that the potential harm resulting from the possibility of more seizures caused by folic acid outweighs any benefit gained by folic acid replacement therapy.[3,16] Also, patients should be monitored for decreased phenytoin concentrations.

References

1. Baylis, E.M.: Influence of folic acid on blood-phenytoin levels, Lancet **1:**62, 1971.
2. Reynolds, E.H.: Effects of folic acid on the mental state and fit-frequency of drug treated epileptic patients, Lancet **1:**1086, 1967.
3. Strauss, R.G., and Bernstein, R.: Folic acid and dilantin antagonism in pregnancy, Qbstet. Gynecol. **44:**345, 1974.
4. MacCosbe, P.E., and Toomey, K.: Interaction of phenytoin and folic acid, Clin. Pharm. **2:**362, 1983.
5. Berg, M.J., and others: Phenytoin and folic acid: individualized drug-drug interaction, Ther. Drug. Monit. **5:**395, 1983.
6. Berg, M.J., and others: Phenytoin and folic acid interaction: a preliminary report, Ther. Drug. Monit. **5:**389, 1983.
7. Maxwell, J.D.: Folate deficiency after anticonvulsant drugs: an effect of hepatic enzyme induction, Br. Med. J. **1:**297, 1972.
8. Norris, J.W., and Pratt, R.F.: A controlled study of folic acid in epilepsy, Neurology **21:**659, 1971.
9. Wells, D.G.: Folic acid and neuropathy in epilepsy, Lancet **1:**146, 1968.
10. Reynolds, E.H.: Anticonvulsants, folic acid and epilepsy, Lancet **1:**1376, 1973.
11. Mattson, R.H., and others: Folate therapy in epilepsy: a controlled study, Arch. Neutrol. **29:**78, 1973.
12. Norris, J.W., and Pratt, R.F.: Folic acid deficiency and epilepsy, Drugs **8:**366, 1974.
13. Rivey, M.P., and others: Phenytoin-folic acid: a review, Drug Intell. Clin. Pharm. **18:**292, 1984.
14. Speidel, B.D., and Meadow, S.R.: Epilepsy, anticonvulsants and congenital malformations, Drugs **8:**354, 1974.
15. Baile, Y., and others: Congenital malformations due to anticonvulsant drugs, Obstet. Gynecol. **45:**439, 1975.
16. Jany, D.: The teratogenic risk of antiepileptic drugs, Epilepsia **16:**159, 1975.
17. Neubauer, C.: Mental deterioration in epilepsy due to folate deficiency, Br. Med. J. **2:**759, 1970.
18. Hoffbrand, A.V., and Neckeles, T.F.: Mechanisms of folate deficiency in patients receiving phenytoin, Lancet **2:**528, 1968.
19. Davis, R.E., and Woodliff, H.J.: Folic acid deficiency in patients receiving anticonvulsant drugs, Med. J. Aust. **2:**1070, 1971.
20. Houlihan, C.M., and others: The effect of phenytoin on the absorption of synthetic folic acid poly-glutanate, Gut **13:**189, 1972.
21. Olesen, O.V., and Jenson, O.N.: The influence of folic acid on phenytoin (DPH) metabolism and the 24-hour fluctuation in urinary output of 5-(p-hydroxyphenyl)-5-phenyl-hydantoin (HPPH), Acta Pharmacol. Toxicol. **28:**265, 1970.
22. Glazko, A.V.: Diphenylhydantoin metabolism a prospective review, Drug Metab. Dispos. **1:**711, 1973.
23. Andreasen, P.B., and others: Folic acid and phenytoin metabolism, Lancet **1:**645, 1971.
24. Jenson, O.N., and Olesen, O.V.: Subnormal serum folate due to anticonvulsive therapy. A double blind study of the effect of folic acid treatment in patients with drug-induced subnormal serum folates, Arch. Neurol. **22:**181, 1970.
25. Ralston, A.J., and others: Effects of folic acid on fit-frequency and behavior in epileptics on anticonvulsants, Lancet **1:**867, 1970.
26. Grant, R.H.E., and Stores, O.P.R.: Folic acid in folate-deficient patients with epilepsy, Br. Med. J. **4:**644, 1970.
27. Richens, A.: Folic acid in epilepsy, Br. Med. J. **1:**109, 1971.
28. Grant, R.H.E., and others: Folic acid in epilepsy, Br. Med. J. **1:**728, 1971.
29. Horwitz, S.J., and others: Relation of abnormal folate metabolism to neuropathy developing during anticonvulsant drug therapy, Lancet **1:**563, 1968.
30. Kariks, J., and others: Serum folic acid and phenytoin levels in permanently hospitalized epileptic patients receiving anticonvulsant drug therapy, Med. J. Aust. **2:**368, 1971.
31. Anonymous: Use of folic acid in pregnancy and in clinical disorders, Med. Lett. Drug Ther. **14:**50, 1972.

Phenytoin–Ibuprofen

3

Summary: The concomitant administration of phenytoin and ibuprofen may increase phenytoin plasma levels and result in phenytoin toxicity. In a case study a patient stabilized on phenytoin began ibuprofen therapy and developed cerebellar ataxia, nystagmus, nausea, and frontal headaches. Phenythoin plasma levels were significantly elevated. When ibuprofen was discontinued, the patient's symptoms resolved in 2 to 3 weeks.[1]

Related Drugs: Phenylbutazone and oxyphenbutazone have been reported to interact with phenytoin (see Phenytoin-Phenylbutazone, p. 264). Other nonsteroidal anti-inflammatory agents (e.g., indomethacin, naproxen, sulindac [see Appendix]) may also increase phenytoin plasma levels; however, documentation is lacking. Documentation is also lacking regarding an interaction between ibuprofen and the other hydantoin anticonvulsants (ethotoin and mephenytoin), although a similar interaction may be expected because of a similar metabolic fate.

Mechanism: It has been suggested that ibuprofen inhibits the hepatic microsomal enzymes responsible for phenytoin metabolism.[1] However, documentation is lacking to support this hypothesis.

Recommendations: The possibility of this interaction should be considered, and the appropriate dosage adjustment of phenytoin should be made when given with ibuprofen, especially when ibuprofen is used in the higher dosage range.[1]

Reference

1. Sandyk, R.: Phenytoin toxicity induced by interaction with ibuprofen, South Afr. Med. J. **65:**592, 1982.

Phenytoin–Imipramine

3

Summary: Imipramine, when administered concurrently with phenytoin, has been reported to cause an increase in phenytoin levels in 2 patients. One patient developed mild signs of phenytoin intoxication, and the phenytoin levels of both patients were reduced once imipramine was withdrawn.[1] One patient was taking nitrazepam and clonazepam, and the other was taking sodium valproate and carbamazepine.[1]

Related Drugs: Nortriptyline has been shown to cause an insignificant increase in phenytoin levels,[2] whereas another study reported nortriptyline had no effect on phenytoin half-life.[3] The action of other antidepressants are varied and conflicting. One study reported that amitriptyline had no effect on phenytoin elimination in 3 patients.[3] The tricyclic antidepressants desipramine, protriptyline, and amoxapine as well as nortriptyline, amitriptyline, and imipramine have been reported to cause seizures in epileptic and nonepileptic patients.[3-10] Plasma levels of nomifensine and mianserin (not currently commercially available) were reduced by phenytoin, but only in combination with phenobarbital or carbamazepine, not with phenytoin alone.[11] Whether the increased incidence of seizures is caused by these agents alone or by concurrent use with phenytoin has not been documented. Because of conflicting results it is difficult to determine whether an interaction would occur between phenytoin and the other tricyclic antidepressants (doxepin and trimipramine) and the tetracyclic antidepressant (maprotiline).

There is no documentation regarding an interaction between imipramine and the other hydantoin anticonvulsants (ethotoin and mephenytoin). However, because of pharmacologic similarity an interaction may be expected.

Mechanism: The mechanism is unknown. However, it has been postulated that imipramine can inhibit the metabolism of phenytoin, which results in its accumulation in the body. It was not reported if the other drugs the patients were taking concurrently affected the interaction.[1]

Recommendations: If imipramine (and possibly other tricyclic or tetracyclic antidepressants) and phenytoin are coadministered, an increase in phenytoin half-life, serum levels, or side effects may occur. If signs and symptoms of phenytoin toxicity develop (e.g., nystagmus, gait ataxia, poor muscle tone, or lethargy), serum phenytoin levels should be determined and doses of phenytoin reduced to establish therapeutic levels. Conversely, patients should be monitored closely for a possible increase in seizure frequency whenever an antidepressant is administered. If such an increase occurs, an increase in anticonvulsant dosage may be required.

References

1. Perucca, E., and Richens, A.: Interaction between phenytoin and imipramine, Br. J. Clin. Pharmacol. **4:**485, 1977.
2. Houghton, G.W., and Richens, A.: Inhibition of phenytoin metabolism by other drugs used in epilepsy, Int. J. Clin. Pharmacol. **12:**210, 1975.
3. Pond, S.M., and others: Effects of tricyclic antidepressants on drug metabolism, Clin. Pharmacol. Ther. **18:**191, 1975.

4. Dallos, V., and Heathfeld, K.: Iatrogenic epilepsy due to antidepressant drugs, Br. Med. J. 4:80, 1969.
5. Davison, K.: EEG activation after intravenous amitryptyline, Electroencephalogr. Clin. Neurophysiol. 19:298, 1965.
6. Gannon, P., and others: Clinical and quantitative electroencephalographical effects of MK940, Arzneimittelforsch. 20:971, 1970.
7. Gelenberg, A.J., and Klerman, G.L.: Preclinical pharmacology of antidepressants: part 2. tricyclics. In Clark, W.G., and Del Guidice, J. editors: Principles of pharmacology. New York, 1968, Academic Press.
8. Ives, T. and Heath, R.: Amitriptyline-induced tonic-clonic seizures in the mentally retarded, Drug Intell. Clin. Pharm. 14:378, 1980.
9. Edwards, J.G.: Antidepressants and convulsions, Lancet 2:1368, 1979.
10. Koval, G., and others: Seizures with amoxapine, Am. J. Psychiatry 139:845, 1982.
11. Nawishy, S., and others: Interactions of anticonvulsant drugs with mianserin and nomifensine, Lancet 2:871, 1981.

Phenytoin–Isoniazid

2

Summary: Isoniazid, when added to the therapy of patients receiving phenytoin, increases the serum phenytoin concentration, which can result in an increased incidence of phenytoin toxicity.[1-5] The interaction is dose dependent and significant at usual therapeutic doses of isoniazid.[6] This interaction appears to be of greater consequence in patients who are genetically slow acetylators of isoniazid.[3,6]

Related Drugs: Isoniazid may interact with other hydantoin anticonvulsants (ethotoin and mephenytoin) because of a similar metabolic fate, although such interactions have not been reported. Two other antitubercular drugs, aminosalicylic acid and cycloserine, interact with phenytoin in vitro,[3] and aminosalicyclic acid may potentiate the isoniazid-phenytoin interaction in humans.[1]

Mechanism: Isoniazid blocks the para-hydroxylation of phenytoin and the conjugation of the principal metabolite 5-(p-hydroxyphenyl)-5-phenylhydantoin in the rat[7-9] and humans.[1]

Recommendations: Patients receiving phenytoin and isoniazid concurrently should have periodic determinations of serum phenytoin concentrations and should be observed closely for signs and symptoms of toxicity (e.g., ataxia, nystagmus).[5,6] Patients known to be slow acetylators of isoniazid should have the phenytoin dosage reduced when isoniazid is added to the regimen. If phenytoin toxicity occurs, phenytoin should be discontinued or the dosage reduced until toxic signs and symptoms subside. Phenytoin may then be reinstituted and the dosage adjusted until therapeutic concentrations are obtained.[10]

References

1. Kutt, H., and others: Depression of parahydroxylation of diphenylhydantoin by antituberculosis chemotherapy, Neurology **16:**594, 1966.
2. Murray, F.J.: Outbreak of unexpected reactions among epileptics taking isoniazid, Am. Rev. Resp. Dis. **86:**729, 1962.
3. Kutt, H., and others: Diphenylhydantoin intoxication. A complication of isoniazid therapy, Am. Rev. Resp. Dis. **101:**377, 1970.
4. Johnson, J., and Freeman, H.L.: Death due to isoniazid and phenytoin, Br. J. Psychiatry **129:**511, 1976.
5. Miller, R.R., and others: Clinical importance of the interaction of phenytoin and isoniazid: a report from the Boston Collaborative Drug Surveillance Program, Chest **75:**356, 1979.
6. Brennan, R.W., and others: Diphenylhydantoin intoxication attendant to slow inactivation of isonazid, Neurology **20:**687, 1970.
7. Kutt, H., and others: Inhibition of diphenylhydantoin metabolism in rats and rat liver microsomes by antitubercular drugs, Neurology **18:**706, 1968.
8. Buttor, H.S., and others: Effect of isoniazid on the metabolism of 14C-diphenylhydantoin in rats, Arch. Int. Pharmacodyn. Ther. **235:**9, 1978.
9. Buttor, H.S.: Isoniazid-induced inhibition in the biotransformation of (14C) diphenylhydantoin in the rat, Res. Commun. Chem. Pathol. Pharmacol. **18:**35, 1977.
10. Kutt, H., and McDowell, F.: Management of epilepsy with diphenylhydantoin sodium dosage regulation for problem patients, J.A.M.A. **203:**969, 1968.

Phenytoin–Levodopa

3

Summary: In a double-blind study, the therapeutic effects of levodopa were inhibitied by the concurrent use of phenytoin. Patients with parkinsonism showed a worsening of symptoms, and a reduction of levodopa-dependent dyskinesias was also noted.[1]

Related Drugs: There are no drugs related to levodopa. A similar interaction may be expected between levodopa and the other hydantoins (ethotoin and mephenytoin) because of pharmacologic similarity; however, documentation is lacking.

Mechanism: The mechanism of this interaction is unknown.

Recommendations: If the concurrent use of levodopa and phenytoin is necessary, a higher dose of levodopa may be required.

Reference

1. Mendez, J.S., and others: Diphenylhydantoin blocking of levodopa effects, Arch. Neurol. **32:**44, 1975.

Phenytoin–Methylphenidate

3

Summary: Methylphenidate raises serum phenytoin concentration and may cause symptoms of phenytoin toxicity (e.g., ataxia, nystagmus) in some children.[1,2] These effects were not seen in controlled studies in adults.[3-5]

Related Drugs: Primidone has been reported to interact with methylphenidate in a similar manner.[1] Although not reported, other hydantoin anticonvulsants (ethotoin and mephenytoin) may also interact with methylphenidate because of a similar metabolic fate.

Mechanism: In vitro studies have shown that methylphenidate is a competitive inhibitor of the hepatic metabolism of phenytoin and other drugs.[6,7]

Recommendations: Serum concentrations of phenytoin should be monitored and the dose altered to bring the anticonvulsant level into the therapeutic range. Although considerable individual variation exists, nystagmus generally appears when the serum phenytoin concentration reaches 20 μg/ml or higher, gait ataxia is observed at concentrations above 30 μg/ml, and lethargy remains constant at levels approaching 40 μg/ml.[8]

References

1. Garrettson, L. K., and others: Methylphenidate interaction with both anticonvulsants and ethyl bis-coumacetate, J.A.M.A. **207:**2053, 1969.
2. Solow, E.B., and Green, J.B.: The simultaneous determination of multiple anticonvulsant drug levels by gas liquid chromatography, Neurology **22:**540, 1972.
3. Mirkin, B.L., and Wright, F.: Drug interactions: effect of methylphenidate on the disposition of diphenyl-hydantoin in man, Neurology **21:**1123, 1971.
4. Kupferberg, H.J., and others: Effect of methylphenidate on plasma anticonvulsant levels, Clin. Pharmacol. Ther. **13:**201, 1972.
5. Oettinger, L.: Interaction of methylphenidate and diphenylhydantoin, Drug Ther. **5:**107, 1976.
6. Perel, J.M., and Black, N.: In vitro metabolism studies with methylphenidate, Fed. Proc. **29:**345, 1970.
7. Hunninghake, D.: Studies of the inhibition of drug metabolism by methylphenidate, Fed. Proc. **29:**345, 1970.
8. Kutt, H., and McDowell, F.: Management of epilepsy with diphenylhydantoin sodium. Dosage regulations for problem patients, J.A.M.A. **203:**969, 1968.

Phenytoin–Nitrofurantoin

Summary: A patient stabilized on phenytoin had a reduction in plasma phenytoin levels after concurrent nitrofurantoin was initiated. The phenytoin dosage had to be increased because 2 seizure episodes occurred; after discontinuation of nitrofurantoin the patient continued on his previous phenytoin therapy without any loss of seizure control.[1]

Related Drugs: There are no reports regarding an interaction between nitrofurantoin and the other hydantoin anticonvulsants (ethotoin and mephenytoin), although a similar interaction may be expected because of a similar metabolic fate. There is also a lack of documentation concerning an interaction between phenytoin and the other nitrofuran, furazolidone. Since the exact mechanism for this interaction is unknown and the metabolic fate of furazolidone and nitrofurantoin differ, it is not possible to predict whether a similar interaction could occur.

Mechanism: The mechanism of this interaction is unknown. However, it has been suggested that impaired phenytoin absorption and increased phenytoin metabolism by nitrofurantoin are responsible.[1]

Recommendations: These agents need not be avoided. However, patients should be monitored for an increase in seizure frequency. If loss of seizure control occurs, the dose of phenytoin may need to be increased or nitrofurantoin may have to be discontinued.

Reference

1. Heipertz, R., and Pilz, H.: Interaction of nitrofurantoin with diphenylhydantoin, J. Neurol. **218:**297, 1978.

Phenytoin–Oral Contraceptive Agents

3

Summary: The concurrent use of oral contraceptive agents with anticonvulsant therapy including phenytoin may result in breakthrough bleeding, spotting, and in some cases loss of contraceptive effect, which resulted in pregnancy.[1-5] However, a clear-cut cause and effect relationship has not been determined. Also, the concomitant use of these agents may lead to loss of seizure control,[6,7] although 1 study involving 20 epileptics failed to confirm this interaction.[8] Another study indicated a tendency for higher plasma phenytoin levels in oral contraceptive users.[9]

Related Drugs: Documentation is lacking regarding an interaction between oral contraceptive agents and the other hydantoin anticonvulsants (ethotoin and mephenytoin), although a similar interaction may be expected because of similar effect on hepatic microsomal enzymes. Besides taking phenytoin, the patients in the previously cited studies were receiving phenobarbital, primidone, or carbamazepine.

Mechanism: It has been suggested that oral contraceptive failure occurs because phenytoin (as well as the other anticonvulsants mentioned) induces hepatic microsomal enzymes, thereby increasing the rate of metabolism of the oral contraceptives.[1-5] The loss of seizure control may result from changes in fluid retention induced by oral contraceptives.[6] It has also been postulated that contraceptive agents affect plasma protein binding of phenytoin or inhibit its metabolism.[7,9] However, in one study no effect of oral contraceptives on phenytoin binding was found.[10]

Recommendations: Patients may need an alternate form of contraception if phenytoin or other anticonvulsants are required. Also, patients should be monitored for loss of seizure control since an increased phenytoin dose may be necessary.

References

1. Kenyon, I.E.: Unplanned pregnancy in an epileptic, Br. Med. J. **1:**686, 1972.
2. Hempel, E., and others: Medikamentose enzyminduktion und hormonale kontrazeption, Zentralbl. Gynakol. **95:**1451, 1973.
3. Janz, D., and Schmidt, D.: Anti-epileptic drugs and failure of oral contraceptives, Lancet **1:**1113, 1974.
4. Laengner, H., and Detering, K.: Antiepileptic drugs and failure of oral contraceptives, Lancet **2:**600, 1974.
5. Coulam, C.B., and Annegers, J.F.: Do anticonvulsants reduce the efficacy? Epilepsia **20:**519, 1979.
6. McArthur, J.: Oral contraceptives and epilepsy (notes and comments), Br. Med. J. **3:**162, 1967.
7. Kutt, H., and McDowell, F.: Management of epilepsy with diphenylhydantoin sodium, J.A.M.A. **203:**969, 1968.
8. Espir, M., and others: Epilepsy and oral contraception, Br. Med. J. **1:**294, 1969.
9. DeLeacy, E.A., and others: Effects of subjects' sex and intake of tobacco, alcohol and oral contraceptives on plasma phenytoin levels, Br. J. Clin. Pharmacol. **8:**33, 1979.
10. Hooper, W.D., and others: Plasma protein binding of diphenylhydantoin. Effects of sex hormones, renal and hepatic disease, Clin. Pharmacol. Ther. **15:**276, 1974.

Phenytoin–Phenobarbital

3

Summary: Phenobarbital may increase, decrease, or cause no change in serum phenytoin concentrations with corresponding changes in toxicity or efficacy.[1-13] However, other evidence indicates that phenobarbital levels may be increased with concomitant phenytoin.[4,7,14,15]

Related Drugs: Primidone has been shown to interact like phenobarbital with phenytoin (see Primidone-Phenytoin, p. 272) in humans.[16-18] Other hydantoin anticonvulsants (ethotoin and mephenytoin) may also interact with phenobarbital because of pharmacologic similarity, although clinical documentation is lacking. There is also no information regarding possible interactions of other barbiturates (e.g., amobarbital, butabarbital, secobarbital [see Appendix]) with phenytoin; however, they may be expected to interact in a similar manner because of similar effect on hepatic enzymes.

Mechanism: Because of conflicting data, the mechanism is difficult to determine. Phenobarbital induces hepatic microsomal enzyme activity, and this increases the rate of metabolism of phenytoin and decreases its half-life. Conversely, the 2 drugs may compete for the hepatic microsomal enzyme system, resulting in inhibition of phenytoin metabolism with an increase in phenytoin half-life.[1-6] In addition, phenobarbital levels may rise, but no mechanism has been postulated regarding this effect.

Recommendations: Concurrent phenytoin and phenobarbital therapy need not be avoided when indicated. However, the unpredictable clinical outcome of the drug interaction requires that the serum phenytoin concentrations be determined when initiating concurrent therapy, and that phenytoin and phenobarbital concentrations be determined periodically thereafter until the serum drug levels are stabilized. A determination of serum phenytoin and phenobarbital concentrations after 3 or 4 weeks of therapy may serve as a good indicator of the quality of the therapeutic regimen.[19]

Serum drug concentrations should be determined at the first sign of phenytoin or phenobarbital toxicity. The recommended serum concentration for phenytoin is 10 to 20 µg/ml[19] and 10 to 30 µg/ml for phenobarbital.[20] If toxicity occurs, phenytoin or phenobarbital should be discontinued or the dosage should be reduced until toxic signs and symptoms disappear. Then the drug can be reinstituted or the dosages can be adjusted until therapeutic concentrations are attained.

References

1. Kutt, H., and others: The effect of phenobarbital on plasma diphenylhydantoin level and metabolism in man and rat liver microsomes, Neurology **19:**611, 1969.
2. Garrettson, L.K., and Dayton, P.G.: Disappearance of phenobarbital and diphenylhydantoin from serum of children, Clin. Pharmacol. Ther. **11:**674, 1970.
3. Kristensen, M., and others: The influence of phenobarbital on the half-life of diphenylhydantoin in man, Acta Med. Scand. **185:**347, 1969.

4. Cucinell, S.A., and others: Drug interactions in man. I. Lowering effect of phenobarbital on plasma levels of bishydroxycoumarin (dicumarol) and diphenylhydantoin (dilantin), Clin. Pharmacol. Ther. **6:**420, 1965.
5. Buchanan, R., and others: The effect of phenobarbital on diphenylhydantoin metabolism in children, Pediatrics **43:**114, 1969.
6. Sotaniemi, E., and others: The clinical significance of microsomal enzyme induction in the therapy of epileptic patients, Ann. Clin. Res. **2:**223, 1970.
7. Morselli, P.L., and others: Interaction between phenobarbital and diphenylhydantoin in animals and in epileptic patients, Ann. N.Y. Acad. Sci. **179:**88, 1971.
8. Diamond, W.D., and Buchanan, R.A.: A clinical study of the effect of phenobarbital on diphenylhydantoin plasma levels, J. Clin. Pharmacol. **10:**306, 1970.
9. Booker, H.E., and others: Concurrent administration of phenobarbital and diphenylhydantoin: lack of an interference effect, Neurology **21:**383, 1971.
10. Izumi, N.: Studies on phenobarbital and diphenylhydantoin in the plasma and phenobarbital in the cerebrospinal fluid. I. The concurrent determination of phenobarbital and diphenylhydantoin in the plasma by ultraviolet spectrophotometry and its clinical application, Acta Paediatr. Jap. **74:**539, 1970.
11. Vapaatalo, H., and Lehtinen, L.: Variations of serum diphenylhydantoin concentrations in epileptic outpatients, Eur. Neurol. **5:**303, 1971.
12. Buchanan, R.A., and Allen, R.J.: Diphenylhydantoin (dilantin) and phenobarbital blood levels in epileptic children, Neurology **21:**866, 1971.
13. Weiss, C.F., and Heffelfinger, J.C.: Serial dilantin levels in mentally retarded children, Am. J. Ment. Defic. **73:**826, 1968-1969.
14. Windorfer, A., and Sauer, W.: Drug interactions during anticonvulsant therapy in childhood: diphenylhydantoin, primidone, phenobarbitone, clonazepam, nitrazepam, carbamazepine and dipropylacetate, Neuropadiatrie **8:**29, 1977.
15. Lambie, D.G., and Johnson, R.: The effects of phenytoin on phenobarbitone and primidone metabolism, J. Neurol. Neurosurg. Psychiatry **44:**148, 1981.
16. Fincham, R.W., and others: The influence of diphenylhydantoin on primidone metabolism, Arch. Neurol. **30:**259, 1974.
17. Wilson, J.T., and Wilkinson, G.R.: Chronic and severe phenobarbital intoxication in a child treated with primidone and diphenylhydantoin, J. Pediatr. **83:**484, 1973.
18. Gallagher, B.B., and others: Primidone, diphenylhydantoin and phenobarbital. Aspects of acute and chronic toxicity, Neurology **23:**145, 1973.
19. Kutt, H., and McDowell, F.: Management of epilepsy with diphenylhydantoin sodium: dosage regulation for problem patients, J.A.M.A. **203:**969, 1968.
20. Svensmark, D., and Buchthal, F.: Accumulation of phenobarbital in man, Epilepsia **4:**199, 1963.

Phenytoin—Phenylbutazone

Summary: Concurrent administration of phenytoin and phenylbutazone may result in a significant increase in the half-life, free fraction, and serum level of phenytoin in some patients.[1-7] This interaction is subject to large individual variability.

Related Drugs: Oxyphenbutazone, [1-6,8] an active metabolite of phenylbutazone, and sulfinpyrazone[9,10] have been reported to interact with phenytoin in a similar manner.

Although this effect has not been documented, other hydantoin anticonvulsants (ethotoin and mephenytoin) may interact with phenylbutazone, oxyphenbutazone, and sulfinpyrazone in a similar manner because of pharmacologic similarity.

Mechanism: Phenylbutazone, oxyphenbutazone, sulfinpyrazone, and phenytoin probably compete for the limited metabolic capacity of the microsomal hydroxylation enzymes in the liver.[11] Since phenytoin metabolism is saturable within the normal therapeutic range,[12] p-hydroxylation is impaired resulting in phenytoin accumulation and intoxication. Phenylbutazone,[5-7] oxyphenbutazone,[5,6] and sulfinpyrazone[9] also displace phenytoin from its protein binding sites, thus resulting in increased free phenytoin concentrations in the plasma, although this may be only a transitory effect. Both mechanisms are associated with large individual variability.

Recommendations: If phenylbutazone, oxyphenbutazone, or sulfinpyrazone and phenytoin are coadministered, an increase in phenytoin half-life, serum levels, or side effects may occur within the first 4 weeks of therapy, particularly when phenylbutazone, oxyphenbutazone, or sulfinpyrazone is added to the drug regimen of a patient previously stabilized on phenytoin. If signs and symptoms of phenytoin toxicity develop (e.g., nystagmus, gait ataxia, poor muscle tone, or lethargy), serum phenytoin levels should be determined and doses of phenytoin reduced to establish therapeutic levels.

References

1. Andreason, P.B., and others: Diphenylhydantoin half-life in man and its inhibition by phenylbutazone: the role of genetic factors, Acta Med. Scand. **193:**561, 1973.
2. Christensen, L.K., and Skovsted, L.: Inhibition of drug metabolism by chloramphenicol, Lancet **2:**1397, 1966.
3. Hansen, J.M., and others: Dicumarol-induced diphenylhydantoin intoxication, Lancet **2:**265, 1966.
4. Lucas, B.G.: Dilantin overdosage, Med. J. Aust. **2:**639, 1968.
5. Kurata, D., and Wilkinson, G.R.: Erythrocyte uptake and plasma binding of diphenylhydantoin, Clin. Pharmacol. Ther. **16:**355, 1974.
6. Lunde, P.K.M., and others: Plasma protein binding of diphenylhydantoin in man: interaction with other drugs and the effect of temperature and plasma dilution, Clin. Pharmacol. Ther. **11:**846, 1970.
7. Neuvonen, P.J., and others: Antipyretic analgesics in patients on antiepileptic drug therapy, Eur. J. Clin. Pharmacol. **15:**263, 1979.
8. Soda, D.M., and Levy, G.: Inhibition of drug metabolism by hydroxylated metabolites: cross-inhibition and specificity, J. Pharm. Sci. **64:**1928, 1975.

9. Pederson, A.K., and others: Clinical pharmacokinetics and potentially important drug interactions of sulphinpyrazone, Clin. Pharmacokinet. **7:**42, 1982.
10. Hansen, J.M., and others: Inhibition of phenytoin metabolism by sulfinpyrazone, World Conference on Clinical Pharmacology and Therapeutics. London, 1980, MacMillan Publishing.
11. Glasko, A.J.: Antiepileptic drugs: biotransformation, metabolism, and serum half-life, Epilepsia **16:**367, 1975.
12. Bochner, F., and others: Effects of dosage increments on blood phenytoin concentration, J. Neurol. Neurosurg. Psychiatry **35:**874, 1972.

Phenytoin–Pyridoxine

3

Summary: Large doses of pyridoxine (200 mg/day) with concurrent phenytoin may cause a marked reduction in phenytoin serum levels. In a study of epileptic patients, some patients showed up to a 50% reduction in phenytoin levels, whereas others were unaffected.[1] It is not known if smaller doses of pyridoxine would have a similar effect on phenytoin levels.

Related Drugs: No documentation is available regarding an interaction between pyridoxine and the other hydantoin anticonvulsants (ethotoin and mephenytoin). However, if the mechanism involves induction of hepatic enzymes by pyridoxine, then a similar interaction may be expected. There are no drugs related to pyridoxine.

Mechanism: The mechanism is unknown; however, it has been postulated that pyridoxine may increase the liver enzyme activity responsible for phenytoin metabolism.

Recommendations: Because not all patients appear to be affected by concurrent pyridoxine and phenytoin, these agents need not be avoided. However, the possibility of an interaction does exist, and patients should be monitored for decreased phenytoin levels or loss of seizure control during concurrent administration.

Reference

1. Hansson, O., and Sillanpaa, M.: Pyridoxine and serum concentrations of phenytoin and phenobarbitone, Lancet **1:**256, 1976.

Phenytoin–Sulfamethizole

Summary: Concurrent administration of phenytoin and sulfamethizole may result in a significant increase in the half-life and serum level of phenytoin in some patients.[1-4] This interaction is subject to large individual variability.

Related Drugs: Sulfadiazine[1,4] and sulfamethoxazole, alone[1,4] and in combination with trimethoprim,[4] have been reported to impair phenytoin metabolism and increase its half-life. Sulfisoxazole[2] does not impair phenytoin metabolism; however, sulfisoxazole[5] has been reported to displace phenytoin from its protein binding sites. Because of the variations in response to different sulfonamides, it is impossible to predict possible interactions of other sulfonamides (sulfapyridine and sulfasalazine) with phenytoin.

Although this effect has not been documented, other hydantoin anticonvulsants (ethotoin and mephenytoin) and other anticonvulsants metabolized by hepatic microsomal hydroxylation (e.g., phenobarbital and primidone) may also interact with sulfamethizole and other sulfonamides in a similar manner.

Mechanism: Sulfamethizole and phenytoin probably compete for the limited metabolic capacity of the microsomal hydroxylation enzymes in the liver.[2,3,6] Since phenytoin metabolism is saturable within the normal therapeutic range,[7] phenytoin p-hydroxylation is impaired with subsequent phenytoin accumulation and intoxication. Sulfisoxazole displaces phenytoin from its protein binding sites,[5] thus resulting in increased free phenytoin concentrations in the plasma. However, the clinical significance of this effect has not been documented. Both mechanisms are associated with large individual variability.

Recommendations: If sulfamethizole and phenytoin are coadministered, an increase in phenytoin half-life, serum levels, or side effects should occur within the first 4 weeks of therapy, particularly when the sulfonamide is added to the drug regimen of a patient previously stabilized on phenytoin. If signs and symptoms of phenytoin toxicity develop (e.g., nystagmus, gait ataxia, poor muscle tone, or lethargy) serum phenytoin levels should be determined and doses of phenytoin reduced to establish therapeutic levels.

References

1. Hansen, J.M., and others: Potentiation of warfarin by co-trimoxazole, Br. Med. J. **2:**684, 1975.
2. Siersbaek-Nelson, K., and others: Sulfamethizole-induced inhibition of diphenylhydantoin and tolbutamide metabolism in man, Clin. Pharmacol. Ther. **14:**148, 1973.
3. Lumholtz, B., and others: Sulfamethizole-induced inhibition of diphenylhydantion, tolbutamide, and warfarin metabolism, Clin. Pharmacol. Ther. **17:**731, 1975.
4. Hansen, J.M., and others: The effect of different sulfonamides on phenytoin metabolism in man, Acta Med. Scand. suppl. **624:**106, 1979.
5. Lunde, P.K.M., and others: Plasma protein binding of diphenylhydantoin in man: interaction with other durgs and the effect of temperature and plasma dilution, Clin. Pharmacol. Ther. **11:**846, 1970.
6. Glasko, A.J.: Antiepileptic drugs: biotransformation, metabolism, and serum half-life, Epilepsia **16:**367, 1975.
7. Bochner, F., and others: Effects of dosage increments on blood phenytoin concentration. J. Neurol. Neurosurg. Psychiatry **35:**874 1972.

Phenytoin–Trimethoprim

2

Summary: In a study involving 7 subjects, concurrent administration of trimethoprim and intravenous phenytoin resulted in an increased phenytoin elimination half-life and a reduced metabolic clearance rate.[1]

Related Drugs: There are no drugs related to trimethoprim. Because of pharmacologic similarity, a similar interaction may be expected between trimethoprim and the other hydantoin anticonvulsants (ethotoin and mephenytoin).

Mechanism: Trimethoprim may inhibit the hepatic metabolism of phenytoin.[1]

Recommendations: Patients should be monitored for increased phenytoin plasma levels since a lower dosage of phenytoin may be necessary during concurrent use of these agents.

Reference

1. Hansen, J.M., and others: The effect of different sulfonamides on phenytoin metabolism in man, Acta Med. Scand. suppl. **624:**106, 1979.

Phenytoin–Valproic Acid

Summary: Concurrent administration of valproic acid and phenytoin will decrease total (bound and unbound) plasma phenytoin concentrations while the percentage of free phenytoin increases.[1-12] The total plasma concentration generally returns to pre–valproic acid levels as combined therapy is continued for several more weeks.

Related Drugs: Reports indicate that ethosuximide does not undergo an interaction with valproic acid.[6,10,13-16] Valproic acid increases trimethadione serum levels,[16,17] but there is no documentation of interactions with the other nonhydantoin anticonvulsants (e.g., methsuximide, phensuximide, paramethadione). The other hydantoin anticonvulsants (ethotoin and mephenytoin) may be expected to interact with valproic acid in a similar manner to phenytoin because they are pharmacologically related. There are no drugs related to valproic acid; however, its sodium salt, sodium valproate, and divalproex sodium, a stable coordination compound containing equal proportions of valproic acid and sodium valproate, would be expected to interact in the same manner as valproic acid.

Mechanism: Valproic acid has separate and opposite effects on phenytoin disposition: (1) it displaces phenytoin from plasma protein binding sites, and (2) it reduces the clearance of the drug by inhibiting its metabolism in the liver. The first effect would be expected to enhance phenytoin elimination, shorten half-life, and increase the systemic clearance of the total drug, whereas the second would be expected to influence each of the above parameters in the opposite direction. The overall result of the interaction will depend on the combination of the two opposing trends, thus providing an explanation for the apparent lack of effect of valproic acid on phenytoin half-life and the major metabolite (HPPH) excretion, as well as for the enhancement of total drug clearance being lower than predicted from the reduction in plasma protein binding.[18]

Recommendations: Surveillance of the patient requiring both phenytoin and valproic acid for seizure control should not be limited solely to the serum concentration of total phenytoin, because measurements may grossly underestimate the concentration of free (active) drug. Dosage adjustments should be determined by clinical signs of over- or underdose. Phenytoin serum levels should be determined before valproic acid is administered. After valproic acid is given, a change in serum concentration of phenytoin is cited to determine any phenytoin dose adjustments that might be necessary. The measurement of free (active) phenytoin levels should provide a better therapeutic guide than total serum concentrations.[5] The serum concentration of free phenytoin should be determined by ultrafiltration methods[19] or by using saliva samples.[3,12] One report shows that free phenytoin concentrations follow a diurnal variation,[20] suggesting that monitoring should occur at the same time each day.

References

1. Bruni, J., and others: Interactions of valproic acid with phenytoin, Neurology **30:**1233, 1980.
2. Brady, A., and others: Valproate may lower serum phenytoin, Lancet **2:**1297, 1976.

3. Mattson, R.H., and others: Valproic acid in epilepsy: clinical and pharmacological effects, Ann. Neurol. **3:**20, 1978.
4. Adams, D.J., and others: Sodium valproate in the treatment of intractable seizure disorders: a clinical and electroencephalographic study, Neurology **28:**152, 1978.
5. Keys, P.A.: Valproic acid: interactions with phenytoin and phenobarbital, Drug Intell. Clin. Pharm. **16:**737, 1982.
6. Wilder, B.J., and others: Valproic acid: interaction with other anticonvulsant drugs, Neurology **28:**892, 1978.
7. Bruni, J., and others: Valproic acid and plasma levels of phenytoin, Neurology **29:**904, 1979.
8. Friel, P.N., and others: Valproic acid-phenytoin interaction, Ther. Drug Monit. **1:**243, 1979.
9. Monks, A., and Richens, A.: Effect of single doses of sodium valproate on serum phenytoin levels and protein binding in epileptic patients, Clin. Pharmacol. Ther. **27:**89, 1980.
10. Gram, L., and others: Valproate sodium: a controlled clinical trial including monitoring of drug levels, Epilepsia **18:**141, 1977.
11. Bruni, J., and Wilder, B.J.: Valproic acid: review of a new antiepileptic drug, Arch. Neurol. **36:**393, 1979.
12. Knott, C., and others: Phenytoin-valproate interaction: importance of saliva monitoring in epilepsy, Br. Med. J. **284:**13, 1982.
13. Gugler, R., and von Unruh, G.E.: Clinical pharmacokinetics of valproic acid, Clin. Pharmacokinet. **5:**67, 1980.
14. Bauer, L.A., and others: Ethosuximide kinetics: possible interaction with valproic acid, Clin. Pharmacol. Ther. **31:**741, 1982.
15. Mattson, R.H., and Cramer, J.A.: Valproic acid and ethosuximide interaction, Ann. Neurol. **7:**583, 1980.
16. Flachs, H., and others: Drug levels of other antiepileptic drugs during concomitant treatment with sodium valproate, Epilepsia **20:**187, 1979.
17. Gram, L., and others: Sodium valproate, relationship between serum levels and therapeutic effect: a controlled study. In Johannssen, S.I., and others, editors: Antiepileptic therapy: advances in drug monitoring. New York, 1980, Raven Press.
18. Perucca, E., and others: Interaction between phenytoin and valproic acid: plasma binding and metabolic effects, Clin. Pharmacol. Ther. **28:**779, 1980.
19. Levy, R.H., and Koch, K.M.: Drug interactions with valproic acid, Drugs **24:**543, 1982.
20. Haidukewych, D., and Rodin, E.A.: Serial free and plasma valproic acid and phenytoin monitoring and drug interactions, Ther. Drug Monit. **3:**303, 1981.

Primidone–Acetazolamide

3

Summary: Concurrent administration primidone and acetazolamide has been reported to decrease or delay the absorption of primidone.[1] When acetazolamide was withdrawn from therapy, primidone absorption was improved.

Related Drugs: Although primidone is metabolized to phenobarbital, an interaction between acetazolamide and long-acting barbiturates often used as anticonvulsants (phenobarbital and mephobarbital) has not been reported. No documentation exists regarding an interaction between acetazolamide and other barbiturates (e.g., amobarbital, butabarbital, secobarbital [see Appendix]). Similarly, no reports have appeared of barbiturate interaction with other carbonic anhydrase inhibitors (ethoxzolamide, dichlorphenamide, and methazolamide).

Mechanism: The mechanism is not known. It does appear that acetazolamide decreases the gastrointestinal absorption of primidone as contrasted to increasing primidone's metabolism.

Recommendations: Patients receiving these agents concomitantly should be monitored for decreases in primidone and/or phenobarbital serum concentrations, or lack of seizure control.

Reference

1. Syversen, G.B., and others: Acetazolamide-induced interference with primidone absorption, Arch. Neurol. **34:**80, 1977.

Primidone–Phenytoin

2

Summary: Concomitant phenytoin therapy increases the plasma concentrations of phenobarbital derived from metabolism of primidone.[1-9] However, concurrent use of phenytoin only slightly decreases primidone plasma concentrations[1-8,10]; likewise, primidone had little influence on phenytoin levels[2,3,10] but may increase phenytoin clearance slightly.[9]

Related Drugs: Ethosuximide had no effect on primidone levels,[1,5] but primidone caused a slight increase in ethosuximide levels.[5] Ethosuximide did not influence phenobarbital derived from primidone.[1,5] Methsuximide increased primidone levels and phenobarbital levels derived from primidone in 4 patients receiving other anticonvulsants.[11] Phenobarbital, when administered as the parent drug, has been shown to interact with phenytoin (see Phenytoin-Phenobarbital, p. 262).

Although documentation is lacking, an interaction may be expected between primidone and the other hydantoin anticonvulsants (ethotoin and mephenytoin) because the other hydantoin anticonvulsants have a similar effect on hepatic enzymes.

Mechanism: Two mechanisms have been proposed. The first suggests that phenytoin induces the microsomal enzymes responsible for the oxidation of primidone to phenobarbital. This hypothesis is supported by the slight decrease seen in primidone levels and a reported increased primidone clearance.[12] It has been postulated that the degree of change in primidone levels indicates that phenytoin inhibits phenobarbital metabolism, excretion, or both thus leading to phenobarbital accumulation.[1,4]

Recommendations: Because these agents are often administered together successfully, their concurrent use need not be avoided. However, patients taking phenytoin and primidone concurrently should be monitored to assure effective anticonvulsant control. Additionally, they may have to be monitored for possible phenobarbital toxicity.

References:

1. Schmidt, D.: The effect of phenytoin and ethosuximide on primidone metabolism in patients with epilepsy, J. Neurol. **209:**115, 1975.
2. Fincham, R.W., and others: The influence of diphenylhydantoin on primidone metabolism, Trans. Am. Neurol. Assoc. **98:**197, 1973.
3. Fincham, R.W., and others: The influence of diphenylhydantoin on primidone metabolism, Arch. Neurol. **30:**259, 1974.
4. Reynolds, E.H., and others: Interaction of phenytoin and primidone, Br. Med. J. **2:**594, 1975.
5. Battino, D., and others: Plasma levels of primidone and its metabolite phenobarbital: effect of age and associated therapy, Ther. Drug Monit. **5:**73, 1983.
6. Callaghan, N., and others: The effect of anticonvulsant drugs which induce liver microsomal enzymes on derived and ingested phenobarbitone levels, Acta Neurol. Scand. **56:**1, 1977.
7. Porro, M.G., and others: Phenytoin: an inhibitor and inducer of primidone metabolism in an epileptic patient, Br. J. Clin. Pharmacol. **14:**294, 1982.

8. Porro, G., and others: In vivo effects of phenytoin on primidone metabolism: an enzymatic induction and/or competitive inhibition?, Pharmacologist **23:**194, 1981.
9. Van der Kleijn, E., and others: Kinetics of drug interactions in the treatment of epilepsy, Int. J. Clin. Pharmacol. **16:**467, 1978.
10. Windorfer, A., and Sauer, W.: Drug interactions during anticonvulsant therapy in childhood: diphenyl-hydantoin, primidone, phenobarbitone, clonazepam, nitrazepam, carbamazepine and dipropyl-acetate, Neuropadiatrie **8:**29, 1977.
11. Browne, T.R., and others: Methsuximide for complex partial seizures: efficacy, toxicity, clinical pharmacology, and drug interactions, Neurology **33:**414, 1983.
12. Cloyd, J.C., and others: Primidone kinetics: effects of concurrent drugs and duration of therapy, Clin. Pharmacol. Ther. **29:**402, 1981.

Valproic Acid–Aluminum Hydroxide, Magnesium Hydroxide

3

Summary: In one study involving 7 healthy volunteers, a 500 mg dose of valproic acid was given with a dose of an aluminum hydroxide–magnesium hydroxide antacid preparation. The bioavailability of valproic acid was significantly increased as the area-under-curve increased by a mean of 12%. There is a potential for increased steady-state serum levels with this interaction; however, none of the reported side effects of valproic acid are serum level dependent. Whether this increase is clinically significant at steady state remains to be determined.[1]

Related Drugs: The same study also reported use of valproic acid concurrently with a calcium carbonate/glycine antacid and an aluminum/magnesium trisilicate antacid. Although there was a trend toward an increase in the valproic acid area-under-curve, the increases did not reach statistical significance.[1] No drugs are related to valproic acid; however, its sodium salt, sodium valproate, and divalproex sodium, a stable coordination compound containing equal proportions of valproic acid and sodium valproate, may be expected to interact similarly.

Mechanism: The mechanism of this interaction is unknown. However, the aluminum/magnesium hydroxide antacid increased the bioavailability of valproic acid because of an increase in F/V (fraction of the dose absorbed/volume of distribution), probably as a result of an increase in the dose absorbed.[1]

Recommendations: Whether this interaction is clinically significant with steady state valproic acid therapy or with smaller amounts of antacids is not known. Since antacids are often recommended to relieve gastrointestinal symptoms common to valproic acid administration (indigestion, nausea and vomiting, cramps, diarrhea, etc.), it is important to monitor patients closely for signs of valproic acid toxicity when antacids are used concurrently.

Reference

1. May, C.A., and others: Effects of three antacids on the bioavailability of valproic acid, Clin. Pharm. **1:**244, 1982.

Valproic Acid–Aspirin

3

Summary: In a study involving 6 epileptic children taking valproic acid, concurrent aspirin led to an increase in serum valproic acid free fraction and an increased half-life. Renal clearance of free valproic acid was found to decrease.[1] In another study involving 5 children, concurrent valproic acid and aspirin resulted in a decrease in free valproic acid clearance although total valproic acid levels did not change significantly.[2] These studies indicate that the therapeutic and toxic effects of valproic acid may be increased. However, 1 study reported that the concurrent use of valproic acid and aspirin leads to an increased excretion of valproic acid and a decreased total salicylate excretion.[3] The clinical significance was not determined.

Related Drugs: No documentation exists regarding an interaction between valproic acid and the other salicylates (e.g., choline salicylate, salicylamide, sodium salicylate [see Appendix]), although because of pharmacologic similarity a similar interaction may be expected. There are no drugs related to valproic acid; however, its sodium salt, sodium valproate, and divalproex sodium, a stable coordination compound containing equal proportions of valproic acid and sodium valproate, would be expected to interact similarly.

Mechanism: Aspirin appears to not only displace valproic acid from serum albumin but also to alter valproic acid metabolism and elimination.[1] It has been suggested that salicylic acid competes for active transport sites in the renal tubules or liver.[2] Regarding the increased valproic acid excretion, it has been suggested that aspirin displaces valproic acid from plasma proteins, thus more unbound valproic acid is available for excretion. However, it has also been suggested that aspirin increases only glucuronide excretion, inhibiting the conjugation of valproic acid.[3] This finding would be more consistent with the results of the other studies, since plasma valproic acid was not measured.

Recommendations: Patients receiving these agents concurrently should be closely monitored for valproic acid toxicity. The dose of valproic acid may have to be decreased.

References

1. Orr, J.M., and others: Interaction between valproic acid and aspirin in epileptic children: serum protein binding and metabolic effects, Clin. Pharmacol. Ther. **31**:642, 1982.
2. Farrell, K., and others: The effect of acetylsalisylic acid on serum free valproate concentrations and valproate clearance in children, J. Pediatr. **101**:142, 1982.
3. Schobben, F., and others: Pharmacokinetics, metabolism and distribution of 2-N-propyl-pentanoate (sodium valproate) and the influence of salicylate comedication. In Meinardi and Rowan, editors: Advances in epileptology. Amsterdam, 1977, Swets and Zectlinger Publishers.

Valproic Acid–Carbamazepine

2

Summary: Concurrent use of carbamazepine and valproic acid results in a decrease in serum valproic acid concentrations.[1-6] Valproic acid may cause an increase in serum carbamazepine concentrations,[5-8] but some studies reported no effect.[9-12]

Related Drugs: Interactions with valproic acid and other anticonvulsants are discussed in other monographs. There are no drugs related to valproic acid; however, its sodium salt, sodium valproate, and divalproex sodium, a stable coordination compound containing equal proportions of valproic acid and sodium valproate, would be expected to interact similarly.

Mechanism: Carbamazepine is thought to induce hepatic microsomal enzymes, thereby enhancing the metabolism of valproic acid.[1,3,4,13] Concomitant valproic acid causes increased carbamazepine epoxide levels,[5,6,11] but does not produce a consistent effect on the parent carbamazepine. It is not clearly determined how valproate reduces the elimination of the epoxide metabolite.

Recommendations: Serum valproic acid determinations may be helpful in assessing the need of changing the valproic acid dosage when carbamazepine is added to or withdrawn from valproate therapy. There is not enough documentation to substantiate a need to reduce carbamazepine dosage in the presence of valproic acid.

References

1. Bowdle, T.A., and others: Effects of carbamazepine on valproic acid kinetics in normal subjects, Clin. Pharmacol. Ther. **26:**629, 1979.
2. Sackellares, J.C., and others: Reduction of steady-state valproic levels by other antiepileptic drugs, Epilepsia **22:**437, 1981.
3. Mihaly, G.W., and others: Single and chronic dose pharmacokinetic studies of sodium valproate in epileptic patients, Eur. J. Clin. Pharmacol. **16:**23, 1979.
4. Reunanen, M.I., and others: Low serum valproic acid concentrations in epileptic patients on combination therapy, Curr. Ther. Res. **28:**456, 1980.
5. Gugler, R., and von Unruh, G.E.: Clinical pharmacokinetics of valproic acid, Clin. Pharmacokinet. **5:**67, 1980.
6. Perucca, E.: Pharmacokinetic interactions with antiepileptic drugs, Clin. Pharmacokinet. **7:**57, 1982.
7. Jeavons, P.M., and Clark, J.E.: Sodium valproate in treatment of epilepsy, Br. Med. J. **2:**584, 1974.
8. Mattson, G.F., and others: Interaction between valproic acid and carbamazepine: an in vitro study of protein binding, Ther. Drug Monit. **4:**181, 1982.
9. Flachs, H., and others: Drug levels of other antiepileptic drugs during concomitant treatment with sodium valproate, Epilepsia **20:**187, 1979.
10. Wilder, B.J., and others: Valproate acid: interaction with other anticonvulsant drugs, Neurology **28:**892, 1978.
11. McKauge, L., and others: Factors influencing simultaneous concentratons of carbamazepine and its epoxide in plasma, Ther. Drug Monit. **3:**63, 1981.
12. Gram, L., and others: Valproate sodium: a controlled clinical trial including monitoring of drug levels, Epilepsia **18:**141, 1977.
13. Levy, R.H., and Koch, K.M.: Drug interactions with valproic acid, Drugs **24:**543, 1982.

Valproic Acid–Clonazepam

3

Summary: Concurrent administration of clonazepam and valproic acid does not appear to cause any alterations in plasma concentrations of either drug.[1-5] However, a few reports do state that absence seizures developed in some patients receiving these agents concomitantly and drowsiness developed in other patients.[6-8]

Related Drugs: Drowsiness occurred in 4 patients receiving nitrazepam* and valproic acid,[9] which rapidly disappeared on nitrazepam reduction. It has been reported that valproic acid increases the free diazepam serum concentration[10] and inhibits diazepam metabolism.[10,11] There is no documentation regarding an interaction between valproic acid and other benzodiazepines (e.g., chlordiazepoxide, flurazepam, triazolam [see Appendix]); however, a similar interaction may be expected as a result of pharmacologic similarity. No drugs are related to valproic acid; however, its sodium salt, sodium valproate, and divalproex sodium, a stable coordination compound containing equal proportions of valproic acid and sodium valproate, would be expected to interact similarly.

Mechanism: The mechanism is not adequately proved. Drowsiness may be the result of an increase in the benzodiazepines' serum levels since 2 reports indicate that valproic acid may inhibit the metabolism of diazepam.[10,11] Also, valproic acid increased the unbound fraction of diazepam from 1.8% to 3.9% in vitro[12] and from 1.75% to 3.36% in vivo.[10]

Recommendations: The incidence of this interaction is expected to be low. Nevertheless, it should be considered a possibility when these agents are used together. If drowsiness occurs, reduction of the clonazepam dosage may be required.

References

1. Wilder, B.J., and others: Valproic acid: interaction with other anticonvulsant drugs, Neurology **28:**892, 1978.
2. Gram, L., and others: Valproate sodium: a controlled clinical trial including monitoring of drug levels, Epilepsia **18:**141, 1977.
3. Gugler, R., and von Unruh, G.E.: Clinical pharmacokinetics of valproic acid, Clin. Pharmacokinet. **5:**67, 1980.
4. Flachs, H., and others: Drug levels of other antiepileptic drugs during concomitant treatment with sodium valproate, Epilepsia **20:**187, 1979.
5. Baruzzi, A., and others: Plasma levels of di-n-propylacetate and clonazepam in epileptic patients, Int. J. Clin. Pharmacol. Biopharm. **15:**403, 1977.
6. Watson, W.A.: Interaction between clonazepam and sodium valproate, N. Engl. J. Med. **300:**678, 1979.
7. Browne, T.R.: Interaction between clonazepam and sodium valproate (reply), N. Engl. J. Med. **300:**678, 1979.
8. Jeavons, P.M., and others: Treatment of generalized epilepsies of childhood and adolescence with sodium valproate ("Epilim"), Dev. Med. Child Neurol. **19:**9, 1977.
9. Jeavons, P.M., and Clark, J.E.: Sodium valproate in treatment of epilepsy, Br. Med. J. **2:**584, 1974.

*Not available in the U.S.

10. Dhillon, S., and Richens, A.: Valproic acid and diazepam interaction in vitro, Br. J. Clin. Pharmacol. **13:**553, 1982.
11. Perucca, E: Pharmacokinetic interactions with antiepileptic drugs, Clin. Pharmacokinet. **7:**57, 1982.
12. Dhillon, S., and Richens, A.: Serum protein binding of diazepam and its displacement by valproic acid in vitro, Br. J. Clin. Pharmacol. **12:**591, 1981.

CHAPTER SIX

Antidepressant Drug Interactions

TABLE 6. Antidepressant Drug Interactions

Drug Interaction	Significance Code	Potential Effects	Recommendations	See Page
Amitriptyline–Chlordiazepoxide	3	Concurrent use may impair motor function and enhance the anticholinergic action of amitriptyline.	Advise patients of possible enhanced CNS depression.	282
Amitriptyline–Disulfiram	3	Concurrent use may cause acute organic brain syndrome including confusion and overt psychotic symptoms.	If signs or symptoms of acute organic brain syndrome develop, one or both drugs may need to be withdrawn.	283
Doxepin–Propoxyphene	3	Doxepin levels may rise to more than twice initial plasma levels, resulting in increased CNS side effects.	Monitor patients for increased CNS effects. Decrease the doxepin dosage or withdraw propoxyphene if needed.	284
Imipramine–Chlorpromazine	3	Concurrent use may increase serum concentrations of either drug.	Monitor for toxicity of both drugs; make dosage adjustments as needed.	285
Imipramine–Cimetidine	3	Cimetidine may alter the clearance of imipramine, resulting in increased serum concentrations and adverse effects.	Reduce the imipramine dosage if adverse effects occur.	287
Imipramine–Epinephrine	1	Epinephrine exerts enhanced cardiovascular effects when given with imipramine.	Avoid concurrent use, but if concomitant therapy is necessary lower the initial dose of epinephrine.	289
Imipramine–Ethinyl Estradiol	3	Patients on ethinyl estradiol may be resistant to imipramine therapy. Concurrent use is associated with a higher incidence of side effects.	Monitor for lack of therapeutic effect or imipramine toxicity, and adjust the dosage if needed.	291
Imipramine–Levodopa	3	Concurrent use may reduce levodopa absorption, although the clinical significance of this is undetermined.	Concomitant use need not be avoided since they have been used successfully and uneventfully. However, levodopa dosage adjustment may be needed.	293
Imipramine–Liothyronine	2	Liothyronine may enhance and accelerate the antidepressant action in euthyroid patients.	Patients who fail to respond to antidepressant therapy should be examined for hypothyroidism and considered for concurrent therapy.	294
Imipramine–Methyltestosterone	3	Concurrent use may cause paranoid reactions that resolve when methyltestosterone is discontinued.	If a paranoid reaction occurs, one or both drugs may need to be withdrawn.	295

Abbreviations: CNS, central nervous system.

TABLE 6. Antidepressant Drug Interactions—cont'd

Drug Interaction	Significance Code	Potential Effects	Recommendations	See Page
Imipramine–Reserpine	3	Reserpine induces a response in patients refractory to tricyclic antidepressant therapy.	Use concurrently in only the most recalcitrant patients, and then only if potential therapeutic gain outweighs the risk of adverse effects.	296
Imipramine–Tranylcypromine	2	Although severe toxic and fatal reactions have occurred with concurrent use, numerous studies report beneficial and uneventful co-therapy.	Use concurrently only in carefully selected patients who have not responded to conventional therapy. Monitor closely.	297
Nortriptyline–Phenobarbital	3	Phenobarbital may decrease serum concentrations of nortriptyline within a few days on initiating co-therapy, although the change in therapeutic activity has not been correlated to the decreased serum levels.	A benzodiazepine may be considered instead of phenobarbital since they do not affect the metabolism of tricyclic antidepressants.	298
Phenelzine–Levodopa	1	Levodopa causes a significant rise in blood pressure, flushing, and palpitations when used with phenelzine. Phenelzine increases dopamine levels in peripheral tissue and brain, and levodopa increases CNS dopamine levels, which may enhance spontaneous motor activity.	Avoid concurrent use. Alternatively a tricyclic antidepressant or a carbidopa-levodopa combination can be given.	299
Tranylcypromine–Phenylpropanolamine	1	Concurrent use may cause abrupt elevation of blood pressure, resulting in a potentially fatal hypertensive crisis.	Patients given tranylcypromine should be instructed to avoid indirect-acting sympathomimetics in any form. Treat marked elevation in blood pressure with phentolamine.	300
Tranylcypromine–Propranolol	4	No clinically significant interaction occurs with these drugs. One study suggests that tranylcypromine be withdrawn at least 2 weeks before propranolol is started, but this is a theoretical consideration.	Concurrent use need not be avoided.	302

Amitriptyline–Chlordiazepoxide

3

Summary: The concurrent administration of amitriptyline and chlordiazepoxide has been reported to cause impairment of motor function in at least 3 patients,[1,2] and chlordiazepoxide may enhance the anticholinergic action of the tricyclic antidepressant.

Related Drugs: No documentation exists concerning a similar interaction between other tricyclic antidepressants (e.g., desipramine, imipramine, nortriptyline [see Appendix]) or the tetracyclic antidepressant (maprotiline) and other benzodiazepines (e.g., clonazepam, diazepam, oxazepam [see Appendix]), although because of pharmacologic similarity, the same interaction may be expected to occur.

Mechanism: The mechanism is unknown. However, it is postulated that the effects of amitriptyline and other tricyclic antidepressants enhance the sedation produced by chlordiazepoxide. Two clinical studies[3,4] measured the effect of a benzodiazepine (chlordiazepoxide, diazepam, or oxazepam) on the serum levels of a tricyclic antidepressant (amitriptyline or nortriptyline). No detectable change in the serum levels of the tricyclic antidepressant occurred.

Recommendations: Although the occurrence of a clinically significant interaction appears uncommon, patients receiving these drugs concurrently should be advised of the possibility of enhanced central nervous system depression. Concurrent administration of these drugs has been suggested[5,6] for the treatment of depression with concurrent anxiety, but the therapeutic efficacy of such treatment in depression has not proved to be superior to the tricyclic antidepressant alone.[7]

References

1. Kane, F.J., and Taylor, T.W.: A toxic reaction to combined elavil-librium therapy, Am. J. Psychiatry **119:**1179, 1963.
2. Abdou, F.A.: Elavil-Librium combination, Am. J. Psychiatry **120:**1204, 1964.
3. Silverman, G., and Braithwaite, R.A.: Benzodiazepines and tricyclic antidepressant plasma levels, Br. Med. J. **3:**18, 1973.
4. Gram, L.F., and others: Influence of neuroleptics and benzodiazepines on metabolism of tricyclic antidepressants in man, Am. J. Psychol. **131:**863, 1974.
5. Kline, N.S.: Psychochemotherapeutic drug combinations, J.A.M.A. **210:**1928, 1969.
6. Hare, H.P.: Comparison of chlordiazepoxide-amitriptyline combination with amitriptyline alone in anxiety-depressive states, J. Clin. Pharmacol. New Drugs **11:**456, 1971.
7. Greenblatt, D.J., and Shader, R.I.: Benzodiazepines in clinical practice, New York, 1974, Raven Press.

Amitriptyline–Disulfiram

3

Summary: Two patients developed acute organic brain syndrome, including confusion and overt psychotic symptoms, when amitriptyline was added to their disulfiram therapy. The symptoms occurred within 1 to 4 weeks after initiation of therapy, and a rapid improvement was seen after withdrawal of one or both agents.[1]

Related Drugs: There are no drugs related to disulfiram. There is a lack of documentation regarding a similar interaction between disulfiram and the other tricyclic antidepressants (e.g., doxepin, imipramine, protriptyline [see Appendix]), however, because of pharmacologic similarity they may be expected to interact in a similar manner.

Mechanism: The mechanism of this interaction is unknown. However, both disulfiram and amitriptyline administration may lead to elevated levels of various monoamines, and potentially to increased dopamine levels, which have been postulated to result in organic brain syndromes and psychoses. It has been suggested that the effects seen in the 2 case studies were potentiated by the combined action of the 2 drugs and the synergistic elevation in dopamine levels.[1]

Recommendations: Although a cause and effect relationship has never been clearly established, if signs or symptoms of acute organic brain syndrome develop it is prudent to discontinue one or both drugs.

Reference

1. Maany, I., and others: Possible toxic interaction between disulfiram and amitriptyline, Arch. Gen. Psychiatry **39:**743, 1982.

Doxepin–Propoxyphene

3

Summary: In a case report, the concurrent use of propoxyphene and doxepin in a patient resulted in doxepin levels that rose to more than twice the initial plasma levels, and the patient became progressively lethargic. Within 5 days after propoxyphene was discontinued, the patient's mental status returned to control levels.[1]

Related Drugs: Documentation is lacking regarding an interaction between propoxyphene and the other tricyclic antidepressants (e.g., amitriptyline, amoxapine, imipramine [see Appendix]) and the tetracyclic antidepressant (maprotiline) although because of pharmacologic similarity a similar interaction may be expected. There is also no documentation regarding a similar interaction between doxepin and the other narcotic analgesics (e.g., codeine, meperidine, morphine [see Appendix]).

Mechanism: It has been suggested that propoxyphene inhibits the hepatic metabolism of doxepin.[1]

Recommendations: Further studies are necessary to confirm the interaction; however, patients should be monitored for increased central nervous system side effects. The dose of doxepin may have to be decreased or propoxyphene may need to be discontinued.

Reference

1. Abernathy, D.R., and others: Impairment of hepatic drug oxidation by propoxyphene, Ann. Intern. Med. **97:**223, 1982.

Imipramine–Chlorpromazine

3

Summary: The concurrent use of imipramine and chlorpromazine may result in increased serum concentrations of either drug.[1-3] The clinical significance of this interaction has not been evaluated.

Related Drugs: Perphenazine, haloperidol (a butyrophenone), and thiothixene (a thioxanthene) have been shown to inhibit the metabolism of imipramine and nortriptyline in humans,[1,2,4] and desipramine has been shown to elevate serum butaperazine concentrations.[3] Various phenothiazines, when added to the regimen of patients receiving either amitriptyline or nortriptyline, caused an increase in the serum concentration of nortriptyline but no effect was shown in the concentration of amitriptyline.[5] Fluphenazine has been shown in 4 patients to increase the plasma concentrations of the parent antidepressant compound and its metabolite (the imipramine/desipramine ratio), exceeding the therapeutic threshold.[6] When nortriptyline was added to the regimen of patients receiving chlorpromazine, serum concentrations of chlorpromazine were increased as were the adverse effects of orthostatic hypotension and tachycardia. However, the therapeutic effect of chlorpromazine was diminished.[7] Because of pharmacologic similarity it is possible that similar effects occur when other phenothiazines (e.g., promazine, thioridazine, trifluoperazine [see Appendix]), the other thioxanthene (chlorprothixene), as well as the dihydroindolone (molindone) and dibenzoxazepine (loxapine) are given concurrently with other tricyclic antidepressants (e.g., amoxapine, doxepin, trimipramine [see Appendix]) or the tetracyclic antidepressant (maprotiline).

Mechanism: The mechanism whereby imipramine increases chlorpromazine concentrations has not been reported. However, perphenazine has been shown to inhibit the hydroxylation and/or glucuronide formation of imipramine, resulting in an increased tissue concentration of imipramine and its metabolites desipramine and iminodibenzyl in rats.[8] It was also demonstrated that perphenazine and chlorpromazine were equally potent with regard to increased tissue concentration of imipramine, presumably by the same mechanism.[8] It has also been suggested that these agents compete for the cytochrome P-450 enzyme system, which metabolizes both compounds in the liver.[6]

Recommendations: Patients should be observed closely for any unexpected toxicities (e.g., extrapyramidal effects, blurred vision, dry mouth, constipation, orthostatic changes, and drowsiness) when receiving imipramine and chlorpromazine concurrently. If adverse effects do occur, the dose of imipramine or chlorpromazine should be adjusted or discontinued.

References

1. Gram, L.F., and Over, K.F.: Drug interaction: inhibiting effect of neuroleptics on metabolism of tricyclic antidepressants in man, Br. Med. J. **1**:463, 1972.
2. Gram, L.F., and others: Influence of neuroleptics and benzodiazepines on metabolism of tricyclic antidepressants in man, Am. J. Psychiatry **131**:863, 1974.

3. El-Yousef, M.K., and Manier, D.H.: Tricyclic antidepressants and phenothiazines, J.A.M.A. **229:**1419, 1974.
4. Nelson, J.C., and Jatlow, P.I.: Neuroleptic effect on desipramine steady-state plasma concentrations, Am. J. Psychiatry **137:**1232, 1980.
5. Vandel, B., and others: Interaction between amitriptyline and phenothiazine in man: effect on plasma concentration of amitriptyline and its metabolite nortriptyline and the correlation with clinical response, Psychopharmacol. Bull. **65:**187, 1979.
6. Siris, S.G., and others: Concomitant flurphenazine decanoate, Am. J. Psychiatry **139:**104, 1982.
7. Loga, S., and others: Interaction of chlorpromazine and nortriptyline in patients with schizophrenia, Clin. Pharmacokinet. **6:**454, 1981.
8. Gram, L.F., and others: Pharmacokinetic interaction between neuroleptics and tricyclic antidepressants in the rat, Acta Pharmacol. Toxicol. **35:**223, 1974.

Imipramine–Cimetidine

3

Summary: Cimetidine may alter the clearance of imipramine, resulting in increased serum concentrations and consequent anticholinergic adverse effects (e.g., blurred vision, dizziness, dry mouth, orthostatic hypotension, urinary retention).[1] A patient on concurrent therapy with these agents was switched to desipramine because of the occurrence of dry mouth and urinary hesitancy. However, the side effects increased and imipramine was again given in place of desipramine, both alone and with cimetidine. In the presence of cimetidine, the elimination half-life increased and clearance of imipramine decreased. Also, the mean concentration of imipramine plus desipramine was higher.[1] In another study involving 6 healthy volunteers, cimetidine increased the half-life of intravenous imipramine by 43% and reduced its clearance by 41%.[2] Similar results were reported in 2 other case studies.[3,4] One patient showed a 58% decrease in imipramine concentration when cimetidine was discontinued.

Related Drugs: In a case report, a patient receiving cimetidine and nortriptyline showed a decreased nortriptyline steady-state serum concentration (from 104 mg/L to 75 mg/L) after the discontinuation of cimetidine. When cimetidine was again administered, the nortriptyline serum concentration increased to 120 mg/L after 6 days.[5] Six volunteers had increased plasma levels of nortriptyline's major metabolite (10-hydroxynortriptyline) after cimetidine pretreatment; however, nortriptyline pharmacokinetics were not significantly affected.[3] Also, a case report describes a male patient who developed breast cancer after concurrent doxepin and cimetidine.[6] It has been suggested that the interaction in this patient resulted from the combined hyperplastic effects of each agent; however, more study is needed. Documentation is lacking regarding an interaction between cimetidine and the other tricyclic antidepressants (e.g., amitriptyline, amoxapine, protriptyline [see Appendix]), although because of pharmacologic similarity a similar interaction may be expected.

There is no documentation regarding a similar interaction between imipramine and the other H_2 receptor antagonist (ranitidine). However, if the mechanism involves inhibition of hepatic metabolism by cimetidine, then ranitidine would not be expected to interact similarly.

Mechanism: It has been postulated that cimetidine suppresses the conversion of imipramine to desipramine,[1] possibly by inhibition of hepatic metabolism. A pharmacokinetic interaction has been supported by a controlled study involving 6 healthy volunteers.[2]

Recommendations: If the anticholinergic adverse effects or toxicity of imipramine become apparent, a decreased dose of imipramine or other tricyclic antidepressants may be necessary. Also, if cimetidine is discontinued in a patient receiving a tricyclic antidepressant, the patient should be monitored for a decreased response to the antidepressant.

References

1. Miller, D.D., and Macklin, M.: Cimetidine–imipramine interaction: a case report, Am. J. Psychiatry **140:**351, 1983.
2. Abernathy, D.R., and others: Imipramine–cimetidine interaction: impairment of clearance and enhanced bioavailability, Clin. Pharmacol. Ther. **33:**237, 1983.
3. Henauer, A.A., and Hollister, L.E.: Cimetidine interaction with imipramine and nortriptyline, Clin. Pharmacol. Ther. **35:**183, 1984.
4. Shapiro, P.A.: Cimetidine–imipramine interaction: case report and comments, Am. J. Psychiatry **141:**152, 1984.
5. Miller, D.D., and others: Cimetidine's effect on steady-state serum nortriptyline concentrations, Drug Intell. Clin. Pharm. **17:**904, 1983.
6. Smedley, H.M.: Malignant breast change in man given two drugs associated with breast hyperplasia, Lancet **2:**638, 1981.

Imipramine–Epinephrine

1

Summary: Epinephrine and other direct-acting sympathomimetic amines exert enhanced cardiovascular effects (e.g., arrhythmias, hypertension, and tachycardia) in individuals concurrently receiving or previously treated with imipramine or other tricyclic antidepressants.

Related Drugs: Other direct and mixed acting sympathomimetic amines have also been reported to interact with tricyclic antidepressants. These include norepinephine, phenylephrine, dopamine, and methoxamine.[1-5]

The pressor effects of the indirect-acting sympathomimetic amines (i.e., amphetamines, ephedrine, methylphenidate, pseudoephedrine, and tyramine) are antagonized by tricyclic antidepressants.[5-9] Maprotiline, a tetracyclic antidepressant, has been shown to cause a 3-fold reduction in tyramine sensitivity in 3 healthy volunteers.[10]

Protriptyline, amitriptyline, and desipramine have also been reported to interact with direct-acting sympathomimetics.[3,5,6] Other tricyclic antidepressants (e.g., amoxapine, trimipramine, nortriptyline [see Appendix]) may be expected to interact in a manner similar to imipramine because of pharmacologic similarity. Maprotiline did not consistently alter the pressor response to norephinephrine infusions in one study.[10]

Mechanism: Epinephrine and other direct-acting sympathomimetic amines would be expected to have an enhanced effect because tricyclic antidepressants block the reuptake of norepinephrine, resulting in an increased concentration at receptor sites.[5,11] Indirect-acting sympathomimetic amines, which require uptake into the adrenergic neuron to produce their effects, are blocked by the tricyclic antidepressants, thus their effect is antagonized.[3,7,9] The cardiovascular effects of mixed-acting sympathomimetics in the presence of tricyclic antidepressants would depend on the ratio of direct to indirect activity.

Recommendations: The concurrent use of epinephrine or other direct acting sympathomimetic amines and tricyclic antidepressants should be avoided. When concurrent therapy is necessary, the initial dose of the sympathomimetic should be lowered, and the patient should be carefully monitored for adverse cardiovascular effects.

References

1. Boakes, A,J., and others: Interactions between sympathomimetic amines and antidepressasnt agents in man, Br. Med. J. **1:**311, 1973.
2. Svedmyr, N.: The influence of a tricyclic antidepressant agent (protriptyline) on some of the circulating effects of noradrenaline and adrenaline in man, Life Sci. **7:**77, 1968.
3. Bonaccorsi, A., and Garattini, S.: Effect of desipramine on directly or indirectly elicited catecholamine pressor responses in rats, J. Pharm. Pharmacol. **18:**443, 1966.
4. Ghose, K.: Assessment of peripheral adrenergic activity and its interactions with drugs in man, Eur. J. Clin. Pharmacol. **17:**233, 1980.

5. Cairncross, K.D.: On the peripheral pharmacology of amitriptyline, Arch. Int. Pharmacodyn. Ther. **154:**438, 1965.
6. Ghose, K., and others: Studies of the interaction of desmethylimipramine with tyramine in man after a single oral dose and its correlation with plasma concentration, Br. J. Clin. Pharmacol. **3:**334, 1976.
7. Jefferson, J.W.: A review of the cardiovascular effects and toxicity of tricyclic antidepressants, Psychosom. Med. **37:**160, 1975.
8. Ragheb, M.: Drug interactions in psychiatric practice, Int. Pharmacopsychiatry **16:**92, 1981.
9. Risch, S.G., and others: Interfaces of psychopharmacology and cardiology—part one, J. Clin. Psychiatry **42:**23, 1981.
10. Briant, R.H., and others: Interaction between guanethidine and maprotiline in man, Br. J. Clin. Pharmacol. **1:**113, 1974.
11. Maxwell, R.A., and others: Molecular features affecting the potency of tricylic antidepressant and structurally related compounds as inhibitors of the uptake of initiated norepinephrine by rabbit aortic strips, J. Pharmacol. Exp. Ther. **166:**320, 1969.

Imipramine–Ethinyl Estradiol

3

Summary: Patients taking ethinyl estradiol have been reported to be relatively resistant to therapy with imipramine.[1,2] Use of the combination has also been associated with an increased incidence of side effects such as headache, hypotension, lethargy, course tremor, urinary retention, and nausea.[1-3]

Related Drugs: Similar reactions have been reported between conjugated estrogens and imipramine[4] but there are no reports with other tricyclic antidepressants (e.g., amitriptyline, desipramine, nortriptyline [see Appendix]) or the tetracyclic antidepressant (maprotiline). However, based on the mechanism a similar interaction may be expected to occur. A study of one patient receiving ethinyl estradiol, norethindrone acetate, and imipramine suggested a decreased first-pass metabolism of imipramine compared to findings in 3 other patients not taking oral contraceptives.[5] Based on pharmacologic similarity, other estrogenic substances (e.g., estradiol, estrone, estropipate [see Appendix]) may be expected to interact in a similar manner with imipramine.

Mechanism: The mechanism of the interaction has not been fully delineated. Long-term use of oral contraceptives in humans has resulted in inhibition of the microsomal enzymes.[6-8] Studies with norethindrone in mice demonstrate added accumulation of imipramine in the brain and other tissues because of impaired metabolism.[9] The interaction may be dose related since contraceptive products containing 30 μg of ethinyl estradiol may not inhibit microsomal enzymes to the same degree as contraceptives containing 50 μg ethinyl estradiol.[10]

It has also been suggested that receptor responses to antidepressants are dependent, at least in part, on baseline hormonal balance.[11]

A third mechanism of action proposed from a study performed in rats suggests that imipramine inhibits the contraceptive's metabolism, enhancing the effect of the estrogens and potentially causing the adverse effects reported.[12,13]

Recommendations: A patient receiving concurrent ethinyl estradiol and imipramine therapy should be observed for lack of effect or enhanced toxicities of imipramine. Should such effects occur, the dose of one of the agents should be adjusted accordingly.

References

1. Prange, A.J., and others: The effect of estrogen on imipramine response in depressed women, presented at the 5th World Congress on Psychiatry, Mexico City, Mexico, November, 1971.
2. Prange, A.J.: Estrogen may well affect response to antidepressants, J.A.M.A. **219**:143, 1972.
3. Khurana, R.C.: Estrogen-imipramine interaction, J.A.M.A. **222**:702, 1972.
4. Orme, M.L.E., and others: Clinical pharmacokinetics of oral contraceptive steroids, Clin. Pharmacokinet. **8**:95, 1983.
5. Gram, L.F., and Christiansen, J.: First-pass metabolism of imipramine in man, Clin. Pharmacol. Ther. **17**:555, 1975.
6. Field, B., and others: Inhibition of hepatic drug metabolism by norethindrone, Clin. Pharmacol. Ther. **25**:196, 1979.
7. Carter, D.E., and others: Effect of oral contraceptives on drug metabolism, Clin. Pharmacol. Ther. **15**:22, 1974.

8. O'Malley, K., and others: Impairment of human drug metabolism by oral contraceptive steroids, Clin. Pharmacol. Ther. **13:**552, 1972.

9. Bellward, G.D., and others: The effects of pretreatment of mice with norethindrone on the metabolism of ^{14}C-imipramine by the liver microsomal drug-metabolizing enzymes, Can. J. Physiol. Pharmacol. **52:**28, 1974.

10. Luscombe, D.K., and John, V.: Influence of age, cigarette smoking and the oral contraceptive on plasma concentrations of clomipramine, Postgrad. Med. J. **56**(suppl. 1):99, 1980.

11. Kendall, D.A., and others: The influence of sex hormones on antidepressant-induced alterations in neurotransmitter receptor binding, J. Neurosci. **2:**254, 1982.

12. Tazi, A., and others: Effect of imipramine on hepatic gamma-glutamyltransferase in female rats. Interaction with contraceptives, Biochem. Pharmacol. **29:**2874, 1980.

13. Somani, S.M., and Khurana, R.C.: Mechanism of estrogen-imipramine interaction, J.A.M.A. **223:**560, 1973.

Imipramine–Levodopa

3

Summary: One study reported a reduction in the absorption of levodopa after the concurrent use of imipramine (100 mg daily for 3 days).[1] However, the clinical significance of this interaction was not determined.

Related Drugs: In another single case report, the concurrent use of amitriptyline, a combination of levodopa-carbidopa, and metoclopramide resulted in an elevated blood pressure, which decreased when all 3 agents were withdrawn.[2] Documentation is lacking regarding an interaction between levodopa and the other tricyclic antidepressants (e.g., doxepin, nortriptyline, protriptyline [see Appendix]) and the tetracyclic antidepressant (maprotiline). However, because all possess some degree of anticholinergic activity, an interaction may be expected to occur.

Mechanism: It has been suggested that imipramine and other tricyclic antidepressants, which possess anticholinergic activity, slow gastric emptying time which in turn allows more time for levodopa to be metabolized in the gastrointestinal tract.[3] This would reduce the amount of levodopa available for absorption. It is not known how the hypertensive reaction occurred with amitriptyline. Metoclopramide or the combination of levodopa-carbidopa may have played a role in this interaction.

Recommendations: Because tricyclic antidepressants have been used successfully and uneventfully for depression in patients with Parkinson's disease,[4-6] the concurrent use of these agents need not to be avoided. However, it is advisable to be aware of a possibility of decreased levodopa levels since a dosage adjustment may be necessary.

References

1. Morgan, J.P., and others: Imipramine-medicated interference with levodopa absorption from the gastrointestinal tract in man, Neurology **25:**1029, 1975.
2. Rampton, D.S.: Hypertensive crisis on a patient given sinemet, metoclopramide, and amitriptyline, Br. Med. J. **3:**607, 1977.
3. Messcha, F.S., and Morgan, J.P.: Imipramine-mediated effects on levodopa metabolism in man, Biochem. Pharmacol. **23:**1503, 1974.
4. Yahr, M.D.: The treatment of parkinsonism—current concepts, Med. Clin. North Am. **56:**1377, 1972.
5. Calne, D.B., and Reid, J.L.: Antiparkinsonian drugs: pharmacological and therapeutic aspects, Drugs **4:**49, 1972.
6. VanWiegren, A., and Wright, J.: Observatons on patients with Parkinson's disease treated with L-dopa. I. Trial and evaluation of L-dopa therapy, South Afr. Med. J. **46:**1262, 1972.

Imipramine–Liothyronine

2

Summary: There is clinical evidence that liothyronine, when added in doses of 25 µg/day to antidepressant therapy, may enhance and accelerate the onset of antidepressant effects in euthyroid patients.[1-4] However, confirmatory studies are needed because liothyronine has failed to potentiate imipramine's action in at least one study,[5] and most studies yielding positive results have been conducted by a single group of investigators.

Related Drugs: Liothyronine has been shown to potentiate the effect of protriptyline and amitriptyline as well as imipramine.[2,6] Therefore, it may also potentiate the action of other tricyclic antidepressants (e.g., desipramine, doxepin, nortriptyline [see Appendix]) and the tetracyclic antidepressant (maprotiline) because of pharmacologic similarity. Although liothyronine has been used for potentiation of antidepressant effects in most studies, similar results may be expected with other thyroid preparations (e.g., levothyroxine, liotrix, thyroid [see Appendix]) based on similar pharmacologic activity.

Mechanism: The mechanism for this interaction is unknown but is thought to involve thyroid enhancement of antidepressant receptor sensitivity. Tricyclic antidepressant plasma levels are not increased by concurrent liothyronine administration.[7]

Recommendations: Since a patient's thyroid function can affect the response to tricyclic antidepressant agents, patients who fail to respond to such drugs should be examined for hypothyroidism. The addition of liothyronine (25 µg/day) to tricyclic antidepressant therapy may be considered in selected patients who do not respond to tricyclic antidepressants alone.

References

1. Wilson, I.C., and others: Thyroid-hormone enhancement of imipramine in nonretarded depression. N. Engl. J. Med. **282:**1063, 1970.
2. Wheatley, D.: Potentiation of amitriptyline by thyroid hormone, Arch. Gen. Psychiatry **26:**229, 1972.
3. Prange, A.J.: Antidepressant effects of thyroid hormone in euthyroid patients, J.A.M.A. **248:**878, 1982.
4. Goodwin, F.K., and others: Potentiation of antidepressant effects by L-triiodothyronine in tricyclic nonresponders, Am. J. Psych. **139:**34, 1982.
5. Feighner, J.P., and others: Hormonal potentiation of imipramine and ECT in primary depression, Am. J. Psych. **128:**1230, 1972.
6. Earle, B.V.: Thyroid hormone and tricyclic antidepressants in resistant depressions, Am. J. Psych. **126:**1667, 1970.
7. Garbutt, J., and others: Effects of triiodothyronine on drug levels and cardiac function in depressed patients treated with imipramine, Am. J. Psych. **136:**980, 1979.

Imipramine–Methyltestosterone

3

Summary: Four or 5 patients developed paranoid reactions after the concurrent use of methyltestosterone and imipramine for the treatment of primary unipolar depression. When methyltestosterone was discontinued, the paranoid reactions cleared.[1]

Related Drugs: Documentation is lacking regarding an interaction between the other tricyclic antidepressants (e.g., amitriptyline, doxepin, nortriptyline [see Appendix]), the tetracyclic antidepressant (maprotiline), and the other androgen derivatives (e.g., fluoxymesterone, nandrolone, testosterone [see Appendix]), although because of pharmacologic similarity a similar interaction may be expected to occur.

Mechanism: The mechanism of this interaction is unknown.

Recommendations: If paranoid reactions occur during concomitant use of imipramine and methyltestosterone, one or both drugs may have to be discontinued.

Reference

1. Wilson, I.C., and others: Methyltestosterone with imipramine in men: conversion of depression to paranoid reaction, Am. J. Psychiatry **131**:71, 1974.

Imipramine–Reserpine

3

Summary: Reserpine has been used to induce a response in patients refractory to tricyclic antidepressant therapy.[1-3] Although most investigators report positive results,[1-3] some have found no improvement.[4] Adverse effects such as hypotension, flushing, diarrhea, and manic reactions have been reported.[1,2,4]

Related Drugs: Desipramine,[1] amitriptyline,[3] and trimipramine[3] have been reported to interact with reserpine. The other tricyclic antidepressants (e.g., doxepin, nortriptyline, protriptyline [see Appendix]) and tetracyclic antidepressant (maprotiline) may react similarly because of pharmacologic similarity, although this has not been documented. No reports have been presented regarding an interaction between imipramine and the other rauwolfia alkaloids (e.g., alseroxylon, deserpidine, rescinnamine [see Appendix]) although they may be expected to interact in a similar manner based on their pharmacologic activity.

Mechanism: The mechanism for this interaction has not been completely elucidated. The onset of action of reserpine is slow since several days are required to deplete existing norepinephrine stores within the nerve ending. However, when reserpine is added to existing imipramine therapy, the initial effect is a release of norepinephrine into the synapse where imipramine inhibits its reuptake into the presynaptic neurons.[5]

Recommendations: These agents should be used concurrently to induce an antidepressant response only in the most recalcitrant patients. Experience with this combination is limited to a few patients, and the risk of adverse effects may outweigh potential therapeutic gains. Also, since reserpine may itself cause depression, this fact should be considered before concurrent administration with imipramine.

References

1. Poldinger, W.: Combined administration of desipramine and reserpine or tetrabenazine in depressive patients, Psychopharmacologia **4:**308, 1963.
2. Haskovek, I., and Rysanek, K.: The action of reserpine in imipramine resistant patients, Psychopharmacologia **11:**18, 1967.
3. Hopkinson, G., and Kenny, F.: Treatment with reserpine of patients resistant to tricyclic antidepressants, Psychiat. Clin. (Basel) **8:**109, 1975.
4. Carney, M.P., and others: Effects of imipramine and reserpine in depression, Psychopharmacologia **14:**349, 1969.
5. Stern, S.L., and Mendels, J.: Drug combinations in the treatment of refractory depression: a review, J. Clin. Psychiatry **42:**368, 1981.

Imipramine–Tranylcypromine

Summary: Although severe toxic and fatal reactions have been reported when tricyclic antidepressant drugs (e.g., imipramine) have been given concurrently with a mono-amine oxidase inhibitor (e.g., tranylcypromine),[1,2] numerous studies in a total of over 600 patients describe beneficial and uneventful concurrent use.[3] Adverse effects of the interaction may include hyperpyrexia, excitability, muscular rigidity, fluctuations in blood pressure, convulsions, and coma.[1-3]

Related Drugs: Although this effect has not been well documented, doxepin, nortriptyline, and protriptyline may interact with monoamine oxidase inhibitors in a manner similar to imipramine.[1] No information exists regarding the other tricyclic antidepressants (e.g., amitriptyline, desipramine, trimipramine [see Appendix]) although they also may interact similarly because of pharmacologic similarity. Since cyclobenzaprine is structurally related to the tricyclic antidepressants, it may react in a similar manner with the monoamine oxidase inhibitors. Other monoamine oxidase inhibitors (e.g., isocarboxazid, pargyline, and phenelzine [see Appendix]) may be expected to interact with imipramine in a manner similar to tranylcypromine based on a similar pharmacologic activity.

Mechanism: Two possible mechanisms have been proposed for this interaction: (1) the monoamine oxidase inhibitor may enhance the effect of the tricyclic antidepressant indirectly through inhibition of microsomal enzymes, and (2) the tricyclic antidepressant may sensitize adrenergic receptors to amines which then accumulate extraneuronally as a result of monoamine oxidase inhibition.[4]

Recommendations: Concurrent use of these drugs should be attempted only in carefully selected, reliable, closely supervised patients who have not responded to any conventional treatment for depression. Most authors recommend that the drugs be given orally and that imipramine and tranylcypromine be avoided.[2,5,6] The tricyclic antidepressant should be administered first, or together with the monoamine oxidase inhibitor, and combined therapy should be initiated at a low dosage after stopping all drugs for 10 to 14 days. Dosage can be increased gradually over a 2 to 3 week period to levels somewhat lower than maximum recommended doses for single drug therapy.[3] Chlorpromazine has been shown to be useful in treating this interaction, possibly because of inhibition of dopamine and serotonin receptors.[2]

References

1. Schuckit, M., and others: Tricyclic antidepressants and monoamine oxidase inhibitors: combination therapy in the treatment of depression, Arch. Gen. Psychiatry **24:**509, 1971.
2. Graham, P.M., and others: Combination monoamine oxidase inhibitor/tricyclic antidepressant interaction, Lancet **2:**440, 1982.
3. Ponto, L.B., and others: Tricyclic antidepressant combination therapy, Am. J. Hosp. Pharm. **34:**954, 1977.
4. Sjoquist, F.: Psychotropic drugs: interaction between monoamine oxidase inhibitors and other substances, Proc. R. Soc. Med. **58:**967, 1965.
5. Stern, S.L., and Mendels, J.: Drug combinations in the treatment of refractory depression: a review, J. Clin. Psychiatry **42:**368, 1981.
6. White, K., and Simpson, G.: Combined MAOI-tricyclic antidepressant treatment: a reevaluation, J. Clin. Psychopharmacol. **1:**264, 1981.

Nortriptyline–Phenobarbital

3

Summary: Limited data indicate that phenobarbital may decrease the serum concentrations of nortriptyline approximately 30% within a few days of initiation of co-therapy.[1]

Related Drugs: Amobarbital,[2,3] pentobarbital,[1,4] and secobarbital[1] have been suggested to interact similarly with nortriptyline; however, the data are limited and unreliable. Desipramine and phenobarbital,[2] and protriptyline and amobarbital[5] undergo a similar interaction.[5]

Although the mechanism is not documented, if it involves stimulation of metabolism by barbiturates, a similar interaction may occur between all other barbiturates (e.g., aprobarbital, butabarital, mephobarbital [see Appendix]), other tricyclic antidepressants (e.g., amitriptyline, imipramine, trimipramine [see Appendix]), and the tetracyclic antidepressant (maprotiline).

Mechanism: Reports suggest that barbiturates can stimulate the metabolism of the tricyclic antidepressants.[1-3,6]

Recommendations: Although the clinical data are limited, they are sufficient to indicate that phenobarbital will decrease serum nortriptyline levels in patients receiving these drugs concurrently. Because the change in therapeutic effect caused by decreased serum nortriptyline levels is not known, the clinical significance of this drug interaction is difficult to assess. If patients are unresponsive to nortriptyline therapy, concurrent barbiturate therapy should be considered as a possible underlying cause.

If additional drugs must be used, the benzodiazepines may be useful in treating anxiety symptoms since they do not affect the metabolism of the tricyclic drugs. Flurazepam, a benzodiazepine, apparently does not affect the metabolism of tricyclic antidepressants: therefore, it may be an alternative to barbiturate co-therapy.

References

1. Alexanderson, B., and others: Steady-state plasma levels of nortriptyline in twins: influence of genetic factors and drug therapy, Br. Med. J. **4:**764, 1969.
2. Silverman, G., and Braithwaite, R.: Interaction of benzodiazepines with tricyclic antidepressants, Br. Med. J. **4:**111, 1972.
3. Burrows, G.D., and Davies, B.: Antidepressants and barbiturates, Br. Med. J. **4:**113, 1971.
4. Asberg, M., and others: Relationship between plasma level and therapeutic effects of nortriptyline, Br. Med. J. **3:**331, 1971.
5. Moody, J.P., and others: Pharmacokinetic aspects of protriptyline plasma levels, Eur. J. Clin. Pharmacol. **11:**51, 1977.
6. Risch, S., and others: Plasma levels of tricyclic antidepressants and clinical efficacy: review of the literature—part 1, J. Clin. Psychiatry. **40:**4, 1979.

Phenelzine–Levodopa

1

Summary: Levodopa (in doses of 50 mg or more) causes a significant rise in blood pressure as well as flushing and palpitations when given to patients receiving phenelzine, a monoamine oxidase inhibitor.[1-5] The interaction may occur within 1 hour after levodopa administration.

Related Drugs: Other monoamine oxidase inhibitors that have been reported to interact with levodopa include isocarboxazid,[1] pargyline,[2] and tranylcypromine.[1] This interaction would also be expected to occur with other agents that possess monoamine oxidase inhibitor activity (furazolidone and procarbazine). There are no drugs related to levodopa.

Mechanism: Phenelzine, like other monoamine oxidase inhibitors, increases the levels of dopamine in the peripheral tissues and the brain. Levodopa also increases the levels of dopamine in the central nervous system, and a marked enhancement of spontaneous motor activity may result.[6] The concurrent administration of carbidopa, a peripheral decarboxylase inhibitor, with levodopa suppresses the hypertensive reaction caused by monoamine oxidase inhibitors, indicating that the reaction is peripherally mediated.[7]

Recommendations: Levodopa and monoamine oxidase inhibitors should not be administered concurrently. If an antidepressant must be used in a patient receiving levodopa, a tricyclic antidepressant should be considered.[8] If a monoamine oxidase inhibitor must be used concurrently with levodopa, a carbidopa-levodopa combination product should be considered instead of levodopa alone.

The effects of monoamine oxidase inhibition usually last 2 weeks after the drug is discontinued; therefore, levodopa should not be given until at least 4 weeks after the monoamine oxidase inhibitor is discontinued.[1]

References

1. Hunter, K.R., and others: Monoamine oxidase inhibitors and l-dopa, Br. Med. J. **3:**388, 1970.
2. Hodge, J.V.: Use of monoamine-oxidase inhibitors, Lancet **1:**764, 1965.
3. McGeer, P.L., and others: Drug induced extrapyramidal reactions. Treatment with diphenhydramine hydrochloride and dihydroxyphenylalanine, J.A.M.A. **177:**665, 1961.
4. Friend, D.G., and others: The action of l-dihydroxyphenylalanine in patients receiving nialimide, Clin. Pharmacol. Ther. **6:**362, 1965.
5. Schilldkraut, J.J., and others: Biochemical and pressor effects of oral d, l-dihydroxyphenylalanine in patients pretreated with antidepressant drugs, Ann. N.Y. Acad. Sci. **107:**1005, 1963.
6. Hornykiewicz, O.: Dopamine (3-hydroxytyramine) and brain function, Pharmacol. Rev. **18:**925, 1966.
7. Teychenne, P.F., and others: Interactions of levodopa with inhibitors of monoamine oxidase and l-aromatic amino acid decarboxylase, Clin. Pharmacol. Ther. **18:**273, 1975.
8. Hunter, K.R., and others: Use of levodopa with other drugs, Lancet **9:**1283, 1970.

Tranylcypromine–Phenylpropanolamine

1

Summary: Indirect acting sympathomimetic amines, such as phenylpropanolamine, may cause abrupt elevation of blood pressure when administered to patients taking tranylcypromine or other monoamine oxidase inhibitors,[1-3] resulting in a potentially fatal hypertensive crisis.

Related Drugs: The other monoamine oxidase inhibitors (isocarboxazid, pargyline, and phenelzine)[4,5] have been reported to interact with other indirect-acting sympathomimetics (amphetamines, ephedrine, methylphenidate, and tyramine).[6,7] Although this effect has not been documented, pseudoephedrine may also be expected to interact similarly. Mixed (direct and indirect) acting sympathomimetics (e.g., metaraminol, phenylephrine [see Appendix]) have also been shown to interact with monoamine oxidase inhibitors depending on their degree of indirect action.[8,9] The direct-acting sympathomimetics epinephrine, isoproterenol, norepinephrine, and methoxamine have not been reported to interact.[7,9-11] Dopamine is metabolized by monoamine oxidase, and its pressor effect is enhanced by monoamine oxidase inhibitors.[9,12] Since procarbazine, an antineoplastic agent, is a weak monoamine oxidase inhibitor, hypertensive reactions may result from its concurrent use with indirect and mixed acting sympathomimetics.[13] Furazolidone, an antibacterial with monoamine oxidase inhibitor action, has also been shown to interact with indirect acting sympathomimetics (see Furazolidone-Amphetamine, p. 362)

Mechanism: The apparent selectivity of the monoamine oxidase inhibitor enhancement of indirect-acting sympathomimetics indicates that monoamine oxidase functions in the regulation of viable stores of active mediator or in the amount released.[14,15] Therefore, the stimulation of norepinephrine release by the indirect-acting adrenergic agents results in an increased amount of the neurotransmitter present at the adrenergic receptor. Other proposed mechanisms suggest that the enhancement results from an inhibition of the hepatic microsomal enzymes that catabolize alpha-methylated amines resistant to monoamine oxidase degradation rather than from an inhibition of monoamine oxidase itself.

Recommendations: Patients receiving monoamine oxidase inhibitors should be instructed to avoid indirect-acting sympathomimetic agents, foods containing tyramine, and nonprescription items with the potential to interact (e.g., cough and cold preparations). Symptoms such as headache, gastrointestinal upset, fever, and visual disturbances should be pointed out as indicators of hypertension caused by such combinations. Marked elevation of blood pressure under these circumstances may be treated by alpha-adrenergic blocking agents like phentolamine (5 mg intramuscularly or intravenously).[9,16,17]

References

1. Cuthbert, M.F.: MAOI's, Br. Med. J. **2**:433, 1968.
2. Cuthbert, M.F., and others: Cough and cold remedies: a potential danger to patients on monoamine oxidase inhibitors, Br. Med. J. **1**:404, 1969.

3. Smookler, S., and Bermudez, A.J.: Hypertensive crisis resulting from an MAO inhibitor and over-the-counter appetite suppressant, Ann. Emerg. Med. **11:**482, 1982.
4. Mason, A.M.S., and Buckle, R.M.: Cold cures and monoamine oxidase inhibitors, Br. Med. J. **1:**845, 1969.
5. Lloyd, J.T.A., and Walker, D.R.H.: Death after dexamphetamine and phenelzine, Br. Med. J. **2:**168, 1965.
6. Krisko, I., and others: Severe hyperpyrexia due to tranylcypromine amphetamine toxicity, Ann. Intern. Med. **70:**559, 1969.
7. Boakes, A.J., and others: Interactions between sympathomimetic amines and antidepressant agents in man, Br. Med. J. **1:**311, 1973.
8. Horber, A.R., and Wynne, N.A.: Hypertensive crisis due to pargyline and metaraminol, Br. Med. J. **2:**460, 1965.
9. Elis, J., and others: Modification by monoamine oxidase inhibitors of the effect of some sympathomimetics on blood pressure, Br. Med. J. **2:**75, 1967.
10. Horwitz, D., and others: Increased blood pressure responses to dopamine and norepinephrine produced by monoamine oxidase inhibitors in man, J. Lab. Clin. Med. **56:**747, 1960.
11. Cuthbert, M.F., and Vere, D.W.: Potentiation of the cardiovascular effects of some catecholamines by a monoamine oxidase inhibitor, Br. J. Pharmacol. **43:**471P, 1971.
12. Hornykiewicz, O.: Dopamine (3-hydroxytyramine) and brain function, Pharmacol. Rev. **18:**925, 1966.
13. Calabresi, P., and Parks, R.E.: Chemotherapy of neoplastic diseases. In Gilman, A.G., Goodman, L.S., and Gilman, A., eds.: The pharmacological basis of therapeutics. New York, 1980, Macmillan Publishing.
14. Goldberg, L.I.: Monoamine oxidase inhibitors: adverse reactions and possible mechanisms, J.A.M.A. **190:**456, 1969.
15. Kopin, I.J.: Biochemical aspects of release of norepinephrine and other amines from sympathetic nerve endings, Pharmacol. Rev. **18:**513, 1966.
16. Bethune, H.C., and others: Vascular crisis associated with monoamine oxidase inhibitors, Am. J. Psychiatry **121:**245, 1964.
17. O'Dea, K., and Rand, M.J.: Interaction between amphetamine and monoamine oxidase inhibitors, Eur. J. Pharmacol. **6:**115, 1969.

Tranylcypromine–Propranolol

4

Summary: Based on available information, it appears that the concomitant administration of tranylcypromine and propranolol does not result in an increase in pressor activity or tachycardia.[1] At this time the interaction is based on theoretical considerations only. One animal study failed to demonstrate any adverse effects resulting from the concurrent use of these agents.[1]

Related Drugs: Documentation is lacking regarding an interaction between other monoamine oxidase inhibitors (isocarboxazid, pargyline, and phenelzine) and other beta-blocking agents (e.g., atenolol, nadolol, pindolol [see Appendix]) as well as with furazolidone and procarbazine, which possess monoamine oxidase inhibitor activity.

Mechanism: The mechanism of this interaction is unknown.

Recommendations: One study suggests that monamine oxidase inhibitors should be discontinued at least 2 weeks before the institution of propranolol therapy,[2] but this is a theoretical consideration only and no clinical interaction has been documented. Therefore, this combination need not be avoided at this time.

References

1. Barrett, A.M., and Callum, V.A.: Lack of interaction between propranolol and mebanazine, J. Pharm. Pharmacol. **20:**911, 1968.
2. Frieden, J.: Propranolol as an antiarrhythmic agent, Am. Heart J. **74:**283, 1967.

Antihypertensive Drug Interactions

*Not available in the U.S.

TABLE 7. Antihypertensive Drug Interactions

Drug Interaction	Significance Code	Potential Effects	Recommendations	See Page
Bethanidine*– Mazindol	2	In 1 patient a single dose of mazindol reversed the antihypertensive action and side effects of bethanidine.	Concomitant use may need to be avoided. Monitor the blood pressure frequently.	307
Captopril– Aspirin	2	Aspirin may decrease the antihypertensive effect of captopril.	Monitor the blood pressure closely. Aspirin may need to be withdrawn.	308
Captopril– Furosemide	2	Severe postural hypotension may occur when furosemide is added to a captopril regimen, especially in sodium-depleted patients.	This interaction is usually transient and should not prevent long-term use of these agents.	309
Captopril– Indomethacin	2	Indomethacin may decrease or abolish the antihypertensive action of captopril.	Avoid concomitant use, but if this is not possible, monitor the blood pressure carefully.	310
Captopril– Probenecid	3	Probenecid may reduce both total body clearance and renal clearance of captopril, although the clinical significance of this is unknown.	Concurrent use need not be avoided, but monitor the blood pressure regularly.	311
Clonidine– Propranolol	1	Rapid blood pressure elevation may occur when clonidine is abruptly withdrawn from cotherapy with propranolol. A similar result may occur when clonidine is abruptly discontinued in the absence of beta-blocking agents.	Substituting labetalol for propranolol has prevented this interaction. Tapering clonidine for 7 days did not prevent the interaction.	312
Clonidine– Rifampin	4	Elimination kinetics of clonidine are not affected by cotherapy with rifampin. This may be significant in patients addicted to narcotics who are receiving clonidine to avert withdrawal symptoms, since rifampin does induce methadone metabolism, resulting in withdrawal symptoms.	Clonidine may be an alternative to methadone for averting narcotic withdrawal, and the concurrent use of rifampin and clonidine need not be avoided.	313
Guanethidine– Alcohol, Ethyl	2	Because of its acute vasodilator effects, alcohol may enhance the orthostatic hypotension and syncope caused by guanethidine.	Caution patients about postural hypotension and that concurrent alcohol may worsen the symptoms.	314

*Not available in the U.S.

Abbreviations: CNS, central nervous system; MAO, monoamine oxidase.

TABLE 7. Antihypertensive Drug Interactions—cont'd

Drug Interaction	Significance Code	Potential Effects	Recommendations	See Page
Guanethidine–Chlorpromazine	1	In doses >100 mg/day, chlorpromazine may reverse the antihypertensive effects of guanethidine after several days of co-therapy.	Avoid concomitant use, but if this is not possible an increased dosage of guanethidine may be needed.	316
Guanethidine–Desipramine	1	Desipramine antagonizes the antihypertensive action of guanethidine within 3-7 days of initial co-therapy.	Avoid concomitant use, but if this is not possible monitor the patient for 1-2 weeks, expecting an increased guanethidine dose.	318
Guanethidine–Dextroamphetamine	2	Dextroamphetamine may decrease the antihypertensive action of guanethidine.	Avoid concomitant use. Clonidine, methyldopa, or a beta-blocking agent may be substituted for guanethidine since they do not interact with dextroamphetamine.	320
Guanethidine–Hydrochlorothiazide	2	Hydrochlorothiazide is often used to reduce sodium and water retention and the associated increased blood volume caused by guanethidine.	Guanethidine dosage may need to be reduced in concurrent therapy.	322
Guanethidine–Minoxidil	2	Minoxidil can potentiate the orthostatic hypotensive action of guanethidine, even when guanethidine is discontinued 3 days before initiating minoxidil therapy.	Guanethidine should be discontinued 1 week before instituting minoxidil therapy.	324
Guanethidine–Phenelzine	2	MAO inhibitors may compromise the antihypertensive efficacy of guanethidine.	Avoid concurrent use. Careful monitoring of blood pressure is required if concomitant use cannot be avoided.	325
Guanethidine–Phenylephrine	2	Systemically administered phenylephrine may antagonize the antihypertensive action of guanethidine resulting in hypertension.	It is important to be aware of a possible decreased pharmacologic response.	326
Methyldopa–Amitriptyline	3	Amitriptyline may antagonize the antihypertensive effects of methyldopa. Limited information indicates that not all tricyclic antidepressants interact with alpha-adrenergic agents.	It is important to monitor blood pressure during concomitant use.	327
Methyldopa–Haloperidol	3	Dementia has occurred within 3 days of initiating co-therapy.	If abnormal CNS symptoms develop, discontinue the haloperidol.	329

TABLE 7. Antihypertensive Drug Interactions—cont'd

Drug Interaction	Significance Code	Potential Effects	Recommendations	See Page
Methyldopa–Levodopa	3	Methyldopa can have opposite effects on levodopa, depending on individual patient response or dosages of the drugs. It can enhance the effect of levodopa, or it can induce parkinsonism.	These agents may be used concomitantly for some patients with parkinsonism. If side effects occur, the methyldopa may need to be withdrawn.	330
Methyldopa–Norepinephrine	2	Methyldopa may increase and prolong the pressor effect of norephinephrine, possibly resulting in a hypertensive episode.	If severe hypertension develops, norepinephrine dosage should be reduced or discontinued.	331
Methyldopa–Phenobarbital	4	An early report that phenobarbital might lower methyldopa blood levels by increasing metabolism has not been confirmed by direct analysis.	No special precautions seem to be warranted.	332
Methyldopa–Propranolol	2	Concurrent use of these agents may result in increased blood pressure.	This interaction may be potentially serious, especially when neurotransmitter release is increased by drugs or clinical events.	333
Prazosin–Indomethacin	2	The concurrent use of these agents may reduce the hypotensive action of prazosin.	Monitor blood pressure carefully and increase the prazosin dosage if necessary.	334
Prazosin–Propranolol	2	Concurrent use may enhance the acute postural hypotensive reaction after the first dose of prazosin.	Advise patients of the risk. Prazosin may be initiated with a dose of 0.5 mg or less when used with propranolol.	335
Reserpine–Ephedrine	2	Reserpine may antagonize the responsiveness to ephedrine.	If a pressor agent is required with reserpine, a direct-acting sympathomimetic (e.g., norepinephrine) is recommended.	336
Reserpine–Halothane	3	Early reports indicated an increased risk of hypotension with co-therapy. However, recent information suggests co-administration may be tolerated without an increased risk of hypotension.	If reserpine is not discontinued before surgery and hypotension does occur, a direct-acting sympathomimetic may be advisable.	337

Bethanidine*—Mazindol

2

Summary: In one report, a single dose of mazindol reversed the antihypertensive effect of bethanidine in a male subject with mild hypertension. In addition, mazindol administration also resulted in the loss of bethanidine-induced side effects (e.g., stuffy nose, snoring, postural giddiness, nocturia).[1]

Related Drugs: Other antihypertensives related to bethanidine (e.g., debrisoquin,* guanadrel, guanethidine [see Appendix]) may be expected to interact similarly because of pharmacologic similarity. Although documentation is lacking, other anorexiants that possess indirect-acting sympathomimetic activity (e.g., diethylpropion, fenfluramine, phentermine [see Appendix]) may also be expected to interact with bethanidine. Phenylpropanolamine, another anorexiant-sympathomimetic, has antagonized the antihypertensive effects of bethanidine.[2] The interactions between guanethidine and indirect-acting sympathomimetics are discussed in another monograph. (See Guanethidine-Dextroamphetamine, p. 320.)

Mechanism: It is postulated that the anorexiants with indirect-acting sympathomimetic activity may either compete with bethanidine for uptake or displace bethanidine from adrenergic neurons.

Recommendations: The concomitant use of these agents may need to be avoided. If concurrent use is required, blood pressure should be monitored frequently.

References

1. Boakes, A.J.: Antagonism of bethanidine by mazindol, Br. J. Clin. Pharmacol.**4:**486, 1977.
2. Misage, J.R., and McDonald, R.H.: Antagonism of hypotensive action of bethanidine by "common cold" remedy, Br. Med. J. **4:**347, 1970.

*Not available in the U.S.

Captopril–Aspirin

2

Summary: In one study, 4 of 8 patients receiving captopril and aspirin showed a decreased antihypertensive effect after a single dose of captopril. These patients had essential hypertension and their sodium was restricted. In the 4 patients who showed decreased effects, the excretion of a metabolite of prostaglandin E_2 was decreased.[1]

Related Drugs: There are no drugs related to captopril. Documentation is lacking regarding an interaction between captopril and the other salicylates (e.g., choline salicylate, salicylamide, sodium salicylate [see Appendix]). However, because all salicylates inhibit prostaglandin synthesis[2] a similar interaction may be expected to occur.

Mechanism: The initial hypotensive effect of captopril is mainly the result of suppression of the renin-angiotensin-aldosterone system by its ability to inhibit the angiotensin converting enzyme. Long-term captopril therapy, on the other hand, may augment the release of endogenous vasodilating prostaglandins.[1,3-6] Aspirin is a known inhibitor of prostaglandin synthesis, and it has been postulated that this effect is responsible for this interaction by interfering with the release of vasodilating prostaglandins enhanced by long-term captopril therapy.[1]

Recommendations: Patients should be closely monitored for blood pressure changes during concurrent use of these agents. If blood pressure control decreases, discontinuation of the aspirin may be necessary.

References

1. Moore, T.J., and others: Contribution of prostaglandins to the antihypertensive action of captopril in essential hypertension, Hypertension **3:**168, 1981.
2. Flower, R.J., and others: Drug therapy of inflamation. In Gilman, A.G., Goodman, L.S., and Gilman, A., editors: The pharmacological basis of therapeutics. New York, 1980, MacMillan Publishing.
3. Abe, K., and others: Indomethacin inhibits the antihypertensive effect of captopril, SQ14225, in low renin hypertension, Tohoku J. Exp. Clin. Med. **132:**117, 1980.
4. Abe, K., and others: Role of prostaglandin in the antihypertensive mechanism of captopril in low renin hypertension, Clin. Sci. **59:**141s, 1980.
5. Ogihara, T., and others: Hormonal responses to long-term converting enzyme inhibition in hypertensive patients, Clin. Pharmacol. Ther. **30:**328, 1981.
6. Fujita, T., and others: Effect of indomethacin on antihypertensive patients, Clin. Exp. Hypertens. **3:**939, 1981.

Captopril–Furosemide

Summary: Severe postural hypotension has been reported when furosemide was added to a captopril regimen.[1,2] A precipitous reduction of blood pressure may be more prevalent in patients who are sodium depleted from concomitant diuretics or those on severe dietary salt restriction or dialysis.[3,4] This hypotensive response is transient and should not be considered significant on subsequent dosing.[4]

Related Drugs: There are no drugs presently available that are related to captopril. Documentation has not appeared in the literature regarding a similar interaction with the other loop diuretics (ethacrynic acid and bumetanide), thiazide diuretics (e.g., benzthiazide, methyclothiazide, polythiazide [see Appendix]), the mercurial diuretic (mersalyl), and other thiazide related diuretics (e.g., chlorthalidone, quinethazone, indapamide [see Appendix]). However, since all diuretics may cause sodium depletion, one might expect a similar interaction to occur.

In addition to the sodium depletion possibility of the potassium-sparing diuretics (amiloride, spironolactone, and triamterene), these agents should be used with the utmost caution when they are administered concurrently with captopril since captopril itself increases serum potassium levels.[2,5,6]

Mechanism: The exact mechanism by which furosemide accentuates the hypotensive effects of captopril is not known. The initial hypotensive effect of captopril is mainly the result of suppression of the renin-angiotensin-aldosterone system by its ability to inhibit the angiotensin converting enzyme. Captopril inhibits the formation of angiotensin II, thereby lowering aldosterone levels with subsequent sodium and water depletion.[4,6] Therefore, furosemide as well as other diuretics that cause sodium and water loss may exaggerate the hypotensive state.

Recommendations: Because the hypotensive response is transient, subsequent doses of captopril and furosemide are not expected to cause a similar contraindication. If the hypotension does occur, the patient should be placed in a supine position and, if necessary, should receive an intravenous infusion of normal saline. Alternatively, to minimize the possibility of hypotension, the diuretics may be discontinued or sodium intake increased 1 week before initiation of captopril therapy.

References

1. Ferguson, R.K., and others: Captopril in severe treatment resistant hypertension, Am. Heart J. **99**:579, 1980.
2. Case, D.B., and others: Clinical experience with blockade of the renin-angiotensin-aldosterone system by an oral converting-enzyme inhibitor (SQ14225, captopril) in hypertensive patients, Prog. Cardiovasc. Dis. **21**:195, 1978.
3. Heel, R.C., and others: Captopril: a preliminary review of its pharmacological properties and therapeutic efficacy, Drugs **20**:409, 1980.
4. Captopril Product Information, E.R. Squibb Co., 1982.
5. MacGregor, G.A., and others: Essential hypertension: effect of an oral inhibitor of angiotensin-converting enzyme, Br. Med. J. **2**:1106, 1979.
6. White, N.J., and others: Captopril and frusemide in severe drug resistant hypertension, Lancet **2**:108, 1980.

Captopril–Indomethacin

2

Summary: Indomethacin may decrease or completely abolish the antihypertensive effect of captopril during concurrent use.[1-6] This effect was seen in low renin hypertensive patients, whereas no marked change in blood pressure was induced by indomethacin in normal renin hypertensive patients.[1-4] One study showed a decrease in the hypotensive effect in sodium restricted patients with essential hypertension.[5] In a study involving 12 healthy volunteers, concomitant indomethacin therapy reversed the hypotensive effect of captopril and also reduced baseline levels of plasma renin activity, angiotensin I concentration, aldosterone, urinary aldosterone excretion, PGE_2 excretion, and heart rate.[6]

Related Drugs: There are no drugs related to captopril. No documentation exists regarding an interaction between captopril and other nonsteroidal anti-inflammatory agents (e.g., ibuprofen, naproxen, piroxicam [see Appendix]) although because of their ability to inhibit prostaglandins to some extent, a similar interaction may be expected to occur.

Mechanism: The initial hypotensive effect of captopril is mainly the result of suppression of the renin-angiotensin-aldosterone system by its ability to inhibit the angiotensin converting enzyme. Long-term captopril therapy, on the other hand, may augment the release of endogenous vasodilating prostaglandins. It has been postulated that indomethacin, which inhibits endogenous prostaglandin synthesis, interferes with the release of vasodilating prostaglandins enhanced by long-term captopril therapy.[1-6]

Recommendations: The concurrent administration of these agents should be avoided. If concomitant use is necessary, blood pressure should be closely monitored.

References

1. Abe, K., and others: Indomethacin inhibits the antihypertensive effect of captopril, SQ 14225, in low renin hypertension, Tohoku J. Exp. Med. **132:**117, 1980.
2. Abe, K., and others: Role of prostaglandin in the antihypertensive mechanism of captopril in low renin hypertension, Clin. Sci. **59:**141s, 1980.
3. Ogihara, T., and others: Hormonal responses to long-term converting enzyme inhibition in hypertensive patients. Clin. Pharmacol. Ther. **30:**328, 1981.
4. Fujita, T., and others: Effect of indomethacin on antihypertensive action of captopril in hypertensive patients, Clin. Exp. Hypertens. **3:**939, 1981.
5. Moore, T.J., and others: Contribution of prostaglandins to the antihypertensive action of captopril in essential hypertension, Hypertension **3:**168, 1981.
6. Witzgall, H., and others: Acute haemodynamic and hormonal effects of captopril are diminished by indomethacin, Clin. Sci. **62:**611, 1982.

Captopril–Probenecid

3

Summary: In one study, the average total body clearance and renal clearance of captopril were reduced in the presence of probenecid. The volume of distribution of captopril during steady state was not altered by probenecid.[1] At this time it has not been possible to relate blood concentrations of either captopril or its metabolites to the lowering of blood pressure in hypertensive patients. Therefore, the clinical significance of this interaction is unknown.

Related Drugs: There are no drugs related to captopril. Documentation is lacking regarding an interaction between captopril and the other uricosuric (sulfinpyrazone); however, a similar interaction may be expected to occur since sulfinpyrazone can also inhibit tubular secretion in the kidney.

Mechanism: Captopril is rapidly eliminated by the kidney, and its clearance exceeds that of glomerular filtration. Captopril is therefore actively secreted into the urine, and tubular secretion is the major mechanism by which it is excreted. It is well known that probenecid can interfere with tubular secretion of drugs into the proximal tubule, and it has been suggested that this mechanism interferes with captopril excretion.[1]

Recommendations: Because it is not clear whether the moderate increase in captopril levels will have any significant effect on the antihypertensive action of captopril, the concurrent use of these agents need not be avoided. However, it is prudent to monitor the patient's blood pressure regularly, and a decrease in the dose of captopril may be necessary.

Reference

1. Singhvi, S.M., and others: Renal handling of captopril: effect of probenecid, Clin. Pharmacol. Ther. **32**:182, 1982.

Clonidine–Propranolol

1

Summary: The acute rapid discontinuation of clonidine from combined therapy with propranolol may produce severe symptoms of sympathetic activity and rapid blood pressure elevations within 24 to 72 hours.[1-4] Symptoms may include tremor, insomnia, nausea, apprehension, flushing, and headaches. The combination may also produce a paradoxic hypertension not part of the pharmacologic activity of either agent when used alone. A rapid blood pressure elevation may also occur when clonidine is abruptly discontinued in the absence of concurrent beta-blocking agents.

Related Drugs: A similar discontinuation syndrome has been reported in patients taking timolol[5] but not labetalol.[6] Although the mechanism is undocumented, if it involves the neutralization of the vasodilatory effect of $beta_2$-adrenergic receptors in the vessels, then the $beta_1$ cardioselective beta blocking agents (atenolol and metoprolol) would not be expected to interact similarly. However, the other noncardioselective beta-blocking agents (nadolol and pindolol) may interact in a manner similar to propranolol.

Mechanism: The beta-blocking action of propranolol neutralizes the vasodilatory effect of $beta_2$-adrenergic receptors. When clonidine is abruptly stopped, neurotransmitters are released and they manifest their alpha-adrenergic receptor activity (vasoconstriction) while the the $beta_2$-adrenergic receptor activity is neutralized.

Recommendations: Attempts to taper the clonidine dosage up to 7 days before discontinuing clonidine while either continuing, discontinuing abruptly, or concurrently tapering propranolol have not avoided the discontinuation syndrome.[7,8] One report showed that substituting labetalol prophylactically when clonidine was abruptly discontinued caused no alterations in blood pressure.[6] It is therefore recommended that labetalol or one of the cardioselective beta-blocking agents may be used preventively or that propranolol therapy be discontinued well in advance of stopping clonidine therapy.

References

1. Houston, M.C.: Clonidine hydrochloride, South. Med. J. **75**:713, 1982.
2. Houston, M.C.: Clonidine hydrochloride: review of pharmacologic and clinical aspects, Prog. Cardiovasc. Dis. **23**:337, 1981.
3. Vernon, C., and Sakula, A.: Fatal rebound hypertension after abrupt withdrawal of clonidine and propranolol, Br. J. Clin. Pract. **33**:112, 1979.
4. Bruce, D.L., and others: Preoperative clonidine withdrawal syndrome, Anesthesiology **51**:90, 1979.
5. Barley, R.R., and Neal, T.J.: Rapid clonidine withdrawal with blood pressure overshoot exaggerated by beta blockade, Br. Med. J. **1**:942, 1976.
6. Rosenthal, T., and others: Use of labetalol in hypertensive patients during discontinuation of clonidine therapy, Eur. J. Clin. Pharmacol. **20**:237, 1981.
7. Strauss, F.G., and others: Withdrawal of antihypertensive therapy: hypertensive crisis in renovascular hypertension, J.A.M.A. **238**:1734, 1977.
8. Cairns, S.A., and Marshall, A.J.: Clonidine withdrawal, Lancet **1**:368, 1976.

Clonidine–Rifampin

4

Summary: The results of a study involving 6 normal volunteers indicates that no change occurred in the elimination kinetics of clonidine during rifampin administration. This may be significant in patients addicted to narcotics who are receiving methadone to avert withdrawal symptoms,[1] since rifampin is known to induce the metabolism of methadone, resulting in withdrawal symptoms (see Methadone-Rifampin, p. 48). In these patients, replacement of methadone with clonidine may be warranted as clonidine has also been used to avert withdrawal symptoms.

Related Drugs: There are no drugs related to rifampin or clonidine.

Mechanism: Because only 50% of clonidine is biotransformed by the liver and the rest is eliminated unchanged by the kidney,[2] rifampin does not appear to induce the metabolism of clonidine as measured by 24 hour urinary d-glucaric acid concentration (UDGA). The UDGA excretion levels are a measurement of enhanced or inhibited microsomal drug metabolizing enzyme activity.[1]

Recommendations: Rifampin has not been shown to alter the elimination of clonidine, and no special precautions need to be taken when these 2 agents are used concomitantly.

References

1. Affrime, M.B., and others: Failure of rifampin to induce the metabolism of clonidine in normal volunteers, Drug Intell. Clin. Pharm. **15:**964, 1981.
2. Lowenthal, D.T., and Affrime, M.B.: Pharmacokinetics of clonidine, J. Cardiovasc. Pharmacol. **2:**529, 1980.

Guanethidine–Alcohol, Ethyl

2

Summary: Alcohol, because of its acute vasodilator effects, may enhance the orthostatic hypotension and syncope caused by guanethidine. No specific studies have been conducted to determine the incidence, severity, or mechanism of the interaction.[1-4]

Related Drugs: Although clinical data are lacking, other drugs pharmacologically related to guanethidine (bethanidine,* debrisoquin,* and guanadrel) may be expected to interact with alcohol in a similar manner.

Mechanism: Alcohol produces vasodilation, which may further inhibit the ability of a patient taking guanethidine to respond to orthostatic changes. The acute ingestion of moderate amounts of alcohol (0.9 to 1.0 g/kg) has been associated with causing a reduction in peripheral vascular resistance with no change in myocardial contractility for up to 90 minutes after alcohol ingestion in patients not receiving guanethidine.[5,6] Chronic alcohol ingestion may be associated with depression of myocardial contractility, cardiac hypertrophy, and QT prolongation.[7,8] Alcohol has also been reported to cause hypertension.[9]

Guanethidine, by reducing the storage and blocking the normal release of norepinephrine, may cause a complete inhibition of the reflex-induced arterial and venous constriction normally seen with standing, rising, or exercising.[1-4]

Recommendations: Patients prescribed guanethidine should be informed of the following: (1) concurrent alcohol ingestion may increase the incidence of guanethidine-induced orthostatic hypotension, dizziness, and syncope, thus alcohol intake should be limited, if possible; (2) these adverse reactions are most likely to occur during hot weather or while standing for long periods, rising rapidly from a sitting or prone position, or exercising; (3) if such symptoms occur, lie, sit, or squat immediately.[2]

References

1. Weiner, N.: Drugs that inhibit adrenergic nerves and block adrenergic receptors. In Gilman, A.G., Goodman, L.S., and Gilman, A., editors: The pharmacological basis of therapeutics, New York, 1980, MacMillan Publishing.
2. Guanethidine. In Heller, W.M., executive director: United States pharmacopeia dispensing information, Easton, PA, 1984, Mack Printing Company.
3. Jandhyala, B.S., and others: Effects of prolonged administration of certain antihypertensive agents, J. Pharm. Sci. **63:**1497, 1974.
4. Stanford, J.R., and Fann, W.E.: Drug interactions with guanidinium antihypertensives, Drugs **13:**57, 1977.
5. Kupari, M.: Acute cardiovascular effect of ethanol. A controlled noninvasive study, Br. Heart J. **49:**174, 1983.
6. Greenberg, B.H., and others: Acute effects of alcohol in patients with congestive heart failure, Ann. Intern. Med. **97:**171, 1982.

*Not available in the U.S.

7. Kino, M., and others: Cardiovascular status in asymptomatic alcoholics, with reference to the level of ethanol consumption, Br. Heart J. **46:**545, 1981.
8. Abelmann, W.H., and Ramirez, A.: Alcoholic cardiovascular disease. In Rothschild, M.A., Oratz, M., and Schreiber, S.S., editors: Alcohol and abnormal protein biosynthesis. Biochemical and clinical, New York, 1975, Pergamon Press.
9. Saunders, J.B., and others: Alcohol-induced hypertension, Lancet **2:**653, 1981.

Guanethidine–Chlorpromazine

1

Summary: Chlorpromazine, in doses greater than 100 mg daily, may reverse the antihypertensive effects of guanethidine.[1-5] A time lag of 3 to 7 days after the initiation of concurrent therapy usually occurs before the blood pressure increases significantly.[1,2] Withdrawal of chlorpromazine may result in a further elevation of blood pressure, which was reported to remain elevated for 12 days in 1 patient.[2]

Related Drugs: Two studies performed in rats found that chlorpromazine, compared to other phenothiazines, was the most competitive inhibitor of norepinephrine uptake into sympathetic nerves.[6,7] Therefore, chlorpromazine may interact with guanethidine to a greater degree than other phenothiazines (e.g., promazine, thioridazine, trifluoperazine [see Appendix]), the thioxanthene (chlorprothixene), and the dibenzoxazepine (loxapine), although because of pharmacologic similarity a similar interaction may be expected. Administration of the butyrophenone antipsychotic (haloperidol) in 3 patients and the other thioxanthene (thiothixene) in 1 patient caused a significant increase in blood pressure previously controlled with guanethidine.[1] The antagonism by haloperidol and thiothixene was not as great as that caused by chlorpromazine.[1]

A clinical trial documented that molindone, a dihydroindolone antipsychotic, does not alter the antihypertensive effects of guanethidine.[8] This is the only psychotropic agent studied that does not interfere in vitro or in vivo with the uptake of norepinephrine into human sympathetic neurons.[4,5]

Bethanidine,* debrisoquin,*[9] and guanadrel are pharmacologically related to guanethidine. Although clinical data are lacking, these drugs may be expected to interact similarly with chlorpromazine.

Mechanism: Guanethidine exerts its antihypertensive effects by competing with norepinephrine for transport into the postganglionic adrenergic neuron. Once there, guanethidine depletes norepinephrine stores and becomes sequestered in neuronal granules.[8,9] The pressor response to adrenergic neuronal activation is therefore reduced.[6,9] Chlorpromazine apparently blocks the transport of guanethidine into the neuron.[8]

Chlorpromazine also possesses alpha-adrenergic blocking activity[9]; therefore, a complete antagonism of guanethidine effect may not occur. The possibility of additive hypotensive effects during the initial days of concurrent guanethidine-chlorpromazine therapy has not been reported in clinical trials.

Recommendations: Because this interaction is clinically significant, patients should not receive chlorpromazine and guanethidine concomitantly, if possible. If concurrent administration is required, patients should be closely monitored for a reversal of the hypotensive effect of guanethidine.[1-8] The dose of guanethidine may have to be increased to maintain the hypotensive effect.

*Not available in the U.S.

Antihypertensive drugs, such as methyldopa, which do not interact with chlorpromazine may be considered as alternatives to guanethidine.[3,10] Also, molindone, which does not appear to alter the antihypertensive effect of guanethidine, may be a suitable alternative to chlorpromazine.

References

1. Janowsky, D.S., and others: Antagonism of guanethidine by chlorpromazine, Am. J. Psychiatry **130:**808, 1973.
2. Fann, W.E., and others: Chlorpromazine reversal of the antihypertensive actions of guanethidine, Lancet **2:**436, 1971.
3. Rankin, G.O., and others: Chlorpromazine interactions with guanethidine and alpha-methyldopa: effects on arterial pressure control and heart rate in renovascular hypertensive rats, Arch. Int. Pharmacodyn. Ther. **260:**130, 1982.
4. Gilder, D.A., and others: A comparison of the abilities of chlorpromazine and molindone to interact adversely with guanethidine, J. Pharmacol. Exp. Ther. **198:**255, 1976.
5. Simpson, L.L.: Combined use of molindone and guanethidine in patients with schizophrenia and hypertension, Am. J. Psychiatry **136:**1410, 1979.
6. Tuck, D., and others: Drug interactions: effect of chlorpromazine on the uptake of monoamines into adrenergic neurons in man, Lancet **2:**492, 1972.
7. Davis, J.M.: Psychopharmacology in the aged: use of psychotropic drugs in geriatric patients, J. Geriatr. Psychiatry **7:**145, 1974.
8. Maxwell, R.A.: Guanethidine after twenty years: a pharmacologist's perspective, Br. J. Clin. Pharmacol. **13:**35, 1982.
9. Nickerson, M., and Collier, B.: Drugs inhibiting adrenergic nerves and structures innervated by them. In Gilman, A.G., Goodman, L.S., and Gilman, A., editors: The pharmacological basis of therapeutics, New York, 1980, MacMillan Publishing.
10. Mitchell, J.R., and others: Guanethidine and related agents. III. Antagonism of drugs which inhibit the norepinephrine pump in man, J. Clin. Invest. **49:**1596, 1970.

Guanethidine–Desipramine

Summary: The antihypertensive effect of guanethidine will be antagonized within 3 to 7 days of initiating desipramine therapy and the antagonism will persist up to 1 week after withdrawal of the medication.[1-5] Continuance of concomitant therapy may demand a large escalation in the dose of guanethidine.[6] The interaction is well documented and clinically significant.

Related Drugs: Amitriptyline, imipramine, protriptyline, nortriptyline, and doxepin (in doses greater than 150 mg daily) have been shown to inhibit the antihypertensive effects of guanethidine.[2,6-10] There is no documentation regarding the other tricyclic antidepressants (amoxapine and trimipramine), although a similar effect may be expected because of pharmacologic similarity. Cyclobenzaprine (a skeletal muscle relaxant) is structurally related to the tricyclic antidepressants and may antagonize the antihypertensive effect of guanethidine.[11] Mianserin,* a tetracyclic antidepressant that does not block the tyramine pressor response, therefore does not block the antihypertensive effects of guanethidine.[12,13] Both bethanidine* and debrisoquin,* which are pharmacologically related to guanethidine, have shown a loss of antihypertensive effect when administered concurrently with tricyclic antidepressants.[3,14] In 1 study, loss of blood pressure was reported in 1 of 6 patients who received concurrent bethanidine* and maprotiline (a tetracycline antidepressant).[15] In another study involving 1 patient, similar results were reported.[16] In the same study 2 patients received guanethidine and 1 received debrisoquin,* and no significant interaction involving blood pressure was demonstrated after concomitant administration of maprotiline.[16] An interaction may be expected to occur between desipramine and guanadrel, which is pharmacologically related to guanethidine; however, no documentation exists.

Mechanism: Guanethidine binds to an "amine pump receptor" and is actively transported by and sequestered in granules, thereby displacing the norepinephrine usually stored in the adrenergic neurons.[3] The amine pump also transports norepinephrine and can be blocked by large bulky molecules such as desipramine and other tricyclic antidepressants. By inhibiting the transport and subsequent accumulation of guanethidine in the neuron, desipramine antagonizes guanethidine's antihypertensive and neuronal blocking effects.[2,3,5] Antagonism of the antihypertensive effect is not immediate but is dependent upon the concentration of guanethidine in the neuron.[17,18]

Recommendations: The concurrent administration of guanethidine and desipramine or other tricyclic antidepressants should be avoided. If co-therapy is selected, the patient should be closely monitored for 1 to 2 weeks, with the expectation that the guanethidine dose may have to be increased. High doses (300 mg) of guanethidine have been successful in overcoming the antidepressant antagonism.[7]

*Not available in the U.S.

Antihypertensive agents such as prazosin, atenolol, or other beta-blockers may be considered as guanethidine substitutes since they do not interact with desipramine. The antidepressant doxepin (in doses less than 150 mg daily) may be substituted for desipramine.[13,14] However, doxepin in this dosage rarely produces an adequate antidepressant effect.[9]

References

1. Mitchell, J.R., and others: Antagonism of the antihypertensive action of guanethidine sulfate by desipramine hydrochloride, J.A.M.A. **202:**973, 1967.
2. Mitchell, J.R., and Oates, J.A.: Guanethidine and related agents. I. Mechanisms of the selective blockade of adrenergic neurons and its antagonism by drugs, J. Pharmacol. Exp. Ther. **172:**100, 1970.
3. Maxwell, R.A.: Guanethidine after twenty years: a pharmacologist's perspective, Br. J. Clin. Pharmacol. **13:**35, 1982.
4. Juul, P., and Sand, O.: Determination of guanethidine in sympathetic ganglia, Acta Pharmacol. Toxicol. **32:**487, 1973.
5. Stone, C.A., and others: Antagonism of certain effects of catecholamine-depleting agents by antidepressant and related drugs, J. Pharmacol. Exp. Ther. **144:**196, 1964.
6. Leishman, A.W.D., and others: Antagonism of guanethidine by imipramine, Lancet **1:**112, 1963.
7. Meyer, J.F., and others: Insidious and prolonged antagonism of guanethidine by amitriptyline, J.A.M.A. **213:**1487, 1970.
8. Evans, B.K., and others: Interaction in vivo between chronically administered guanethidine and imipramine, Gen. Pharmacol. **10:**79, 1979.
9. Fann, W.E., and others: Doxepin: effects on transport of biogenic amines in man, Psychopharmacologica **22:**111, 1971.
10. Hattab, J.R.: The cardiovascular effect of Ludiomil in comparison with tricyclic antidepressants, Psychopharmacologica **29:**191, 1978.
11. Merck Sharp & Dohme: Flexeril® product information. In Angel, J.E., publisher: Physician's desk reference. Oradell, NJ, 1983, Medical Economics Co.
12. Coppen, A., and others: Effect of mianserin hydrochloride on peripheral uptake mechanisms for noradrenaline and 5-hydroxytryptamine in man, Br. J. Clin. Pharmacol. **5:**(suppl.):13, 1978.
13. Burgess, C.D., and Turner, P.: Cardiovascular responses to mianserin hydrochloride: a comparison with tricyclic antidepressants, Br. J. Clin. Pharmacol. **5:**(suppl.): 21, 1978.
14. Stafford, J.R., and Fann, W.E.: Drug interactions with guanethidine antihypertensives, Drugs **13:**57, 1977.
15. Briant, R.H., and George, C.F.: The assessment of potential drug interactions with a new tricyclic antidepressant drug, Br. J. Clin. Pharmacol. **1:**113, 1974.
16. Smith, A.J., and Bant, W.P.: Interactions between post-ganglionic sympathetic blocking drugs and antidepressants, J. Int. Med. Res. **3**(suppl. 2):55, 1975.
17. Ober, K.F., and Wang, R.I.H.: Drug interactions with guanethidine, Clin. Pharmacol. Ther. **14:**190, 1973.
18. Gulati, D.D., and others: Antagonism of adrenergic neuron blockade in hypertensive subjects, Clin. Pharmacol. Ther. **7:**510, 1966.

Guanethidine–Dextroamphetamine

2

Summary: The concurrent use of guanethidine and dextroamphetamine may result in a decrease in the antihypertensive effect of guanethidine.[1-4]

Related Drugs: Bethanidine,[5*] debrisoquin,[6*] and guanadrel[7] are pharmacologically related to guanethidine and also show a potential for decreased antihypertensive effect when used with dextroamphetamine. Several other indirect acting sympathomimetics, which are chemically and pharmacologically similar to the amphetamines, show a similar effect when used with guanethidine. These include methamphetamine[1] and to a lesser extent ephedrine,[1,2,4] methylphenidate,[1] and mephentermine.[2,4]

Phenylpropanolamine is also related chemically and pharmacologically to the amphetamines and has antagonized the effects of bethanidine.[8] The interaction of other direct and mixed (direct and indirect) acting sympathomimetics (direct: e.g., epinephrine, norepinephrine [see Appendix]; mixed: e.g., dopamine, metaraminol [see Appendix]) with guanethidine are discussed in another monograph. (See Guanethidine-Phenylephrine, p. 326.)

Mechanism: The antihypertensive effect of guanethidine is primarily the result of its ability to block the release of norepinephrine from the sympathetic nerve endings. This blockade is apparently dependent on its active transport into the nerve terminal.[9]

Amphetamines and related agents exert their pharmacologic effect on the periphery primarily by causing the release of norepinephrine from sympathetic neurons. The indirect acting sympathomimetics have a strong affinity for the same site within the nerve ending as that occupied by guanethidine.[10] This affinity is sufficiently great to displace guanethidine if it is present or to inhibit its uptake into the nerve ending when guanethidine is administered after amphetamine.[2,4,10,11] The rapid onset of amphetamine-induced reversal suggests a direct effect on vasoconstrictor receptors in addition to competition for the transport mechanism.[3,12]

Recommendations: The reversal of guanethidine's effect by dextroamphetamine, and its resultant effect on blood pressure, suggest that the 2 drugs should not be administered concurrently.

If dextroamphetamine and antihypertensive therapy are indicated for the treatment of a given patient, clonidine, methyldopa, or a beta-blocking agent whose effect has not been reported to be antagonized by dextroamphetamine should be considered.

In addition, since the effect of guanethidine on blood pressure is known to last for several days after discontinuation,[13] the effects of amphetamines on blood pressure must be monitored even after guanethidine discontinuation because these patients may quickly revert to pretreatment levels of blood pressure. One should also note that this prolonged antihypertensive effect of guanethidine may also enhance

---

*Not available in the U.S.

the effect of alternative forms of blood pressure control, even after drug therapy has been altered.

References

1. Gulati, O.D., and others: Antagonism of adrenergic neuron blockade in hypertensive subjects, Clin. Pharmacol. Ther. **7:**510, 1966.
2. Day, M.D.: Effect of sympathomimetic amines on the blocking action of guanethidine, bretylium and xylocholine, Br. J. Pharmacol. **18:**421, 1962.
3. Ober, K.F., and Wang, R.I.H.: Drug interactions with guanethidine, Clin. Pharmacol. Ther. **14:**190, 1973.
4. Day, M.D., and Rand, M.J.: Antagonism of guanethidine by dextroamphetamine and other related sympathomimetic amines, J. Pharm. Pharmacol. **14:**541, 1962.
5. Feagin, O.T., and others: Uptake and release of guanethidine and bethanidine by the adrenergic neuron, J. Clin. Invest. **48:**23a, 1969.
6. Abbs, E.T., and Dodd, M.G.: The relation between the adrenergic neurone-blocking and noradrenaline-depleting actions of some guanidine derivatives, Br. J. Pharmacol. **51:**237, 1974.
7. Hylorel®, Product Information, Pennwalt Corp., May, 1983.
8. Misage, J.R., and McDonald, R.H.: Antagonism of hypotensive action of bethanidine by "common cold" remedy, Br. Med. J. **4:**347, 1970.
9. Boura, A.L.A., and Green, A.F.: Adrenergic neurone blocking agents, Ann. Rev. Pharmacol. **5:**183, 1965.
10. Day, M.D., and Rand, M.J.: Evidence for a competitive antagonism of guanethidine by dextroamphetamine, Br. J. Pharmacol. **20:**17, 1963.
11. Flegin, O.T., and others: The mechanism of reversal of the effect of guanethidine by amphetamines in cat and man, Br. J. Pharmacol. **39:**253P, 1970.
12. Gokhale, S.D., and others: Antagonism of the adrenergic neuron blocking action of guanethidine by certain antidepressant and antihistamine drugs, Arch. Int. Pharmacodyn. Ther. **160:**321, 1966.
13. Nies, A.S.: Cardiovascular disorders. I. Hypertension. In Melmon, K.L. and Morrelli, H.F., editors: Clinical pharmacology: basic principles in therapeutics. Second edition, New York, 1978, MacMillan Publishing.

Guanethidine–Hydrochlorothiazide

Summary: Concurrent hydrochlorothiazide and guanethidine therapy reduces the sodium and water retention and increased blood volume, which occur with long-term guanethidine administration. Optimal antihypertensive therapy is achieved at minimal doses of each agent with a potential reduction in the incidence of adverse effects such as orthostatic and exercise-induced hypotension.[1-7] This beneficial interaction is of clinical significance.

Related Drugs: Other diuretics that possess antihypertensive properties because of their ability to reduce sodium and water retention may be expected to undergo a similar interaction with guanethidine. These include other thiazide diuretics (e.g., chlorothiazide, methyclothiazide, polythiazide [see Appendix]), loop diuretics (bumetanide, ethacrynic acid, and furosemide), thiazide related diuretics (e.g., chlorthalidone, indapamide, metolazone [see Appendix]) and spironolactone, a potassium-sparing diuretic. Other potassium-sparing diuretics (amiloride and triamterene) have little or no antihypertensive effect.[1]

Bethanidine,*[8] debrisoquin,* and guanadrel are pharmacologically related to guanethidine and may be expected to interact with hydrochlorothiazide in a similar manner.

Mechanism: The mechanism of the antihypertensive action of the thiazide diuretics has not been fully delineated. The thiazides appear to initially cause fluid and sodium depletion with resultant reduction in peripheral vascular resistance with long-term use.[1]

Guanethidine produces its antihypertensive effect by blocking the uptake of norepinephrine into the neuron and reducing the tissue stores of norepinephrine.[1,9] Long-term use of guanethidine results in a progressive resistance to its antihypertensive effect because of increasing sodium retention and edema formation, which cannot be reversed with larger doses of guanethidine.[1] These symptoms may be reversed with concomitant hydrochlorothiazide therapy.[1-7]

Recommendations: The addition of hydrochlorothiazide to long-term guanethidine therapy may result in the need to reduce the dose of guanethidine. The thiazide diuretic will enhance the antihypertensive effect of guanethidine. Patients should be informed of the possible occurrence of dizziness or syncope from the enhanced antihypertensive effect of the combination therapy.

References

1. Weiner, M.: Drugs that inhibit adrenergic nerves and block adrenergic receptors. In Gilman, A.G., Goodman, L.S., and Gilman, A., editors: The pharmacological basis of therapeutics, New York, 1980, MacMillan Publishing.
2. Maronde, R.F., and others: Comparison of guanethidine and guanethidine plus a thiazide diuretic, Am. J. Med. Sci. **242:**228, 1961.
3. Gerber, J.G., and others: Antihypertensive pharmacology, West. J. Med. **132:**430, 1980.

*Not available in the U.S.

4. Moses, C.: Drug treatment of mild hypertension: adverse consequences, Ann. N.Y. Acad. Sci. **304:**84, 1978.
5. Kohler, C., and others: The effect of guanethidine and hydrochlorothiazide on blood pressure and vascular tyrosine hydroxylase activity in the spontaneously hypertensive rat, Eur. J. Pharmacol. **42:**161, 1977.
6. Reader, R.: Therapeutic trials in mild hypertension ongoing throughout the world, Ann. N.Y. Acad. Sci. **304:**309, 1978.
7. Brown, W.J., Jr., and Brown, F.K.: The use of guanethidine and hydrochlorothiazide in the long-term treatment of essential hypertension, Curr. Ther. Res. **17:**544, 1975.
8. Ramirez, E.A., and others: Multiclinic controlled trial of bethanidine and guanethidine in severe hypertension, Circulation **55:**519, 1977.
9. Maxwell, R.A.: Guanethidine after twenty years: a pharmacologist's perspective, Br. J. Clin. Pharmacol. **13:**35, 1982.

Guanethidine–Minoxidil

Summary: The coadministration of guanethidine and minoxidil may result in a profound orthostatic hypotension.[1,2] The potentiation still occurs even if guanethidine is discontinued 3 days before initiation of minoxidil therapy.[3]

Related Drugs: Although this effect has not been documented, drugs that are pharmacologically related to guanethidine (bethanidine*, debrisoquin,* and guanadrel) may be expected to produce a similar hypotensive episode with minoxidil. There are no drugs related to minoxidil.

Mechanism: The exact mechanism by which this occurs is not known. Guanethidine is known to cause orthostatic hypotension. Minoxidil alone does not have such an effect but can accentuate the guanethidine effect.

Recommendations: It is recommended that guanethidine be discontinued at least one week before initiation of minoxidil, if possible. If not possible, it is suggested that minoxidil therapy be started in a hospital setting and that the patient remain in the hospital until the severe orthostatic effects dissipate or until the patient learns how to avoid activities that produce these effects.

References

1. Smith, G.H.: Minoxidil, Drug Intell. Clin. Pharm. **14:**477, 1980.
2. Miller, D.D., and Love, D.W.: Evaluation of monoxidil, Am. J. Hosp. Pharm. **37:**808, 1980.
3. Lowenthal, D.T., and others: Radioimmunoassay, pharmacokinetics and pharmacodynamics for minoxidil in chronic renal failure, Clin. Res. **24:**475A, 1976.

Guanethidine–Phenelzine

2

Summary: Addition of a monoamine oxidase (MAO) inhibitor to guanethidine may result in a compromise in the antihypertensive effectiveness of guanethidine.[1] Reports of substantiated increases in blood pressure in humans receiving MAO inhibitors while on guanethidine are lacking.

Related Drugs: Tranylcypromine has shown similar antagonism of guanethidine in animals.[1] Although this effect is undocumented, other monoamine oxidase inhibitors (isocarboxazid and pargyline) may be expected to interact similarly. Drugs that are pharmacologically related to guanethidine (bethanidine*, debrisoquin,* and guanadrel) may have potential to interact in the same manner.

Mechanism: It is postulated that monoamine oxidase inhibitors antagonize guanethidine's hypotensive effect by interfering with catecholamine depletion caused by guanethidine within the adrenergic neuron.[2]

Recommendations: To avoid any risk in compromise of blood pressure control, MAO inhibitors should not be added to any antihypertensive regimen including guanethidine. Careful monitoring of blood pressure is required if this combination cannot be avoided.

References

1. Day, M.D.: Effect of sympathomimetic amines on the blocking action of guanethidine, bretylium and xylocholine, Br. J. Pharmacol. **18:**421, 1962.
2. Woolsey, N.L., and Nies, A.S.: Guanethidine, N. Engl. J. Med. **295:**1053, 1976.

*Not available in the U.S.

Guanethidine–Phenylephrine

Summary: Systemically administered direct and mixed acting sympathomimetics may antagonize the hypotensive effects of patients pretreated with guanethidine, resulting in hypertension.[1,2] This interaction is not documented with topical phenylephrine.

Related Drugs: The drugs that are pharmacologically related to guanethidine (bethanidine*, debrisoquin,* and guanadrel) may also show potential to interact in the same manner. Other sympathomimetics (direct acting: e.g., epinephrine, methoxamine, norepinephrine [see Appendix]; mixed acting: dopamine and metaraminol) when administered systemically may show an effect similar to phenylephrine, although data are limited and controversial. Interactions between indirect-acting sympathomimetics (e.g., dextroamphetamine, methamphetamine, ephedrine [see Appendix]) and guanethidine are discussed in another monograph. (See Guanethidine-Dextroamphetamine, p. 320.)

Mechanism: Guanethidine initially blocks the release of norepinephrine from sympathetic neurons and during continued administration can cause a depletion of neuronal norepinephrine.[3] Prolonged interference of nerve impulses increases the reactivity of effector cells to direct stimulation, which may produce an acute increase in sensitivity to direct and mixed acting sympathomimetics. This type of supersensitivity may be related to the ability of guanethidine to indirectly interfere with the adrenergic neuron amine uptake mechanism and/or to a direct sensitizing action of the drug on the adrenergic receptor.[4-8]

Recommendations: A compromise in blood pressure control may occur when direct or mixed-acting sympathomimetic agents are used by patients who are receiving or have recently received guanethidine. The concurrent use of these agents should be avoided.

References

1. Gulati, O.D., and others: Antagonism of adrenergic neuron blockade in hypertensive subjects, Clin. Pharmacol. Ther. **7:**510, 1966.
2. Ober, K.F., and Wang, R.I.H.: Drug interactions with guanethidine, Clin. Pharmacol. Ther. **14:**190, 1973.
3. Boura, A.L.A., and Green, A.F.: Adrenergic neuron blocking agents, Ann. Rev. Pharmacol. **5:**183, 1965.
4. Hertting, G., and others: Effect of drugs on the uptake and metabolism of H^3-norepinephrine, J. Pharmacol. Exp. Ther. **134:**146, 1961.
5. Iverson, L.L.: Catecholamines uptake processes, Br. Med. Bull. **29:**130, 1973.
6. Trendelenburg, U.: Classification of sympathomimetic amines, Handbook Exp. Pharmacol. **33:**336, 1972.
7. Maxwell, R.A.: Concerning the mode of action of guanethidine and some derivatives in augmenting vasomotor action of adrenergic amines in vascular tissues of the rabbit, J. Pharmacol. Exp. Ther. **148:**320, 1965.
8. Abboud, F.M., and others: Early potentiation of the vasoconstrictor action of norepinephrine by guanethidine, Proc. Soc. Exp. Biol. Med. **110:**489, 1962.

*Not available in the U.S.

Methyldopa–Amitriptyline

Summary: In a single case report, loss of blood pressure control occurred when amitriptyline was added to a methyldopa regimen.[1]

Related Drugs: In a controlled study in 3 patients, methyldopa was reported not to interact with desipramine.[2] Similarly, the antihypertensive effects of methyldopa were not antagonized in 5 normotensive patients pretreated with desipramine.[3] Clonidine, whose mechanism of action is very similar to methyldopa, has been reported to interact with tricyclic antidepressants.[4] In a controlled trial, desipramine attentuated the antihypertensive and sedative response to clonidine in both hypertensive[5] and depressed patients.[6] Imipramine has also been reported to antagonize the antihypertensive effects of clonidine in 3 cases.[7-9] Tricyclic antidepressants interfere with the antihypertensive effects of both clonidine[10-12] and methyldopa[12-14] in animals.

Another centrally active antihypertensive agent with properties similar to clonidine and methyldopa, guanabenz, may be expected to interact similarly with the other tricyclic antidepressants (e.g., amoxapine, doxepin, nortriptyline [see Appendix]) though no such interactions have yet been reported.

In a controlled study of 11 patients, the tetracyclic antidepressant mianserin* was shown to have no interaction with the antihypertensive action of clonidine or methyldopa.[15] The concurrent use of maprotiline, another tetracyclic antidepressant, and clonidine was not associated with an altered response to clonidine in a study involving 8 healthy volunteers.[16]

Mechanism: Although the exact mechanism of this interaction has not been established, there is evidence that tricyclic antidepressants have anti–alpha-adrenergic properties in the central nervous system.[6] Since methyldopa and clonidine depend on central alpha-adrenergic stimulation for their action,[4] it would follow that the tricyclic antidepressants could directly antagonize their effect.

Recommendations: Based on the information available, it would seem that the interaction between methyldopa and amitriptyline is unlikely to occur in most patients; however, it is prudent to monitor blood pressure if tricyclic antidepressants are added to methyldopa therapy. The interaction between clonidine and desipramine is more firmly established and appears to occur regularly, although it can be overcome by increasing the dose of clonidine.[17] Patients who receive tricyclic antidepressants in combination with clonidine should have their blood pressure closely monitored during the first several days of combined therapy. Alternatively, the tetracyclic antidepressant maprotiline may be substituted for the tricyclic antidepressant if clonidine therapy is chosen.

---

*Not available in the U.S.

References

1. White, A.G.: Methyldopa and amitriptyline, Lancet **2:**441, 1965.
2. Mitchell, J.R., and others: Guanethidine and related agents. III. Antagonism by drugs which inhibit the norepinephrine pump in man, J. Clin. Invest. **49:**1596, 1970.
3. Reid, J.L., and others: The effect of desmethylimipramine on the pharmacological actions of alpha methyldopa in man, Eur. J. Clin. Pharmacol. **16:**75, 1979.
4. Blaschke, T.F., and Melmon, K.L.: Antihypertensive agents and the drug therapy of hypertension. In Gilman, A.G., Goodman, L.S., and Gilman, A., editors: The pharmacological basis of therapeutics, New York, 1980, Macmillan Publishing.
5. Briant, R.H., and others: Interaction between clonidine and desipramine in man, Br. Med. J. **1:**522, 1973.
6. Checkley, S.A., and others: A pilot study of the mechanism of action of desipramine, Br. J. Psychiatry **138:**248, 1983.
7. Conolly, M.E., and others: In: Conolly, M.E., editor: Catapres in hypertension, London, 1969, Butterworth's Publishing.
8. Coffler, D.E.: Antipsychotic drug interaction, Drug Intell. Clin. Pharm. **10:**114, 1976.
9. Hui, K.K.: Hypertensive crisis induced by interaction of clonidine with imipramine, J. Am. Geriatr. Soc. **31:**164, 1983.
10. van Zwieten, P.A.: The reversal of clonidine-induced hypotension by protriptyline and desipramine, Pharmacology **14:**227, 1976.
11. van Spanning, H.W., and van Zwieten, P.A.: The interference of tricyclic antidepressants with the central hypotensive effect of clonidine, Eur. J. Pharmacol. **24:**402, 1973.
12. van Zwieten, P.A.: Interaction between centrally acting hypotensive drugs and tricyclic antidepressants, Arch. Int. Pharmacodyn. Ther. **12:**214, 1975.
13. van Spanning, H.W., and van Zwieten, P.A.: The interaction between alpha-methyldopa and tricyclic antidepressants, Int. J. Clin. Pharmacol. Biopharm. **11:**65, 1975.
14. Kale, A.K., and Satoskar, R.S.: Modification of the central hypotensive effect of alpha-methyldopa by reserpine, imipramine and tranylcypromine, Eur. J. Pharmacol. **9:**120, 1970.
15. Elliot, H.L., and others: Assessment of the interaction between mianserin and centrally-acting anti-hypertensive drugs, Br. J. Clin. Pharmacol. **15**(suppl. 2):323S, 1983.
16. Gundert-Remy, U., and others: Lack of interaction between the tetracyclic anti-depressant maprotiline and the centrally acting anti-hypertensive drug clonidine, Eur. J. Clin. Pharmacol. **25:**595, 1983.
17. Raftos, J.: Clonidine in the treatment of severe hypertension, Med. J. Aust. **1:**786, 1973.

Summary: Three cases have been reported where dementia occurred within 3 days after haloperidol was added to an existing methyldopa regimen.[1,2] Symptoms cleared within 3 days after haloperidol was discontinued.[1] Another report describes side effects of somnolence and dizziness in a study of combined therapy for 4 weeks.[3]

Related Drugs: Although no documentation exists, other antipsychotics such as the phenothiazines (e.g., chlorpromazine, thioridazine, trifluoperazine [see Appendix]), thioxanthenes (chlorprothixene and thiothixene), as well as the dihydroindolone (molindone) and dibenzoxazepine (loxapine) may be expected to interact in a similar manner with methyldopa because of pharmacologic similarity to haloperidol, an antipsychotic butyrophenone. There are no drugs related to methyldopa.

Mechanism: The mechanism is unknown. However, it has been postulated that this interaction results from an additive inhibition of dopamine in the central nervous system.[1]

Recommendations: The reports suggest that the concurrent use of these agents can lead to abnormal central nervous system symptoms. Although the incidence may be low, it is important to be aware of this possible interaction. Should central nervous system symptoms occur, discontinuation of haloperidol should resolve the reaction.

References

1. Thornton, W.E.: Dementia induced by methyldopa with haloperidol, N. Engl. J. Med. **294:**1222, 1976.
2. Nadel, I., and Wallach, M.: Drug interaction between haloperidol and methyldopa, Br. J. Psychiatry **135:**484, 1979.
3. Chouinard, G., and others: Potentiation of haloperidol by alpha-methyldopa in treatment of schizophrenic patients, Curr. Ther. Res. **15:**473, 1973.

Methyldopa–Levodopa

3

Summary: Concurrent administration of levodopa and methyldopa can result in increased therapeutic effectiveness of either drug or adverse effects depending on individual patient response or the dose of either drug used. Methyldopa has been reported to both cause and relieve parkinsonism.

Although methyldopa has been found to inhibit the therapeutic response to levodopa,[1,2] it has also been used to reduce the maintenance dose of levodopa in normotensive patients.[3,4]

Related Drugs: There are no drugs related to levodopa or methyldopa.

Mechanism: Methyldopa may enhance the antiparkinsonian effects of levodopa by preventing its extracerebral decarboxylation,[5,6] thus enabling the active moiety to be present in greater concentration for transport to the central nervous system.[7] Conversely, methyldopa's central inhibition of dopa decarboxylase may reduce cerebral dopamine, resulting in a parkinsonian-like syndrome.[8,9] Additive or synergistic hypotensive effects have also been described when the 2 drugs are administered concurrently.[10] This is presumably the result of an enhanced pharmacologic effect.

Recommendations: Although several reports indicate that concurrent use of levodopa and methyldopa may produce a beneficial effect on the symptoms of parkinsonism without increasing the risk of adverse drug reactions,[3,10] the possibility that this combination influences the therapeutic response to levodopa in certain patients should be considered. The occurrence of side effects such as vomiting and drowsiness induced by either drug may require a dose reduction or discontinuation of methyldopa.[4]

References

1. Cotzias, G.C., and others: L-dopa in Parkinson's syndrome (letter), N. Engl. J. Med. **281:**272, 1969.
2. Kofman, O.: Treatment of Parkinson's disease with L-dopa. A current appraisal, Can. Med. Assoc. J. **104:**483, 1971.
3. Fermaglich, J., and O'Doherty, D.S.: A second generation of L-dopa therapy, Neurology **21:**408, 1971.
4. Mones, R.J.: Evaluation of alpha-methyldopa and alpha-methyldopa hydrazine with L-dopa therapy, N.Y. State J. Med. **74:**47, 1974.
5. Clark, W.G., and Pogrund, R.S.: Inhibition of dopa decarboxylase in vitro and in vivo, Circ. Res. **9:**721, 1961.
6. Smith, S.E.: The pharmacological actions of 3,4-dihydroxyphenyl-alpha-methylalanine (alpha-methyldopa) an inhibitor of 5-hydroxytryptophan decarboylase, Br. J. Pharmacol. **15:**319, 1960.
7. Pletscher, A., and Bartholini, G.: Selective rise in brain dopamine by inhibition of extracerebral levodopa decarboxylation, Clin. Pharmacol. Therap. **12:**344, 1971.
8. Peaston, M.J.T.: Parkinsonism associated with alpha-methyldopa therapy, Br. Med. J. **2:**168, 1964.
9. Vaidya, R.A., and others: Galactorrhea and parkinson-like syndrome: an adverse effect of alpha-methyldopa, Metabolism **19:**1068, 1970.
10. Gibberd, F.B., and Small, E.: Interaction between levodopa and methyldopa, Br. Med. J. **2:**90, 1973.

Methyldopa–Norepinephrine

Summary: The pressor effect of norepinephrine was found to increase and to be prolonged with the concurrent administration of methyldopa.[1,2] A possible hypertensive episode may result.

Related Drugs: Other direct-acting sympathomimetics (e.g., epinephrine, isoproterenol, methoxamine [see Appendix]) may interact similarly with methyldopa, although documentation is lacking. The pressor effect of tyramine, an indirect-acting sympathomimetic, was found to increase in 12 hypertensive patients receiving methyldopa.[1,3] A severe hypertensive reaction was reported in a patient receiving phenylpropanolamine, a mixed-acting sympathomimetic, with methyldopa and oxprenolol*.[4] There is no other documentation regarding an interaction between methyldopa and other mixed and indirect-acting sympathomimetics (mixed: e.g., metaraminol, phenylephrine [see Appendix]; indirect: e.g., amphetamine, ephedrine [see Appendix]); however because of pharmacologic similarity an interaction may be expected to occur.

Mechanism: The mechanism of action of methyldopa, although not conclusively demonstrated, is attributed to its metabolite, alpha-methylnorepinephrine. This metabolite lowers arterial pressure by stimulation of central inhibitory alpha-adrenergic receptors, false neurotransmission, and/or reduction of plasma renin activity.[5] Alpha-methylnorepinephrine has a weaker pressor activity (alpha-adrenergic) than norepinephrine. The mechanism involved in this interaction is probably the additive effect between the false transmitter and the normal transmitter at the same alpha receptor sites. Another proposed mechanism is related to the fact that methyldopa's metabolites are not substrates for monoamine oxidase, therefore facilitating their access to alpha-adrenergic receptor sites.[3]

Recommendations: It is important to be aware of a possible interaction between methyldopa and norepinephrine or other sympathomimetics (direct, indirect, and mixed acting), which may lead to hypertension. Phentolamine or another alpha-adrenergic blocking agent may be useful if hypertension does occur. It may also be necessary to discontinue the sympathomimetic amine. The norepinephrine dose should initially be reduced when used concurrently with methyldopa, and one study suggests beginning with one-tenth the usual dose.[2]

References

1. Dollery, C.T., and others: Haemodynamic studies with methyldopa: effect on cardiac output and response to pressor amines, Br. Heart J. **25:**670, 1963.
2. Dollery, C.T.: Physiological and pharmacological interactions of antihypertensive drugs, Proc. R. Soc. Med. **58:**983, 1965.
3. Pettinger, W., and others: Enhancement by methyldopa of tyramine sensitivity in man, Nature **200:**1107, 1963.
4. McLaren, E.H.: Severe hypertension produced by interaction of phenylpropanolamine with methyldopa and oxprenolol, Br. Med. J. **2:**283, 1976.
5. Aldomet® product information, Merck Sharp and Dohme, Feb., 1982.

*Not available in the U.S.

Summary: Indirect evidence obtained from measurement of catecholamine level changes suggested that barbiturate therapy could result in lowered methyldopa blood levels.[1] However, subsequent studies utilizing a more specific assay that directly measured methyldopa and metabolite levels failed to confirm an interaction between methyldopa and barbiturates.[2,3]

Related Drugs: Other barbiturates (e.g., amobarbital, butabarbital, secobarbital [see Appendix]) might be expected to act in a similar manner to phenobarbital because of pharmacologic similarity. There are no drugs related to methyldopa.

Mechanism: Although the mechanism has not been established, it has been postulated that phenobarbital administration to patients receiving methyldopa increases methyldopa metabolism, resulting in decreased serum methyldopa levels.[1]

Recommendations: The clinical significance of the potential interaction between methyldopa and phenobarbital has not been substantiated. Therefore, it appears that no dosage adjustments or additional precautions are necessary when these 2 agents are administered concurrently.

References

1. Kaldor, A., and others: Enhancement of methyldopa metabolism with barbiturate, Br. Med. J. **3:**518, 1971.
2. Kristensen, M., and others: Barbiturates and methyldopa metabolism, Br. Med. J. **1:**49, 1973.
3. Kristensen, M., and others: Plasma concentration of alpha-methyldopa and its main metabolite, methyldopa-o-sulfate during long-term treatment with alpha-methyldopa with special reference to possible interaction with other drugs given simultaneously, Clin. Pharmacol. Ther. **14:**140, 1973.

Methyldopa–Propranolol

2

Summary: In a case report, a patient receiving both methyldopa and hydralazine exhibited increased blood pressure when intravenous propranolol was given during crisis treatment.[1]

Related Drugs: Propranolol effectively blocks the peripheral vasodilator (beta$_2$) effect of sympathomimetics with alpha and beta agonist activity, allowing the expression of the alpha-adrenergic properties. Therefore, other nonselective beta blocking agents (nadolol, pindolol, and timolol) would be expected to interact in a similar manner with methyldopa. However, cardioselective (beta$_1$) adrenergic blocking agents (atenolol and metoprolol) do not substantially inhibit the peripheral vasodilator effect (beta$_2$) of the alpha- and beta-adrenergic sympathomimetic agents, and therefore would not be expected to interact with methyldopa to a similar degree.[2]

One patient receiving methyldopa and oxprenolol* had a severe hypertensive episode after taking a cold preparation that contained phenylpropanolamine and acetaminophen.[3]

Mechanism: Methyldopa is metabolized to alpha-methylnorepinephrine in central adrenergic neurons and replaces the normal neurotransmitter, norepinephrine. Alpha-methylnorepinephrine has a weaker pressor activity (alpha receptor) but a greater vasodilator activity (beta receptor) than norepinephrine. Beta-blocking agents, when administered concurrently, would block the beta receptor activity allowing the alpha receptor activity (pressor effect) to occur unopposed, resulting in hypertension.

Recommendations: These interactions are potentially serious. It would seem prudent to consider the possibility of this interaction in patients taking methyldopa and beta-adrenergic blocking agents, especially when a drug or clinical situation may cause an increased release of the neurotransmitter.

References

1. Nies, A.S., and Shand, D.G.: Hypertensive response to propranolol in a patient treated with methyldopa—a proposed mechanism, Clin. Pharmacol. Ther. **14**:823, 1973.
2. Weiner, N.: Drugs that inhibit adrenergic nerves and block adrenergic receptors. In Gilman, A.G., Goodman, L.S., and Gilman, A., editors: The pharmacological basis of therapeutics. New York, 1980, Macmillan Publishing.
3. McLaren, E.H.: Severe hypertension produced by interaction of phenylpropanolamine with methyldopa and oxprenolol, Br. Med. J. **2**:283, 1976.

*Not available in the U.S.

Prazosin–Indomethacin

2

Summary: The concurrent use of prazosin and indomethacin may reduce the hypotensive effect of prazosin. In a study involving 9 healthy volunteers, in 4 of 9 subjects indomethacin considerably attenuated prazosin-induced hypotension. The effect of prazosin in the other 5 subjects was not influenced by indomethacin.[1]

Related Drugs: There are no drugs related to prazosin. Documentation is lacking regarding a similar interaction with the other nonsteroidal anti-inflammatory agents (e.g., ibuprofen, naproxen, sulindac [see Appendix]). However, if the mechanism involves prostaglandin inhibition, these agents may interact similarly since they also inhibit prostaglandins to some extent.

Mechanism: Indomethacin prevented the rise in plasma renin activity that is seen following administration of prazosin. There is some evidence that this suppression by indomethacin is directly related to the extent of prostaglandin synthetase inhibition.[1]

Recommendations: Patients' blood pressure should be closely monitored during concurrent use of these agents. An increased prazosin dose may be necessary.

Reference

1. Rubin, P., and others: Studies on the clinical pharmacology of prazosin. II. The influence of indomethacin and of propranolol on the action and disposition of prazosin, Br. J. Clin. Pharmacol. **10:**33, 1980.

Prazosin–Propranolol

2

Summary: The concurrent use of prazosin and propranolol may enhance the acute postural hypotensive reaction after the first dose of prazosin.[1,2] In a double-blind crossover study involving 8 healthy subjects, the severity and duration of the orthostatic hypotension were significantly increased during concomitant use of these agents.[1] Similar results were reported in the study involving 6 hypertensive patients, 3 of whom were taking propranolol.[2]

Related Drugs: An exaggerated hypotensive effect was also seen with concurrent prazosin and alprenolol.*[3] Documentation is lacking regarding an interaction between prazosin and the other beta-blocking agents (e.g., atenolol, nadolol, pindolol [see Appendix]), although because of pharmacologic similarity a similar interaction may be expected to occur. There are no drugs related to prazosin.

Mechanism: The most drastic side effect of prazosin is the first dose phenomenon. This is a syncope caused by severe hypotension and impaired venous return. These orthostatic symptoms develop only when the compensatory tachycardia is not maintained and bradycardia dramatically supervenes. It has been postulated that the compensatory responses of the heart after the first dose of prazosin is blocked by the beta-blockade produced by propranolol.[1,3] Pharmacokinetics do not appear to play a role.[3] Also, no unusually marked blood pressure decrease was observed when the first dose of a beta-blocking agent was given to a patient on long-term prazosin, indicating that the first dose response is involved in this interaction.[3]

Recommendations: Patients should be advised of the increased risk involved with the first dose of prazosin, especially when it is added to a beta-blocking agent. Initiation of prazosin treatment with a dose of 0.5 mg or less has been suggested.[2,3]

References

1. Elliott, H.L., and others: Immediate cardiovascular responses to oral prazosin—effects of concurrent beta-blockers, Clin. Pharmacol. Ther. **29:**303, 1981.
2. Graham, R.M., and others: Prazosin: the first-dose phenomenon, Br. Med. J. **2:**1293, 1976.
3. Seideman, P., and others: Prazosin first dose phenomenon during combined treatment with a beta-adrenoreceptor blocker in hypertensive patients, Br. J. Clin. Pharmacol. **13:**865, 1982.

*Not available in the U.S.

Reserpine–Ephedrine

2

Summary: The indirect sympathomimetic action of ephedrine may be antagonized as a result of depletion of norepinephrine from adrenergic vesicles by reserpine. Since clinical exposure to reserpine may produce a partial or complete catecholamine depletion, variable responses to ephedrine can be anticipated.

Related Drugs: Other sympathomimetic agents with indirect action such as amphetamine, methylphenidate, tyramine, and phenylpropanolamine may also be expected to interact with reserpine in a similar manner.[1] Although no documentation exists, other rauwolfia alkaloids (e.g., alseroxylon, deserpidine, rescinnamine [see Appendix]) may also be expected to interact with ephedrine because of pharmacologic similarity. There is no documentation regarding an interaction between reserpine and mixed acting sympathomimetics (dopamine, metaraminol, and phenylephrine) but the occurence of an interaction would probably depend on the degree of direct and indirect activity. Documentation is also lacking regarding an interaction between reserpine and direct acting sympathomimetics (e.g., epinephrine, methoxamine, norepinephrine [see Appendix]), but because they exert their action directly on the adrenergic receptor and do not depend on neuronal release, a similar interaction would not be expected.

Mechanism: Reserpine depletes the peripheral vascular adrenergic nerve endings of catecholamines and reduces their intraneuronal storage.[2] Ephedrine stimulates the adrenergic receptor site directly and also indirectly by promoting the release of norepinephrine from its storage vesicles in the sympathetic nerve endings.[3] When reserpine is given before ephedrine, it may antagonize the indirect action of ephedrine, resulting in a decreased cardiovascular response to this sympathomimetic.[2]

Recommendations: Patients receiving reserpine who are not responsive to therapeutic doses of ephedrine should be switched to a direct acting sympathomimetic agent such as norepinephrine or phenylephrine. The direct acting adrenergic agents will bypass the vesicle depletion action of reserpine and initiate the desired hypertensive action. Should norepinephrine be used, the added reuptake action of this agent will partially restore normal catecholamine activity. Smaller doses of direct acting sympathomimetics may be sufficient since the vasculature in reserpine treated patients is often more sensitive to these drugs.[4]

References

1. Burn, J.H., and Rand, M.J.: The action of sympathomimetic amines in animals treated with reserpine, J. Physiol. **144**:314, 1958.
2. Trendelenburg, U.: Supersensitivity and subsensitivity to sympathomimetic amines, Pharmacol. Rev. **15**:225, 1963.
3. Snedden, J.M., and Turner, P.: Ephedrine mydriasis in hypertension and the response to treatment, Clin. Pharmacol. Ther. **10**:64, 1969.
4. Smessaert, A.A., and Hicks, R.G.: Problems caused by rauwolfia drugs during anesthesia and surgery, N.Y. State J. Med. **61**:2399, 1961.

Reserpine–Halothane

Summary: Several studies have suggested that concurrent administration of halothane in patients receiving reserpine may be tolerated without increased risk of hypotension.[1-4] This is contrary to earlier reports[5,6] which recommend discontinuing reserpine therapy in hypertensive patients 1 or 2 weeks preoperatively before receiving anesthesia. One study comparing the results in patients undergoing elective surgery whose reserpine therapy had been discontinued before anesthesia with results in patients from emergency cases in which reserpine had not been discontinued found no significant differences in the incidence of intraoperative hypotension between the 2 groups.[4]

Related Drugs: Although the occurrence of a drug interaction is doubtful, a decrease in blood pressure has been associated with the use of other general anesthetic agents and rauwolfia alkaloids. Such anesthetic agents include cyclopropane,[1,5] ether,[1,2] methoxyflurane,[1] and nitrous oxide.[2,5,6] Although this effect is undocumented, other anesthetic agents (e.g., enflurane, ethyl chloride, isoflurane [see Appendix]) may be expected to interact similarly with reserpine. Other rauwolfia alkaloids (e.g., alseroxylon, deserpidine, rescinnamine [see Appendix]) may be expected to interact with halothane and other general anesthetics in a similar manner because of pharmacologic similarity.

Mechanism: Halothane produces direct myocardial depression[7,9] and an increased parasympathetic activity with a resultant reduction in heart rate and myocardial depression.[10] In addition, halothane may also affect catecholamine activity through central nervous system depression of sympathetic activity,[11] sympathetic blockade,[12] or reduction of the effect of catecholamines on myocardial and vascular smooth muscle.[13] It has been postulated that halothane added to the catecholamine depleting action of reserpine[14,15] causes enhanced depressant effects on the heart, resulting in decreased cardiac output and hypotension. Recent studies indicate that these effects may not occur any more often in patients taking reserpine than in those administered halothane alone.[1-4]

Recommendations: Clinical evidence indicates that long-term reserpine therapy is not a contraindication to anesthesia and surgery.[1-3] However, patients on reserpine therapy should be observed for any unexpected hypotensive episodes during administration of halothane, particularly when there is associated blood loss, excessive speed of induction of anesthesia, surgical manipulation, position change, or excessive amount of anesthetic agents used. If reserpine is not withdrawn before surgery and if hypotension does occur, an exacerbated effect may be noticed since the endogenous catecholamines have already been chronically depleted by reserpine. Therefore, the use of an indirect-acting sympathomimetic agent would be ineffective, and a direct-acting sympathomimetic agent would be required to treat the hypotension.[4,14]

References

1. Katz, R.L., and others: Anesthesia, surgery and rauwolfia, Anesthesiology **25:**142, 1964.
2. Munson, W.M., and Jenicek, J.A.: Effect of anesthetic agents on patients receiving reserpine therapy, Anesthesiology **23:**741, 1962.
3. Alper, M.H., and others: Pharmacology of reserpine and its implications for anesthesia, Anesthesiology **24:**524, 1963.
4. Ominsky, A.J., and Wolman, H.: Hazards of general anesthesia in the reserpinized patients, Anesthesiology **30:**443, 1969.
5. Smessaert, A.A., and Hick, R.G.: Problems caused by rauwolfia drugs during anesthesia and surgery, N.Y. State J. Med. **61:**2399, 1961.
6. Ziegler, C.H., and Lovette, J.B.: Operative complications after therapy with reserpine and reserpine compounds, J.A.M.A. **176:**916, 1961.
7. Flacke, W., and Alper, M.H.: Actions of halothane and norepinephrine in the isolated mammalian heart, Anesthesiology **23:**793, 1962.
8. Goldberg, A.H., and Ullrick, W.C.: Effects of halothane on isometric contractions of isolated heart muscle, Anesthesiology **28:**838, 1967.
9. Shimosato, S., and Etsten, B.: Performance of digitalized heart during halothane anesthesia, Anesthesiology **24:**41, 1963.
10. Laver, M.B., and Turndorf, H.: Atrial activity and systemic blood pressure during anesthesia in man, Circulation **23:**63, 1963.
11. Price, H.L., and Price, M.L.: Has halothane a predominant circulatory action? Anesthesiology **27:**764, 1966.
12. Garfield, J.M., and others: A pharmacological analysis of ganglionic actions of some general anesthetics, Anesthesiology **29:**79, 1968.
13. Price, M.L., and Price, H.L.: Effects of general anesthetics on contractile responses of rabbit aortic strips, Anesthesiology **23:**16, 1962.
14. Weiner, N.: Drugs that inhibit adrenergic nerves and block adrenergic receptors. In Gilman, A.G., Goodman, L.S., and Gilman, A., editors: The pharmacological basis of therapeutics. New York, 1980, Macmillan Publishing.
15. Chidsey, C.A., and others: Myocardial norepinephrine concentration in man: effects of reserpine and of congestive heart failure, N. Engl. J. Med. **269:**653, 1963.

CHAPTER EIGHT

Anti-infective Drug Interactions

*Not available in the U.S.

*This combination is not available in the U.S.

TABLE 8. Anti-infective Drug Interactions

Drug Interaction	Significance Code	Potential Effects	Recommendations	See Page
Acyclovir–Probenecid	3	Probenecid decreases the elimination rate of parenteral acyclovir. The clinical significance is unknown.	Necessary dosage adjustments of acyclovir should be made.	347
Ampicillin–Allopurinol	3	Concurrent use may result in an increased incidence of drug-induced skin rash when compared to the use of either drug alone.	One or both drugs may need to be discontinued if a rash develops.	348
Ampicillin–Oral Contraceptive Agents	2	Concurrent use may cause breakthrough bleeding and loss of contraceptive protection in some patients.	Since prediction of who will be affected by this interaction is not possible, an alternative form of contraception is advisable during co-therapy.	349
Cefoperazone–Alcohol, Ethyl	2	Cephalosporins with the methyltetrazolethiol side chain may produce a disulfiram-like reaction when combined with alcohol.	Abstention from alcohol during and for several days after cefoperazone therapy is advisable.	351
Cephaloridine*–Furosemide	2	Cephaloridine nephrotoxicity may be enhanced by concurrent furosemide.	Avoid concurrent use, but if this is not possible, monitor renal function regularly.	353
Cephalothin–Colistimethate	2	Concurrent use has been associated with an increased risk of nephrotoxicity.	Monitor renal function closely.	355
Cephalothin–Probenecid	2	Probenecid raises and prolongs serum concentrations of cephalothin, increasing potential nephrotoxicity. Significance varies according to the nephrotoxic potential of the individual cephalosporin.	Cephalothin dosage should be reduced. Monitor renal function.	356
Chloramphenicol–Phenobarbital	3	Phenobarbital may decrease chloramphenicol serum concentration.	Chloramphenicol dosage may need to be increased.	358
Doxycycline–Carbamazepine	2	Long-term carbamazepine therapy may reduce the antimicrobial effectiveness of doxycycline.	A noninteracting tetracycline may be substituted for doxycycline.	359
Doxycycline–Phenobarbital	2	Phenobarbital may reduce serum levels, half-life, and urinary excretion of doxycycline.	It may be advisable to increase the doxycycline dosage or substitute a noninteracting tetracycline.	360

*Not available in the U.S.

Abbreviations: CNS, central nervous system; GI, gastrointestinal; IM, intramuscular; IV, intravenous; MAO, monoamine oxidase.

TABLE 8. Anti-infective Drug Interactions—cont'd

Drug Interaction	Significance Code	Potential Effects	Recommendations	See Page
Doxycycline–Phenytoin	2	Phenytoin may decrease the half-life of doxycycline, resulting in lower serum levels and inadequate antibiotic activity.	It has been suggested to double the daily dose of doxycycline.	361
Furazolidone–Amphetamine	1	Concurrent use may result in a hypertensive crisis because furazolidone has MAO inhibitor activity. This hazard is increased by prolonged use.	Avoid the concomitant use of furazolidone and amphetamines, tyramine containing food, and other indirect and mixed acting sympathomimetics.	362
Gentamicin–Carbenicillin	1	Carbenicillin significantly reduces the activity of gentamicin in patients with renal failure. This interaction is not seen in patients with normal renal function.	Adjust dosages of both agents for patients with renal failure.	363
Gentamicin–Cephalothin	2	Concurrent use is associated with an increased risk of nephrotoxicity, acute renal failure, and acquired Fanconi syndrome.	Monitor closely for signs of nephrotoxicity.	365
Gentamicin–Polymyxin B	2	Since both agents may cause nephrotoxicity and neuromuscular blockade, concurrent use may increase the risk of developing these effects.	One study reported no effect with concurrent use; however, it is recommended that co-therapy be avoided.	367
Griseofulvin–Phenobarbital	3	Phenobarbital reduces serum levels of griseofulvin.	If clinical response is inadequate, increase the griseofulvin dosage.	368
Isoniazid–Aluminum Hydroxide	3	Large doses of aluminum hydroxide may decrease peak serum levels and delay or decrease isoniazid absorption.	Administer isoniazid at least 1 hour before antacid administration.	369
Isoniazid–Disulfiram	3	Concurrent use may result in adverse CNS effects, although variables in the studies make the significance difficult to determine.	Monitor for CNS effects and reduce or discontinue the disulfiram if needed.	370
Isoniazid–Meperidine	3	Concurrent use may produce lethargy and hypotension within 20 minutes of an IM meperidine dose.	Discontinue the meperidine if symptoms occur. Morphine may be substituted for meperidine since it was shown not to interact.	371
Isoniazid–Prednisolone	3	Prednisolone may significantly reduce isoniazid plasma levels. The greatest decrease appears to occur in rapid acetylators.	Isoniazid dosage may need to be increased.	372

TABLE 8. Anti-infective Drug Interactions—cont'd

Drug Interaction	Significance Code	Potential Effects	Recommendations	See Page
Isoniazid–Pyridoxine	4	Some studies indicate that pyridoxine may neutralize the anti-tubercular activity of isoniazid. However, co-therapy is often used for preventing isoniazid-induced pyridoxine deficiency and appears to cause no problems.	Concurrent use need not be avoided.	373
Isoniazid–Rifampin	2	Hepatotoxicity has occurred from concurrent use. Onset and severity may be increased in infants and children, although other risk factors have also been suggested.	Advise patients of signs and symptoms of hepatitis and monitor frequently.	374
Kanamycin–Ethacrynic Acid	1	Concurrent use may increase the incidence of ototoxic effects, especially in patients with decreased renal function.	Avoid concomitant use of these agents. If concurrent use is necessary, use caution, reduce dosages, and monitor eighth cranial nerve function.	375
Ketoconazole–Aluminum Hydroxide, Magnesium Hydroxide	3	Antacids may decrease the peak ketoconazole concentration and area-under-curve.	Administer these agents several hours apart.	377
Ketoconazole–Cyclosporine	2	Ketoconazole increases cyclosporine blood levels. Concurrent use may increase the risk of nephrotoxicity since cyclosporine alone is nephrotoxic.	Avoid concurrent use, but if ketoconazole is necessary another immunosuppressive agent should be used or cyclosporine dosage reduced with frequent assessment of drug levels and renal function.	378
Lincomycin–Erythromycin	3	Erythromycin may theoretically antagonize lincomycin activity by blocking access to the ribosomal binding site.	Avoid concurrent use if possible since this combination may offset any therapeutic advantage.	379
Lincomycin–Kaolin	1	Kaolin reduces the GI absorption of lincomycin.	If diarrhea develops due to the lincomycin, kaolin should be avoided or given at least 2 hours before the lincomycin.	380
Metronidazole–Disulfiram	2	Concurrent use may lead to acute psychoses or confusion.	Avoid concurrent use, but if this is not possible monitor closely and discontinue one or both drugs if needed.	381

TABLE 8. Anti-infective Drug Interactions—cont'd

Drug Interaction	Significance Code	Potential Effects	Recommendations	See Page
Metronidazole–Phenobarbital	3	Metronidazole failed to eradicate vaginal trichomoniasis in a patient taking phenobarbital, although the infection subsided when metronidazole dosage was increased.	Monitor for lack of antimicrobial response and increase metronidazole dosage if needed.	382
Nitrofurantoin–Probenecid	3	Probenecid, particularly in high doses, may decrease the renal clearance and increase serum levels of nitrofurantoin. Increased nitrofurantoin levels have been associated with polyneuropathies.	Avoid concomitant use if possible, especially in patients with renal dysfunction.	383
Nitrofurantoin–Propantheline	3	Propantheline may cause increased nitrofurantoin absorption and excretion, possibly resulting in increased therapeutic efficacy and adverse effects.	Concurrent use need not be avoided, but administer as far apart as possible.	384
Penicillin–Aspirin	3	Large doses of aspirin (3 g/day) may significantly increase penicillin concentrations and half-life.	Possible toxicities from high dose aspirin therapy may outweigh possible benefits of this interaction.	385
Penicillin–Chloramphenicol	4	Bacteriostatic action of chloramphenicol may antagonize penicillin's bactericidal action. Prolonged half-life and elevated chloramphenicol have also been reported.	Concurrent use need not be avoided since there is no evidence that significant antagonism occurs.	386
Penicillin–Chlortetracycline	2	Chlortetracycline may antagonize the bactericidal action of penicillin. Increased incidence of mortality, reinfection, and secondary infection has been reported.	There appears to be no justification for concurrent use.	387
Penicillin–Erythromycin	3	Concurrent use may cause synergism, antagonism, or no alteration of the combined antibacterial effect, depending on several varied factors (e.g., type of organism, susceptibility, inoculum effect).	If used concurrently, check both the minimum inhibitory concentration and minimum bactericidal concentration to ensure a synergistic bactericidal effect.	388
Penicillin–Probenecid	3	Probenecid may induce higher and more sustained serum penicillin levels.	Complications result from increased antibiotic levels; therefore, it may be advisable to reduce the penicillin dosage and monitor drug levels.	390

TABLE 8. Anti-infective Drug Interactions—cont'd

Drug Interaction	Significance Code	Potential Effects	Recommendations	See Page
Polymyxin B– Prochlorpera- zine	2	Concurrent use may cause severe apnea since both agents possess neuromuscular blocking activity.	Use cautiously and with ventilatory assistance available.	391
Rifampin– Aminosalicylic Acid	4	Bentonite, an excipient in aminosalicylic acid granules, decreases the bioavailability and pharmacologic activity of rifampin.	Administering these agents 8-12 hours apart may prevent this interaction.	392
Rifampin– Oral Contra- ceptive Agents	1	Rifampin decreases the elimination half-life and reduces the bioavailability of contraceptive steroids, which may increase the incidence of menstrual disorders and pregnancies.	Since it is unpredictable who will be affected by this interaction, an alternative form of contraception is recommended.	393
Rifampin– Prednisolone	2	Rifampin may decrease the corticosteroid activity of prednisolone.	Prednisolone dosage may need to be increased.	395
Rifampin– Probenecid	4	Data are conflicting on the increased therapeutic benefits of co-therapy.	The advantage of concurrent therapy is of questionable value.	396
Sulfametha- zine, Trimeth- oprim*–Cy- closporine	3	IV trimethoprim and sulfamethazine resulted in undetectable levels of cyclosporine in 1 patient. When the antibiotics were given orally, the trough cyclosporine levels increased. It was not determined whether the route of administration or the drugs themselves were responsible for this interaction.	An increase in the cyclosporine dose, oral route for the antibiotics, or an alternative antibiotic may be necessary.	397
Sulfasalazine– Ampicillin	3	Ampicillin may affect the extent of sulfasalazine absorption, thus reducing its bioavailability.	Monitor for loss of sulfasalazine efficacy.	398
Tetracycline— Aluminum Hy- droxide	1	Antacids containing aluminum hydroxide or other divalent ions significantly decrease the GI absorption of tetracycline.	Give antacids at least 2 hours after tetracycline.	399
Tetracycline– Cimetidine	3	Cimetidine may reduce the mean peak plasma concentration, area-under-curve, and urinary excretion of tetracycline. This may occur only with the capsule form of tetracycline.	Monitor for decreased tetracycline effect. Increase antibiotic dosage or change to the oral solution if needed.	401

*This combination is not available in the U.S.

TABLE 8. Anti-infective Drug Interactions—cont'd

Drug Interaction	Significance Code	Potential Effects	Recommendations	See Page
Tetracycline–Ferrous Sulfate	1	Concurrent use interferes with the absorption of both drugs, leading to decreased serum levels of both agents.	Ferrous salts should be given not less than 3 hours before or 2 hours after tetracycline.	402
Tetracycline–Oral Contraceptive Agents	2	Tetracycline decreases the urinary excretion and increases fecal excretion of ethinyl estradiol. Contraceptive failures have been reported.	Since it is unpredictable who will be affected by this interaction, an alternative form of contraception is recommended.	403
Tetracycline–Sodium Bicarbonate	4	Decreased tetracycline absorption has been reported in an earlier study, although recent studies indicate sodium bicarbonate does not affect tetracycline disposition.	It may be advisable to give these agents 2 to 3 hours apart.	404
Troleandomycin–Oral Contraceptive Agents	2	Concurrent use of these agents has caused jaundice. Withdrawal of the drugs produced recovery within 1 month for most patients.	Women taking oral contraceptives should avoid troleandomycin.	405
Vidarabine–Allopurinol	2	Concurrent use has caused severe neurotoxicity.	Caution is advised when used concurrently.	406

Acyclovir–Probenecid

3

Summary: The oral administration of probenecid caused a 32% decrease in the elimination rate of parenterally administered acyclovir in 3 volunteers.[1]

Related Drugs: Acyclovir disposition has not been studied with other uricosuric agents, such as sulfinpyrazone, which inhibit the renal tubular reabsorption of uric acid, although a similar interaction may be expected to occur based on the mechanism for this interaction. There are no drugs related to acyclovir.

Mechanism: Acyclovir is eliminated predominantly by urinary excretion, by both glomerular filtration and tubular secretion.[2] Probenecid blocks the tubular secretion of acyclovir accounting for the decline in renal clearance.[1]

Recommendations: Until further information concerning this interaction is available, the clinical significance is difficult to assess. However, when acyclovir is used parenterally with probenecid, the resulting reduced elimination of acyclovir should be considered and any necessary dosage adjustments made.

References

1. Laskin, O.L., and others: Effects of probenecid on the pharmacokinetics and elimination of acyclovir in humans, Antimicrob. Agents Chemother. **21:**804, 1982.
2. Blum, M.R., and others: Overview of acyclovir pharmacokinetic disposition in adults and children, Am. J. Med. **73:**186, 1982.

Ampicillin–Allopurinol

3

Summary: The concurrent use of allopurinol and ampicillin may result in an increased incidence of drug-induced skin rash when compared to the use of either drug alone.[1,2]

Related Drugs: Similar results were reported in patients receiving both allopurinol and amoxicillin.[2] Documentation is lacking regarding a similar interaction between allopurinol and the other penicillins (e.g., bacampicillin, hetacillin, penicillin [see Appendix]). However, since both bacampicillin and hetacillin are converted to ampicillin in vivo, a similar interaction with allopurinol may be expected to occur. There are no drugs related to allopurinol.

Mechanism: The mechanism of this interaction is unknown. A higher incidence of penicillin allergy has been reported in asymptomatic hyperuricemic patients,[3] therefore it was not determined if the increased rash incidence is the result of a drug-drug interaction or an ampicillin-hyperuricemia interaction.[2,3]

Recommendations: The concurrent use of these agents need not be avoided; however, one or both drugs may have to be discontinued if a rash develops.

References

1. Boston Colaborative Drug Surveillance Program: Excess of ampicillin rashes associated with allopurinol or hyperuricemia, N. Engl. J. Med. **286:**505, 1972.
2. Jick, H., and Porter, J.B.: Potentiation of ampicillin skin reactions by allopurinol or hyperuricemia, J. Clin. Pharmacol. **21:**456, 1981.
3. Fessel, W.J., and others: Correlates and consequences of asymptomatic hyperuricemia, Arch. Intern. Med. **132:**44, 1973.

Ampicillin–Oral Contraceptive Agents

Summary: Ampicillin given to pregnant women resulted in lowered urinary estrogen excretion[1,6] in some women as soon as 3 days after ampicillin therapy began. Some reports state that plasma estrogen concentrations are lowered when ampicillin is given,[1,2,6] whereas others report no effect.[3,4] Within 2 days after termination of antibiotic therapy, estrogen levels returned to preantibiotic levels.

In women taking oral contraceptive products, concurrent ampicillin has caused breakthrough bleeding and a loss of contraception protection.[7,8] It was found that ampicillin decreased the urinary excretion of estrogens[1] but had little effect on serum levels.[9-11]

Related Drugs: Phenoxymethylpenicillin (penicillin V) produced similar alterations in urinary estrogen excretion and plasma levels in 6 pregnant women.[12] Oral contraceptive failures have been further reported for amoxicillin and penicillin G.[13] Although specific information is lacking concerning other penicillins (e.g., cloxacillin, methicillin, oxacillin [see Appendix]), it would seem that all penicillins may cause a similar effect because they are pharmacologically related.

Mechanism: The mechanism is unknown. However, estrogens and progestogens are extensively excreted in the bile principally as glucoronide conjugates. Subsequently, they undergo enterohepatic circulation where bacterial hydrolysis occurs, allowing for reabsorption of the oral contraceptive through the bowel wall and eventual urinary excretion. Treatment with the antibiotics destroys the gut flora and prevents steroid reabsorption, resulting in lower than normal concentrations of the contraceptive and excretion via the feces rather than the urine.[14,15]

Recommendations: The majority of women may take these agents concomitantly without risk, but there seems no way to predict who will be affected.

Some prescribers may choose to warn patients that spotting and breakthrough bleeding are signs of diminished contraceptive effectiveness and additional alternative forms of contraception should be used. Others may choose to recommend an alternative contraception method during concurrent use.

References

1. Trybuchowski, H.: Effect of ampicillin on the urinary output of steroidal hormones in pregnant and non-pregnant women, Clin. Chim. Acta **45:**9, 1973.
2. Willman, K., and Pulkkinen, M.O.: Reduced maternal plasma and urinary estriol during ampicillin treatment, Am. J. Obstet. Gynecol. **109:**893, 1971.
3. Sybulski, S., and Maughan, G.B.: Effect of ampicillin administration on estradiol, estriol, and cortisol levels in maternal plasma and on estriol levels in urine, Am. J. Obstet. Gynecol. **124:**349, 1976.
4. Boehm, F.H., and others: The effect of ampicillin administration on urinary estriol and serum estradiol in the normal pregnant patient, Am. J. Obstet. Gynecol. **119:**98, 1974.
5. Tikkanen, M.J., and others: Effects of antibiotics on oestrogen metabolism, Br. Med. J. **2:**369, 1973.
6. Adlercreutz, H., and others: Effect of ampicillin administration on plasma conjugated and unconjugated estrogen and progesterone levels in pregnancy, Am. J. Obstet. Gynecol. **128:**266, 1977.

7. Roberton, Y.R., and Johnson, E.S.: Interactions between oral contraceptives and other drugs: a review, Curr. Med. Res. Opin. **3:**647, 1976.
8. Dossetor, J.: Drug interactions with oral contraceptives, Br. Med. J. **4:**467, 1975.
9. Friedman, C.I., and others: The effect of ampicillin on oral contraceptive effectiveness, Obstet. Gynecol. **55:**33, 1980.
10. Back, D.J., and others: The effects of ampicillin on oral contraceptive steroids in women, Br. J. Clin. Pharmacol. **14:**43, 1982.
11. Joshi, J.V., and others: A study of interaction of low-dose combination oral contraceptive with ampicillin and metronidazole, Contraception **22:**643, 1980.
12. Pulkkinen, M., and Willman, K.: Maternal oestrogen levels during penicillin treatment, Br. Med. J. **4:**48, 1971.
13. Back, D.J., and others: Interindividual variation and drug interactions with hormonal steroid contraceptives, Drugs **21:**46, 1981.
14. True, R.J.: Interaction between antibiotics and oral contraceptives, J.A.M.A. **247:**1408, 1982.
15. Rubin, D.F.: Antibiotics and oral contraceptives, Arch. Dermatol. **117:**189, 1981.

Cefoperazone–Alcohol, Ethyl

2

Summary: A disulfiram-like reaction including such symptoms as flushing, tachycardia, bronchospasm, sweating, nausea, and vomiting may occur in patients ingesting alcohol and receiving cefoperazone.[1-5] The reaction has been reported in patients who had been receiving the antibiotic periodically or continuously before alcohol ingestion. This effect has occurred within 30 minutes of alcohol ingestion.

Related Drugs: Patients receiving moxalactam[6,7] or cefamandole[8,9] have also exhibited this reaction. These cephalosporins, like cefoperazone, have a methyltetrazolethiol side chain that closely resembles part of the disulfiram molecule. It is expected that cefametazole* and cefmenoxime,* which also have such a side chain, will interact with alcohol.[10]

No interaction was found with cephalothin, cephradine, cefoxitin, cefazolin, or cefotaxime in animal studies,[11,12] or ceftizoxime, cefonicid, and cefsulodin* in human studies.[13] These cephalosporins do not have the methyltetrazolethiol side chain.

Mechanism: Disulfiram-like reactions (flushing, tachycardia, dyspnea, hyperventilation, pounding headache) are caused when disulfiram interferes with acetaldehyde dehydrogenase activity, and acetaldehyde subsequently accumulates. It has been suggested that the cephalosporins with the methyltetrazolethiol side chain interfere with the alcohol metabolizing enzyme aldehyde dehydrogenase activity, resulting in elevated concentrations of acetaldehyde. Such a relationship was found in one subject.[14] It is unclear at this time whether a dose-response relationship exists or how long the enzyme inhibition persists.[12] It has been suggested that this interaction is not seen unless the antibiotic is given *before* alcohol ingestion.[10,14] Specific host factors may also play a role in predisposing certain individuals to this reaction.[10,13]

Recommendations: Patients receiving cefoperazone or the other cephalosporins with a methyltetrazolethiol side chain should be warned of the possible interaction with concurrent alcohol. It is suggested that patients abstain from alcoholic beverages during and several days after antibiotic therapy.

References

1. Foster, T.S., and others: Disulfiram-like reaction associated with a parenteral cephalosporin, Am. J. Hosp. Pharm. **37:**858, 1980.
2. Reeves, D.S., and Davies, A.J.: Antabuse effect with cephalosporins, Lancet **2:**540, 1980.
3. McMahon, F.G.: Disulfiram-like reaction to a cephalosporin, J.A.M.A. **243:**2397, 1980.
4. Porpaaczy, P.: Interaction between cephalosporins and alcohol (letter), Infection **9:**210, 1981.
5. Keimmerich, B., and Lode, H.: Interaction between cephalosporins and alcohol (letter), Infection **9:**110, 1981.
6. Neu, H.C., and Prince, A.S.: Interaction between moxalactam and alcohol, Lancet **1:**1422, 1980.
7. Brown, K.R., and others: Theophylline elixir, moxalactam, and a disulfiram reaction, Ann. Intern. Med. **97:**621, 1982.

*Not available in the U.S.

8. Portier, H., and others: Interaction between cephalosporins and alcohol, Lancet **2:**263, 1980.

9. Drummer, S., and others: Antabuse-like effect of beta-lactam antibiotics, N. Engl. J. Med. **303:**1417, 1980.

10. Platt, R.: Adverse effects of third-generation cephalosporins, J. Antimicrob. Chemother. **10**(suppl. C):135, 1982.

11. Buening, M.K., and Wold, J.S.: Ethanol-moxalactam interactions in vivo, Rev. Infect. Dis. **4**(suppl.):555, 1982.

12. Buening, M.K., and others: Disulfiram-like reaction to beta-lactams, J.A.M.A. **245:**2027, 1981.

13. McMahon, F.G., and Noveck, R.J.: Lack of disulfiram-like reactions with ceftizoxime, J. Antimicrob. Chemother. **10**(suppl. C):129, 1982.

14. Elenbaas, R.M., and others: On the disulfiram-like activity of moxalactam, Clin. Pharmacol. Ther. **32:**347, 1982.

Cephaloridine*–Furosemide

Summary: Cephaloridine nephrotoxicity may be enhanced by concurrent furosemide administration, but reports are complicated because of concurrent administration of other drugs.[1-6] Furosemide increased the half-life of cephaloridine approximately one-fourth[7] with a corresponding decrease in cephaloridine clearance.[8,9]

Related Drugs: Animal studies indicate that furosemide enhances the nephrotoxicity of cephacetrile[10] and cephalothin.[11] Cephalexin and cephapirin in animals[12] and cefoxitin in humans[13] appear not to be nephrotoxic when administered with furosemide. Cefazolin also appears to be less nephrotoxic than cephaloridine.[14] Other cephalosporins (e.g., cefaclor, cefotaxime, moxalactam [see Appendix]) vary in their potential to interact with furosemide.

In cephaloridine-treated mice, ethacrynic acid increased renal damage while chlorothiazide did not.[2] There is no documentation regarding a similar interaction with the other loop diuretic (bumetanide). No other reports have appeared involving an interaction between cephaloridine and the thiazide diuretics (e.g., hydrochlorothiazide, methyclothiazide, polythiazide [see Appendix]), and thiazide related diuretics (e.g., chlorthalidone, metolazone, indapamide [see Appendix]).

Mechanism: The mechanism is not established but several possibilities have been proposed. An additive stimulation of renin release by both agents might lead to acute renal failure.[2,5] Also, furosemide inhibits water reabsorption into the tubular cell, which may lead to a higher concentration of cephaloridine and enhance its precipitation in the proximal convoluted tubule, leading to nephrotoxicity.[12,15] Another possibility is that natriuresis induced by furosemide, which reduces intravascular space, may lead to higher concentration of cephaloridine in plasma and tissue.[12]

Recommendations: Concurrent use of furosemide and cephaloridine should be avoided in patients with even mild preexisting renal disease or impaired renal function, the elderly, and those receiving other nephrotoxic drugs. Use of a less nephrotoxic cephalosporin may be preferable if this combination is required, and renal function should be monitored regularly.

References

1. Foard, R.D.: Cephaloridine and the kidney, Prog. Antimicrob. Anticancer Chemother. **1**:597, 1969.
2. Dodds, M.G., and Foard, R.D.: Enhancement by potent diuretics of renal tubular necrosis induced by cephaloridine, Br. J. Pharmacol. **40**:227, 1970.
3. Simpson, I.J.: Nephrotoxicity and acute renal failure associated with cephalothin and cephaloridine, N. Z. Med. J. **74**:312, 1971.
4. Kleinknecht, D., and others: Nephrotoxicity of cephaloridine, Ann. Intern. Med. **80**:421, 1974.
5. Lawson, D.H., and others: The nephrotoxicity of cephaloridine, Postgrad. Med. J. **46**(suppl.):36, 1970.
6. Busuttil, A.A., and others: Possible cephaloridine nephrotoxicity in a neonate, Lancet **1**:264, 1973.
7. Lawson, D.H., and others: Furosemide interactions: studies in normal volunteers, Clin. Res. **24**:3, 1976.

*Not available in the U.S.

8. Norrby, R., and others: Interaction between cephaloridine and furosemide in man, Scand. J. Infect. Dis. **8**:209, 1976.

9. Tilstone, W.J., and others: Effects of furosemide on glomerular filtration rate and clearance of practolol, digoxin, cephaloridine, and gentamicin, Clin. Pharmacol. Ther. **22**:389, 1977.

10. Luscombe, D.K., and Nicholls, P.J.: Possible interaction between cephacetrile and frusemide in rabbits and rats, J. Antimicrob. Chemother. **1**:67, 1972.

11. Lawson, D.H., and others: Effect of furosemide on antibiotic-induced renal damage in rats, J. Infect. Dis. **126**:593, 1972.

12. Linton, A.L., and others: Relative nephrotoxicity of cephalosporin antibiotics in an animal model, Can. Med. Assoc. J. **107**:414, 1972.

13. Trollfors, B.: Effects on renal function of treatment with cefoxitin alone or in combination with furosemide, Scand. J. Infect. Dis. **13**(suppl.):73, 1978.

14. Silverblatt, F., and others: Nephrotoxicity of cephalosporin antibiotics in experimental animals, J. Infect. Dis. **128**:5367, 1973.

15. Boyd, J.F., and others: The nephrotoxic effect of cephaloridine and its polymers, Int. J. Clin. Pharmacol. **7**:307, 1973.

Cephalothin–Colistimethate

2

Summary: Concurrent use of cephalothin and colistimethate has been associated with an increased risk of nephrotoxicity.[1,2] Four cases of acute renal failure have been attributed to concurrent use of these antibiotics.[1]

Related Drugs: Although there is no specific documentation, other cephalosporins (e.g., cephalexin, cefamandole, moxalactam [see Appendix]) may interact in a similar manner with colistimethate or other polypeptide antibiotics (bacitracin, capreomycin, and polymyxin B) when used concurrently based on pharmacologic similarity.

Mechanism: The mechanism of the interaction is unknown, but it has been suggested that cephalothin interferes with the renal excretion of colistimethate.[2]

Recommendations: Renal function should be closely monitored if these drugs are used together or sequentially.[2] It has been recommended that the colistimethate dosage be determined according to kidney function rather than body weight.[1,2]

References

1. Adler, S., and Segel, D.P.: Nonoliguric renal failure secondary to sodium colistimethate: a report of four cases, Am. J. Med. Sci. **262:**109, 1971.
2. Koch-Weser, J., and others: Adverse effects of sodium colistimethate: manifestations and specific reaction rates during 317 courses of therapy, Ann. Intern. Med. **72:**875, 1970.

Cephalothin–Probenecid

2

Summary: Ample documentation shows that concurrent administration of probenecid and a cephalosporin results in higher and prolonged serum cephalosporin concentrations, as shown with cephalothin.[1-3]

Related Drugs: Other cephalosporins that have increased serum levels with concurrent probenecid are cefazolin,[4] cephacetrile,[5,6] cephaloglycin,[7,8] cephalexin,[9-14] cephradine,[15-17] cefoxitin,[18-20] cefadroxil,[21] cefaclor,[16] cefamandole,[22] and ceftizoxime.[23] Probenecid does not significantly affect the elimination of moxalactam.[24] Other cephalosporins (cephapirin and cefotaxime) would be expected to interact with probenecid in a manner similar to cephalothin.

Mechanism: Two mechanisms have been proposed for the enhanced cephalosporin levels with concurrent probenecid, and they resemble the mechanism proposed for the same interaction seen with penicillin. Since cephalosporins are removed from the circulation largely by the kidneys, it is suggested that probenecid competes with the antibiotic for active renal secretion by the proximal tubule. It has also been suggested that the volume of distribution of the cephalosporin is restricted by probenecid.[25-27]

Recommendations: Concurrent use of a cephalosporin and probenecid will increase and prolong the serum levels of the cephalosporin. These elevated serum levels can increase the potential nephrotoxicity of the cephalosporins and the dosage should be reduced. The degree of significance of this interaction will vary depending on the nephrotoxic potential of the individual cephalosporin.

References

1. Tuano, S.B., and others: Cephaloridine versus cephalothin: relation of the kidney to blood level differences after parenteral administration, Antimicrob. Agents Chemother. **1966:**101, 1967.
2. Kaplan, K., and others: Cephaloridine: antimicrobial activity and pharmacologic behavior, Am. J. Med. Sci. **253:**667, 1967.
3. Kump, J., and others: Cephaloridine in the treatment of streptococcal endocarditis: a preliminary evaluation, South. Med. J. **62:**461, 1969.
4. Duncan, W.C.: Treatment of gonorrhea with cefazolin plus probenecid, J. Infect. Dis. **120:**398, 1974.
5. Westenfelder, S.R., and others: Pharmacokinetics of a new cephalosporin, cephacetrile, in patients with normal and impaired renal function, Infection **1:**157, 1973.
6. Wise, R., and Reeves, D.S.: Pharmacological studies of cephacetrile in human volunteers, Curr. Med. Res. Opin. **2:**249, 1974.
7. Pitt, J., and others: Antimicrobial activity and pharmacological behavior of cephaloglycine, Antimicrob. Agents Chemother. **1967:**630, 1968.
8. Applestein, J.M., and others: In vitro antimicrobial activity and human pharmacology of cephaloglycin, Appl. Microbiol. **16:**1006, 1968.
9. Thornhill, T.S., and others: In vitro antimicrobial activity and human pharmacology of cephalexin, a new orally absorbed cephalosporin C antibiotic, Appl. Microbiol. **17:**457, 1969.
10. Meyers, B.R., and others: Cephalexin-microbiological effects and pharmacologic parameters in man, Clin. Pharmacol. Ther. **10:**810, 1969.

11. Taylor, W.A., and Holloway, W.J.: Cephalexin in the treatment of gonorrhea, Int. J. Clin. Pharmacol. Ther. Toxicol. **6**:7, 1972.

12. Sales, J.E., and others: Cephalexin levels in human bile in presence of biliary tract disease, Br. Med. J. **3**:441, 1972.

13. Regamey, C., and others: Pharmacokinetics of parenteral sodium cephalexin in comparison with cephalothin and cefazolin, Infection **2**:132, 1974.

14. Oller, L.Z., and others: Cephaloridine and cephalexin in venereological practice, Postgrad. Med. J. **46**:99, 1970.

15. Mischler, T.W., and others: Influence of probenecid and food on the bioavailability of cephradine in normal male subjects, J. Clin. Pharmacol. **14**:604, 1974.

16. Welling, P.G., and others: Probenecid: an unexplained effect on cephalosporin pharmacology, Br. J. Clin. Pharmacol. **8**:491, 1979.

17. Roberts, D.H., and others: Pharmacokinetics of cephradine given intravenously with and without probenecid, Br. J. Clin. Pharmacol. **11**:561, 1981.

18. Reeves, D.S., and others: The effect of probenecid on the pharmacokinetics and distribution of cefoxitin in healthy volunteers, Br. J. Clin. Pharmacol. **11**:353, 1981.

19. Goodwin, C.S., and others: Effects of rate of infusion and probenecid on serum levels, renal excretion, and tolerance of intravenous doses of cefoxitin in humans: comparison with cephalothin, Antimicrob. Agents Chemother. **6**:338, 1974.

20. Bent, A.J., and others: Effect of probenecid on serum cefoxitin concentrations, J. Antimicrob. Chemother. **3**:627, 1977.

21. Marino, E.L., and Deminquez-Gil, A.: The pharmacokinetics of cefadroxil associated with probenecid, Int. J. Clin. Pharmacol. Ther. Toxicol. **19**:506, 1981.

22. Griffith, R.S., and others: Effect of probenecid on the blood levels and urinary excretion of cefamandole, Antimicrob. Agents Chemother. **11**:809, 1977.

23. LeBel, M., and others: Effect of probenecid on the pharmacokinetics of ceftizoxime, J. Antimicrob. Chemother. **12**:147, 1983.

24. Professional Product Information, Moxalactam, Eli Lilly Co., 1980.

25. Gilbaldi, M., and Schwartz, M.A.: Apparent effect of probenecid on the distribution of penicillins in man, Clin. Pharmacol. Ther. **9**:345, 1968.

26. Gibaldi, M., and others: Modification of penicillin distribution and elimination by probenecid, Int. J. Clin. Pharmacol. Ther. Toxicol. **3**:182, 1970.

27. Barza, M., and Weinstein, L.: Some determinants of the distribution of penicillins and cephalosporins in the body. Practical and theoretical considerations, Ann. N.Y. Acad. Sci. **235**:613, 1974.

Chloramphenicol–Phenobarbital

3

Summary: Concurrent administration of these agents has resulted in significantly decreased chloramphenicol serum concentrations in infants and children.[1-5] Also, a case has been reported where phenobarbital clearance was reduced approximately 40%[6] in a young adult patient receiving these agents plus phenytoin.

Related Drugs: No studies have been reported regarding an interaction between chloramphenicol and other barbiturates (e.g., amobarbital, butabarbital, secobarbital [see Appendix]); however, these other barbiturates may be expected to interact similarly because of their ability to induce hepatic microsomal enzymes.

Mechanism: Ninety percent of chloramphenicol is inactivated by the liver and the decline in chloramphenicol levels may be the result of induction of hepatic microsomal enzymes by phenobarbital. It is not clear why the phenobarbital clearance was decreased in the one patient, but it suggests that chloramphenicol may inhibit phenobarbital metabolism.

Recommendations: It will be necessary to carefully monitor patients who receive these agents concomitantly. Chloramphenicol dosage may need to be significantly increased within a few days of initiating combined therapy. The possible rise in phenobarbital concentrations may cause sedation or other toxic symptoms, thereby necessitating a decreased phenobarbital dosage.

References

1. Bloxham, R.A., and others: Chloramphenicol and phenobarbitone—a drug interaction, Arch. Dis. Child. **54:**76, 1979.
2. Krasinski, K., and others: Pharmacologic interactions among chloramphenicol, phenytoin and phenobarbital, Pediatr. Infect. Dis. **1:**232, 1982.
3. Rylance, G.W.: Chloramphenicol and phenobarbitone—a drug interaction, Arch. Dis. Child. **54:**563, 1979.
4. Durbin, G.M., and Winterborn, M.H.: Chloramphenicol and phenobarbitone: a drug interaction, Arch. Dis. Child. **54:**564, 1979.
5. Powell, D.A., and others: Interactions among chloramphenicol, phenytoin and phenobarbital in a pediatric patient, J. Pediatr. **98:**1001, 1981.
6. Koup, J.R., and others: Interaction of chloramphenicol with phenytoin and phenobarbital, Clin. Pharmacol. Ther. **24:**571, 1978.

Doxycycline–Carbamazepine

Summary: The intravenous or oral administration of doxycycline to patients receiving long-term carbamazepine therapy will result in a reduction of approximately 45% in the half-life of doxycycline, thereby reducing the antimicrobial effectiveness of doxycycline.[1-4] An average doxycycline half-life of 15.1 hours was reported in 9 control patients and an average of 8.4 hours in 5 patients receiving carbamazepine.[1]

Related Drugs: For tetracycline, methacycline, oxytetracycline, demeclocycline, and chlortetracycline, half-lives and quantity excreted in the urine have not been shown to be affected by the concurrent long-term administration of carbamazepine.[1,4] There is a lack of data concerning whether this interaction occurs with minocycline, which like doxycycline is partially inactivated by hepatic metabolism.

Mechanism: The exact mechanism for the interaction is unknown since the metabolic pathway of doxycycline has not been delineated.[5] Doxycycline may be partially metabolized by conjugation and secreted into the gastrointestinal tract by some route other than biliary secretion. Carbamazepine is known to induce these liver enzymes and possibly accelerate the metabolism of doxycycline.[4,6,7]

Recommendations: To maintain adequate serum levels of doxycycline, the antibiotic should be given every 12 hours to patients on long-term therapy with carbamazepine,[4] or another noninteracting tetracycline product may be used.

References

1. Penttila, O., and others: Interaction between doxycycline and some antiepileptic drugs, Br. Med. J. **2:**470, 1974.
2. Neuvonen, P.J., and Penttila, O.: Interaction between doxycline and barbiturates, Br. Med. J. **1:**535, 1974.
3. Johannessen, S.I.: Antiepileptic drugs: pharmacokinetic and clinical aspects, Ther. Drug Monit. **3:**17, 1981.
4. Neuvonen, P.J., and others: Effect of antiepileptic drugs on the elimination of various tetracycline derivatives, Eur. J. Clin. Pharmacol. **9:**147, 1975.
5. Cunha, B.A., and others: Doxycycline, Ther. Drug Monit. **4:**115, 1982.
6. von Schach, W.M., and Twomey, T.M.: The disposition of doxycycline by man and the dog, Chemotherapy **16:**217, 1971.
7. Remmer, H.: Induction of drug metabolizing enzyme system in the liver, Eur. J. Clin. Pharmacol. **5:**116, 1972.

Doxycycline–Phenobarbital

Summary: Doxycycline serum levels, half-life, and urinary excretion may be reduced by concurrent administration of phenobarbital. This effect may last for several days after discontinuion of therapy with the barbiturate.[1-3]

Related Drugs: Other tetracyclines that are eliminated by both renal and hepatic mechanisms (e.g., oxytetracycline, chlortetracycline, methacycline) have not been documented to be affected by phenobarbital[3] or other barbiturates. Amobarbital and pentobarbital have also been reported to decrease the half-life of doxycycline, and other barbiturates (butabarbital, secobarbital, mephobarbital [see Appendix]) may be expected to interact similarly because of their ability to induce hepatic enzymes. There is lack of data concerning whether this interaction occurs with minocycline, which like doxycycline is partially inactivated by hepatic metabolism; however, a similar interaction may be expected to occur based on the mechanism.

Mechanism: Reductions in doxycycline half-life resulting from phenobarbital administration have been attributed to metabolic induction of hepatic microsomal enzymes resulting in enhanced doxycycline elimination.

Recommendations: A higher dosage of doxycycline or normal dosage of a noninteracting tetracycline derivative should be used during concurrent adminstration with phenobarbital.[1-3]

References

1. Neuvonen, P.J., and Pentilla, O.: Interaction between doxycycline and barbiturates, Br. Med. J. **1:**535, 1974.
2. Pentilla, O., and others: Interaction between doxycycline and some anticonvulsant drugs, Br. Med. J. **2:**470, 1974.
3. Neuvonen, P.J., and others: Effect of antiepileptic drugs on the elimination of various tetracycline derivatives, Eur. J. Clin. Pharmacol. **9:**147, 1975.

Doxycycline–Phenytoin

2

Summary: The concurrent use of doxycycline and phenytoin may result in a decreased half-life of doxycycline, an effect that can occur for several days after the discontinuation of the interacting agent.[1,2] This may result in lower serum levels of doxycycline and an inadequate antibacterial effect.

Related Drugs: Other tetracycline derivatives (e.g., chlortetracycline, oxytetracyline, methacycline [see Appendix]) were shown to be unaffected by these anticonvulsants.[2] There is lack of data concerning whether this interaction occurs with minocycline, which like doxycycline is partially inactivated by hepatic metabolism; however, an interaction may be expected to occur based on the mechanism. Information does not exist on whether this interaction can occur with the other hydantoin anticonvulsants (mephenytoin and ethotoin), although a similar interaction may be expected to occur because of similar effects on hepatic microsomal enzymes.

Mechanism: The decrease in half-life of doxycycline has been attributed to the induction of microsomal enzymes by phenytoin, although displacement of doxycycline from plasma protein may also contribute to the increased turnover.[1-3]

Recommendations: The clinical response to doxycycline in patients receiving concurrent anticonvulsants should be monitored closely. It has been suggested that doxycycline's daily dose be doubled.[2]

References

1. Penttila, O., and others: Interaction between doxycycline and some antiepileptic drugs, Br. Med. J. **2:**470, 1974.
2. Neuvonen, P.J., and others: Effect of antiepileptic drugs on the elimination of various tetracycline derivatives, Eur. J. Clin. Pharmacol. **9:**147, 1975.
3. Neuvonen, P.J., and Penttila, O.: Interaction between doxycycline and barbiturates, Br. Med. J. **1:**535, 1974.

Furazolidone–Amphetamine

Summary: The antibacterial action of furazolidone is accompanied by progressive and generalized monoamine oxidase inhibition, and concurrent administration of amphetamine could result in a hypertensive crisis. Since the monoamine oxidase inhibitory action of furazolidone is cumulative, this hazard is increased by prolonged use, especially if the therapy extends beyond the recommended 5 days.[1]

Related Drugs: Tyramine has been reported to interact with furazolidone,[1] and tyramine containing foods (e.g., chocolate, cheeses, wine) may also interact. Other sympathomimetics (e.g., indirect: methylphenidate, phenylpropanolamine [see Appendix]) may have the potential for interacting with furazolidone. The primary direct acting sympathomimetics including epinephrine, isoproterenol, norepinephrine, and methoxamine do not interact with furazolidone.[1] Other monoamine oxidase inhibitors (e.g., isocarboxazid, phenelzine, pargyline [see Appendix]) have also been shown to interact with indirect acting sympathomimetics (see Tranylcypromine–Phenylpropanolamine, p. 300). Procarbazine, which also possesses monoamine oxidase inhibitor activity, may be expected to interact similarly.

Mechanism: Although it is used as an antibacterial agent, furazolidone has monoamine oxidase inhibitor activity in humans.[1] The inhibition of monoamine oxidase by furazolidone is thought to be caused by the result of a metabolite.[2] Amphetamine is an indirect-acting sympathomimetic amine, promoting the release of norepinephrine from adrenergic neurons. Inhibition of monoamine oxidase by furazolidone causes a supersensitivity to amphetamine apparently because of an increased amount of norepinephrine released at the adrenergic neuron terminals.[3]

Recommendations: Tyramine containing foods, amphetamines, other indirect acting sympathomimetic agents, and mixed acting sympathomimetics are contraindicated in patients receiving furazolidone.

References

1. Pettinger, W.A., and others: Inhibiton of monoamine oxidase in man by furazolidone, Clin. Pharmacol. Ther. **9:**442, 1968.
2. Stern, I.J., and others: The anti-monoamine oxidase effects of furazolidone, J. Pharmacol. Exp. Ther. **156:**492, 1967.
3. Pettinger, W.A., and Oates, J.A.: Supersensitivity to tyramine during monoamine oxidase inhibition in man, Clin. Pharmacol. Ther. **9:**341, 1968.

Gentamicin–Carbenicillin

1

Summary: Concurrent parenteral gentamicin and carbenicillin are reportedly more effective against certain susceptible organisms than either drug alone.[1-5] However, gentamicin activity can be significantly diminished if mixed with carbenicillin in vitro. A similar inactivation can occur in patients with renal failure since carbenicillin can reduce serum gentamicin levels[1,10,12] and half-life.[10,13] No such interaction was found to occur in a patient with normal renal function.[1]

Related Drugs: Carbenicillin and ticarcillin have been reported to cause the in vitro inactivation of sisomicin,*[9] netilmicin,[14] tobramycin,[9,15] and amikacin.[9,14] This has also been reported for ticarcillin and gentamicin.[9,10] The other aminoglycosides (e.g., kanamycin, neomycin, streptomycin [see Appendix]) may undergo a similar in vitro inactivation. Serum levels of penicillin V have been reduced in patients receiving neomycin.[16] Ampicillin and penicillin G decrease gentamicin activity when mixed in vitro.[8,11] The possibility of a similar interaction with the aminoglycosides may exist with other extended spectrum penicillins (e.g., mezlocillin, piperacillin, azlocillin) or other penicillins (e.g., nafcillin, oxacillin, cloxacillin [see Appendix]).

Mechanism: Semisynthetic penicillins chemically interact with aminoglycosides forming biologically inactive amides. The reaction moieties are the amino groups of the aminoglycosides and the beta-lactam rings of the penicillins.[17] The decreased penicillin V levels found with concurrent neomycin are probably related to a reversible malabsorption syndrome.[16]

Recommendations: To prevent in vitro inactivation, the antibiotics should not be mixed in infusion fluids. There apparently is no contraindication for using these agents together in patients with normal renal function. For patients with renal failure who are to receive these agents, the dosage of the aminoglycoside and the penicillin must be adjusted for renal impairment and the serum levels of both agents should be monitored.[12] Concurrent use of neomycin and orally administered penicillins should be avoided.

References

1. Eykyn, S., and others: Gentamicin plus carbenicillin, Lancet **1:**545, 1971.
2. Kluge, R.M., and others: The carbenicillin-gentamicin combination against Pseudomonas aeruginosa. Correlation of effect with gentamicin sensitivity, Ann. Intern. Med. **81:**584, 1974.
3. Smith, C.B., and others: Use of gentamicin in combination with other antibiotics, J. Infect. Dis. **119:**370, 1969.
4. Nunnery, A.W., and others: Carbenicillin: in vivo synergism and combined therapy, J. Infect. Dis. **122:**78, 1970.
5. Klastersky, J.: Carbenicillin plus gentamicin, Lancet **1:**653, 1971.
6. McLaughlin, J.E., and others: Clinical and laboratory evidence for the inactivation of gentamicin by carbenicillin, Lancet **1:**261, 1971.
7. Levison, M.E., and Kaye, D.: Carbenicillin plus gentamincin, Lancet **2:**45, 1971.
8. Lynn, B.: Carbenicillin plus gentamicin, Lancet **1:**653, 1971.

*Not available in the U.S.

9. Holt, H.A., and others: Interactions between aminoglycoside antibiotics and carbenicillin or ticarcillin, Infection **4**:109, 1976.
10. Davies, M., and others: Interactions of carbenicillin and ticarcillin with gentamicin, Antimicrob. Agents Chemother. **7**:431, 1975.
11. Riff, L., and Jackson, G.G.: Gentamicin plus carbenicillin, Lancet **1**:592, 1971.
12. Weibert, R., and others: Carbenicillin inactivation of aminoglycosides in patients with severe renal failure, Trans. Am. Soc. Artif. Intern. Organs **22**:439, 1976.
13. Riff, L.J., and Jackson, G.G.: Laboratory and clinical conditions for gentamicin inactivation by carbenicillin, Arch. Intern. Med. **130**:887, 1972.
14. Pickering, L.K., and Gearhart, P.: Effect of time and concentration upon inactivation between gentamicin, tobramycin, netilmicin or amikacin and carbenicillin or ticarcillin, Antimicrob. Agents Chemother. **15**:592, 1979.
15. Chow, M.S., and others: In vivo inactivation of tobramycin by ticarcillin, J.A.M.A. **247**:658, 1982.
16. Cheng, S.H., and White, A.: Effect of orally administered neomycin on the absorption of penicillin V, N. Engl. J. Med. **267**:1296, 1962.
17. Perenyi, T., and others: Uber die Wechselwirkun, de Penizilline and aminoglykosid-Antibiotika, Int. J. Clin. Pharmacol. Ther. Toxicol. **10**:50, 1974.

Gentamicin–Cephalothin

2

Summary: Concurrent use of gentamicin and cephalothin has been associated with an increased risk of nephrotoxicity and acute renal failure[1-10] and the development of an acquired Fanconi syndrome.[11] Gentamicin[12-14] and cephalothin[1,15-19] have been shown to cause nephrotoxicity when used individually; therefore, this interaction may be the additive effect of these agents.

Related Drugs: Tobramycin co-therapy with cephalothin has an increased risk of nephrotoxicity.[20] In 11 patients taking cytotoxic drugs for leukemia, hypokalemia developed in 9 receiving gentamicin and cephalexin.[21] Other aminoglycosides (e.g., amikacin, kanamycin, netilmicin [see Appendix]), which are known to increase the risk of nephrotoxicity when used alone, may interact similarly with cephalothin and other cephalosporins (e.g., cefamandole, cephapirin, moxalactam [see Appendix]).

Mechanism: The exact mechanisms by which gentamicin and cephalothin cause nephrotoxicity are not known. Gentamicin appears to primarily affect the proximal tubule causing mild azotemia with a transient rise in blood urea nitrogen.[22,23] Cephalothin may cause acute tubular necrosis.[19] These actions may be additive when these agents are used in combination[5] or there may be a mutual enhancement of toxicity.

Recommendations: Patients receiving these drugs concurrently should be observed and monitored closely for signs of nephrotoxicity. High doses of either antibiotic given over an extended period should be avoided.

   If the concurrent use of these drugs is chosen, dosage should be based on creatinine clearance.

References

1. Fillastre, J.P., and Kleinknecht, D.: Acute renal failure associated with cephalosporin therapy, Am. Heart J. **89:**809, 1975.
2. Plager, J.E.: Association of renal injury with combined cephalothin-gentamicin therapy among patients severely ill with malignant disease, Cancer **37:**1937, 1976.
3. Noone, P., and others: Experience in monitoring gentamicin therapy during treatment of serious gram-negative sepsis, Br. Med. J. **1:**477, 1974.
4. Tvedegaard, E.: Interaction between gentamicin and cephalothin as cause of acute renal failure, Lancet **2:**581, 1976.
5. Cabanillas, F., and others: Nephrotoxicity of combined cephalothin gentamicin regimen, Arch. Intern. Med. **135:**850, 1975.
6. Bobrow, S.N., and others: Anuria and acute tubular necrosis associated with gentamicin and cephalothin, J.A.M.A. **222:**1546, 1972.
7. Fillastre, J.P., and others: Acute renal failure associted with combined gentamicin and cephalothin therapy, Br. Med. J. **2:**395, 1973.
8. Kleinknecht, D., and others: Acute renal failure after high doses of gentamicin and cephalothin, Lancet **1:**1129, 1973.
9. Wade, J.C., and others: Cephalothin plus an aminoglycoside is more nephrotoxic than methicillin plus an aminoglycoside, Lancet **2:**604, 1978.

10. Noone, P., and others: Renal failure in combined gentamicin and cephalothin therapy, Br. Med. J. **2:**777, 1973.
11. Schwartz, J.H., and others: Fanconi syndrome associated with cephalothin and gentamicin therapy, Cancer **41:**769, 1978.
12. Falco, F.G., and others: Nephrotoxicity of aminoglycosides and gentamicin, J. Infect. Dis. **119:**406, 1969.
13. Jackson, G.G.: Gentamicin, Practitioner **198:**855, 1967.
14. Abramowicz, M., and Edelmann, C.M.: Nephrotoxicity of anti-infective drugs, Clin. Pediatr. **7:**389, 1968.
15. Thomas, B.L.: Renal function and cephalothin, N. Engl. J. Med. **280:**505, 1969.
16. Pickering, M.J., and others: Declining renal function associated with administration of cephalothin, South. Med. J. **63:**426, 1970.
17. Burton, J.R., and others: Acute renal failure during cephalothin therapy, J.A.M.A. **229:**679, 1974.
18. Pasternak, D.P., and Stephens, B.G.: Reversible nephrotoxicity associated with cephalothin therapy, Arch. Intern. Med. **135:**599, 1975.
19. Carling, P.C., and others: Nephrotoxicity associated with cephalothin administration, Arch. Intern. Med. **135:**797, 1975.
20. Tobias, J.S., and others: Severe renal dysfunction after tobramycin/cephalothin therapy, Lancet **1:**425, 1976.
21. Young, G.P., and others: Hypokalaemia due to gentamicin/cephalexin in leukaemia, Lancet **2:**855, 1973.
22. Kahn, T., and Stein, R.: Gentamicin and renal failure, Lancet **1:**498, 1972.
23. Wilfert, J.N., and others: Renal insufficiency associated with gentamicin therapy, J. Infect. Dis. **124**(suppl.):148, 1971.

Gentamicin—Polymyxin B

Summary: Since both gentamicin and polymyxin B may cause nephrotoxicity and neuromuscular blockade,[1] the combination of the 2 drugs may place the patient at increased risk of developing these side effects. There is also a report of combined therapy with gentamicin and polymyxin that did not result in nephrotoxicity.[2]

Related Drugs: The combination of kanamycin and polymyxin resulted in an apneic episode in a single case report, which was attributed to the combined neuromuscular blocking effects of both drugs.[3] Among the aminoglycoside antibiotics, neomycin, streptomycin, and kanamycin appear to have the greatest potential for causing neuromuscular blockade[4]; gentamicin and tobramycin are less likely to cause the problem.[5] The potential for other aminoglycosides (amikacin, netilmicin, and paromomycin) to cause neuromuscular blockade also exists. All of the aminoglycosides are potentially nephrotoxic, as are the polypeptide antibiotics (bacitracin, capreomycin, and colistimethate).

Mechanism: The aminoglycoside and polypeptide antibiotics may produce reversible neuromuscular blockade at the myoneural end-plate[2,6] and nephrotoxicity by a direct toxic effect on renal tubules.[1] Because the combined or sequential use of 2 aminoglycosides may result in increased toxicity[1] and the aminoglycosides and polymyxins may enhance the neuromuscular blockade of other agents,[2] it is proposed that the toxicities of these 2 groups of drugs is additive.

Recommendations: With rare exception, the combination of these 2 drugs can, and should, be avoided because of the availability of safer, less toxic combinations. If the interaction does occur, the patient should be supported, as necessary, until the effects dissipate.

References

1. Kucers, A., and Bennett, N.M.: The use of antibiotics. Philadelphia, 1979, J.B. Lippincott Company.
2. Williams, B.B., and others: Severe combined nephrotoxicity of BL-P1654 and gentamicin, J. Infect. Dis. **130:**694, 1974.
3. Pittinger, C.B., and others: Antibiotic-induced paralysis, Anesth. Analg. (Cleve.) **49:**487, 1970.
4. Argov, Z., and Mastaglia, F.L.: Disorders of neuromuscular transmission caused by drugs, N. Engl. J. Med. **301:**409, 1979.
5. Hudgson, P.: Adverse drug reactions in the neuromuscular apparatus, Adv. Drug React. Ac. Pois. Rev. **1:**35, 1982.
6. McQuillen, M.P., and others: Myasthenic syndrome associated with antibiotics, Arch. Neurol. **18:**402, 1968.

Griseofulvin–Phenobarbital

3

Summary: Serum levels of orally administered griseofulvin are lowered by concurrent administration of phenobarbital.[1-4] It is unknown at the present time if the effect of phenobarbital on serum griseofulvin is sufficient to modify therapeutic response.

Related Drugs: The effect of concurrent administration of other barbiturates (e.g., amobarbital, butabarbital, secobarbital [see Appendix]) on serum griseofulvin levels has not been studied. However, barbiturates as a class may interact in a similar manner because they are related pharmacologically.

Mechanism: The mechanism of this interaction is unclear. Initially, increased metabolism of the griseofulvin as a result of enzyme induction by concurrent phenobarbital administration was shown in rats.[3] In normal volunteers the interaction did not occur when the phenobarbital was administered parenterally. Decreased absorption of griseofulvin was noted when phenobarbital was administered orally.[1] Decreased absorption has also been demonstrated in rats and did not occur with a suspension formulation of griseofulvin.[4]

Recommendations: The clinical course of patients taking griseofulvin and phenobarbital concurrently should be closely followed. If the clinical response is inadequate, the dose of griseofulvin may need to be increased.

References

1. Riegilman, S., and others: Griseofulvin-phenobarbital interaction in man, J.A.M.A. **213:**426, 1970.
2. Busfield, D., and others: An effect of phenobarbitone on blood levels of griseofulvin in man, Lancet **2:**1042, 1963.
3. Busfield, D., and others: An effect of phenobarbitone on griseofulvin metabolism in the rat, Br. J. Pharmacol. **22:**137, 1964.
4. Jamali, F., and Axelson, J.E.: Griseofulvin-phenobarbital interaction: A formulation-dependent phenomenon, J. Pharm. Sci. **67:**466, 1978.

Isoniazid–Aluminum Hydroxide

3

Summary: The simultaneous administration of large doses of aluminum hydroxide may decrease the peak serum levels and delay or decrease the absorption of isoniazid.

Related Drugs: In 1 study of this interaction aluminum hydroxide and an aluminum-magnesium compound (magaldrate) were used. The effect with magaldrate was less pronounced and more variable.[1] It is difficult to determine whether an interaction would occur between isoniazid and other antacids (e.g., aluminum carbonate, magnesium hydroxide, calcium carbonate [see Appendix]). There are no drugs related to isoniazid.

Mechanism: Aluminum hydroxide delays gastric emptying and causes retention of isoniazid in the stomach.[2] Because isoniazid is absorbed primarily in the small intestine, lower peak serum concentrations result from its retention in the stomach.

Recommendations: Single high doses of isoniazid are more effective in arresting tuberculosis than the same amount of drug in divided doses.[3,4] Although the clinical significance of this interaction is not known, high peak serum concentrations of isoniazid appear to be important in antitubercular therapy. Therefore isoniazid should be administered at least 1 hour before antacid administration.

References

1. Hurwitz, A., and Schlozman, D.L.: Effects of antacids on gastrointestinal absorption of isoniazid in rat and man, Am. Rev. Resp. Dis. **109:**41, 1974.
2. Hava, M., and Hurwitz, A.: The relaxing effect of aluminum and lanthanum on rat and human gastric smooth muscle in vitro, Eur. J. Pharmacol. **7:**156, 1973.
3. Fox, W.: General considerations in intermittent drug therapy of pulmonary tuberculosis, Postgrad. Med. J. **47:**729, 1971.
4. Hudson, L.D., and Sharbara, J.A.: Twice weekly tuberculosis therapy, J.A.M.A. **223:**139, 1973.

Isoniazid–Disulfiram

3

Summary: The concurrent use of isoniazid and disulfiram has been reported to result in adverse central nervous system (CNS) effects such as irritability, nausea, dizziness, lethargy, uncoordination, and disorientation in a total of 11 patients.[1] However, the lack of a consistent temporal relationship of the onset and resolution of signs and symptoms to disulfiram administration, the concurrent use of other psychotropic medications, and the possible contribution of underlying disease states makes the true significance of this interaction difficult to determine.

Related Drugs: There are no drugs related to isoniazid or disulfiram.

Mechanism: The mechanism for the development of CNS effects with the concurrent use of isoniazid and disulfiram has not been established. It has been postulated that the combination of isoniazid and disulfiram results in altered dopamine metabolism in the brain, resulting in an accumulation of methylated byproducts of dopamine.[1] However, effects from concurrent medications, underlying diseases, or disulfiram itself cannot be ruled out in the cases reported.

Recommendations: Since a series of case reports in one article[1] constitutes the literature pertaining to this interaction, the exact incidence and severity of the interaction cannot be established. One additional patient receiving isoniazid, rifampin, and disulfiram was reported to experience no toxic effects.[2] Until further documentation is provided, patients receiving isoniazid and disulfiram concurrently should be monitored for the occurrence of CNS effects such as dizziness, irritability, lethargy, and uncoordination. If these signs or symptoms occur, dosage reduction or discontinuation of disulfiram should be considered.[1]

References

1. Whittington, H.G., and Grey, L.: Possible interaction between disulfiram and isoniazid, Am. J. Psychiatry **125:**1725, 1969.
2. Rothstein, E.: Rifampin with disulfiram, J.A.M.A. **219:**1216, 1972.

Isoniazid–Meperidine

3

Summary: One patient became lethargic and hypotensive within 20 minutes after an intramuscular dose of meperidine while on triple antitubercular treatment that included isoniazid. This patient had previously received meperidine without concurrent isoniazid with no report of any adverse reactions. When meperidine was switched to morphine, the patient continued to receive isoniazid without any further symptoms.[1]

Related Drugs: There are no drugs related to isoniazid. Documentation is lacking regarding a similar interaction between isoniazid and the other narcotic analgesics (e.g., codeine, methadone, oxycodone [see Appendix]).

Mechanism: The mechanism of this interaction is unknown.

Recommendations: Patients should be monitored for adverse reactions during concurrent use of these agents. If lethargy or hypotension occurs, meperidine may need to be discontinued. Also, since morphine was shown not to interact in this particular patient, it may be considered as a suitable alternative to meperidine.

Reference

1. Gannon, R., and others: Isoniazid, meperidine and hypotension, Ann. Intern. Med. **99:**415, 1983.

Isoniazid–Prednisolone

3

Summary: Isoniazid plasma levels were significantly lower after concurrent predniso-lone as compared to administration of isoniazid alone in a study involving 26 patients. The decrease was greater in patients who were rapid acetylators (40%) than in those who were slow acetylators (25%).[1] The addition of rifampin reduced the effect of prednisolone on isoniazid. The clinical effect of this interaction has not been studied.

Related Drugs: Documentation is lacking regarding an interaction between isoniazid and the other corticosteroids (e.g., hydrocortisone, prednisone, triamcinolone [see Appendix]), although because they are pharmacologically related, a similar interaction may be expected to occur. There are no drugs related to isoniazid.

Mechanism: Although the exact mechanism of this interaction is not known, it has been suggested that prednisolone increases the hepatic metabolism and/or renal clearance of isoniazid.

Recommendations: If concurrent administration of isoniazid and prednisolone is necessary, the dose of isoniazid may need to be increased.

Reference

1. Sarma, G.R., and others: Effect of prednisolone and rifampin on isoniazid metabolism in slow and rapid inactivators of isoniazid, Antimicrob. Agents Chemother. **18:**661, 1980.

Isoniazid–Pyridoxine

Summary: Some in vitro and in vivo studies have indicated that pyridoxine may neutralize the antitubercular activity of isoniazid.[1-4] However, this antagonism has not been a problem in humans, and currently pyridoxine is prescribed with isoniazid for prevention of isoniazid-induced pyridoxine deficiency and peripheral neuropathy.[5,6]

Related Drugs: There are no drugs related to isoniazid or pyridoxine.

Mechanism: The mechanism by which pyridoxine would inhibit isoniazid's antitubercular effect has not been satisfactorily elucidated.[1-4]

Recommendations: Concurrent administration of pyridoxine and isoniazid does not reduce the effectiveness of isoniazid in eradicating tubercle bacilli. The use of concurrent pyridoxine-isoniazid therapy is currently advocated.[5,6]

References

1. Pope, H.: The neutralization of isoniazid activity in mycobacterium tuberculosis by certain metabolites, Am. Rev. Tuberc. **73:**735, 1956.
2. McCune, R., and others: The delayed appearance of isoniazid antagonism by pyridoxine in vivo, Am. Rev. Tuberc. **76:**1100, 1957.
3. Beggs, W.H., and Jenne, J.W.: Mechanism for the pyridoxal neutralization of isoniazid action in mycobacterium tuberculosis, J. Bacteriol. **94:**793, 1967.
4. Boone I., and others: Effect of pyridoxal on uptake of C^{14} activity from labeled isoniazid by mycobacterium tuberculosis, Am. Rev. Tuberc. **76:**568, 1957.
5. Anon, Drugs for tuberculosis, Med. Lett. Drugs Ther. **24:**17, 1982.
6. Mandel, G.L., and Sande, M.A.: Drugs used in the chemotherapy of tuberculosis and leprosy. In Gilman, A.G., Goodman, L.S., Gilman, A., editors: The pharmacological basis of therapeutics. New York, 1980, Macmillan Publishing.

Isoniazid–Rifampin

2

Summary: Rifampin is frequently combined with isoniazid to treat tuberculosis since combination chemotherapy is more effective and reduces infectivity and the development of resistant organisms.[1] However, hepatotoxicity has been reported to occur more frequently when rifampin and isoniazid are administered concurrently.[2-3] Although the majority of cases have occurred in adults, several reports have indicated that the rapidity of onset and severity of liver toxicity may be increased when the combination is administered to infants and children.[4-7] Several other risk factors have been suggested, including high dose of isoniazid, previous general anesthesia, female patients, and administration of additional enzyme-inducing drugs.[6]

Related Drugs: There are no drugs related to rifampin or isoniazid.

Mechanism: The pharmacokinetic parameters of isoniazid and rifampin have been compared, both alone and in combination, and the results provide no evidence of a kinetic interaction. The pattern of absorption, metabolism, and excretion of each drug administered alone was not found to be different than concurrent administration, both in normal subjects and in those with liver disease.[8,9] However, it has been postulated that liver damage caused by isoniazid is related to formation of hepatotoxic metabolites and is enhanced by enzyme-inducing drugs. Rifampin is known to be a liver enzyme inducer, a fact that could account for the potentiating toxic effects when it is administered concurrently with isoniazid.[6] This may also be related to the fact that fast acetylators hydrolyze much more isoniazid to potentially toxic metabolites than do slow acetylators, and there may be a relationship between susceptibility of liver toxicity and rapid acetylators.[10]

Recommendations: Patients should be made aware of the signs and symptoms of hepatitis when taking rifampin and isoniazid and should be frequently monitored for liver toxicity.

References

1. Zimmer, B.L., and others: In vitro synergistic activity of ethambutol, isoniazid, kanamycin, rifampin and streptomycin against mycobacterium avium-intracellular complex, Antimicrob. Agents Chemother. **22:**148, 1982.
2. Lal, S., and others: Effect of rifampicin and isoniazid on liver function, Br. Med. J. **1:**148, 1972.
3. Pessayre, D., and others: Isoniazid-rifampin fulminant hepatitis. A possible consequence of the enhancement of isoniazid hepatotoxicity by enzyme induction, Gastroenterology **72:**284, 1977.
4. Casteels-VanDaele, M., and others: Hepatotoxicity of rifampicin and isoniazid in children, J. Pediatr. **86:**739, 1975.
5. Llorens, J., and others: Pharmacodynamic interference between rifampin and isoniazid, Chemotherapy **24:**97, 1978.
6. Bistritzer, T., and others: Isoniazid-rifampin-induced fulminant liver disease in an infant, J. Pediatr. **97:**480, 1980.
7. Thulasimany, M.: Increased incidence of hepatitis induced by isoniazid-rifampin combination in children, J. Pediatr. **100:**174, 1982.
8. Acocella, G., and others: Kinetics of rifampin and isoniazid administered alone and in combination to normal subjects and patients with liver disease, Gut **13:**47, 1972.
9. Boman, G.: Serum concentration and half-life of rifampicin after simultaneous oral administration of aminosalicylic acid or isoniazid, Eur. J. Clin. Pharmacol. **7:**217, 1974.
10. Mitchell, J.R., and others: Isoniazid liver injury: clinical spectrum, pathology and probable pathogenesis, Ann. Intern. Med. **84:**181, 1976.

Kanamycin–Ethacrynic Acid

Summary: Concurrent administration of kanamycin and ethacrynic acid may result in an increased incidence of ototoxic effects, especially in patients with decreased renal function. Permanent hearing loss involving cranial nerve damage has been reported after administration of these 2 agents.[1]

Related Drugs: Ethacrynic acid and other aminoglycoside antibiotics including gentamicin,[2] neomycin,[3] streptomycin,[4-6] tobramycin,[7] and netilmicin[8] have been reported to interact in a similar manner. Amikacin has not been reported to cause deafness but ototoxicity has been attributed to its administration.[8] Bumetanide and furosemide have been reported to interact with the aminoglycosides as well, resulting in transient to permanent hearing problems.[1,9-13] An interaction between kanamycin and bumetanide has also been shown to occur in an animal study.[14]

Mechanism: Both the aminoglycosides and ethacrynic acid have been individually reported to cause hearing damage[5], consequently, a possible synergistic ototoxic effect may be involved. Another hypothesis involves reduced antibiotic clearance resulting in elevated blood concentrations of the antibiotic.[15]

Recommendations: The concurrent use of these agents should be avoided whenever possible. Extreme caution as well as dose reduction and continuous monitoring of eighth cranial nerve function should be followed if concurrent administration is necessary.

References

1. Asakuma, S., and Snow, J.B.: Effects of furosemide and ethacrynic acid on the cochlear direct current potential in normal and kanamycin-treated guinea pigs, Otolargyngol. Head Neck Surg. **88:**188, 1980.
2. Meriwether, W.D., and others: Deafness following standard intravenous dose of ethacrynic acid, J.A.M.A. **216:**795, 1971.
3. Matz, G.J., and others: Ototoxicity of ethacrynic acid, Arch. Otolaryng. **90:**60, 1969.
4. Schneider, W.J., and Becker, E.L.: Acute transient hearing loss after ethacrynic acid therapy, Arch. Intern. Med. **177:**715, 1966.
5. Mathog, R.H., and Klein, W.J., Jr.: Ototoxicity of ethacrynic acid and aminoglycoside antibiotics in uremia, N. Engl. J. Med. **280:**1223, 1969.
6. Johnson, A.H., and Hamilton, C.A.: Kanamycin ototoxicity—possible potentiation by other drugs, South. Med. J. **63:**511, 1970.
7. Geddes, A.M., and others: Clinical and laboratory studies with tobramycin, Chemotherapy **20:**245, 1974.
8. Tally, F.P., and others: Amikacin therapy for severe gram-negative sepsis, Ann. Intern. Med. **83:**484, 1975.
9. Schwartz, G.H., and others: Ototoxicity induced by furosemide, N. Engl. J. Med. **282:**1413, 1970.
10. Lloyd-Mostyn, R.H., and Lord, I.J.: Ototoxicity of intravenous furosemide, Lancet **2:**1156, 1971.
11. Tuzel, I.H.: Comparison of adverse reactions to bumetanide and furosemide, J. Clin. Pharmacol. **21:**615, 1981.
12. Brummet, R.E., and others: Comparative ototoxicity of bumetanide and furosemide when used in combination with kanamycin, J. Clin. Pharmacol. **21:**628, 1981.

13. Santi, P.A., and others: Kanamycin and bumetanide ototoxicity: anatomical, physiological, and behavioral correlates, Hear. Res. **7**:261, 1982.
14. Ohtani, I., and others: Interaction of bumetanide and kanamycin, Otorhinolaryngology **40**:216, 1978.
15. Lawson, D.H., and others: Effect of furosemide on the pharmacokinetics of gentamicin in patients, J. Clin. Pharmacol. **22**:254, 1982.

Ketoconazole–Aluminum Hydroxide, Magnesium Hydroxide

3

Summary: Simultaneous administration of an antacid containing aluminum hydroxide and magnesium hydroxide decreased peak ketoconazole concentrations and 8-hour area-under-curve approximately 40% in 4 patients.[1]

Related Drugs: There is a report of sodium bicarbonate and aluminum oxide interfering with the resorption of orally administered ketoconazole.[2] Although other antacids may also interfere with ketoconazole's absorption, specific documentation is lacking. Cimetidine, though not considered an antacid, also increases gastric pH, and ketoconazole plasma levels have been shown to be reduced with concurrent cimetidine administration.[2] A similar interaction may be expected to occur with the other available H_2 receptor antagonist (ranitidine).

Mechanism: It has been shown that ketoconazole requires an acidic media for predictable dissolution to occur,[2] and solubility decreases as pH increases.[3] The antacid, as well as the H_2 receptor antagonists, presumably increases the intragastric pH, thereby decreasing dissolution and subsequent absorption.

Recommendations: A prudent regimen would be to administer the 2 agents as far apart as possible. Since there is no information regarding how long antacids affect intragastric pH, antacids should be administered after ketoconazole dosages.

References

1. Brass, C., and others: Disposition of ketoconazole, an oral antifungal, in humans, Antimicrob. Agents Chemother. **21:**151, 1982.
2. Van der Meer, J.W.M., and others: The influence of gastric acidity on the bioavailability of ketoconazole, J. Antimicrob. Chemother. **6:**552, 1980.
3. Carlson, J.A., and others: Effect of pH on disintegration and dissolution of ketoconazole tablets, Am. J. Hosp. Pharm. **40:**1334, 1983.

Ketoconazole–Cyclosporine

2

Summary: The concurrent use of cyclosporine and ketoconazole has led to increased cyclosporine blood levels as reported in several studies.[1-6] Creatinine concentrations also rose, and both creatinine and cyclosporine concentrations gradually decreased when ketoconazole was withdrawn from therapy.[6] In 1 report patients on concomitant therapy showed a decrease in the percentage of the cell-bound cyclosporine concentration, while the plasma bound cyclosporine concentration increased.[4] Because cyclosporine alone is nephrotoxic,[7-9] the combination of these agents may lead to an increased risk of nephrotoxicity.

Related Drugs: There are no drugs related to cyclosporine. Amphotericin B, another antifungal agent, has also been shown to increase cyclosporine concentrations.[10,11] In 1 study, renal failure persisted for prolonged periods of time even after amphotericin B had been discontinued for 14 to 17 days.[11]

Mechanism: The mechanism of this interaction has not been fully elucidated. However, several mechanisms have been suggested such as an increase in cyclosporine absorption,[5] competition for hepatic biotransformation,[6] competition for cell binding sites,[4] ketoconazole-induced inhibition of hepatic metabolism,[2] or competition for an excretion pathway.[1]

Recommendations: The concurrent use of these agents should be avoided if possible. If ketoconazole therapy is necessary, either cyclosporine should be replaced with another immunosuppressive agent or a dosage reduction should be made accompanied by frequent assessment of serum cyclosporine concentration and renal function.[6]

References

1. Daneshmend, T.K.: Ketoconazole-cyclosporin interaction, Lancet **2:**1342, 1982.
2. Ferguson, R.M., and others: Ketoconazole, cyclosporin metabolism, and renal transplantation, Lancet **2:**882, 1982.
3. Morgenstein, G.R., and others: Cyclosporin interaction with ketoconazole and melphalan, Lancet **2:**1342, 1982.
4. Smith, J.M., and others: Interaction of CyA and ketoconazole, Clin. Sci. **64:**67p, 1983.
5. Gluckman, E., and others: Nephrotoxicity of cyclosporin A in bone-marrow transplantation, Lancet **1:**144, 1981.
6. Dieperink, H., and Moller, J.: Ketoconazole and cyclosporin, Lancet **2:**1217, 1982.
7. Calne, R.Y., and others: Cyclosporin A in cadaveric organ transplantation, Br. Med. J. **282:**934, 1981.
8. Sweny, P., and others: Sixteen months experience with cyclosporin A in human kidney transplantations, Transplant. Proc. **13:**365, 1981.
9. Sweny, P., and others: Nephrotoxicity of cyclosporin A, Lancet **1:**663, 1981.
10. Kennedy, M.S., and others: Cyclosporin A: Clinical pharmacologic aspects of a novel immunosuppressant, Clin. Res. **29**(2):273A, 1981.
11. Tutschka, P.J., and others: Cyclosporin A in allogenic bone marrow transplantation: preclinical and clinical studies. In Cyclosporin A, Proc. Internat. Conference on cyclosporine, Cambridge (U.K), Sept. 1981. New York, 1982, Elsevier, pp. 519-538.

Lincomycin–Erythromycin

3

Summary: Erythromycin, because of its greater affinity for the 50S ribosomal unit of the bacterial cell, can theoretically antagonize the activity of lincomycin by blocking access to the ribosomal binding site.[1-4]

Related Drugs: The other macrolide antibiotics (oleandomycin and troleandomycin) as well as chloramphenicol may also have the potential for interfering with the activity of lincomycin or its structural analog clindamycin since they all bind to the 50S ribosomal unit.

Mechanism: Chloramphenicol, erythromycin, and lincomycin bind to the 50S portion of the ribosomal unit.[2] This results in bacterial cell death. Since only one antibiotic molecule can combine with the 50S ribosomal unit,[3,4] the presence of more than one antibiotic results in competition for the binding site. Since erythromycin has greater affinity for the 50S ribosomal unit than lincomycin, erythromycin could block the effects of lincomycin by displacing it from the binding site or by preventing binding.[5-7]

Recommendations: Although there are insufficient data to conclude that an interaction occurs between lincomycin and erythromycin, the clinician should be aware of the possibility of the development of cross interference. This may offset any therapeutic advantage of combining these agents. If possible, concurrent use of lincomycin and erythromycin should be avoided.

References

1. Igarashi, K., and others: Comparative studies on the mechanism of action of lincomycin, streptomycin, and erythromycin, Biochem. Biophys. Res. Commun. **37:**499, 1969.
2. Weinstein, L.: Modes of action of antibiotics on bacteria and man, N.Y. State J. Med. **72:**2166, 1972.
3. Garrett, E.R., and others: Kinetics and mechanisms of action of drugs on micro-organisms. XI: Effect of erythromycin and its supposed antagonism with lincomycin on the microbial growth of escherichia coli, J. Pharm. Sci. **59:**1448, 1970.
4. Mao, J.C.H.: The stoichiometry of erythromycin binding to ribosomal particles of staphylococcus aureus, Biochem. Pharmacol. **16:**2441, 1967.
5. Chang, F.N., and Weisblum, B.: The specificity of lincomycin binding to ribosomes, Biochemistry **6:**836, 1967.
6. Kabins, S.A.: Interactions among antibiotics and other drugs, J.A.M.A. **219:**206, 1972.
7. Weisblum, B.: Pneumococcus resistant to erythromycin and lincomycin, Lancet **1:**843, 1967.

Lincomycin–Kaolin

1

Summary: When given simultaneously, kaolin reduces the gastrointestinal absorption of lincomycin by as much as 90%.[1-3] Because there is a relatively high incidence of diarrhea among patients receiving lincomycin therapy[4] and many antidiarrheal products contain kaolin as the active ingredient, this interaction is clinically significant.

Related Drugs: Although clindamycin is structurally related to lincomycin, it was reported that kaolin had no effect on the extent of clindamycin absorption, but it markedly reduced its absorption rate.[5]

Mechanism: The exact mechanism by which kaolin interferes with the absorption of lincomycin from the gastrointestinal tract is unknown. The physical coating action of kaolin on the intestinal mucosa and kaolin's adsorbent property may be responsible.

Recommendations: In patients receiving lincomycin who require antidiarrheal therapy, products that do not contain kaolin should be considered. When a kaolin-containing product must be used, it should be given at least 2 hours before lincomycin.

References

1. Wagner, J.G.: Aspects of pharmacokinetics and biopharmaceutics in relation to drug activity, Am. J. Pharm. **141:**5, 1969.
2. Wagner, J.G.: Design and data analysis of biopharmaceutical studies in man, Can. J. Pharm. Sci. **1:**55, 1966.
3. Wagner, J.G.: Pharmacokinetics. 1. Definitions, modeling and reasons for measuring blood levels and urinary excretion, Drug Intell. Clin. Pharm. **2:**38, 1968.
4. Geddes, A.M., and others: Lincomycin hydrochloride: clinical and laboratory studies, Br. Med. J. **2:**670, 1964.
5. Albert, K.S., and others: Pharmacokinetic evaluation of a drug interaction between kaolin-pectin and clindamycin, J. Pharm. Sci. **67:**1579, 1978.

Metronidazole–Disulfiram

Summary: In a study involving hospitalized alcoholics receiving disulfiram, 6 of 29 patients who received metronidazole concurrently developed acute psychoses or confusion. Of these 6, 5 had paranoid delusions and 3 experienced visual and auditory hallucinations. This reaction was not reported in the 29 patients who received placebo with disulfiram.[1]

Related Drugs: There are no drugs related to metronidazole or disulfiram.

Mechanism: The mechanism of this interaction is unknown. However, it has been postulated that metronidazole has an attenuated disulfiram effect. This is reinforced by data that demonstrate that each of these agents selectively inhibits not only the oxidase site of xanthine oxidase activity but the function of alcohol dehydrogenase as well. Since disulfiram has been associated with psychotic behavior in some patients, this interaction has been attributed to a combined toxicity with metronidazole.[2]

Recommendations: Until further clinical studies are done, the administration of these agents should be avoided if possible. If concomitant use is necessary, patients should be closely monitored, and one or both drugs may need to be discontinued if symptoms occur.

References

1. Rothstein, E., and Clancy, D.D.: Toxicity of disulfiram combined with metronidazole, N. Engl. J. Med. **280**:1006, 1969.
2. Goodhue, W.W.: Disulfiram-metronidazole (well-identified) toxicity, N. Engl. J. Med. **280**:1482, 1969.

Metronidazole–Phenobarbital

3

Summary: Metronidazole failed to eradicate vaginal trichomoniasis in a patient taking concurrent phenobarbital. When the dose of metronidazole was increased, the infection subsided.[1]

Related Drugs: Although documentation is lacking, a similar interaction may be expected to occur between metronidazole and the other barbiturates (e.g., amobarbital, pentobarbital, secobarbital [see Appendix]) because of similar effects on hepatic enzyme induction.

Mechanism: It has been suggested that phenobarbital, a known hepatic enzyme inducer, increases the hepatic metabolism of metronidazole. In this study the patient was reported to have an increased amount of hydroxymetronidazole (a metabolite of metronidazole) and an increased half-life of metronidazole.

Recommendations: Patients on metronidazole therapy should be observed for a lack of antimicrobial response during the concurrent administration of phenobarbital. An increased dose of metronidazole may be necessary.

Reference

1. Mead, P.B., and others: Possible alteration of metronidazole metabolism by phenobarbital, N. Engl. J. Med. **306:**1490, 1982.

Nitrofurantoin–Probenecid

3

Summary: Concurrent administration of probenecid, particularly in high doses, decreases the renal clearance of nitrofurantoin and increases the serum levels of the anti-infective agent.[1] Increased nitrofurantoin serum levels have been associated with the onset of polyneuropathies including degeneration of sensory and motor nerves[1-3] and the formation of toxic immune complexes.[4] Decreased renal clearance produces urinary nitrofurantoin levels below the minimum inhibitory concentration of susceptible urinary tract infections.[1-5]

Related Drugs: Uricosuric agents such as sulfinpyrazone may have an effect on nitrofurantoin excretion similar to that of probenecid.[6]

Mechanism: Renal tubular secretion of nitrofurantoin and its apparent inhibition by probenecid was demonstrated in dogs and chickens.[7] Tubular secretion of nitrofurantoin is also thought to occur in humans. Probenecid is known to inhibit the tubular secretion of many compounds and presumably exerts the same effect with nitrofurantoin.

Recommendations: The significance of this interaction is difficult to determine for several reasons. Reports of a nitrofurantoin-probenecid interaction in clinical practice have been sparse. Second, the lower doses of probenecid frequently used in clinical practice would not exert as great an effect on nitrofurantoin excretion and systemic accumulation as the doses of 500 to 1000 mg every 2 hours used experimentally.[1]

An additional factor for consideration involves renal dysfunction. Systemic accumulation and decreased urinary excretion of nitrofurantoin occurred in patients in whom serum creatinine levels were greater than about 2.5 to 3 mg% (normal, 0.6 to 1.2 mg%).[1] Thus, patients with decreased renal efficiency may not be good candidates for nitrofurnatoin therapy.

An increase in nitrofurantoin dosage in an attempt to enhance urine levels would only serve to increase the likelihood of systemic accumulation and the adverse effects associated with increased serum levels. Thus, concurrent administration of these drugs should be avoided whenever possible.

References

1. Hubmann, R., and Bremer, G.: Die ausscheidung von Furadantin bei manifester niereninsuffizienz, Med. Welt. **19**:1039, 1965.
2. Hoyest, M., and Zachara, E.: A case of polyneuritis during long-term treatment with nitrofurantoin, Pol. Tyg. Lek. **23**:1978, 1968.
3. Mudge, G.H.: Inhibitors of tubular transport of organic compounds. In Gilman, A.G., Goodman, L.S., and Gilman, A., editors: The pharmacologic basis of therapeutics, New York, 1980, MacMillan Publishing.
4. Witte, K., and others: Immunology of adverse drug reactions, Pharmacotherapy **2**:54, 1982.
5. Hawes, E.M.: Pharmacokinetic drug-drug interaction update. Part 3: renal excretion, Can. J. Hosp. Pharm. **33**:90, 1980.
6. Schirmeister, J., and others: Renal handling of nitrofurantoin in man, Antimicrob. Agents Chemother. **5**:223, 1966.
7. Buzard, J.A., and others: Renal tubular transport of nitrofurantoin, Am. J. Physiol. **202**:1136, 1962.

Nitrofurantoin–Propantheline

3

Summary: In a crossover study involving 6 subjects, the concurrent use of nitrofurantoin and propantheline caused a statistically significant increase in nitrofurantoin absorption and excretion as compared with the control.[1] An increase in therapeutic efficacy and adverse effects of nitrofurantoin may be expected.

Related Drugs: There are no drugs related to nitrofurantoin. Documentation is lacking regarding an interaction with the other anticholinergics (e.g., atropine, dicyclomine, methantheline [see Appendix]); however, based on pharmacologic similarity, an interaction may be expected to occur.

Mechanism: It has been suggested that propantheline decreases gastric emptying time because of its ability to reduce gastric motility.[1] This may increase nitrofurantoin bioavailability by allowing an increased dissolution of nitrofurantoin before absorption in the small intestine.

Recommendations: The concurrent use of these agents need not be avoided. However, it is prudent to separate the administration of these drugs by as much time as possible.

Reference

1. Jaffe, J.M.: Effect of propantheline on nitrofurantoin absorption, J. Pharm. Sci. **64:**1729, 1975.

Penicillin–Aspirin

3

Summary: Limited clinical data indicate that large doses of aspirin (3 g/day) significantly increase penicillin serum concentrations and half-life.[1] The study was conducted in 11 patients with arteriosclerotic disorders who were given penicillin G before and after 5 to 7 days of aspirin.[1] The clinical effects of the increase were not determined.

Related Drugs: Aspirin has reduced the serum protein binding of cloxacillin, dicloxacillin, nafcillin, and oxacillin.[2] Reports of the clinical effect of such displacement are lacking.

There appear to be no reports of the other salicylates (e.g., choline salicylate, salicylamide, sodium salicylate [see Appendix]) affecting the disposition of penicillin. However, if the mechanism of the interaction involves the acetyl group of aspirin covalently binding to lysine residue on albumin and affecting protein binding of other drugs, then only those salicylates that contain an acetyl group would be expected to interact.

Mechanism: The exact mechanism of this interaction is unclear, but it may involve 2 separate effects. Aspirin may displace penicillin from its protein binding sites. The acetyl group of aspirin binds covalently to lysine residues on albumin, resulting in an altered secondary structure. This altered structure may result in altered protein binding to other drugs.[3,4] Another possible mechanism involves competition of the 2 drugs for the same renal secretory sites in the proximal tubule.[1,5-7]

Recommendations: The limited clinical data prevent definite assessment of the clinical significance of this drug interaction. Concurrent use of high doses of aspirin has been suggested to increase the clinical benefits of penicillin,[4] but the possible toxicities resulting from high-dose aspirin administration discourage such therapy.

References

1. Kampmann, J.: Effect of some drugs on penicillin half-life in blood, Clin. Pharmacol. Ther. **13:**516, 1972.
2. Kunin, C.M.: Clinical pharmacology of the new penicillins. II. Effect of drugs that interfere with binding to serum proteins, Clin. Pharmacol. Ther. **7:**180, 1966.
3. Hawkins, D., and others: Structural changes in human serum albumin induced by ingestion of acetylsalicylic acid, J. Clin. Invest. **48:**536, 1969.
4. Moskowitz, B., and others: Salicylate interaction with penicillin and secobarbital binding sites on human serum albumin, Clin. Toxicol. **6:**247, 1973.
5. Suffness, M.: Potential drug interactions and adverse effects related to aspirin, Drug Intell. Clin. Pharm. **8:**694, 1974.
6. Robinson, D.S.: Pharmacokinetic mechanisms of drug interactions, Postgrad. Med. **57:**55, 1975.
7. Hayes, A.H.: Therapeutic implications of drug interactions with acetaminophen and aspirin, Arch. Intern. Med. **41:**301, 1981.

Penicillin–Chloramphenicol

4

Summary: The bacteriostatic action of chloramphenicol may antagonize the bactericidal action of penicillin, as suggested by in vitro and in vivo animal studies.[1-5] However, another study indicated that the concurrent use of these agents resulted in a prolonged half-life and elevated levels of chloramphenicol.[6] Human data indicate that administration of the 2 drugs simultaneously does not compromise clinical effectiveness in many situations.[7,8] Several variables such as the organisms involved and the doses used can affect the potential interaction.

Related Drugs: Concurrent administration of chloramphenicol and ampicillin was found to be superior to chloramphenicol alone in patients with typhoid.[9] Another study compared concomitant chloramphenicol and procaine penicillin to chloramphenicol alone in 700 patients with gonorrhea, and concurrent treatment again was found to be superior.[10] There is no documentation regarding an interaction between chloramphenicol and other penicillins (e.g., cloxacillin, dicloxacilin, oxacillin [see Appendix]); however, because of their bactericidal action, a similar interaction may be expected to occur. There are no drugs related to chloramphenicol.

Mechanism: Penicillin inhibits cell wall synthesis. Chloramphenicol, however, inhibits protein synthesis, which may mask the bactericidal action of penicillin.

Recommendations: There is no unequivocal clinical evidence that chloramphenicol causes any significant antagonism of the bactericidal effect of penicillin. Therefore, concurrent use of these antiobiotics need not be avoided in the limited circumstances where such therapy is indicated.

References

1. Wallace, J.F., and others: Studies on the pathogenesis of meningitis. VI. Antagonism between penicillin and chloramphenicol in experimental pneumococcal meningitis, J. Lab. Clin. Med. **70:**408, 1967.
2. Jawetz, E., and others: The combined action of penicillin with streptomycin or chloromycetin on enterococci in vitro, Science **3:**254, 1950.
3. Jawetz, E., and others: Studies on antibiotic synergism and antagonism, Arch. Intern. Med. **87:**349, 1951.
4. Yourassowsky, E., and Monsieur, R.: Antagonism limit of penicillin G and chloramphenicol against Neisseria meningitides, Arzneimittel Forsch. **21:**1385, 1971.
5. Ardalan, P.: Zur Frage des Antagonismus von Penicillin and Chloramphicolus klinischer sicht, Prax. Klin. Pneumol. **23:**772, 1969.
6. Windorfer, A., and others: Studies of concentration of chloramphenicol in serum and cerebrospinal fluid of neonates, infants, and small children: reciprocal reactions between chloramphenicol, penicillin, and phenobarbitone, Eur. J. Pediatr. **124:**129, 1977.
7. Jawetz, E.: The use of combinations of antimicrobial drugs, Ann. Rev. Pharmacol. **8:**151, 1968.
8. Crofton, J.: Some principles in the chemotherapy of bacterial infections, Br. Med. J. **2:**137, 1969.
9. De Ritis, F., and others: Chloramphenicol combined with ampicillin in treatment of typhoid, Br. Med. J. **4:**17, 1972.
10. Gjessing, H.C., and Odegaard, K.: Oral chloramphenicol alone and with intramuscular procaine penicillin in the treatment of gonorrhea, Br. J. Vener. Dis. **43:**133, 1967.

Penicillin–Chlortetracycline

2

Summary: Tetracycline derivatives may antagonize the bactericidal action of penicillin G under conditions such as meningitis where rapid bacterial kill is desired.[1-6] Increased incidence of mortality,[3,4] reinfection,[5] and secondary infections[6] have been reported in patients receiving combinations of chlortetracycline and penicillin G.

Related Drugs: Penicillin G is the only penicillin for which there is documented antagonism by a tetracycline preparation.[3,5] Antagonism of the action of all other penicillins (e.g., penicillin V, oxacillin, cloxacillin [see Appendix]) might be expected based on their common mechanism of action. The evidence primarily involves the antagonism of the action of penicillin by chlortetracycline, but there are also data to suggest a similar effect by oxytetracycline and tetracycline.[4] All tetracyclines (e.g., demeclocycline, doxycycline, minocycline [see Appendix]) may be expected to interact in a similar manner with penicillin because of pharmacologic similarity.

Mechanism: Spheroplast formation, a preceding step in the lysis of bacteria exposed to penicillin, is inhibited by bacteriostatic agents such as tetracyclines.[1] Antagonism, however, is not always apparent to the same degree[2] and precise mechanisms of antagonism are not defined.

Recommendations: Tetracycline may cause a clinically significant antagonism of penicillin in situations where rapid bactericidal activity is necessary (e.g., pneumococcal meningitis). There is no clinical evidence supporting a penicillin-tetracycline interaction with infections where rapid bacterial kill is not critical. Even in those cases where no antagonism occurs, there is no justification for concurrent use of penicillin and tetracycline.

References

1. Chang, T.W., and Weinstein, L.: Inhibitory effects of other antibiotics on bacterial morphological changes induced by penicillin G, Nature **211:**763, 1966.
2. Speck, R.S., and others: Studies on antibiotic synergism and antagonism, Arch. Intern. Med. **88:**68, 1951.
3. Lepper, M.H., and Dowling, H.F.: Treatment of pneumoccocic meningitis with penicillin compared with penicillin plus aureomycin, Arch. Intern. Med. **88:**489, 1951.
4. Olsson, R.A., and others: Pneumococcal meningitis in the adult. Clinical, therapeutic, and prognostic aspects in forty three patients, Ann. Intern. Med. **55:**545, 1961.
5. Strom, J.: The question of antagonism between penicillin and chlortetracycline, illustrated by therapeutical experiments in scarlatina, Antibiot. Med. **1:**6, 1955.
6. Ahern, J.J., and Kirby, W.M.: Lack of interference of aureomycin with penicillin in treatment of pneumococcic pneumonia, Arch. Intern. Med. **91:**197, 1953.

Penicillin–Erythromycin

3

Summary: Concomitant usage of penicillin and erythromycin may result in synergism, antagonism, or no alteration of the combined antibacterial effect. This action appears to be dependent on several factors including type of microorganism involved and its susceptibility to these antibiotics,[1] the inoculum effect,[2-4] the relative concentrations of the 2 antibiotics used,[1,5-7] and the time of incubation.[4]

Related Drugs: Of the penicillin analogs, penicillin G,[1,3,5-11] penicillin V,[8,12] ampicillin,[4,13,14] and methicillin[1,3,15] have been documented to interact in vitro and in vivo with erythromycin. Cephalosporins have chemical and pharmacologic properties related to those of the penicillins[16] and may be expected to interact with erythromycin in a similar manner since this interaction has occurred between erythromycin and cephaloridine.[15]

Mechanism: Beta-lactams such as the penicillins exert their bactericidal effect by combining with receptors known as penicillin-binding proteins. The resultant effect is an inhibition of bacterial cell wall synthesis, leaving the actual formation of the cytoplasm undisturbed.[5,16] Erythromycin exerts a bacteriostatic effect by affecting the formation of the cytoplasm via inhibition of cellular protein and enzyme synthesis. This effect results in decreased bacterial cytoplasmic growth and a decreased susceptibility to cellular lysis induced by bactericidal drugs such as penicillin.[5,17]

Recommendations: Penicillins should not be used routinely in combination with erythromycin. Although concurrent administration has revealed synergism, indifference[12] and antagonism[5,11] have also been reported and are most likely the result of differences in microorganisms studied and their related susceptibilities to these antibiotics. If these drugs are used concurrently, both the minimum inhibitory concentration and the minimum bactericidal concentration should be checked to ensure a synergistic bactericidal effect.[14]

References

1. Garrod, L.P., and Waterworth, P.M.: Methods of testing combined antibiotic bactericidal action and the significance of the results, J. Clin. Pathol. **15:**328, 1967.
2. Waterworth, P.M.: Apparent synergy between penicillin and erythromycin or fusidic acid, Clin. Med. **70:**941, 1963.
3. Roberts, C.E., and others: Synergism of erythromycin and penicillin against resistant staphylococci: mechanism and relation to synthetic penicillins, Antimicrob. Agents Chemother. Annual, p. 831, 1962.
4. Finland, M., and others: Synergistic action of ampicillin and erythromycin against Nocardia asteroides: effect of time of incubation, Antimicrob. Agents Chemother. **5:**344, 1974.
5. Manten, A. and Terra, J.I.: The antagonism between penicillin and other antibiotics in relation to drug concentration, Chemotherapia **8:**21, 1964.
6. Oswald, E.J., and others: Antibiotic combinations: an in vitro study of antistaphylococcal effects of erythromycin plus penicillin, streptomycin, or tetracycline, Antimicrob. Agents Chemother. Annual, p. 904, 1961.
7. Barber, M.: Drug combinations in antibacterial chemotherapy, Proc. R. Soc. Med. **58:**990, 1965.

8. Chang, T.W., and Weinstein, L.: Inhibitory effects of other antibiotics on bacterial morphologic changes induced by penicillin G, Nature **211:**763, 1966.
9. Herrell, W.E., and others: Erythrocillin: a new approach to the problem of antibiotic-resistant staphylococci, Antibiot. Med. Clin. Therap. **7:**637, 1960.
10. Allen, N.E., and Epp, J.K.: Mechanism of penicillin-erythromycin synergy on antibiotic resistant Staphylococcus aureus, Antimicrob. Agents Chemother. **13:**849, 1978.
11. Manten, A.: Synergism and antagonism between antibiotic mixtures containing erythromycin, Antibiot. Chemother. **4:**1228, 1954.
12. Strom, J.: Penicillin and erythromycin singly and in combination in scarlatina fever and the interference between them, Antibiot. Chemother. **11:**694, 1961.
13. Bach, M.C., and others: Pulmonary nocariosis: therapy with minocycline and with erythromycin plus ampicillin, J.A.M.A. **224:**1378, 1973.
14. Robinson, L., and Fonseca, K.: Value of the minimum bactericidal concentration of antibiotics in the management of a case of recurrent Streptococcus bovis septicemia, J. Clin. Pathol. **35:**879, 1982.
15. Gronroos, J.A.: Changes in the susceptibility of staphylococci during passages in combination of erythromycin and various penicillin derivatives and cephaloridine, Curr. Ther. Res. **8:**879, 1982.
16. Mandell, G.L., and Sande, M.A.: Antimicrobial agents: penicillins and cephalosporins. In Gilman, A.G., Goodman, L.S., and Gilman, A., editors: The pharmacological basis of therapeutics, New York, 1980, Macmillan Publishing.
17. Sande, M.A., and Mandell, G.L.: Antimicrobial agents: miscellaneous antibacterial agents, antifungal and antiviral agents. In Gilman, A.G., Goodman, L.S., and Gilman, A., editors: The pharmacological basis of therapeutics, New York, 1980, Macmillan Publishing.

Penicillin–Probenecid

3

Summary: Concurrent administration of penicillin and probenecid results in higher and more sustained serum penicillin levels.

Related Drugs: Several other penicillin analogs have also been reported to interact with probenecid. These include amoxicillin,[1] ampicillin,[2] azlocillin,[3] carbenicillin,[4] cloxacillin,[5] methicillin,[6] mezlocillin,[7] nafcillin,[8] oxacillin,[6] piperacillin,[9] and ticarcillin.[10] All other penicillins (e.g., bacampicillin, cyclacillin, dicloxacillin [see Appendix]) may also be expected to interact in a similar manner with probenecid.

Mechanism: Two mechanisms have been proposed to explain this interaction. One possibility is that probenecid actively competes with other weak organic acids for the renal transport process and thus diminishes tubular secretion of such compounds (e.g., penicillins).[11] A second possibility is that probenecid decreases the apparent volume of distribution of the penicillins, resulting in a larger penicillin fraction in the central (plasma and extracellular water) compartment.[12]

Recommendations: Complications during concurrent administration of these drugs result from increased antibiotic levels and are encountered most frequently during long-term treatment. It may be advisable to reduce the dosage of penicillin when probenecid is combined with the antibiotic and to monitor the penicillin serum levels.

References

1. Sutherland, R., and others: Amoxycillin: a new semi-synthetic penicillin, Br. Med. J. **3:**13, 1972.
2. Treatment and prevention of syphilis and gonorrhea, Med. Lett. Drugs Ther. **13:**85, 1971.
3. Leroy, A., and others: Pharmacokinetics of azlocillin in healthy subjects, Scand. J. Infect. Dis. **29**(suppl.):49, 1981.
4. Standiford, H.C., and others: Clinical pharmacology of carbenicillin compared with other penicillins, J. Infect. Dis. **122**(suppl.):S9, 1970.
5. Nauta, E.H., and others: Effect of probenecid on the apparent volume of distribution and elimination of cloxacillin, Antimicrob. Agents Chemother. **6:**300, 1974.
6. Simon, H.J., and Rantz, L.A.: The newer penicillins. I. Bacteriological and clinical pharmacological investigations with methicillin and oxacillin, Ann. Intern. Med. **57:**335, 1962.
7. Verbist, L., and others: Mezlocillin pharmacokinetics, Arzneimmittel Forsch. **29:**1962, 1979.
8. Klein, J.O., and Finland, M.: Nafcillin, Am. J. Med. Sci. **246:**44/10, 1963.
9. Tjandramaga, T.B., and others: Piperacillin: human pharmacokinetics after intravenous and intramuscular administration, Antimicrob. Agents Chemother. **14:**829, 1978.
10. Davies, B.E., and others: Pharmacokinetics of ticarcillin in man, Eur. J. Clin. Pharmacol. **23:**167, 1982.
11. Weiner, I.M., and others: On the mechanism of action of probenecid on renal tubular secretion, Bull. Johns Hopkins Hosp. **106:**333, 1960.
12. Gibaldi, M., and Schwartz, M.A.: Apparent effect of probenecid on the distribution of penicillins in man, Clin. Pharmacol. Ther. **9:**345, 1968.

Polymyxin B–Prochlorperazine

2

Summary: In 1 case report, a patient who received intravenous polymyxin B experienced severe apnea after the concurrent administration of prochlorperazine.[1]

Related Drugs: A similar interaction was documented after the concurrent administration of colistin and promethazine.[2] Although documentation is lacking a similar interaction may be expected to occur between the other polypeptide antibiotics (bacitracin, capreomycin, and colistimethate) and the other phenothiazines (e.g., chlorpromazine, thioridazine, trifluopromazine [see Appendix]) because of pharmacologic similarity.

Mechanism: It has been shown in humans that colistin and the other polypeptide antibiotics possess a neuromuscular blocking activity on the intercostal muscles that can produce apnea at higher than therapeutic doses.[3] Also, prochlorperazine and other phenothiazines have been shown to have some neuromuscular blocking activity.[4] Therefore, the development of apnea in these patients may result from a synergistic neuromuscular blockade, although this has not been clearly demonstrated.

Recommendations: Caution should be used when concurrently administering polymyxin B and prochlorperazine, or other polypeptide antibiotics and phenothiazines. Ventilatory assistance should be made available.

References

1. Pohlmann, G.: Respiratory arrest associated with intravenous administration of polymyxin B, J.A.M.A. **196:**181, 1966.
2. Anthony, M.A., and Louis, D.L.: Apnea due to intramuscular colistin therapy, Ohio Med. J. **62:**336, 1966.
3. Sabawala, P.B., and Dillon, J.B.: The action of some antibiotics on the human intercostal nerve-muscle complex, Anesthesiology **20:**659, 1959.
4. Regan, A.G., and Aldrete, J.A.: Prolonged apnea after administration of promazine hydrochloride following succinylcholine infusion, Anesth. Analg. (Cleve.) **46:**315, 1967.

Rifampin–Aminosalicylic Acid

4

Summary: Aminosalicylic acid granules have been reported to decrease the bioavailability and subsequent pharmacologic activity of rifampin.[1-3] Subsequent studies found that the reduction was caused by bentonite, an excipient in the aminosalicylic acid granules, which decreased absorption by rapidly adsorbing rifampin.[4]

Related Drugs: There are no drugs related to rifampin or aminosalicylic acid.

Mechanism: Rifampin was shown to adsorb onto bentonite in vitro. Aminosalicylic acid tablets prepared without bentonite did not affect rifampin bioavailability in humans. Placebo tablets containing bentonite, without aminosalicylic acid, produced a decrease in rifampin bioavailability. Because adsorption is a characteristic of bentonite, it is likely that physical adsorption of rifampin is the mechanism in vivo as well.[4]

Recommendations: It may not be possible to know if a granule formulation contains bentonite. However, it was demonstrated that separating the administration of these 2 agents by 8 to 12 hours prevented the interaction.[1]

References

1. Boman, G., and others: Drug interaction: decreased serum concentrations of rifampicin when given with P.A.S., Lancet **1**:800, 1971.
2. Boman, G., and others: Pharmacokinetic interactions between the tuberculostatics rifampicin, para-amino salicylic acid and isoniazid, Acta Pharmacol. Toxicol. **28**(suppl. 1):15, 1970.
3. Boman, G.: Serum concentration and half-life of rifampicin after simultaneous oral administration of amino salicylic acid or isoniazid, Eur. J. Clin. Pharmacol. **7**:217, 1974.
4. Boman, G., and others: Mechanism of the inhibitory effect of P.A.S. granules on the absorption of rifampicin: adsorption of rifampicin by an excipient, bentonite, Eur. J. Clin. Pharmacol. **8**:293, 1975.

Rifampin–Oral Contraceptive Agents

1

Summary: Concurrent administration of rifampin and oral contraceptive agents results in an increased incidence of menstrual disorders[1-5] and pregnancies.[2,4,6,7] Rifampin decreases the elimination half-life and reduces the bioavailability of the contraceptive steroids.[8-13]

Related Drugs: There are no drugs related to rifampin.

Mechanism: Two mechanisms may be operative, both of which would explain the contraceptive failures reported. Estrogens and progestogens are extensively excreted in the bile, principally as glucuronide conjugates. Subsequently, they undergo entero-hepatic circulation where bacterial hydrolysis occurs, allowing for reabsorption of the oral contraceptive through the bowel wall and eventual urinary excretion. Treatment with the antibiotics destroys the gut flora and prevents steroid reabsorption resulting in lower than normal concentrations of the contraceptive.

Rifampin is a known microsomal enzyme inducer, and studies in human liver biopsies indicate that the hydroxylation of estrogens is increased 4-fold with rifampin pretreatment.[14-16]

Recommendations: The evidence strongly suggests that women taking these agents have a high possibility of breakthrough bleeding, pregnancy, or both. Although some women may take these agents concomitantly without risk, there is no way to predict who will be affected.

Some prescribers may choose to warn patients that spotting and breakthrough bleeding are signs of diminished contraceptive effectiveness, and additional alternative forms of contraception should be used. Others may choose to recommend an alternative contraception method during concurrent use.

References

1. Reimers, D., and Jezek, A.: The simultaneous use of rifampicin and other antituberculosis agents with oral contraceptives, Prax. Klin. Pneumol. **25:**255, 1971.
2. Nocke-Finck, L., and others: Effect of rifampicin on the menstrual cycle and on oestrogen excretion in patients taking oral contraceptives, Dtsch. Med. Wochenschr. **98:**1521, 1973.
3. Altschuler, S.L., and Valenteen, J.W.: Amenorrhea following rifampin administration during oral contraceptive use, Obstet. Gynecol. **44:**771, 1974.
4. Reimers, D.: Rifampicin, "pill" do not go well together, J.A.M.A. **227:**608, 1974.
5. Cohn, H.D.: Rifampicin and the pill, J.A.M.A. **228:**828, 1974.
6. Skolnick, J.F., and others: Rifampin, oral contraceptives, and pregnancy, J.A.M.A. **236:**1382, 1976.
7. Breckenridge, A.M., and others: Interactions between oral contraceptives and other drugs, Pharmacol. Ther. **7:**617, 1979.
8. Back, D.J., and others: The effect of rifampicin on norethisterone pharmacokinetics, Eur. J. Clin. Pharmacol. **15:**193, 1979.
9. Joshi, J.V., and others: A study of interaction of a low-dose combination oral contraceptive and anti-tubercular drugs, Contraception **21:**617, 1980.
10. Back, D.J., and others: The effect of rifampicin on the pharmacokinetics of ethrylestradiol in women, Contraception **21:**135, 1980.

11. Bolt, H.M., and others: Interaction of rifampicin treatment with pharmacokinetic and metabolism of ethinyloestradiol in man, Acta Endocrinol. **85:**189, 1977.
12. Back, D.J., and others: The pharmacokinetics of norethisterone during single and multiple dosing in women and changes caused by rifampicin, Acta Endocrinol. **212**(suppl.):149, 1977.
13. Back, D.J., and others: Interindividual variation and drug interactions with hormonal steroid contraceptives, Drugs **21:**46, 1981.
14. Bolt, H.M., and others: Rifampicin and oral contraception, Lancet **1:**1280, 1974.
15. Bolt, H.M., and others: Effect of rifampicin treatment on the metabolism of oestradiol and 17alpha-ethinyl-oestradiol by human liver microsomes, Eur. J. Clin. Pharmacol. **8:**301, 1975.
16. Burt, H.M.: Interaction between oral contraceptives and other drugs, Br. Med. J. **280:**1230, 1980.

Rifampin–Prednisolone

2

Summary: It has been reported that prednisolone disposition is altered by antituberculosis co-therapy that included rifampin, resulting in a decreased corticosteroid activity.[1,2] Rifampin was further implicated in the decreased serum area-under-curve and increased clearance of prednisolone.[3] Another study reported that rifampin significantly decreased prednisolone elimination half-life and bioavailability, while volume of distribution remained unaffected.[4]

Related Drugs: Similar changes in corticosteroid disposition have been reported for cortisone acetate,[5,6] fludrocortisone,[5] cortisol (hydrocortisone),[7] and methylprednisolone.[8] Although not reported, a similar interaction may be expected to occur with the other corticosteroids (e.g., betamethasone, prednisone, triamcinolone [see Appendix]) based on a similar metabolic fate. There are no drugs related to rifampin.

Mechanism: Antituberculosis therapy that included rifampin increased cortisol production rates,[5] increased urinary 6-hydroxycortisol excretion,[7] and decreased prednisolone half-life[1,3] and area-under-curve.[3] These changes are consistent with a mechanism where rifampin induces the hepatic metabolizing enzymes leading to an increased metabolism of the steroid.

Recommendations: A reduced corticosteroid activity may be expected when rifampin is coadministered, necessitating an increased steroid dose. One approximation is to double the daily steroid dose when rifampin therapy is initiated.[8] Patients stabilized on both agents may require a steroid dosage decrease when rifampin is discontinued.

References

1. Hendrickse, W., and others: Rifampicin-induced non-responsiveness to corticosteroid treatment in nephrotic syndrome, Br. Med. J. **1**:306, 1979.
2. Van Marle, W., and others: Concurrent steroid and rifampicin therapy, Br. Med. J. **1**:1020, 1979.
3. McAllister, W.A.C., and others: Rifampin reduces effectiveness and bioavailability of prednisolone, Br. Med. J. **286**:923, 1983.
4. Powell-Jackson, P.R., and others: Adverse effect of rifampin administration on steroid-dependent asthma, Am. Rev. Resp. Dis. **128**:307, 1983.
5. Edwards, O.M., and others: Changes in cortisol metabolism following rifampicin therapy, Lancet **2**:549, 1974.
6. Maisey, D.N., and others: Rifampicin and cortisone replacement therapy, Lancet **2**:896, 1974.
7. Yamada, S., and Iwai, K.: Induction of hepatic cortisol-6-hydroxylase by rifampin, Lancet **2**:366, 1976.
8. Buffington, G.A., and others: Interaction of rifampin and glucocorticords, J.A.M.A. **236**:1958, 1976.

Rifampin–Probenecid

4

Summary: Rifampin and probenecid have been the subject of conflicting data designed to evaluate whether the addition of probenecid to rifampin therapy would add any therapeutic benefit.[1-3]

Related Drugs: There are no drugs related to rifampin. It is not known if an interaction occurs between rifampin and the other uricosuric (sulfinpyrazone).

Mechanism: The mechanism of action of a possible synergistic effect after concomitant administration of these 2 agents is not clearly understood. One theory is that both agents compete at the plasma membrane, which results in an increase in peak serum rifampin levels of 86% after oral probenecid.[1] However, other reports have since appeared which demonstrate the fact that individual patient variations could cause the serum levels of rifampin to increase and that changes in the rate of metabolism by the liver could be the factor.[2]

Recommendations: At this point, there appears to be no advantage of adding probenecid to rifampin therapy with the goal of increasing rifampin's plasma levels or decreasing its rate of metabolism.

References

1. Kenwright, S., and Levi, A.J.: Impairment of hepatic uptake of rifamycin antibiotics by probenecid, and its therapeutic implications, Lancet **2**:1401, 1973.
2. Fallon, R.J., and others: Probenecid and rifampin serum levels, Lancet **2**:792, 1975.
3. Allen, B.W., and others: Probenecid and serum rifampin, Lancet **2**:1309, 1975.

Sulfamethazine ⟩ Cyclosporine
Trimethoprim*

3

Summary: In a patient stabilized on cyclosporine for 7 months, the concurrent administration of intravenous trimethoprim and sulfamethazine resulted in undetectable cyclosporine serum levels within 7 days. Graft rejection was evident in this patient during this time, and trough cyclosporine serum levels decreased despite an increase in the cyclosporine dose. When the administration of the antibiotics was switched to the oral route, the trough levels increased.[1] It was not determined whether the route of administration or the drugs themselves were responsible for this interaction. It is also not known if either drug alone would result in the same interaction.

Related Drugs: There are no drugs related to cyclosporine. Because it was not determined whether sulfamethazine alone would result in a similar interaction, it is not known whether other sulfonamides (e.g., sulfacytine, sulfasalazine, sulfisoxazole [see Appendix]) would interact similarly with cyclosporine. Nephrotoxicity was observed in 6 renal transplant patients receiving cyclosporine after administration of trimethoprim or trimethoprim and sulfamethoxazole.[2]

Mechanism: The mechanism of this interaction is unknown.

Recommendations: Patients should be observed for a decrease in cyclosporine serum levels. Until further studies are done, an increase in the cyclosporine dose, use of an alternative antibiotic, or the use of the oral rather than the intravenous route of administration for the antibiotics may be necessary.

References

1. Wallwork, J., and others: Cyclosporine and intravenous sulphadimedine and trimethoprim, Lancet **1:**366, 1983.
2. Thompson, J.F., and others: Nephrotoxicity of trimethoprim and cotrimoxazole in renal allograft recipients treated with cyclosporine, Transplantation **36:**204, 1983.

*This combination is not available in the U.S.

Sulfasalazine–Ampicillin

Summary: After a 5 day course of ampicillin therapy in 5 healthy men, the area under the plasma level time curve for sulfapyridine (a metabolite of sulfasalazine) was significantly lower. Ampicillin affected only the extent of absorption, reducing the availability of sulfasalazine. The time to onset of absorption, time of maximum plasma levels, and absorption and disposition half-lives were not significantly changed.[1]

Related Drugs: There is no documentation regarding an interaction between sulfasalazine and the other penicillins (e.g., amoxicillin, bacampicillin, hetacillin [see Appendix]) although due to pharmacologic similarity a similar interaction may be expected to occur. Based on the proposed mechanism, it is difficult to determine whether an interaction would occur between ampicillin and the other sulfonamides (e.g., sulfadiazine, sulfisoxazole, sulfamethoxazole [see Appendix]).

Mechanism: The mechanism of this interaction is unknown. Sulfasalazine is metabolized in the colon to form sulfapyridine and 5-aminosalicylate (the therapeutically active metabolite). Because ampicillin affects only the extent of absorption of sulfapyridine, this would result in reduced 5-aminosalicylate at the site of action.[1]

Recommendations: Sulfasalazine is often used in the management of inflammatory bowel disease. Therefore, patients receiving this drug should be monitored for loss of therapeutic efficacy when ampicillin is added to their therapy.

Reference

1. Day, J.M., and Houston, J.B.: Effect of ampicillin upon the bioavailability of sulphapyridine following oral administration of sulphasalazine in man, Br. J. Clin. Pharmacol. **11:**423, 1981.

Tetracycline–Aluminum Hydroxide

Summary: Concurrent administration of aluminum hydroxide containing antacids or products containing divalent ions (magnesium or calcium) and tetracycline significantly decreases the gastrointestinal absorption of tetracycline.[1]

Related Drugs: Demeclocycline,[2,3] methacycline,[4] chlortetracycline,[5] and oxytetracycline[4,6] have been reported to interact with aluminum hydroxide and/or dairy products (e.g., cottage cheese, milk). Doxycycline has been reported to interact with aluminum hydroxide[3] but absorption is only slightly decreased with dairy products.[3,4] It is claimed that minocycline absorption is not notably influenced by food and dairy products, but aluminum, calcium, and magnesium ions in the concentration found in antacid preparations may impair absorption.[7] Since sucralfate is an aluminum salt of a sulfated disaccharide, it may prevent absorption of tetracycline.

Magnesium-aluminum hydroxide gel has been shown to decrease the tetracycline area under the serum concentration time curve by nearly 90%.[8] Bismuth subsalicylate, an ingredient in some antidiarrheal mixtures, has been shown to decrease tetracycline absorption.[9] Bismuth subsalicylate has also been reported to decrease the bioavailability of doxycycline.[10]

Simultaneous administration of tetracycline with dicalcium phosphate (40 mg calcium) or tetracycline with other common excipients showed 25% to 50% lower tetracycline serum levels in the presence of calcium.[6]

Mechanism: Tetracycline forms relatively insoluble chelates with divalent and trivalent metallic ions.[11] Aluminum ions form the most stable complexes, whereas magnesium and calcium ions form weaker complexes.[12]

Recommendations: Simultaneous use of antacids containing aluminum, calcium, or magnesium ions or dairy products containing calcium along with tetracycline or its analogs should be avoided. If antacids are indicated, they should be given at least 2 hours after tetracycline administration to allow the maximum amount of tetracycline to be absorbed. Because there are no data to predict the length of time the antacid will affect tetracycline absorption, administration of the antacid before tetracycline should be avoided.

References

1. Penttila, O., and others: Effect of zinc sulphate on the absorption of tetracycline and doxycycline in man, Eur. J. Clin. Pharmacol. **9:**131, 1975.
2. Scheiner, J., and Altemeier, W.A.: Experimental study of factors inhibiting absorption and effective therapeutic levels of declomycin, Surg. Gynecol. Obstet. **114:**9, 1962.
3. Rosenblatt, J.E., and others: Comparison of in vitro activity and clinical pharmacology of doxycycline with other tetracyclines, Antimicrob. Agents Chemother. **6:**134, 1966.
4. Mattila, M.J., and others: Interference of iron preparations and milk with the absorption of tetracyclines, Excerpta Medica Int. Cong. Ser. **254:**128, 1971.
5. Waisbren, B.A., and Hueckel, J.S.: Reduced absorption of Aureomycin caused by aluminum hydroxide gel (Amphojel), Proc. Soc. Exp. Biol. Med. **73:**73, 1950.

6. Boger, W.P., and Gavin, J.J.: An evaluation of tetracycline preparations, N. Engl. J. Med. **261**:827, 1959.
7. Minocin package insert and personal communication with manufacturer representative, Lederle Laboratories, Pearl River, NY, 1983.
8. Garty, M., and Hurwitz, A.: Effect of cimetidine and antacids on gastrointestinal absorption of tetracycline, Clin. Pharmacol. Ther. **28**:203, 1980.
9. Albert, K.A., and others: Decreased tetracycline bioavailability caused by a bismuth subsalicylate antidiarrheal mixture, J. Pharm. Sci. **68**:586, 1979.
10. Ericsson, C.D., and others: Influence of subsalicylate bismuth on absorption of doxycycline, J.A.M.A. **247**:2266, 1982.
11. Albert, A., and Rees, C.W.: Avidity of the tetracyclines for the cations of metals, Nature **177**:433, 1956.
12. Chin, T.F., and Lach, J.L.: Drug diffusion and bioavailability: tetracycline metallic chelation, Am. J. Hosp. Pharm. **32**:625, 1975.

Summary: The concurrent use of tetracycline and cimetidine resulted in a reduction in the mean peak tetracycline plasma concentration, a decrease in the area-under-curve, and a reduction in 72 hour urinary tetracycline excretion. However, tetracycline kinetics were not significantly altered on the fifth day of concomitant use.[1] Another study showed a reduction in the bioavailability of tetracycline in the capsule form, but cimetidine had no affect on the availability of the oral solution.[2] Another study failed to show any effect of concurrent cimetidine on tetracycline bioavailability.[3]

Related Drugs: No documentation exists regarding an interaction between cimetidine and the other tetracyclines (e.g., doxycycline, minocycline, oxytetracycline [see Appendix]) or between tetracycline and the other H_2 receptor antagonist (ranitidine). However, if the mechanism involves an increased gastric pH, then both H_2 receptor antagonists and the tetracyclines may be expected to interact in a similar manner.

Mechanism: The mechanism of this interaction is unknown. However, it has been suggested that dissolution of the capsule form of tetracycline depends on gastric acidity. Cimetidine, by raising gastric pH, may inhibit the dissolution of tetracycline to some extent. When some of the undissolved tetracycline reaches the small intestine, the alkaline environment may further reduce its bioavailability.[2]

Recommendations: Further studies are needed to elucidate this interaction; however, patients should be monitored for a decrease in the efficacy of tetracycline. The dose of tetracycline may need to be increased. Alternatively, the use of the oral solution of tetracycline, which was shown not to interact,[2] may be considered.

References

1. Fisher, P., and others: Effect of cimetidine on the absorption of orally administered tetracycline, Br. J. Clin. Pharmacol. **9:**153, 1980.
2. Cole, J.J., and others: Interaction of cimetidine with tetracycline absorption, Lancet **2:**536, 1980.
3. Garty, M., and Hurwitz, A.: Effect of cimetidine and antacids on gastrointestinal absorption of tetracycline, Clin. Pharmacol. Ther. **28:**203, 1980.

Tetracycline–Ferrous Sulfate

1

Summary: The concurrent oral administration of ferrous sulfate (40 to 120 mg Fe^{+2}) and tetracycline causes an interference with the absorption of tetracycline from the gastrointestinal tract and vice versa, leading to significantly decreased serum levels of the antibiotic[1-3] and ferrous ion.[4,5] Studies have shown that tetracycline absorption is decreased 50% to 90%[1-3,5] while ferrous ion absorption is decreased 50%.[5] In one report however, tetracycline did not affect ferrous absorption.[6]

Related Drugs: The absorption of other tetracycline analogs, doxycycline,[1,7] methacycline,[1] and oxytetracycline[1] is decreased with concurrent administration of ferrous salts. Theoretically, other tetracycline analogs (e.g., demeclocycline, chlortetracycline, minocycline [see Appendix]) can be expected to interact similarly.

Ferrous salts such as the gluconate and fumarate have been shown to interact with tetracycline.[3] Ferrous lactate might also be expected to interact in a similar manner.

Mechanism: Ferric and ferrous ions have been shown to form chelates with tetracyclines in vitro.[8] Chelation is also likely to be the in vivo mechanism for the significantly reduced bioavailability of tetracycline in the presence of ferrous sulfate. It has also been shown that concurrent administration of ferrous sulfate decreases the half-life of doxycycline in humans after intravenous[7] and oral[9] administration. It is suggested that this interaction is caused by the interruption of the enterohepatic recycling pathway for doxycycline disposition.

Recommendations: Ferrous sulfate should not be given simultaneously with tetracycline or tetracycline analogs. When it is necessary for patients to receive both agents orally, this interaction may be avoided by administering the ferrous sulfate not less than 3 hours before or 2 hours after tetracycline.[2]

References

1. Neuvonen, P.J., and others: Interference of iron with the absorption of tetracyclines in man, Br. Med. J. **4:**532, 1970.
2. Gothoni, G., and others: Iron-tetracycline interaction: effect of time interval beween the drugs, Acta Med. Scand. **191:**409, 1972.
3. Neuvonen, P.J., and Turakka, H. Inhibitory effect of various iron salts on the absorption of tetracycline in man, Eur. J. Clin. Pharmacol. **7:**357, 1974.
4. Heinrich, H.C., and Oppitz, K.H.: Tetracycline inhibits iron absorption in man, Naturwissenschaften **60:**524, 1973.
5. Neuvonen, P.J., and others: Inhibition of iron absorption by tetracycline, Br. J. Clin. Pharmacol. **2:**94,1975.
6. Greenberger, N.J.: Absorption of tetracyclines: interference by iron, Ann. Intern. Med. **74:**792, 1971.
7. Neuvonen, P.J., and Penttila, O.: Effect of oral ferrous sulfate on the half-life of doxycycline in man, Eur. J. Clin. Pharmacol. **7:**361, 1974.
8. Albert, A., and Rees, C.W.: Avidity of the tetracyclines for the cations of metals, Nature **177:**433, 1956.
9. Venho, V.M., and others: Modification of the pharmacokinetics of doxycycline in man by ferrous sulfate or charcoal, Eur. J. Clin. Pharmacol. **14:**277, 1978.

Tetracycline–Oral Contraceptive Agents

Summary: The concurrent use of tetracycline and oral contraceptive agents has led to contraceptive failure in a few women.[1-3] One report stated that tetracycline decreased urinary excretion and increased fecal excretion of ethinyl estradiol.[4]

Related Drugs: Four cases of contraceptive failure with concurrent oxytetracycline have been reported, but inadequate information was given for critical evaluation.[2,3] The other tetracycline derivatives, (e.g., chlortetracycline, doxycycline, minocycline [see Appendix]) may be expected to have a similar interaction with oral contraceptive agents because of pharmacologic similarity.

Mechanism: Estrogens and progestogens are extensively excreted in the bile, principally as glucuronide conjugates. Subsequently, they undergo enterohepatic circulation where bacterial hydrolysis occurs allowing for reabsorption of the oral contraceptive through the bowel wall and eventual urinary excretion. Treatment with the antibiotics destroys the gut flora and prevents steroid reabsorption, resulting in lower than normal concentrations of the contraceptive and excretion via the feces rather than the urine.[5]

Recommendations: The majority of women may take these agents concomitantly without risk, but there seems no way to predict who will be affected.

Some prescribers may choose to warn patients that spotting and breakthrough bleeding are signs of diminished contraceptive effectiveness, and additional alternative forms of contraception should be used. Others may choose to recommend an alternative contraceptive method during concurrent use.

References

1. Bacon, J.F., and Shenfield, G.M.: Pregnancy attributable to interation between tetracycline and oral contraceptives, Br. Med. J. **280:**293, 1980.
2. Back, D.J., and others: Interindividual variation and drug interactions with hormonal steroid contraceptives, Drugs **21:**46, 1981.
3. Stockley, I.H.: Tetracycline and oral contraceptives, J. Am. Acad. Dermatol. **7:**279, 1982.
4. Swenson, L., and others: Effect of antibiotics on fecal/urinary excretion of ethinyl estradiol, an oral contraceptive, Gastroenterology **78:**1332, 1980.
5. Hudson, C.P., and Callen, J.P.: The tetracycline–oral contraceptive controversy, J. Am. Acad. Dermatol. **7:**269, 1982.

Tetracycline–Sodium Bicarbonate

4

Summary: Two reports indicate that sodium bicarbonate given with tetracycline does not significantly affect tetracycline disposition.[1,2] These are in contrast to an earlier report, which showed that tetracycline absorption was reduced approximately 50%.[3]

Related Drugs: There appear to be no reports of the effect of sodium bicarbonate on any other tetracycline analog (e.g., doxycycline, minocycline, oxytetracycline [see Appendix]).

Mechanism: The mechanism is not clearly established. It has been suggested that tetracycline dissolves slower at higher intragastric pH.[3] When tetracycline was fully dissolved before ingestion, sodium bicarbonate had no effect on its disposition. Also, the increased intragastric pH may influence the absorption of tetracycline by some mechanism not yet investigated.

Recommendations: The incidence of the tetracycline–sodium bicarbonate interaction is not known, and there is conflicting evidence regarding the occurrence of adverse effects. A cautious regimen would be to administer the drugs as far apart as possible. There is no documentation whether this interaction will occur when tetracycline is administered in a liquid dosage form.

References

1. Garty, M., and Hurwitz, A.: Effect of cimetidine and antacids on gastrointestinal absorption of tetracycline, Clin. Pharmacol. Ther. **28:**203, 1980.
2. Kramer, P.A., and others: Tetracycline absorption in elderly patients with acholorhydria, Clin. Pharmacol. Ther. **23:**467, 1978.
3. Barr, W.H., and others: Decrease of tetracycline absorption in man by sodium bicarbonate, Clin. Pharmacol. Ther. **12:**779, 1971.

Troleandomycin—Oral Contraceptive Agents

2

Summary: The use of troleandomycin in 27 women taking oral contraceptive agents has caused jaundice.[1,2] Intense pruritus occurred within 2 to 15 days after troleandomycin was added, and jaundice followed the pruritus 2 to 5 days later. Withdrawal of medications produced recovery within 1 month for most patients but required more than 2 months in the others.

Related Drugs: Documentation is lacking describing a similar interaction with the other macrolide antibiotics (e.g., erythromycin and oleandomycin).

Mechanism: The explanation for jaundice associated with troleandomycin is not known. Needle liver biopsy in 8 patients showed that cholestasis was the only histologic lesion.

Recommendations: The large number of cases of cholestasis in women taking both troleandomycin and oral contraceptives strongly suggests a marked cholestatic effect of this association; therefore, women taking oral contraceptives should avoid taking troleandomycin.

References

1. Miguet, J.P., and others: Jaundice from troleandomycin and oral contraceptives, Ann. Intern. Med. **92**:434, 1980.
2. Rollux, R., and others: Jaundice by interaction of troleandomycin and contraceptive pills, Nouv. Presse. Med. **8**:1694, 1979.

Summary: Two patients who received allopurinol and vidarabine (adenine arabinoside) concurrently developed severe neurotoxicity consisting of coarse, rhythmic tremors of extremities and facial muscles and impaired mentation, on the fourth day of vidarabine treatment.[1] Seventeen additional patients who had received these 2 agents concomitantly for at least 4 days were studied retrospectively. Five of the 17 had reported adverse reactions, including anemia, nausea, pain, itching, and tremors.[1]

Related Drugs: There are no drugs related to allopurinol or vidarabine.

Mechanism: Mammalian cells convert adenine arabinoside (vidarabine) to hypoxanthine arabinoside, the major metabolic product. Some hypoxanthine arabinoside is then metabolized by xanthine oxidase to form xanthine arabinoside.[2] Inhibition of xanthine oxidase by allopurinol could therefore increase the drug levels of hypoxanthine arabinoside considerably.[1] These increased levels can be expected to produce adverse effects since vidarabine toxicity is dose dependent.[3,4]

Recommendations: Until further information concerning this interaction is available, caution is warranted when these 2 drugs are used simultaneously.

References

1. Friedman, H.M., and Grasela, T.: Adenine arabinoside and allopurinol—possible adverse drug interaction, N. Engl. J. Med. **304:**423, 1981.
2. Connor, J.D., and others: Susceptibility in vitro of several large DNA viruses to the antiviral activity of adenine arabinoside and its metabolite, hypoxanthine arabinoside: relation to human pharmacology. In Pavan-Langston, D., Buchanan, R.A., Alford, C.A., editors: Adenine arabinoside: an antiviral agent. New York, 1975, Raven Press, pp. 177-96.
3. Ross, A.H., and others: Toxicity of adenine arabinoside in humans, J. Infect. Dis. **133:**A192, 1976.
4. Lauter, C.B., and others: Microbiologic assays and neurological toxicity during use of adenine arabinoside in humans, J. Infect. Dis. **134:**75, 1976.

CHAPTER NINE

Antineoplastic Drug Interactions

TABLE 9. Antineoplastic Drug Interactions

Drug Interaction	Significance Code	Potential Effects	Recommendations	See Page
Carmustine–Cimetidine	2	Concomitant use may have an additive bone marrow depressant effect.	If bone marrow depression develops, discontinue the cimetidine.	410
Cyclophosphamide–Allopurinol	2	Allopurinol may increase the toxicity and enhance bone marrow depression of cyclophosphamide, although there are conflicting reports.	Monitor for signs of bone marrow depression (leukopenia, thrombocytopenia, and pancytopenia).	411
Cyclophosphamide, Fluorouracil, Methotrexate–Hydrochlorothiazide	3	Concurrent use resulted in granulocytopenia in 1 study. More studies are needed to determine the responsible agent.	Monitor neutrophil counts closely and lower the dose or withdraw the hydrochlorothiazide if neutropenia develops.	412
Lomustine–Theophylline	3	Concurrent use resulted in epistaxis and thrombocytopenia in 1 patient.	There is insufficient evidence to indicate that these agents should not be used together.	413
Mercaptopurine–Allopurinol	1	Allopurinol significantly increases the pharmacologic and toxic effects of mercaptopurine.	Reduce the initial mercaptopurine to ⅓ or ¼ the usual recommended dose with subsequent adjustments according to clinical response and/or toxicity.	414
Methotrexate–Alcohol, Ethyl	3	Alcohol may increase the hepatotoxicity of methotrexate.	Advise patients to avoid alcohol consumption while taking methotrexate.	415
Methotrexate–Aspirin	1	Aspirin may elevate and prolong methotrexate serum levels, increasing the potential for toxicity.	Avoid concurrent use. Acetaminophen should be substituted for aspirin if possible.	416
Methotrexate–Cytarabine	3	Cytarabine given before methotrexate enhances the cell-kill effects of methotrexate, and methotrexate given first enhances the cell-kill action of cytarabine.	Routine monitoring of chemotherapy is indicated since the effects of this co-therapy are unpredictable.	417
Methotrexate–Leucovorin	1	Methotrexate toxicity can be greatly reduced by consecutive administration of leucovorin.	This beneficial interaction can be achieved only if leucovorin is given 6 hours before or after methotrexate and continued for 48-72 hours or until methotrexate clearance is complete.	419
Methotrexate–Neomycin	2	Neomycin may reduce the absorption, area-under-curve, and cumulative 72 hour urinary excretion of methotrexate.	An increased methotrexate dosage may be necessary.	421

TABLE 9. Antineoplastic Drug Interactions—cont'd

Drug Interaction	Significance Code	Potential Effects	Recommendations	See Page
Methotrexate– Probenecid	1	Probenecid significantly increases methotrexate serum levels as much as 3- to 4-fold.	Concurrent use need not be avoided, although methotrexate dosage may need to be decreased.	422
Methotrexate– Sodium Bicarbonate	3	Sodium bicarbonate may increase the renal elimination of methotrexate, although the clinical significance of this is undetermined.	Although the combination may be used in high dose methotrexate therapy, it is important to monitor for decreased levels.	423
Methotrexate– Sulfisoxazole	3	Sulfisoxazole decreases the plasma protein binding and renal clearance of methotrexate. Although no cases have been reported, toxicity from increased serum levels of unbound methotrexate may occur.	Caution should be exercised during concurrent use.	424

Carmustine–Cimetidine

2

Summary: Clinical evidence suggests that concomitant cimetidine and carmustine have an additive bone marrow depressant effect.[1-3] Although patients were receiving other medications and/or irradiation, the additive effect was clearly demonstrated when compared to control patients.

Related Drugs: There are no published reports of an additive effect between the other antineoplastic nitrosoureas (streptozocin and lomustine) and cimetidine. Because of a lack of available information, it is unknown whether ranitidine would interact similarly when used concomitantly with carmustine. However, if the mechanism involves inhibition of hepatic metabolism by cimetidine, then ranitidine would not be expected to interact similarly.

Mechanism: The mechanism has not been established. Both drugs have bone marrow suppressant properties, which would appear to be additive during co-therapy. However, 2 authors suggest that cimetidine inhibits the metabolism of carmustine.[4,5]

Recommendations: Patients receiving these agents concurrently should be monitored for the appearance of bone marrow suppression. If suppression is detected, cimetidine should be discontinued.

References

1. Selker, R.G., and others: Bone-marrow depression with cimetidine plus carmustine, N. Engl. J. Med. **299:**834, 1978.
2. Volkin, R.L., and others: Potentiation of carmustine-cranial irradiation-induced myelosuppression by cimetidine, Arch. Intern. Med. **142:**243, 1982.
3. Klotz, S.A., and Kay, B.F.: Cimetidine and agranulocytosis, Ann. Intern. Med. **88:**579, 1978.
4. Feagin, O.T.: Alternative mechanisms for severe neutropenia, Arch. Intern. Med. **142:**1971, 1982.
5. Dorr, R.T.: Interaction of CMT-augmentation of cyclophosphamide in mice, Arch. Intern. Med. **142:**1971, 1982.

Cyclophosphamide–Allopurinol

2

Summary: The concurrent administration of cyclophosphamide and allopurinol may enhance the bone marrow depression induced by cyclophosphamide.[1] However, in another study in which allopurinol was used with chemotherapeutic agents including cyclophosphamide, a higher increase in toxicity was not observed.[2]

Related Drugs: No specific interactions have been reported with other alkylating agents (e.g., carmustine, chlorambucil, lomustine [see Appendix]). There are no drugs related to allopurinol.

Mechanism: The mechanism is unknown; however, allopurinol does affect liver microsomal enzyme systems and cyclophosphamide undergoes hepatic microsomal oxidation to form metabolites. Decreased cyclophosphamide clearance with longer plasma half-life has been observed in 1 study,[3] whereas increased metabolite formation or decreased renal clearance of metabolites has been postulated by others.[4]

Recommendations: The routine prophylactic use of allopurinol to prevent hyperuricemia may not be advisable during chemotherapy with alkylating agents. Patients who receive these drugs concurrently should be monitored for signs of bone marrow depression (leukopenia, thrombocytopenia, and pancytopenia).

References

1. Boston Collaborative Drug Surveillance Program: Allopurinol and cytotoxic drugs: interaction in relation to bone marrow depression, J.A.M.A. **227:**1036, 1974.
2. Stolbach, L., and others: Evaluation of bone marrow toxic reactions of patients treated with allopurinol, J.A.M.A. **247:**334, 1982.
3. Bagley, C.M., and others: Clinical pharmacology of cyclophosphamide, Cancer Res. **33:**226, 1973.
4. Witten, J., and others: The pharmacokinetics of cyclophosphamide in man after treatment with allopurinol, Acta Pharmacol. Toxicol. **46:**392, 1980.

Cyclophosphamide		3
Fluorouracil	Hydrochlorothiazide	
Methotrexate		

Summary: The concurrent use of hydrochlorothiazide and a cancer chemotherapy combination including cyclophosphamide, fluorouracil, and methotrexate resulted in granulocytopenia in 1 study. The most consistent change in the neutrophil count was observed during the period of maximal myelosuppresion from the chemotherapy.[1] The antineoplastic agent(s) responsible for this interaction could not be evaluated within the study design.

Related Drugs: The same interaction was shown to occur with chlorothiazide and trichlormethiazide as well.[1] Because they are pharmacologically related, a similar interaction may be expected to occur with all the thiazide diuretics (e.g., flumethiazide, methyclothiazide, polythiazide [see Appendix]) and thiazide related diuretics (e.g., chlorthalidone, indapamide, metolazone [see Appendix]) although documentation is lacking.

Mechanism: The mechanism is unknown. More detailed pharmacologic studies are needed to identify the agent responsible for this hematologic phenomenon and to detail the mechanism of action. It is uncertain whether it is dose or time related.[1]

Recommendations: Patient's neutrophil counts should be monitored closely during concurrent use of these agents. If neutropenia develops, the dose of the thiazide diuretic may need to be lowered or the drug discontinued.

Reference

1. Orr, L.E.: Potentiation of myelosuppression from cancer chemotherapy and thiazide diuretics, Drug Intell. Clin. Pharm. **15:**967, 1981.

Lomustine–Theophylline

3

Summary: A case was reported where a patient receiving theophylline and undergoing treatment with lomustine for medulloblastoma developed epistaxis and thrombocytopenia 3 weeks after the third cycle of chemotherapy.[1] It is also possible that this effect results solely from the antineoplastic agent alone.

Related Drugs: There have been no reports of similar interactions with theophylline and other alkylating agents (e.g., busulfan, chlorambucil, melphalan [see Appendix]). A synergistic effect was reported with theophylline and carmustine in mice.[2] Although this effect has not been documented, other theophylline derivatives (aminophylline and oxtriphylline) may be expected to interact similarly because of pharmacologic similarity. Dyphylline, a theophylline derivative which is not converted to theophylline in vivo[3,4] but shares similar pharmacologic action, may also be expected to interact with lomustine.

Mechanism: The mechanism is unknown, but it has been suggested that theophylline inhibits the phosphodiesterase activity in blood platelets, thus increasing the cyclic AMP levels, which disrupts normal platelet function.[1] However, the theory of phosphodiesterase inhibition is based upon in vitro studies that used concentrations that would be toxic in vivo.[5]

Recommendations: Available evidence is insufficient to indicate that theophylline cannot be used concurrently with lomustine, although one should be aware that thrombocytopenia and myelotoxicity are possible during combined therapy with these agents.

References

1. Zeltzer, P.M., and Ferg, S.A.: Theophylline induced lomustine toxicity, Lancet **2:**960, 1979.
2. DeWys, W.D., and Bathina, S.: Synergistic antitumor effect of cyclic AMP elevation (induced by theophylline) and cytotoxic drug treatment, Proc. Am. Assoc. Cancer Res. **19:**104, 1978.
3. Gisclon, L.G., et al.: Pharmacokinetics of orally administered dyphylline, Am. J. Hosp. Pharm. **36:**1179, 1979.
4. Simons, K.J. and Simons, F.E.K.: Urinary excretion of dyphylline in humans, J. Pharm. Sci. **68:**1327, 1979.
5. Hendeles, L., and Weinberger, M.: Theophylline, a "state of the art" review, Pharmacotherapy **3:**5, 1983.

Mercaptopurine–Allopurinol

1

Summary: The concurrent administration of mercaptopurine and allopurinol has resulted in a clinically significant increase in the pharmacologic and toxic effects of mercaptopurine.[1-4] One study showed a 500% increase in the peak plasma concentration of oral mercaptopurine after allopurinol pretreatment. However, the kinetics of intravenous mercaptopurine were not affected by pretreatment with allopurinol.[4]

Related Drugs: Azathioprine, which is metabolized to 6-mercaptopurine, has been shown in 1 study to interact with allopurinol in the same manner as mercaptopurine.[5] Thioguanine is also related to mercaptopurine but is metabolized differently and should not interact with allopurinol.[6] There are no drugs related to allopurinol.

Mechanism: Mercaptopurine is metabolized to the inactive metabolite 6-thiouric acid by enzymatic oxidation, which is catalyzed by the enzyme xanthine oxidase.[5,7] Xanthine oxidase is primarily located in the liver and intestinal mucosa.[4] Allopurinol inhibits the action of xanthine oxidase, thereby reducing the rate at which oral mercaptopurine is inactivated, resulting in higher blood levels of mercaptopurine.[8] One study showed that allopurinol inhibits the first-pass metabolism of oral mercaptopurine but has no effect on the intravenous form, which is rapidly distributed to body tissues, and only a fraction of the dose reaches the liver and intestine.[4]

Recommendations: The initial dose of oral mercaptopurine should be reduced to one-third or one-fourth of the presently recommended dosage level when allopurinol (200 to 300 mg orally) is administered concurrently.[1] Subsequent adjustments of mercaptopurine dosages should be made on the basis of clinical response and/or toxicity. Alternatively, the intravenous form of mercaptopurine may be considered since it is not affected by allopurinol. In this case, a dose reduction is not necessary.[4]

References

1. Rundles, R.W., and others: Effects of a xanthine oxidase inhibitor on thiopurine metabolism, hyperuricemia and gout, Trans. Assoc. Am. Physicians **76:**126, 1963.
2. Vogler, W.R., and others: Metabolic and therapeutic effects of allopurinol in patients with leukemia and gout, Am. J. Med. **40:**548, 1966.
3. Hitchings, G.H.: Summary of informal discussion on the role of purine antagonists, Cancer Res. **23:**1218, 1963.
4. Zimm, S., and others: Inhibition of first-pass metabolism in cancer chemotherapy: interaction of 6-mercaptopurine and allopurinol, Clin. Pharmacol. Ther. **34:**810, 1983.
5. Elion, G.B., and others: The fate of 6-mercaptopurine in mice, Ann. N.Y. Acad. Sci. **60:**297, 1954.
6. Calabresi, P., and Parks, R.E.: Chemotherapy of neoplastic diseases. In Gilman, A.G., Goodman, L.S., and Gilman, A., editors: The pharmacological basis of therapeutics. New York, 1980, MacMillan Publishing.
7. Hamilton, L., and Elion, G.B.: The fate of 6-mercaptopurine in man, Ann. N.Y. Acad. Sci. **60:**304, 1954.
8. Elion, G.B., and others: Relationship between metabolic fates and antitumor activities of thiopurines, Cancer Res. **23:**1207, 1963.

Methotrexate–Alcohol, Ethyl

3

Summary: The possibility that concurrent methotrexate therapy and ethyl alcohol consumption leads to greater incidence of hepatotoxicity has been suggested by 2 reports.[1,2] The evidence implicating a significant contribution of ethyl alcohol to cirrhosis and hepatic fibrosis during long-term methotrexate therapy is neither clear nor extensive. Hepatotoxicity may be more directly attributed to the actions of methotrexate itself.[3,4]

Related Drugs: Benzyl alcohol used as a preservative in some methotrexate preparations has been implicated as a contributor to neurologic side effects when methotrexate is administered intrathecally. Suggested causes of the complication include direct hypersensitivity reactions related to methotrexate or benzyl alcohol.[5] Benzyl alcohol may also be found as a preservative in other antineoplastic preparations. Preservative free parenteral preparations should be used for this particular route of administration.

Mechanism: A specific mechanism for a methotrexate and ethyl alcohol interaction is not known. In a study of methotrexate transport across intestinal segments in vitro, it was observed that high concentrations of ethyl alcohol weakly inhibited transport.[6] It is possible that transport from hepatocytes is also inhibited by ethyl alcohol, leading to higher intrahepatic concentrations of methotrexate.

Recommendations: Because of the possibility that ethyl alcohol may increase the hepatotoxic potential of methotrexate, patients receiving this drug should be advised to minimize consumption of products containing ethyl alcohol.

References

1. Almeyda, J., and others: Drug reactions XV. Methotrexate, psoriasis and the liver, Br. J. Dermatol. **85:**302, 1971.
2. Pai, S.H., and others: Severe liver damage caused by treatment of psoriasis with methotrexate, N.Y. State J. Med. **73:**2582, 1973.
3. Dahl, M.G.C., and others: Methotrexate hepatotoxicity in psoriasis—comparison of different dose regimens, Br. Med. J. **1:**654, 1972.
4. Tobias, H., and Auerbach, R.: Hepatotoxicity of long-term methotrexate therapy for psoriasis, Arch. Intern. Med. **132:**391, 1973.
5. Baum, E.S., and Holton, C.P.: Intrathecal methotrexate, Lancet **1:**308, 1972.
6. Strum, W.B.L.: Characteristics of the transport of peptoylglutamate and amethopterin in rat jejunum, J. Pharmacol. Exp. Ther. **216:**329, 1981.

Methotrexate–Aspirin

1

Summary: The concurrent administration of methotrexate and aspirin (300 to 640 mg) may result in elevated or prolonged serum concentrations of free methotrexate, which may increase the potential for methotrexate toxicity.[1-5]

Related Drugs: All salicylates (e.g., choline salicylate, sodium salicylate, salicylamide [see Appendix]) and their combination products may be expected to interact with methotrexate based on pharmacologic similarity, although no documentation exists. There are no drugs related to methotrexate.

Mechanism: Two mechanisms acting simultaneously may be responsible for this interaction. Aspirin is highly plasma protein bound and is capable of displacing methotrexate from plasma proteins in vitro.[1-3] Methotrexate and aspirin have a common elimination pathway where aspirin competes with and inhibits methotrexate elimination, leading to an increase in serum methotrexate concentrations and half-life.[2,5]

Recommendations: Administration of aspirin should be avoided in patients receiving methotrexate when an acceptable alternative drug is available. Acetaminophen has been used concurrently with methotrexate without causing an increase in methotrexate toxicity.[6] If concurrent administration is necessary, the patient should be observed closely for methotrexate toxicity.[2,7]

References

1. Calabresi, P., and Parks, R.E.: Antiproliferative agents and drugs used for immuno suppression. In Gilman, A.G., Goodman, L.S., and Gilman, A., editors: The pharmacological basis of therapeutics. New York, 1980, MacMillan Publishing.
2. Liegler, D.G., and others: The effect of organic acids on renal clearance of methotrexate in man, Clin. Pharmacol. Ther. **10:**849, 1969.
3. Dixon, R.L., and others: Plasma protein binding of methotrexate and its displacement by various drugs, Fed. Proc. **24:**454, 1965.
4. Mandel, M.A.: Synergistic effect of salicylates on methotrexate toxicity, Plast. Reconstr. Surg. **57:**733, 1976.
5. Baker, H.: Intermittent high dose oral methotrexate therapy in psoriasis, Br. J. Dermatol. **82:**65, 1970.
6. Dahl, M.G.C., and others: Methotrexate hepatotoxicity in psoriasis—comparison of different dosage regimens, Br. Med. J. **1:**654, 1972.
7. Douglas, I.C.D., and Price, L.A.: Bone marrow toxicity of methotrexate: a reassessment, Br. J. Haematol. **24:**625, 1973.

Methotrexate–Cytarabine

Summary: Administration of cytarabine 48 hours before initiation of methotrexate therapy enhances the cell-kill effects of methotrexate.[1,2] Conversely, the cell-kill effects of cytarabine can be enhanced when methotrexate is administered at least 10 minutes before the initiation of cytarabine therapy.[3,4] The combination has also been reported to be antagonistic in vitro and in animals, but not in humans.[5-7]

Unfortunately, data to support the theories of synergistic or antagonistic effects of concomitant therapy with these drugs are still inconclusive.

Related Drugs: Methotrexate and cytarabine are antineoplastic antimetabolites. However, it is not known whether a similar interaction would occur with the other antineoplastic antimetabolites (e.g., fluorouracil, mercaptopurine, thioguanine [see Appendix]).

Mechanism: Many factors are involved in the mechanism of the interaction of these 2 chemotherapeutic agents. These include the order of administration of the agents, the time interval between administration of the 2 drugs, as well as the complexities of the enzyme-substrate system within a given patient. Thus the exact outcome of the interaction can be variable from patient to patient.

This interaction is theorized to occur via the ability of methotrexate to increase the conversion of deoxyuridylate (dUMP) to deoxythymidylate (dTMP) with a resultant buildup in deoxycytidine triphosphate (dCTP). Cytarabine's effectiveness has been theorized to be decreased by this buildup of dCTP.

Alternatively, increased cell kill has been noted when methotrexate pretreated cells were exposed to cytarabine. This effect is attributed to methotrexate increasing the phosphorylation of cytarabine and thus increasing the levels of cytarabine nucleosides. These increased levels of cytarabine nucleosides may then act to increase the incorporation of cytarabine into the DNA fraction with resultant higher cell kill.

Recommendations: The clinical data to support these observations of mutual enhanced effect of methotrexate and cytarabine are inconclusive. Patient populations tested were often heterogeneous, other antineoplastic agents were used concurrently, doses and administration times of the 2 drugs varied, and statistical analyses of the results of various studies were not carried out.

If a synergistic effect of these drugs is desired, such as in treatment of certain forms of leukemia, cytarabine should be administered either 48 hours before or at least 10 minutes after initiation of therapy with methotrexate.

Because synergism does not occur in all patients[2] and antagonism[5,6] is also possible, routine monitoring of chemotherapy (e.g., determining the percentage of immature and abnormal cell forms present in the bone marrow) would be the best method to determine the unpredictable course of concurrent use of these drugs.

References

1. Lampkin, B.C., and others: Synchronization and recruitment in acute leukemia, J. Clin. Invest. **50:**2204, 1971.

2. Cooper, L.E., and others: The effect of drug-induced alteration in the growth fraction of the clinical response in adult acute leukemia, Clin. Res. **19**:38, 1971.
3. Levitt, M., and others: Combination sequential chemotherapy in advanced reticulum cell sarcoma, Cancer **29**:630, 1972.
4. Skeel, R.T., and others: Development of a combination chemotherapy program for adult acute leukemia, CAM and CAM-L, Cancer **32**:76, 1973.
5. Tattersall, M.H.N., and Harrop, K.R.: Combination chemotherapy: the antagonism of methotrexate and cytarabine, Eur. J. Cancer **9**:229, 1973.
6. Tattersall, M.H.N., and others: Interaction of methotrexate and cytarabine, Lancet **2**:1378, 1972.
7. Grindey, G.B., and Nichol, C.A.: Interaction of drugs inhibiting different steps on the synthesis of DNA, Cancer Res. **32**:527, 1972.

Methotrexate–Leucovorin

Summary: In vitro,[1] animal,[2-4] and human studies[5-15] indicate that methotrexate toxicity can be greatly reduced by consecutive administration of leucovorin within 6 hours.[16] Several studies suggest that "leucovorin rescue" could be accomplished while most of the therapeutic effectiveness of methotrexate against tumors was apparently maintained.[2,3]

Related Drugs: There are no drugs related to methotrexate or leucovorin.

Mechanism: Methotrexate is a folic acid antagonist that combines with dihydrofolate reductase, thereby blocking folate metabolism. The synthesis of thymidylic acid from deoxyuridylic acid, which requires tetrahydrofolate ordinarily supplied by the metabolism of folic acid, is thus blocked, causing an inhibition of nucleic acid synthesis necessary for cell replication.

Leucovorin is an active metabolite of folic acid. Leucovorin supplies tetrahydrofolate, which bypasses the dihydrofolate reductase enzymatic step and negates the effect of methotrexate. This action allows nucleic acid synthesis and other biochemical processes to resume.[17]

Recommendations: The evidence shows that leucovorin reverses methotrexate-induced inhibition of folic acid antagonism. Beneficial results in some diseases are obtained by intramuscular or intravenous methotrexate administration followed by intramuscular leucovorin. The optimal interval between the administration of the 2 drugs is 6 hours or less. Effective leucovorin doses have ranged from 4 to 12 mg. Methotrexate dosage can be greater than usual (up to 600 mg/kg) when consecutive leucovorin administration is used.[16]

References

1. Groff, J.P., and Blakely, R.L.: Rescue of human lymphoid cells from the effects of methotrexate in vitro, Cancer Res. **38:**3847, 1978.
2. Sandberg, J.S., and Goldin, A.: The use of leucovorin orally in normal and leukemic L1210 mice to prevent the toxicity and gastrointestinal lesions caused by high doses of methotrexate, Cancer Res. **30:**1276, 1970.
3. Goldin, A., and others: Eradication of leukemic cells (L1210) by methotrexate and methotrexate plus citrovorum factor, Nature **212:**1548, 1966.
4. Canellos, G.P., and others: The effect of treatment with cytotoxic agents on mouse spleen dihydrofolate reductase activity, Cancer Res. **27:**784, 1967.
5. Ambinder, E.P., and others: High dose methotrexate followed by citrovorum factor reversal in patients with advanced cancer, Cancer **43:**1177, 1979.
6. Isacoff, W.H., and others: Pharmacokinetics of high-dose methotrexate and citrovorum factor rescue, Cancer Treat. Rep. **61:**1665, 1977.
7. Capizzi, R.L., and others: Methotrexate therapy of head and neck cancer: improvement in therapeutic index by the use of leucovorin rescue, Cancer Res. **30:**1782, 1970.
8. Djerassi, I., and others: Long-term remissions in childhood acute leukemia: use of infrequent infusions of methotrexate; supportive roles of platelet transfusions and citrovorum factor, Clin. Pediatr. **5:**502, 1966.
9. Hryniuk, W.M., and Bertino, J.R.: Treatment of leukemia with large doses of methotrexate and folinic acid: clinical-biochemical correlates, J. Clin. Invest. **48:**2140, 1969.

10. Jaffe, N.: Progress report on high-dose methotrexate (NSC-740) with citrovorum rescue in the treatment of metastatic bone tumors, Cancer Chemother. Rep. **58**:275, 1974.

11. Drakoff, I.: Combination chemotherapy, Hosp. Form. **16**:298, 1981.

12. Hande, K.R.: Randomized study of high-dose versus low-dose methotrexate in the treatment of extensive small cell lung cancer, Am. J. Med. **73**:413, 1982.

13. Roenigk, H.H.,Jr., and others: Methotrexate for psoriasis in weekly oral doses, Arch. Dermatol. **99**:86, 1969.

14. Cipriano, A.P., and others: Failure of leucovorin rescue in methotrexate treatment of psoriasis, Arch. Dermatol. **101**:651, 1970.

15. Peck, S.M., and others: Studies in bullous diseases: treatment of pemphigus vulgaris with immunosuppressives (steroids and methotrexate) and leucovorin calcium, Arch. Dermatol. **103**:141, 1971.

16. Penta,J.S.: Overview of protocols on clinical studies of high-dose methotrexate (NSC-740) with citrovorum factor (NSC-3590) rescue, Cancer Chemother. Rep. (part 3) **6**:7, 1975.

17. Mitchell, M.S., and others: Effectiveness of high-dose infusions of methotrexate followed by leucovorin in carcinoma of the head and neck, Cancer Res. **28**:1088, 1968.

Methotrexate–Neomycin

2

Summary: In 1 study, the concurrent use of oral neomycin and methotrexate resulted in a reduced methotrexate absorption. The methotrexate area-under-curve was reduced by 50% as well as the cumulative 72 hour urinary excretion of methotrexate.[1]

Related Drugs: Paromomycin (in combination with vancomycin, polymyxin B and nystatin) also reduced the absorption of methotrexate from 44% to 69% in cancer patients.[2] The other oral aminoglycoside, kanamycin, has been reported to increase methotrexate plasma levels.[1] Based on the proposed mechanism, the parenteral aminoglycosides (e.g., amikacin, gentamicin, tobramycin [see Appendix]) would not be expected to interact similarly with methotrexate, although documentation is lacking. There are no drugs related to methotrexate.

Mechanism: Neomycin is known to produce malabsorption of many drugs, and this may be the mechanism here as well. Paromomycin has also been reported to produce malabsorption syndromes.[3] Kanamycin, however, may be less potent in causing malabsorption. Kanamycin also reduces intestinal bacteria (as do the others) that degrade methotrexate to inactive metabolites in the gut,[1,4] and this may increase the amount of unmetabolized methotrexate available for absorption. Further study is needed to clarify the exact mechanism for this interaction.

Recommendations: Patients should be monitored during concurrent use of these agents. An increased dose of methotrexate may be necessary, or in the case of kanamycin, the dose of methotrexate may need to be reduced.

References

1. Shen, D.D., and Azarnoff, D.: Clinical pharmacokinetics of methotrexate, Clin. Pharmaco. **3:**1, 1978.
2. Cohen, M.H., and others: Effect of oral prophylactic broad spectrum nonabsorption antibiotics on the gastrointestinal absorption of nutrients and methotrexate in small cell bronchogenic carcinoma patients, Cancer **38:**1556, 1976.
3. Keusch, G.T., and others: Malabsorption due to paromomycin, Arch. Intern. Med. **125:**273, 1970.
4. Bleyer, W.A.: The clinical pharmacology of methotrexate, Cancer **41:**36, 1978.

Methotrexate–Probenecid

1

Summary: The concurrent use of methotrexate and probenecid leads to a marked increase in methotrexate serum levels. These levels have been shown to be 3 to 4 times higher in patients 24 hours after methotrexate administration than in those who had not received probenecid.[1-4] The cerebrospinal fluid (CSF) levels of methotrexate were elevated as well, although the CSF half-life was not prolonged.[3]

Related Drugs: There are no drugs related to methotrexate. Documentation is lacking regarding a similar interaction between methotrexate and sulfinpyrazone. However, if the mechanism involves inhibition of renal tubular transport, then a similar interaction may be expected to occur.

Mechanism: Animal studies have shown that probenecid inhibits the excretion of methotrexate by the renal and biliary routes.[5-7] Inhibition of renal tubular transport appears to be the primary mechanism involved in humans since the role of biliary excretion is unclear.

Recommendations: Although the concurrent use of these agents need not be avoided, it is important to monitor methotrexate plasma levels and lower its dose when necessary.

References

1. Aherne, G.W., and others: Prolongation and enhancement of serum methotrexate concentrations by probenecid, Br. Med. J. **1:**1097, 1978.
2. Israili, Z.H., and others: The interaction of methotrexate and probenecid in man and dog, Am. Assoc. Cancer Res. **19:**194, 1978.
3. Howell, S.B., and others: Effect of probenecid on cerebrospinal fluid methotrexate kinetics, Clin. Pharmacol. Ther. **26:**641, 1979.
4. Aherne, G.W., and others: The interaction between methotrexate and probenecid in man, Br. J. Pharmacol. **6:**369, 1978.
5. Bourke, R.S., and others: Inhibition of renal tubular transport of methotrexate by probenecid, Cancer Res. **35:**110, 1975.
6. Kates, R.E., and others: Increased methotrexate toxicity due to concurrent probenecid administration, Biochem. Pharmacol. **25:**1485, 1976.
7. Kates, R.E., and Tozer, T.N.: Biliary secretion of methotrexate in rats and its inhibition by probenecid, J. Pharm. Sci. **65:**1348, 1976.

Methotrexate–Sodium Bicarbonate

3

Summary: In a study involving 11 patients, sodium bicarbonate increased the renal elimination of methotrexate.[1] The clinical significance of this interaction remains to be determined.

Related Drugs: There are no drugs related to methotrexate. If the mechanism deals with urinary alkalinization, then other agents capable of alkalinizing the urine (e.g., calcium carbonate, magnesium hydroxide, potassium bicarbonate) may be expected to interact similarly, although specific documentation is lacking.

Mechanism: Hydration and urinary alkalinization are used after high dose methotrexate therapy to prevent urinary precipitation of methotrexate.[2] However, a urinary pH greater than 8.0 may result in a significant increase in the urinary elimination rate of methotrexate,[3] and sodium bicarbonate can cause a significant alkalinization of the urine with a pH greater than 7.0.[1] This may result in an increased methotrexate elimination because of an increased ionization of the weak acid in the renal tubule, which can reduce its reabsorption back into the blood and result in enhanced urinary excretion.

Recommendations: Although urinary alkalinization with an agent such as sodium bicarbonate is used in high-dose methotrexate therapy, it is important to monitor the patient for decreased methotrexate levels.

References

1. Sand, T.E., and Jacobsen, S.: Effect of urine pH and flow on renal clearance of methotrexate, Eur. J. Clin. Pharmacol. **19:**453, 1981.
2. Stoller, R.G., and others: Pharmacokinetics of high dose methotrexate, Cancer Chemother. Rep. **6:**19, 1975.
3. Nerinberg, A., and others: High dose methotrexate with citrovorum factor rescue: predictive value of serum methotrexate concentrations and corrective measures to avert toxicity, Cancer Treat. Rep. **61:**779, 1977.

Methotrexate–Sulfisoxazole

Summary: Methotrexate plasma protein binding and renal clearance are decreased by the concurrent administration of sulfisoxazole.[1] Displacement from binding sites can be clinically important since methotrexate therapeutic levels are very close to the toxic levels. These changes may result in methotrexate toxicity as a result of increased serum levels of unbound methotrexate, although none has been reported.

Related Drugs: Sulfamethoxypyridazine* was shown to increase methotrexate toxicity in mice.[2] Sulfamethoxazole also inhibits methotrexate elimination.[3] Other sulfonamides (e.g., sulfamethizole, sulfasalazine, sulfapyridine [see Appendix]) have not been investigated but would be expected to have an effect like that of sulfisoxazole because of pharmacologic similarity. There are no drugs related to methotrexate.

Mechanism: Methotrexate is approximately 50% bound to plasma proteins,[4] and sulfonamides can displace this binding in vitro.[5,6] The mechanism by which sulfisoxazole inhibits the renal clearance of methotrexate is not known.

Recommendations: Although there are no reports of toxicity directly attributable to this interaction, caution should be exercised when the combination of these 2 drugs is administered. The patient should be closely observed for hematologic abnormalities produced by methotrexate toxicity.

References

1. Leigler, D.G., and others: The effect of organic acid on renal clearance of methotrexate in man, Clin. Pharmacol. Ther. **10**:849, 1969.
2. Dixon, R.L.: The interaction between various drugs and methotrexate, Toxicol. Appl. Pharmacol. **12**:308, 1968.
3. Gleckman, R., and others: Trimethoprim-sulfamethoxazole, Am. J. Hosp. Pharm. **36**:893, 1979.
4. Calabresi, P., and Parks, R.E.: Antiproliferative agents and drugs used for immuno suppression. In Gilman, A.G., Goodman, L.S., and Gilman, A., editors: The pharmacological basis of therapeutics. New York, 1980, MacMillan Publishing.
5. Dixon, R.L., and others: Plasma protein binding of methotrexate and its displacement by various drugs, Fed. Proc. **24**:454, 1965.
6. Brodie, B.B.: Displacement of one drug by another from carrier or receptor sites, Proc. R. Soc. Med. **58**:946, 1965.

*Not available in the U.S.

CHAPTER TEN

Antipsychotic and Antianxiety Drug Interactions

TABLE 10. Antipsychotic and Antianxiety Drug Interactions

Drug Interaction	Significance Code	Potential Effects	Recommendations	See Page
Chlorproma-zine–Alcohol, Ethyl	2	Concurrent use may intensify the CNS depression of each drug. Alcohol reportedly precipitates extrapyramidal reactions in patients taking phenothiazines by inducing temporary brain dysfunction.	Warn patients receiving phenothiazines that alcohol may enhance CNS depression and should be used with caution.	430
Chlorproma-zine–Aluminum Hydroxide, Magnesium Hydroxide	3	Antacids may alter the absorption of chlorpromazine when taken simultaneously; however, the clinical effects have not been determined.	Antacids should be given 1 hour before or 2 hours after chlorpromazine.	431
Chlorproma-zine–Amphetamine	2	These agents are pharmacologic antagonists and exert opposed effects on monoaminergic function in the central and peripheral nervous systems.	Concurrent use should be restricted to treating amphetamine overdose.	432
Chlorproma-zine–Benztropine	2	Benztropine has been used to manage the antipsychotic-induced EPS. The anticholinergic activity of benztropine antagonizes the increased cholinergic activity, which is secondary to the dopamine receptor blockade by chlorpromazine.	Short-term benztropine therapy may effectively deal with drug-induced parkinsonism.	434
Chlorproma-zine–Diazoxide	2	Concurrent use of chlorproma-zive and oral diazoxide may lead to severe hyperglycemia and diabetic precoma.	Monitor blood glucose levels closely and decrease diazoxide dosage if needed.	436
Chlorproma-zine–Levodopa	3	These agents have the potential for antgonizing the effects of each other, but the interaction is unpredictable.	Observe patients closely for a decreased effect of either agent.	437
Chlorproma-zine–Lithium Carbonate	2	Lithium decreases plasma chlorpromazine levels. Neurotoxic and somnambulistic episodes have also been reported.	Dosage adjustments of one or both drugs may be necessary. It is preferable to use 1 agent alone.	438
Chlorproma-zine–Phenobarbital	3	Long-term phenobarbital therapy may decrease serum chlorpromazine levels. The significance of the interaction has not been determined.	If chlorpromazine effectiveness decreases, an increase in dosage may be necessary.	439

Abbreviations: CNS, central nervous system; IM, intramuscular; EPS, extrapyramidal syndrome.

TABLE 10. Antipsychotic and Antianxiety Drug Interactions—cont'd

Drug Interaction	Significance Code	Potential Effects	Recommendations	See Page
Chlorpromazine–Piperazine	3	A single case of convulsions after the concurrent use of these agents has been reported. Chlorpromazine could cause exaggerated extrapyramidal effects when used with piperazine.	Concurrent use need not be avoided, but monitor patients for development of seizure disorders.	440
Diazepam–Alcohol, Ethyl	2	Concurrent use of these agents enhances disruption of psychomotor performance and increases CNS depression.	Warn patients to avoid alcohol. The use of a short-acting benzodiazepine in place of diazepam may minimize the interaction's effects.	441
Diazepam–Cimetidine	2	Cimetidine significantly impairs elimination and increases absorption of diazepam, potentiating the sedative effects.	Substitute a benzodiazepine that undergoes phase II metabolism (e.g., oxazepam). Ranitidine may be a suitable alternative for cimetidine.	443
Diazepam–Disulfiram	3	Disulfiram reduces diazepam clearance by inhibiting phase I metabolism. This interaction has been associated with enhanced sedation.	Benzodiazepines undergoing phase II metabolism (e.g., oxazepam) may be a better choice for co-therapy.	445
Diazepam–Isoniazid	3	Isoniazid significantly prolonged the half-life and decreased diazepam clearance in 1 study.	A decreased diazepam dosage may be necessary.	446
Diazepam–Levodopa	3	Diazepam may diminish the antiparkinson effect of levodopa, but the interaction is infrequent and is subject to individual variation.	The incidence is too limited to recommend avoiding the concurrent use of these agents.	447
Diazepam–Oral Contraceptive Agents	3	Oral contraceptives may reduce the clearance and prolong the elimination half-life of diazepam, thus increasing the effects of diazepam.	Monitor patients and adjust the diazepam dosage if necessary.	448
Diazepam–Rifampin	3	Rifampin may significantly decrease the half-life and increase the clearance of diazepam.	Increased diazepam dosage may be necessary when receiving concomitant rifampin either alone or in a drug combination.	449
Fluphenazine–Clonidine	3	Concurrent use of these agents led to acute organic brain syndrome in 1 patient. Neurologic symptoms cleared within 72 hours after withdrawing clonidine.	Clonidine may need to be discontinued. Hydralazine, which does not interact with fluphenazine, may be an alternative antihypertensive.	450

TABLE 10. Antipsychotic and Antianxiety Drug Interactions—cont'd

Drug Interaction	Significance Code	Potential Effects	Recommendations	See Page
Lithium Carbonate–Acetazolamide	1	Acetazolamide may increase the urinary excretion of lithium. Forced alkaline diuresis has been used to treat lithium intoxication.	It is important to measure lithium serum levels since a higher dose of lithium carbonate may be necessary.	451
Lithium Carbonate–Carbamazepine	2	Concurrent use may lead to neurotoxicity with plasma concentrations of both agents within their therapeutic range, although other studies have reported no interaction.	Close monitoring for neurotoxic symptoms may be necessary.	452
Lithium Carbonate–Chlorothiazide	1	Chlorothiazide may enhance the cardiotoxic and neurotoxic effects of lithium through decreased lithium clearance.	Although concurrent use should be avoided, when cotherapy is necessary observe closely for lithium toxicity. Potassium-sparing diuretics may be suitable alternatives to chlorothiazide.	453
Lithium Carbonate–Diazepam	3	Concurrent use may cause hypothermia, which is not seen with either drug alone.	Concurrent use need not be avoided. If hypothermia occurs one or both drugs may need to be withdrawn.	455
Lithium Carbonate–Haloperidol	2	Concurrent use has caused a wide variety of encephalopathic syndromes, and some cases of permanent brain damage and irreversible dyskinesias have been reported. This interaction may be dose-related.	It used concurrently during an acute manic stage, conservative lithium dosage is recommended.	456
Lithium Carbonate–Indomethacin	2	Indomethacin increases lithium plasma concentrations, and lithium toxicity has been observed.	Avoid concurrent use, but if this is not possible monitor lithium levels and adjust the dosage if needed.	458
Lithium Carbonate–Mazindol	2	Lithium intoxication was observed in 1 patient who was also taking mazindol. Dieting decreases caloric/sodium intake, which prompts the kidney to reabsorb lithium as well as sodium.	Adequate sodium intake should be ensured during concomitant use. Reduced lithium dosage may be required.	459
Lithium Carbonate–Methyldopa	3	Methyldopa may exacerbate the CNS response to lithium or increase the brain uptake of lithium, thus resulting in signs of lithium toxicity.	If signs of lithium toxicity occur, the lithium dosage may need decreasing or methyldopa may need to be withdrawn.	460
Lithium Carbonate–Metoprolol	2	Metoprolol may lead to objective and subjective improvement of lithium-induced tremors.	Concomitant use may be beneficial for patients with bronchospastic problems since metoprolol is a cardioselective beta blocking agent.	461

TABLE 10. Antipsychotic and Antianxiety Drug Interactions—cont'd

Drug Interaction	Significance Code	Potential Effects	Recommendations	See Page
Lithium Carbonate—Norepinephrine	3	Lithium may decrease the pressor response to norepinephrine, and patients may show a decreased norepinephrine sensitivity after lithium treatment.	A higher norepinephrine dose may be necessary to achieve the desired pressor response.	462
Lithium Carbonate—Phenytoin	3	Phenytoin has caused symptoms of lithium toxicity in some patients. The interaction appears reversible when one or both agents are withdrawn.	Observe closely for signs of lithium toxicity and adjust lithium dosage if needed.	463
Lithium Carbonate—Potassium Iodide	2	Concurrent use may enhance the hypothyroid and goiterogenic effects of either drug.	If hypothyroidism develops, institute thyroid preparations and discontinue iodine-containing drugs. Withdrawing lithium is not necessary.	464
Lithium Carbonate—Tetracycline	2	Tetracycline may increase serum lithium concentrations, leading to lithium toxicity characterized by drowsiness, slurred speech, tremors, and thirst.	Caution should be exerted with concurrent use. Lithium dosage may need to be decreased.	465
Lithium Carbonate—Theophylline	2	Reduced lithium levels and worsening of manic symptoms may occur after increasing doses of theophylline.	Monitor lithium levels and therapeutic response closely. Increase the lithium dosage if required.	466
Lithium Carbonate—Thioridazine	2	Concurrent use may cause reversible neurotoxic and/or somnambulistic episodes. It is not clearly established if the symptoms observed are an additive effect of both agents or a potentiation of the effect of just 1 agent.	Conservative doses of both drugs are warranted if used together. It is preferable to use only 1 agent if possible.	467
Perphenazine—Disulfiram	3	In a case study, concurrent use of these agents led to subtherapeutic plasma perphenazine levels. Increasing the perphenazine dose did not improve symptoms; however, switching from oral to IM perphenazine resulted in clinical improvement.	Disulfiram may need to be discontinued, or switching to the parenteral route of perphenazine may avoid the interaction.	468

Chlorpromazine–Alcohol, Ethyl

2

Summary: Concurrent use of chlorpromazine and alcohol may cause an intensification of the central nervous system (CNS) depression of each drug.[1-3] Alcohol may also precipitate extrapyramidal reactions in patients taking chlorpromazine or other phenothiazines.[4,5]

Related Drugs: Thioridazine may produce less marked CNS depression in combination with alcohol than chlorpromazine.[6] Other phenothiazines (e.g., mesoridazine, promazine, trifluoperazine [see Appendix]), thioxanthenes (chlorprothixene and thiothixene), as well as the butyrophenone (haloperidol), dihydroindolone (molindone), and dibenzoxazepine (loxapine) may be expected to interact in a similar manner with alcohol since they are pharmacologically related.

Mechanism: The exact mechanism whereby chlorpromazine produces added CNS depression with alcohol is not established. It has been proposed that alcohol precipitates extrapyramidal reactions in patients on phenothiazines by inducing a temporary brain dysfunction that results in a lower threshold of resistance to the neurotoxic side effects of the drugs.[4]

Recommendations: Patients receiving chlorpromazine should be warned that alcohol ingestion may produce enhanced CNS depression. Concurrent use may impair their ability to drive an automobile and operate hazardous machinery.[6] Oral prescription and nonprescription products containing alcohol, as well as alcoholic beverages, should be used with caution.

References

1. Sutherland, V.C., and others: Cerebral metabolism in problem drinkers under the influence of alcohol and chlorpromazine hydrochloride, J. Appl. Physiol. **15:**189, 1960.
2. Morselli, P.L., and others: Further observations on the interaction between ethanol and psychotropic drugs, Arzneimittel Forsch. **21:**20, 1971.
3. Fazekas, J.F., and others: Influence of chlorpromazine and alcohol on cerebral hemodynamics and metabolism, Am. J. Med. Sci. **230:**128, 1955.
4. Lutz, E.G.: Neuroleptic-induced akathisia and dystonia triggered by alcohol, J.A.M.A. **236:**2422, 1976.
5. Freed, E.: Alcohol-triggered-neuroleptic-induced tremor, rigidity and dystonia, Med. J. Aust. **2:**44, 1981.
6. Milner, G., and Landauer, A.A.: Alcohol, thioridazine, and chlorpromazine effects on skills related to driving behavior, Br. J. Psychiatry **118:**351, 1971.

Chlorpromazine–Aluminum Hydroxide, Magnesium Hydroxide

3

Summary: Chlorpromazine absorption from the gastrointestinal tract may be altered by the simultaneous administration of antacids. Gel antacids containing aluminum and magnesium salts have been reported to decrease or to have no effect on chlorpromazine levels.[1-4]

Related Drugs: Other phenothiazines (e.g., thioridazine, triflupromazine, trifluoperazine [see Appendix]), thioxanthenes (chlorprothixene and thiothixene), as well as the butyrophenone (haloperidol), dihydroindolone (molindone), and dibenzoxazepine (loxapine) may be expected to interact in a similar manner based on pharmacologic similarity. Chelation of promazine by magnesium ions has occurred in vitro.[5] Trisilicate gel antacids have been shown to decrease chlorpromazine levels whereas calcium carbonate–glycine antacids do not.[3]

Mechanism: Administration of aluminum and magnesium containing antacids decreases the gastrointestinal absorption and serum levels of chlorpromazine, probably because of adsorption of chlorpromazine by the antacid.[2] There are no data to support the theory that alkalinization of the urine by antacids affects chlorpromazine excretion.[6]

Recommendations: It is not known whether the individual agents (magnesium hydroxide and aluminum hydroxide) alone have an effect on chlorpromazine absorption, but documentation[1-3] indicates the combination of ingredients did alter chlorpromazine absorption. Therefore, until further clinical evidence is available, antacid products containing aluminum hydroxide and magnesium hydroxide, or those containing magnesium trisilicate should be administered 1 hour before or 2 hours after chlorpromazine administration.

References

1. Forrest, F.M., and others: Modification of chlorpromazine metabolism by some other drugs frequently administered to psychiatric patients, Biol. Psychiatry **2:**53, 1970.
2. Fann, W.E., and others: Chlorpromazine: effects of antacids on its gastrointestinal absorption, J. Clin. Pharmacol. **13:**388, 1973.
3. Pinell, O.C., and others: Drug-drug interaction of chlorpromazine and antacid (abstract), Clin. Pharmacol. Ther. **23:**125, 1978.
4. Inoue, F.: Antipsychotic drugs: adverse reactions and drug interactions, Can. Pharm. J. **115:**456, 1982.
5. Rajan, K.S., and others: Studies on the metal chelation of chlorpromazine and its hydroxylated metabolites. In I.S. Forrest, and others, editors: The phenothiazines and structurally related drugs. New York, 1974. Raven Press.
6. Gibaldi, M., and others: Effect of antacids on pH of urine, Clin. Pharmacol. Ther. **16:**520, 1974.

Chlorpromazine–Amphetamine

Summary: Chlorpromazine and amphetamine are pharmacologic antagonists. These 2 drugs exert opposing effects on monoaminergic function in the central and peripheral nervous system. This antagonistic relationship has been utilized clinically in the management of amphetamine overdosage.[1] Inclusion of either agent in a therapeutic regimen of the other could prove counterproductive. The amphetamines may antagonize the antipsychotic effect of the phenothiazine.

Related Drugs: Chlorpromazine is a multifunctional antagonist to several neurotransmitters. Other phenothiazines (e.g., promazine, thioridazine, trifluoperazine [see Appendix]) exhibit somewhat different potencies in their ability to interfere with the actions of norepinephrine or dopamine,[2,3] the neurotransmitters generally believed involved in the stimulatory actions of amphetamine. Thus one would presume that other phenothiazine derivatives such as the thioxanthenes (chlorprothixene and thiothixene) as well as the dihydroindolone (molindone) and dibenzoxazepine (loxapine) would also exhibit antagonism of amphetamine actions with varying degrees of potency. Other antipsychotic agents such as haloperidol, a butyrophenone, which possess dopamine blocking activity and significant alpha-adrenergic blocking activity, may also effectively antagonize the actions of amphetamine.[4]

Other indirect-acting sympathomimetic agents (e.g., ephedrine, methylphenidate, tyramine [see Appendix]) as well as direct and mixed-acting sympathomimetics (direct: e.g., epinephrine, isoproterenol, norepinephrine [see Appendix]; mixed: e.g., metaraminol, phenylephrine, phenylpropanolamine [see Appendix]), which characteristically produce central and peripheral stimulation would logically be expected to undergo antagonism by chlorpromazine.

Mechanism: The precise mechanism involved in the antagonism of amphetamine by chlorpromazine is not known but appears to involve quite complex pharmacodynamic interplay with monoaminergic effector and control mechanisms. Both norepinephrine and dopamine neuronal systems are believed to contribute to the spectrum of stimulation produced by amphetamine through its ability to release catecholamines and/or block their reuptake. Chlorpromazine is capable of blocking postsynaptic monoamine receptors and also appears to antagonize amphetamine directly through a presynaptic mechanism.[5] Reports have appeared that describe an inhibition of amphetamine metabolism in animals by low doses of chlorpromazine, leading to enhanced amphetamine action.[6] The clinical significance of this effect is unclear.

Recommendations: Simultaneous use of chlorpromazine and amphetamine should be restricted to treating amphetamine overdose cases. A dose of 1 mg/kg intramuscularly has been recommended. This may be followed by 0.5 mg/kg intramuscularly after 30 minutes if necessary to control recurrence of excitement.[1] Conversely, overdosage with chlorpromazine generally is best managed with supportive measures alone.

References

1. Espelin, D.E., and Done, A.K.: Amphetamine poisoning. Effectiveness of chlorpromazine, N. Engl. J. Med. **278:**1361, 1968.
2. Peroutka, S.J., and others: Neuroleptic drug interactions with norepinephrine alpha-receptor binding sites in rat brain, Neuropharmacol. **16:**549, 1977.
3. Creese, I., and others: Dopamine receptor binding predicts clinical and pharmacological potencies of antischizophrenic drugs, Science **192:**481, 1976.
4. Angrist, B., and others: The antagonism of amphetamine-induced symptomatology by a neuroleptic, Am. J. Psychiatry **131:**817, 1974.
5. Boakes, R.J., and others: Interactions of (+)− amphetamine and chlorpromazine on neurons in the lower brain stem of the rat, Br. J. Pharmacol. **67:**165, 1979.
6. Sulser, F., and Dingell, J.V.: Potentiation and blockade of the central action of amphetamine by chlorpromazine, Biochem. Pharmacol. **17:**634, 1968.

Chlorpromazine–Benztropine

Summary: An interaction between the antidopaminergic agent chlorpromazine and the anticholinergic drug benztropine is used with considerable clinical success in managing certain movement disorders resulting from the antipsychotic induced extrapyramidal syndrome (EPS). Those particular forms of the EPS that are most responsive to amelioration via benztropine therapy are: pseudoparkinsonism, perioral tremor ("rabbit syndrome"),[1] and acute dystonia. Akathisia is generally less responsive to anticholinergic medication and tardive dyskinesia is probably worsened by benztropine. One study reported that benztropine reversed the therapeutic effects of chlorpromazine in schizophrenic patients.[2]

Related Drugs: Virtually all antipsychotic drugs are able to induce the EPS to varying extents. Those antipsychotics that possess the greatest anticholinergic activity (e.g., thioridazine, a phenothiazine) may tend to cause minimal EPS, whereas the most potent, purest dopamine blocker (e.g., haloperidol, a butyrophenone) tends to cause a high frequency of extrapyramidal syndrome side effects.[3] Benztropine and trihexyphenidyl both have been shown to reverse the effects of haloperidol.[2] The concurrent use of atropine and chlorpromazine or promazine led to marked central nervous system depressant activity.[4] Two reports showed that concomitant chlorpromazine and trihexyphenidyl resulted in lower chlorpromazine plasma levels.[5,6] One study, however, reported that perphenazine with biperiden or orphenadrine did not result in any significant interaction.[7] Other phenothiazines (e.g., fluphenazine, mesoridazine, trifluoperazine [see Appendix]), thioxanthenes (chlorprothixene and thiothixene) as well as the dihydroindolone (molindone) and dibenzoxazepine (loxapine) may be expected to interact in a similar manner with benztropine since they are pharmacologically related.

Other anticholinergic drugs commonly used in the treatment of parkinsonism (e.g., chlorphenoxamine, cycrimine, procyclidine [see Appendix]) may be effective in treating chlorpromazine induced parkinsonism. Trihexyphenidyl is commonly used in this manner and a study has suggested that ethopropazine may prove to be a superior agent because of reduced central and peripheral toxicity.[8]

Mechanism: Chlorpromazine induced parkinsonism and presumably dystonia, perioral tremor, and possibly akathisia appear to arise from a functional increase of cholinergic activity secondary to dopamine receptor blockade.[9] Anticholinergic actions of benztropine tend to restore a balance between these systems. In contrast, tardive dyskinesia is thought to arise from dopaminergic supersensitivity secondary to chronic receptor blockade and benztropine could further disrupt normal acetylcholine/dopamine interplay.

Recommendations: Use of benztropine should probably be reserved to treat those responsive aspects of extrapyramidal syndrome that can arise during chlorpromazine therapy. Clinical evidence suggests that relatively short-term treatment (3 to 4 months) with benztropine may suffice to effectively deal with drug-induced parkinsonism.[10] Refractory EPS cases may be a result of suboptimal serum concentrations of anticholinergic medication.[9] Additive anticholinergic actions of benztropine and chlorpromazine may be hazardous in angle closure glaucoma or in individuals hyperresponsive to parasympathetic blockade.

References

1. Sovner, R., and DiMascio, A.: The effect of benztropine mesylate in the rabbit syndrome and tardive dyskinesia, Am. J. Psychiatry **134:**1301, 1977.
2. Singh, M.M., and Kay, S.R.: Therapeutic antagonism between anticholinergic antiparkinsonism agents and neuroleptics in scizophrenia, Neuropsychobiology **5:**74, 1979.
3. Snyder, S.H., and others: Antischizophrenic drugs and brain cholinergic receptors, Arch. Gen. Psychiatry **31:**58, 1974.
4. Gershon, S., and others: Interaction between some anticholinergic agents and phenothiazines, Clin. Pharmacol. Ther. **6:**749, 1965.
5. Rivera-Calimlim, L., and others: Effects of mode of management on plasma chlorpromazine in psychiatric patients, Clin. Pharmacol. Ther. **14:**978, 1973.
6. Rivera-Calimlim, L., and others: Clinical response and plasma levels: effect of dose, dosage schedules, and drug interactions on plasma chlorpromazine levels, Am. J. Psychiatry **133:**6, 1976.
7. Hansen, L.B., and others: Plasma levels of perphenazine and its major metabolites during simultaneous treatment with anticholinergic drugs, Br. J. Clin. Pharmacol. **7:**75, 1979.
8. Chouinard, G., and others: Ethopropazine and benztropine in neuroleptic induced parkinsonism, J. Clin. Psychiatry **40:**147, 1979.
9. Tune, L.E., and others: Management of extrapyramidal side effects induced by neuroleptics, Johns Hopkins Med. J. **148:**149, 1981.
10. DiMascio, A.L.: Toward a more rational use of drugs in psychiatry, Drug Ther. **1:**23, 1971.

Chlorpromazine–Diazoxide

2

Summary: In a single case report, a child on long-term oral diazoxide and bendroflumethiazide treatment developed severe hyperglycemia and a diabetic precoma after a single dose of chlorpromazine.[1]

Related Drugs: There are no drugs related to diazoxide. Although no documentation exists, other phenothiazines (e.g., promazine, thioridazine, trifluoperazine [see Appendix]), the thioxanthenes (chlorprothixene and thiothixene) as well as the butyrophenone (haloperidol), dihydroindolone (molindone), and dibenzoxazepine (loxapine), may be expected to interact in a similar manner with diazoxide since they are pharmacologically related.

Mechanism: The mechanism of this interaction is unknown. However, chlorpromazine alone has been reported to result in hyperglycemia.[2-5]

Summary: Patients' blood glucose should be closely monitored if chlorpromazine and diazoxide are to be used concurrently. The dose of diazoxide may need to be decreased.

References

1. Aynsley-Green, A., and Illig, R.: Enhancement by chlorpromazine of hyperglycemic action of diazoxide, Lancet **2:**658, 1975.
2. Hiles, B.W.: Hyperglycemia and glycosuria following chlorpromazine therapy, J.A.M.A. **162:**1651, 1956.
3. Arneson, G.A.: Phenothiazine derivatives and glucose metabolism, J. Neuropsychiatry **5:**181, 1964.
4. Schwarz, L., and others: Blood sugar levels in patients treated with chlorpromazine, Am. J. Psychiatry **125:**253, 1968.
5. Kornyi, C., and others: Chlorpromazine-induced diabetes, Dis. Nerv. System **29:**827, 1968.

Chlorpromazine–Levodopa

3

Summary: Although the clinical effects of concurrent administration of these drugs are unpredictable, levodopa and chlorpromazine may antagonize each other when these drugs are administered together.

Related Drugs: Other phenothiazines (e.g., promazine, thioridazine, trifluoperazine [see Appendix]), thioxanthenes (chlorprothixene and thiothixene), as well as the butyrophenone (haloperidol), dihydroindolone (molindone), and dibenzoxazepine (loxapine) may be expected to interact in a similar manner with levodopa because of pharmacologic similarity. There are no drugs related to levodopa.

Mechanism: This interaction can be explained on the basis of chlorpromazine and levodopa having opposing actions at central dopaminergic receptor sites. Phenothiazines exert therapeutic and adverse effects by inhibiting stimulation of dopamine receptors in the brain. Levodopa increases synaptic dopamine concentrations and enhances stimulation of dopamine receptors.

Recommendations: The effect of levodopa and chlorpromazine on each other is unpredictable. In instances where no alternative drugs are available and both drugs must be used, the patient should be observed closely for a deterioration in levodopa's growth hormone stimulating[1] or antiparkinson[2,3] effects, or a decrease in the therapeutic effect of chlorpromazine.[4]

References

1. Mims, R.B., and others: Inhibition of l-dopa induced growth hormone stimulation by pyridoxine and chlorpromazine, J. Clin. Endocrinol. Metab. **40:**256, 1975.
2. Duvoisin, R.C.: Diphenidol for levodopa-induced nausea and vomiting, J.A.M.A. **221:**1408, 1972.
3. Campbell, J.B.: Long-term treatment of Parkinson's disease with levodopa, Neurology **20:**18, 1970.
4. Yaryura-Tobias, J.A., and others: Action of l-dopa in drug-induced extrapyramidalism, Dis. Nerv. Syst. **31:**60, 1970.

Chlorpromazine–Lithium Carbonate

2

Summary: Concurrent lithium carbonate has decreased plasma chlorpromazine levels an average of 40% in subjects[1] and 70% in psychiatric patients.[2,3] Neurotoxic and/or somnambulistic episodes have also been reported during concomitant use.[4] It was not clearly established if these episodes were the result of concomitant use or of either agent alone. One study suggests that there may be some correlation between plasma chlorpromazine levels and clinical improvement, indicating a decreased therapeutic response may occur with low chlorpromazine levels.[3]

Related Drugs: There are no drugs related to lithium carbonate. However, in 1 study using lithium citrate, there was a 15% increase in the lithium excretion rate in patients simultaneously treated with chlorpromazine.[5] Interactions between lithium carbonate and other antipsychotics are discussed in other monographs (see Lithium Carbonate–Haloperidol, p. 456, and Lithium Carbonate–Thioridazine, p. 467).

Mechanism: The mechanism is unknown. However, it has been postulated that the decreased chlorpromazine plasma concentrations could be the result of a lithium-induced delay in gastric emptying leading to a decreased bioavailability of chlorpromazine. Also, the decreased levels could result from a decreased chlorpromazine absorption as a result of a lithium-induced reduction in gastrointestinal membrane permeability.[1] Chlorpromazine may facilitate the urinary excretion of lithium.[5,6]

Recommendations: It may be preferable to use only one agent alone. However, if combination therapy is elected, the possibility of these interactions warrant conservative use of both agents. Dosage adjustment of one or both agents might be necessary.

References

1. Rivera-Calimlim, L., and others: Effect of lithium on plasma chlorpromazine levels, Clin. Pharmacol. Ther. **23:**451, 1978.
2. Kerzner, B., and Rivera-Calimlim, L.: Lithium and chlorpromazine (CPZ) interaction, Clin. Pharmacol. Ther. **19:**109, 1976.
3. Rivera-Calimlim, L., and others: Clinical response and plasma levels: effect of dose, dosage schedules, and drug interactions on plasma chlorpromazine levels, Am. J. Psychiatry **133:**646, 1976.
4. Charney, D.S., and others: Somnambulistic-like episodes secondary to combined lithium-neuroleptic treatment, Br. J. Psychiatry **135:**418, 1979.
5. Sletten, I., and others: The effect of chlorpromazine on lithium excretion in psychiatric subjects, Curr. Ther. Res. **8:**441, 1966.
6. Pakes, G.E.: Lithium toxicity with phenothiazine withdrawal, Lancet **2:**701, 1979.

Chlorpromazine–Phenobarbital

3

Summary: The long-term administration of phenobarbital may decrease serum chlorpromazine levels,[1-3] but the significance of this interaction has not been determined, since no change in therapeutic response is documented.

Related Drugs: Chlorpromazine, when administered as preanesthetic medication, may enhance the action of ultra-short acting barbiturates (e.g., methohexital, thiamylal, thiopental [see Appendix]), which may lead to an increased sleep duration or a more rapid induction of sleep or anesthesia.[4,5] Because the barbiturates induce hepatic enzymes, the other barbiturates (e.g., amobarbital, butabarbital, secobarbital [see Appendix]) may be expected to act in a manner similar to phenobarbital.

Promazine has been reported to interact with barbiturates in an animal study.[6] Other phenothiazines (e.g., mesoridazine, thioridazine, trifluoperazine [see Appendix]), thioxanthenes (chlorprothixene and thiothixene), as well as the butyrophenone (haloperidol), dihydroindolone (molindone), and dibenzoxazepine (loxapine) may be expected to interact in a similar manner with phenobarbital because of pharmacologic similarity.

Mechanism: Phenobarbital is a known enzyme inducer. Therefore the metabolism of chlorpromazine may be increased by induction of hepatic microsomal enzymes, which would explain the decreased serum chlorpromazine levels.

Chlorpromazine depresses the central nervous system in many areas, and the sedative action of barbiturates is primarily the result of depression of the ascending reticular arousal system.[7] It is probable that the enhanced action of the ultra-short acting barbiturates is produced by a synergistic action on the same central nervous system sites.

Recommendations: Since long-term administration of barbiturates might decrease the effectiveness of chlorpromazine by decreasing serum levels, the dosage of chlorpromazine may need to be increased. However, if the barbiturate is discontinued, chlorpromazine toxicity may result and the dose would have to be readjusted.

References

1. Loga, S., and others: Interactions of orphenadrine and phenobarbitone with chlorpromazine: plasma concentrations and effects in man, Br. J. Clin. Pharmacol. **2:**197, 1975.
2. Dundee, J.W., and Scott, W.E.B.: The effect of phenothiazine derivatives on thiobarbiturate narcosis, Anesth. Analg. (Cleve.) **37:**12, 1958.
3. Sadove, M.S., and others: The potentiating action of chlorpromazine, Curr. Res. Anesth. Analg. **35:**165, 1956.
4. Forrest, F.M., and others: Modification of chlorpromazine metabolism by some other drugs frequently administered to psychiatric patients, Biol. Psychiatry **2:**53, 1970.
5. Curry, S.H., and others: Factors affecting chlorpromazine plasma levels in psychiatric patients, Arch. Gen. Psychiatry **22:**209, 1970.
6. Tonuma, E.: Some ataractic drugs as adjuvants to thiopental sodium anesthesia in small animals, Can. Vet. J. **7:**128, 1966.
7. Magoun, H.W.: Symposium on sedative and hypnotic drugs, Baltimore, 1954, Williams and Wilkins.

Chlorpromazine–Piperazine

Summary: Although there has been a single report of an adverse interaction leading to convulsions after the concurrent use of chlorpromazine and piperazine,[1] little evidence suggests that this interaction is of major clinical significance. Other studies have either failed to confirm an interaction[2] or extremely high doses of piperazine were necessitated to cause interactions in animals.[3]

Related Drugs: There is a lack of documentation concerning a similar interaction with other phenothiazines (e.g., promazine, thioridazine, trifluoperazine [see Appendix]), thioxanthenes (chlorprothixene and thiothixene), the butyrophenone (haloperidol), dihydroindolone (molindone), or the dibenzoxazepine (loxapine). There are no drugs related to piperazine.

Mechanism: The precise manner whereby chlorpromazine and piperazine may interact is not known. However, chlorpromazine alone does lower the seizure threshold[4] and given in combination with piperazine can cause exaggerated extrapyramidal effects including convulsions.[1]

Recommendations: From analysis of the data available regarding the potential interaction between chlorpromazine and piperazine, this combination appears devoid of serious risk. Individuals receiving this combined therapy should be carefully monitored for any manifestations of seizure disorders. Renal dysfunction may impair elimination of piperazine and potentially enhance the ability of this drug to elicit toxicity or interact with chlorpromazine.[4]

References

1. Boulos, B.M., and David, L.E.: Hazard of simultaneous administration of phenothiazine and piperazine, N. Engl. J. Med. **28:**1245, 1969.
2. Armbrecht, B.H.: Reaction between piperazine and chlorpromazine, N. Engl. J. Med. **282:**1490, 1970.
3. Sturman, G.: Interaction between piperazine and chlorpromazine, Br. J. Pharmacol. **50:**153, 1974.
4. Rollo, I.M.: Drugs used in the chemotherapy of helminthiasis. In Gilman, A.G., Goodman, L.S., and Gilman, A., editors: The pharmacological basis of therapeutics. New York, 1980, MacMillan Publishing.

Diazepam–Alcohol, Ethyl

Summary: A large body of clinical data indicates a definite interaction between diazepam and ethyl alcohol, which leads to enhanced disruption of psychomotor performance and increased central nervous system depression.

Related Drugs: There is evidence that temazepam and the other short-acting benzodiazepines (e.g., alprazolam, halazepam, triazolam) tend to result in less profound alcohol interactions.[1] Reports have been conflicting regarding the actions of chlordiazepoxide when combined with alcohol.[2] Differences in time of exposure, dosage, and response parameters have been used to explain both inconsistent findings with chlordiazepoxide as well as the inability to directly compare the other benzodiazepines (e.g., diazepam, flurazepam, lorazepam [see Appendix]).

Mechanism: There appears to be an unknown pharmacodynamic mechanism causing additive central nervous system depressant effects with benzodiazepines and alcohol. Various studies have also implicated a potential role of pharmacokinetic factors such as altered diazepam absorption,[3] altered distribution,[4] or decreased elimination[5,6] leading to higher concentrations of diazepam in the brain, but conflicting reports render the interpretation of kinetic data difficult.[7] The extent of the interaction depends on the dosage of diazepam and alcohol as well as the time interval between exposure to these drugs. Maximum effects arise if both are administered within 90 minutes and appear 30 minutes after alcohol consumption. Effects persist up to 3 hours after exposure[8] and can occur if alcohol is consumed 9 to 11 hours after diazepam. Mechanistic studies may be further handicapped by the fact that benzodiazepines may have active metabolites and that patient characteristics such as age play a major role in modifying actions of diazepam.[9]

Recommendations: All patients receiving benzodiazepines for any indication must be informed of the fact that alcohol consumption will probably result in significantly decreased psychomotor performance with its associated risks. When it is possible, use of a short acting member of the benzodiazepine family may minimize the potential for extreme alcohol interactions. Although the direct toxicologic manifestations of this interaction may not be particularly hazardous in nonoverdosage situations, operation of an automobile or machinery could profoundly increase the significance of this interaction. Based on the extensive use of diazepam and the popularity of alcohol consumption, it is possible that this interaction occurs frequently. It is notable that subjects suffering from this interaction-induced psychomotor impairment may fail to perceive their disability.[2] Patients taking diazepam must be informed of the potentially serious results of diazepam and alcohol interactions. Situations in which suicide or drug abuse is of concern may render diazepam therapy ill advised since alcohol tends to greatly increase central nervous system depression of diazepam in acute overdosage.[10]

References

1. Lehmann, W., and Liljenberg, B.: Effect of temazepam and temazepam-ethanol on sleep, Eur. J. Clin. Pharmacol. **20:**201, 1981.
2. Ascione, F.J.L.: Benzodiazepines with alcohol, Drug Ther. **8:**58, 1978.
3. Hayes, S.L., and others: Ethanol and oral diazepam absorption, N. Engl. J. Med. **298:**188, 1977.
4. Thiessen, J.J., and others: Plasma protein binding of diazepam and tolbutamide in chronic alcoholics, J. Clin. Pharmacol. **16:**345, 1976.
5. Desmond, P.V., and others: Short-term ethanol administration impairs the elimination of chlordiaz-epoxide (Librium®) in man, Eur. J. Clin. Pharmacol. **18:**275, 1980.
6. Sellers, E.M., and others: Intravenous diazepam and oral ethanol interactions, Clin. Pharmacol. Ther. **28:**638, 1980.
7. Greenblatt, D.J., and others: Plasma diazepam and desmethyldiazepam concentration during long-term diazepam therapy, Br. J. Clin. Pharmacol. **1:**35, 1981.
8. Linoila, M., and others: Effect of treatment with diazepam or lithium and alcohol on psychomotor skills related to driving, Eur. J. Clin. Pharmacol. **7:**33, 1974.
9. Harvey, S.C.: Hynotics and sedatives. In Gilman, A.G., Goodman, L.S., and Gilman, A., editors: The pharmacological basis of therapeutics. New York, 1980, MacMillan Publishing.
10. Divoll, M., and others: Benzodiazepine overdosage: plasma concentrations and clinical outcome, Psychopharmacology **73:**381, 1981.

Diazepam–Cimetidine

Summary: Cimetidine has been found to increase the absorption[1] and significantly impair the elimination of diazepam when coadministered, resulting in a potentiation of the sedative effects of diazepam.[2-6] Diazepam's elimination half-life was reported to increase 34% to 155% in subjects in 4 different studies,[3-5,7] while the total plasma clearance decreased 33% to 51%. This would cause an increase in serum diazepam levels resulting in the increased incidence of diazepam side effects. This interaction has been observed with single[3,5,7] and multiple[4] diazepam dosing and with short term[3,5] cimetidine administration.

Related Drugs: Chlordiazepoxide, which is metabolized by phase I (N-dealkylation or hydroxylation) reactions as is diazepam, has been shown to undergo a similar interaction with cimetidine.[8,9] Cimetidine has been reported to impair the clearance of both alprazolam and triazolam. Alprazolam's major metabolic pathway in humans involves hepatic microsomal oxidative reactions yielding hydroxylated metabolites (phase I).[10] Cimetidine prolonged the elimination half-life of alprazolam while reducing its clearance and volume of distribution (not significant) but had no effect on the peak plasma alprazolam concentration.[11] Also, cimetidine significantly increased the triazolam area-under-curve, increased the peak plasma concentration (not significantly), and had no effect on the elimination half-life.[11] Other benzodiazepines with primary metabolic pathways dependent on phase I (N-dealkylation or hydroxylation) reactions (flurazepam, clonazepam, clorazepate, halazepam, and prazepam) would be expected to undergo a similar interaction.[2,12-14] Although cimetidine had no effect on nitrazepam* peak serum levels, volume of distribution, or time to peak levels, it consistently decreased nitrazepam clearance leading to a prolonged elimination half-life.[15] The elimination of oxazepam,[16-20] lorazepam,[16,18-20] and temazepam[13,21] benzodiazepines with primary metabolic pathways dependent on phase II (glucuronidation) reactions, is not altered by cimetidine; however, lorazepam absorption is enhanced with concomitant cimetidine.[1]

In a study involving 6 healthy volunteers, ranitidine did not significantly affect the mean elimination half-life or apparent volume of distribution of diazepam. However, it significantly reduced steady state plasma levels and increased plasma clearance.[22] In another study, ranitidine was shown not to affect the half-life, clearance, or volume of distribution of intravenous diazepam, and ranitidine also had no effect on lorazepam kinetics.[23]

Mechanism: It is proposed that cimetidine inhibits hepatic microsomal drug metabolism, causing a reduction in the hepatic elimination of diazepam.[3,5] More specifically, cimetidine is thought to impair the phase I reactions[2] responsible for the hepatic N-dealkylation of both diazepam and chlordiazepoxide and the hydroxylation of diazepam.[10,24] It is expected that benzodiazepines undergoing phase II reactions (glucuronidation) as a main route of elimination will not be affected by the concurrent administration of cimetidine.[2,13]

*Not available in the U.S.

Recommendations: If patients receiving cimetidine become candidates for benzodiazepine therapy, a prudent choice would be oxazepam, lorazepam, or one of the other benzodiazepines whose metabolism is unaltered by cimetidine. If diazepam and cimetidine must be given concurrently, the patient should be closely monitored for clinically significant side effects resulting from elevated diazepam serum levels, and dosage adjustment should be made when indicated. Ranitidine may be an alternative agent to use with concomitant diazepam therapy.

References

1. McGowan, W.A.W., and Dundee, J.W.: The effect of intravenous cimetidine on the absorption of orally administered diazepam and lorazepam, Br. J. Clin. Pharmacol. **14:**207, 1982.
2. Mangini, R.J.: Clinically important cimetidine drug interactions, Clin. Pharmacy **1:**433, 1982.
3. Klotz, U., and Reimann, I.: Delayed clearance of diazepam due to cimetidine, N. Engl. J. Med. **302:**1012, 1980.
4. Klotz, U., and Reimann, I.: Elevation of steady-state diazepam levels by cimetidine, Clin. Pharmacol. Ther. **30:**513, 1981.
5. Klotz, U., and others: Cimetidine/diazepam interaction, Lancet **2:**699, 1979.
6. Dasta, J., and others: Diazepam-cimetidine interaction—a preliminary report, Drug Intell. Clin. Pharm. **14:**633, 1980.
7. Gough, P.A., and others: Influence of cimetidine on oral diazepam elimination with measurement of subsequent cognitive change, Br. J. Clin. Pharmacol. **14:**739, 1982.
8. Desmond, P.V., and others: Cimetidine impairs elimination of chlordiazepoxide (Librium) in man, Ann. Intern. Med. **93:**266, 1980.
9. Patwardhan, R.V., and others: Lack of tolerance and rapid recovery of cimetidine-inhibited chlordiazepoxide (Librium) elimination, Gastroenterology **81:**547, 1981.
10. Fawcett, J.A., and Kravitz, H.M.: Alprazolam: pharmacokinetics, clinical efficacy, and mechanism of action, Pharmacotherapeutics **2:**243, 1982.
11. Abernathy, D.R., and others: Cimetidine impairs the clearance of alprazolam and triazolam, Psychopharmacology **80:**275, 1983.
12. Ruffalo, R.L., and others: Cimetidine-benzodiazepine drug interaction, Am. J. Hosp. Pharm. **38:**1365, 1981.
13. Ruffalo, R.L., and Thompson, J.F.: More on cimetidine-benzodiazepine drug interactions, South. Med. J. **75**(3):382, 1982.
14. Ruffalo, R.L., and Thompson, J.F.: Effect of cimetidine on the clearance of benzodiazepines, N. Engl. J. Med. **303:**753, 1980.
15. Ochs, H.R., and others: Cimetidine may decreae clearance of drugs mebabolized by nitroreduction, Clin. Pharmacol. Ther. **34:**227, 1983.
16. Patwardhan, R.V., and others: Cimetidine spares the glucoronidation of lorazepam and oxazepam, Gastroenterology **79:**912, 1980.
17. Klotz, U., and Reimann, I.: Influence of cimetidine on the pharmacokinetics of desmethyldiazepam and oxazepam, Eur. J. Clin. Pharmacol. **18:**517, 1980.
18. Greenblatt, D.J., and Shader, R.I.: Pharmacokinetic understanding of antianxiety drug therapy, South. Med. J. **71**(suppl. 2):2, 1978.
19. Ruffalo, R.L., and others: Diazepam-cimetidine drug interaction: a clinically significant effect, South. Med. J. **74:**1075, 1981.
20. Abernethy, D.R., and others: Differential effect of cimetidine on drug oxidation (antipyrine and diazepam) vs. conjugation (acetaminophen and lorazepam): prevention of acetaminophen toxicity by cimetidine, J. Pharmacol. Exp. Ther. **224:**508, 1983.
21. Schwarz, H.J.: Pharmacokinetics and metabolism of temazepam in man and several animal species, Br. J. Clin. Pharmacol. **8:**23S, 1979.
22. Klotz, V., and others: Effects of ranitidine on the steady state pharmacokinetics of diazepam, Eur. J. Clin. Pharmacol. **24:**357, 1983.
23. Abernathy, D.R., and others: Ranitidine noninteraction with benzodiazepine oxidation or conjugation, Clin. Pharmacol. Ther. **33:**216, 1983.
24. Rendic, S, and others: Interaction of cimetidine with liver microsomes, Xenobiotica **9:**555, 1979.

Diazepam–Disulfiram

3

Summary: Concurrent use of diazepam in patients receiving disulfiram may lead to enhanced sedation. Coadministration of these agents to either healthy subjects or alcoholic patients resulted in a decrease in diazepam clearance attributed to an increase in diazepam's half-life.[1,2] However, the importance of the interaction may in part be offset by the development of tolerance to benzodiazepines[1] resulting from long-term administration.

Related Drugs: Chlordiazepoxide clearance was decreased approximately 50%,[1,2] while disulfiram had little influence on oxazepam[1,2] or lorazepam[2] since they are metabolized by phase II metabolic pathways to inactive products.[1,2] Although no documentation exists, the other benzodiazepine with primary metabolic pathways dependent on phase II reactions (temazepam) may be expected to act similarly to oxazepam and lorazepam. There appear to be no reports of a similar interaction with other benzodiazepines (e.g., clorazepate, flurazepam, prazepam [see Appendix]). However, since their primary metabolic pathway is dependent on phase I reactions and they are metabolized to an active form as is diazepam, a similar interaction may be expected.

Mechanism: Chlordiazepoxide and diazepam are biotransformed initially by phase I N-demethylation and then phase II glucuronidation. The nonglucuronide metabolites of each drug are pharmacologically active. Disulfiram has been reported to inhibit hepatic mixed function oxidase catalyzed N-demethylation and C-hydroxylation of chlordiazepoxide and diazepam as well as the glucuronidation of the metabolites so formed. Sedation by the benzodiazepines has been correlated with the plasma concentration of the drug. Since steady-state drug concentrations are directly dependent on half-life and inversely dependent on clearance, both of which were shown to be affected by disulfiram (plasma clearance decreased 41% to 54%, half-life increased 37% to 84%), accumulation of chlordiazepoxide and diazepam would be expected and would result in increased sedation.[1,2] In contrast, oxazepam and lorazepam undergo only phase II glucuronidation to a pharmacologically inactive metabolite, and their disposition is altered only minimally by disulfiram.[1,2]

Recommendations: Present documentation suggests that the benzodiazepines that undergo N-demethylation, including diazepam, will be affected by disulfiram. It may be necessary to reduce the dosage of these particular benzodiazepines if concurrent use with disulfiram is required. An alternative may be to use oxazepam, lorazepam, or any other benzodiazepine that does not undergo N-demethylation. It is also important to realize that drowsiness is one of the most common side effects of disulfiram, and this may lead to an additive effect with use of benzodiazepines.[1]

References

1. Macleod, S.M., and others: Interaction of disulfiram with benzodiazepines, Clin. Pharmacol. Ther. **24:**583, 1978.
2. Sellers, E.M., and others: Differential effects on benzodiazepine disposition by disulfiram and ethanol, Arzneimittel Forsch. **30:**882, 1980.

Diazepam–Isoniazid

3

Summary: A single intravenous dose of diazepam was given during a 10 day isoniazid (180 mg/day) trial period to 9 healthy volunteers.[1] Isoniazid significantly prolonged the diazepam half-life from an average of 34 hours to 45 hours and decreased the diazepam clearance by approximately 25% as compared to the control value.

Related Drugs: There are no drugs related to isoniazid. One controlled study indicated that isoniazid impairs triazolam oxidation and results in increased systemic availability after oral administration.[2] The other benzodiazepines metabolized by phase I (N-demethylation or hydroxylation) reactions (e.g., chlordiazepoxide, flurazepam, halazepam [see Appendix]) as well as diazepam and triazolam may be expected to interact similarly with isoniazid if the mechanism involves inhibition of hepatic enzymes by isoniazid; however, documentation is lacking. It has not been determined if the benzodiazepines that are dependent on phase II (glucuronidation) metabolism (lorazepam, oxazepam, and temazepam) would interact in a similar manner.

Mechanism: The decrease in diazepam clearance would be consistent with the known ability of isoniazid to inhibit hepatic microsomal drug metabolism.

Recommendations: The reduction in diazepam clearance is small but may necessitate a decreased diazepam dosage in some patients.

References

1. Ochs, H.R., and others: Diazepam interaction with antituberculosis drugs, Clin. Pharmacol. Ther. **29:**671, 1981.
2. Ochs, H.R., and others: Interaction of triazolam with ethanol and isoniazid, Clin. Pharmacol. Ther. **33:**241, 1983.

Summary: Concurrent administration of diazepam and levodopa may result in a diminished antiparkinson effect of levodopa in selected parkinsonian patients.[1-3] Clinical data are insufficient to predict a dose-related effect. The occurrence of this interaction is infrequent and subject to large individual variability.

Related Drugs: Chlordiazepoxide and nitrazepam* have been reported both to antagonize[1,4-6] and to exert no effect[1] on levodopa. Flurazepam[7] and oxazepam[1] have been used concurrently with levodopa without causing any loss in antiparkinson activity. Because of the variations in response to different benzodiazepines, it is difficult to predict possible interactions of other benzodiazepines (e.g., clorazepate, lorazepam, triazolam [see Appendix]) with levodopa. Although not documented, levodopa-carbidopa (a combination product) may interact with benzodiazepines in a similar manner.

Mechanism: The mechanism of the interaction between the benzodiazepines and levodopa is not known. However, benzodiazepines are known to increase the brain's acetylcholine content,[8] thereby possibly antagonizing the beneficial dopamine-mediated response to levodopa.[9]

Recommendations: Clinical data about this drug interaction are insufficient to recommend avoiding the concurrent use of levodopa and benzodiazepines. However, one should be alert for evidence of worsening parkinsonism in patients previously stabilized on levodopa who are receiving this drug combination.

References

1. Hunter, K.R., and others: Use of levodopa with other drugs, Lancet **2**:1283, 1970.
2. Brogden, R.N., and others: Levodopa: a review of its pharmacological properties and therapeutic use with particular reference to parkinsonism, Drugs **2**:262, 1971.
3. Wodak, J., and others: Review of 12 months' treatment with levodopa in Parkinson's disease, with remarks on unusual side effects, Med. J. Aust. **2**:1277, 1972.
4. Mackie, L.: Drug antagonism, Br. Med. J. **2**:651, 1971.
5. Schwartz, G.A., and Fahn, S.: Newer medical treatments in Parkinsonism, Med. Clin. North Am. **54**:773, 1970.
6. Yosselson-Superstine, S., and Lipman, A.G.: Chlordiazepoxide interaction with levodopa, Ann. Intern. Med. **96**:259, 1982.
7. Kales, A., and others: Sleep in patients with Parkinson's disease and normal subjects prior to and following levodopa administration, Clin. Pharmacol. Ther. **12**:397, 1970.
8. Domino, E.F., and Wilson, A.E.: Psychotropic drug influences on brain acetylcholine utilization, Psychopharmacologia **25**:291, 1972.
9. Klawans, H., and others: Theoretical implications of the use of levodopa in Parkinsonism, Acta Neurol. Scand. **46**:409, 1970.

*Not available in the U.S.

Diazepam–Oral Contraceptive Agents

3

Summary: In one study involving 16 women, a single 10 mg dose of diazepam was given by intravenous infusion to 8 women not on oral contraceptives and 8 women who were taking oral contraceptives for at least 3 months. The mean diazepam clearance was 67% lower and the mean elimination half-life was 47% longer in the oral contraceptive users. There was no difference in percentage of unbound drug or volume of distribution between the 2 groups. The clinical result may be an increased effect of diazepam in patients receiving contraceptives.[1]

Related Drugs: In 1 study, the total clearance of chlordiazepoxide was lower and the elimination half-life was longer in users of oral contraceptives.[2] Other studies show oral contraceptives markedly impair clearance and prolong the half-life of diazepam or chlordiazepoxide, but statistical validation was lacking.[3,4] A similar interaction may be expected with the other benzodiazepines that undergo oxidative degradation (e.g., clorazepate, flurazepam, triazolam [see Appendix]). There are conflicting reports regarding an interaction between oral contraceptives and the benzodiazepines metabolized by glucuronidation (lorazepam, oxazepam, and temazepam). One study found their clearance to be greater in oral contraceptive users,[2] whereas another study showed no difference in metabolism.[5]

Mechanism: Because diazepam is oxidatively metabolized by the liver, it has been suggested that estrogens (a component of many oral contraceptives) may bind to cytochrome P-450 and decrease the amount of this hepatic oxidative drug-metabolizing enzyme system that is implicated in diazepam oxidation. This finding has been demonstrated in animals.[1]

Recommendations: Although a direct relation between the plasma concentration of diazepam and its clinical effect is not clearly established, patients who are taking oral contraceptives should be closely monitored for increased diazepam effects. A dosage adjustment may be necessary in some patients.[1]

References

1. Abernathy, D.R., and others: Impairment of diazepam metabolism by low-dose estrogen-containing oral-contraceptive steroids, N. Engl. J. Med. **306:**791, 1982.
2. Patwardhan, R.H., and others: Differential effects of oral contraceptive steroids on the metabolism of benzodiazepines, Hepatology **3:**248, 1983.
3. Roberts, R.K., and others: Disposition of chlordiazepoxide: sex differences and effects of oral contraceptives, Clin. Pharmacol. Ther. **25:**826, 1979.
4. Giles, H.G., and others: Disposition of intravenous diazepam in young men and women, Eur. J. Clin. Pharmacol. **20:**207, 1981.
5. Abernathy, D.R., and others: Lorazepam and oxazepam kinetics in women on low-dose oral contraceptives, Clin. Pharmacol. Ther. **33:**628, 1983.

Diazepam–Rifampin

3

Summary: In a study involving 7 patients with tuberculosis, the concurrent administration of diazepam with rifampin, isoniazid, and ethambutol resulted in a significantly shorter mean half-life and a 3-fold increase in clearance of diazepam as compared to control subjects. Diazepam volume of distribution and protein binding were nearly identical between both groups. Since isoniazid alone was shown to prolong the elimination half-life of diazepam (see Diazepam-Isoniazid, p. 446), and ethambutol alone did not significantly affect diazepam, it was concluded that rifampin caused the increased clearance and reduced half-life of diazepam.[1]

Related Drugs: The other benzodiazepines metabolized by phase I (N-demethylation or hydroxylation) reactions (e.g., chlordiazepoxide, flurazepam, triazolam [see Appendix]), as is diazepam, may be expected to similarly interact with rifampin if the mechanism involves induction of hepatic enzymes by rifampin; however, documentation is lacking. It has not been determined if the benzodiazepines dependent on phase II (glucuronidation) metabolism (lorazepam, oxazepam, and temazepam) would interact in a similar manner. There are no drugs related to rifampin.

Mechanism: Because rifampin is a known enzyme inducer, it has been postulated that the reduced half-life and increased clearance of diazepam result from induction of hepatic microsomal enzymes by rifampin.[1]

Recommendations: It has been suggested that patients receiving rifampin, either alone or in a drug combination, may have markedly enhanced diazepam clearance, and therefore may require higher doses of diazepam.[1]

Reference

1. Ochs, H.R., and others: Diazepam interaction with antituberculosis drugs, Clin. Pharmacol. Ther. **29:**671, 1981.

Fluphenazine–Clonidine

3

Summary: In 1 patient receiving clonidine and chlorthalidone, administration of fluphenazine led to acute organic brain syndrome (delirium, clouded consciousness, agitation, etc.) within 10 days. When clonidine was discontinued, the neurologic symptoms cleared within 72 hours. The symptoms reappeared when the patient was again administered clonidine.[1]

Related Drugs: There are no drugs related to clonidine. Other phenothiazines (e.g., chlorpromazine, mesoridazine, thioridazine [see Appendix]), the thioxanthenes (chlorprothixene and thiothixene), as well as the dibenzoxazepine (loxapine) and dihydroindolone (molindone) may interact in a similar manner because of pharmacologic similarity. A similar interaction did not occur in the patient described when haloperidol, a butyrophenone antipsychotic, was used.[1]

Mechanism: It has been postulated that clonidine, a potent alpha-adrenergic agonist, when combined with fluphenazine, a potent dopamine blocker, results in a relative adrenergic dominance.[1]

Recommendations: Since the discontinuation of clonidine caused the neurologic symptoms to disappear, this is the course of action suggested in patients developing such symptoms. In this patient, hydralazine was substituted for clonidine with no similar interaction.[1]

Reference

1. Allen, R.M., and Flemenbaum, A.: Delirium associated with combined fluphenazine-clonidine therapy, J. Clin. Psychiatry **40:**236, 1979.

Lithium Carbonate—Acetazolamide

1

Summary: One study involving 6 subjects showed that the concurrent use of a single dose of both lithium carbonate and acetazolamide caused a 27% to 31% increase in the urinary excretion of lithium.[1] In 1 case report, a patient recovered from lithium toxicity within a few hours after receiving acetazolamide, sodium bicarbonate, potassium chloride, and mannitol.[2]

Related Drugs: There is a lack of documentation regarding an interaction between lithium carbonate and the other carbonic anhydrase inhibitors (dichlorphenamide, ethoxzolamide, and methazolamide), although since they are pharmacologically related, a similar interaction may be expected to occur.

Mechanism: It has been postulated that acetazolamide increases the renal excretion of lithium, either by alkalinization of the urine or by impairing the proximal tubular reabsorption of lithium. Forced alkaline diuresis has been used to treat lithium intoxication.[3,4]

Recommendations: It is important to measure lithium serum levels during concurrent use of these agents. A higher dose of lithium carbonate may be necessary.

References

1. Thomsen, K., and Schou, M.: Renal lithium excretion in man, Am. J. Physiol. **215:**823, 1968.
2. Horowitz, L.C., and Fisher, G.V.: Acute lithium toxicity, N. Engl. J. Med. **281:**1369, 1969.
3. Forrest, J.: Forced alkaline diuresis for lithium intoxication, Postgrad. Med. J. **51:**189, 1975.
4. McSwiggan, C.: Interaction of lithium and bicarbonate, Med. J. Aust. **1:**38, 1978.

Lithium Carbonate–Carbamazepine

2

Summary: Three reports discuss the development of neurotoxicity during concurrent administration of lithium and carbamazepine.[1-3] In all of these cases the neurotoxicity developed despite normal therapeutic plasma levels of lithium and carbamazepine. Another report indicates that 3 patients with acute mania who were poorly controlled on lithium or carbamazepine therapy alone responded well to combination therapy with these agents without any signs of neurotoxicity.[4]

Related Drugs: There no drugs related to lithium carbonate or carbamazepine.

Mechanism: The mechanism is unknown. However, it has been suggested that lithium inhibits vasopressin-stimulated adenylcyclase causing the distal renal tubule to become insensitive to antidiuretic hormone (ADH). Carbamazepine has been reported to have a direct action on the renal tubule resulting in an increase in renal responsiveness to endogenous ADH. The increased incidence of neurotoxic symptoms may be related to the combined, mutual effect of the 2 agents on sodium metabolism.[2,5]

Recommendations: Although there is a substantial lack of clinical documentation of this interaction, 1 report cites that patients may take these agents together without ill effects.[4] However, close monitoring for neurotoxic symptoms (e.g., unsteady gait, ataxia, horizontal nystagmus, hyperflexia of the limbs, or occasional muscle fasiculation) may be necessary.

References

1. Chaudhry, R.P., and Waters, B.G.H.: Lithium and carbamazepine interaction: possible neurotoxicity, J. Clin. Psychiatry **44:**30, 1983.
2. Ghose, K.: Interaction between lithium and carbamazepine, Br. Med. J. **280:**1122, 1980.
3. A possible adverse carbamazepine–lithium carbonate interaction, Int. Drug Ther. Newsletter **17:**10, 1982.
4. Lipinski, J.R., and Pope, H.G.: Possible synergistic action between carbamazepine and lithium carbonate in the treatment of three acutely manic patients, Am. J. Psychiatry **139:**948, 1982.
5. Perucca, E., and Richens, A.: Interaction between lithium and carbamazepine, Br. Med. J. **280:**863, 1980.

Lithium Carbonate–Chlorothiazide

1

Summary: Concurrent administration of lithium carbonate and prolonged chlorothiazide therapy may result in enhanced cardiotoxicity and neurotoxicity because of lithium.[1-3]

Related Drugs: Any thiazide diuretic that promotes or enhances the excretion of both sodium and potassium could be expected to interact with lithium. Bendroflumethiazide and hydroflumethiazide have effects similar to chlorothiazide on sodium and potassium excretion and have been shown to decrease[1] or not increase lithium excretion.[2] Furosemide, chlorthalidone, and the combinations hydrochlorothiazide-triamterene and hydrochlorothiazide-amiloride have also been shown to increase lithium serum concentrations.[4-10] However, lithium serum concentrations were not affected to the same extent by furosemide as by hydrochlorothiazide.[11]

The following diuretics may be expected to interact with lithium in a similar manner: other loop diuretics (bumetanide and ethacrynic acid), the mercurial diuretic (mersalyl), other thiazides (e.g., benzthiazide, methyclothiazide, polythiazide [see Apendix]) and other thiazide related diuretics including chlorthalidone, quinethazone, metolazone, and indapamide. Spironolactone and triamterene, potassium-sparing diuretics, had no effect on lithium disposition.[12] Amiloride, also a potassium-sparing diuretic, was shown to increase the clearance of lithium in an animal study.[13]

Mechanism: Chlorothiazide causes diuresis by inhibiting renal tubular absorption of sodium and increasing the urinary excretion of chloride, sodium, potassium, and water.[3,14] Since lithium is primarily reabsorbed with sodium in the proximal renal tubule (which is not significantly affected by the thiazide diuretics) and very little is reabsorbed in the distal renal tubule (where the thiazide diuretics exert their main action), long-term thiazide administration may lead to an increase in the reabsorption of lithium and a subsequent decrease in lithium clearance. This may result in higher concentrations of lithium and cause lithium toxicity.[15-18] Chlorothiazide may increase lithium-induced intracellular depletion of potassium and may cause myocardial irritability and premature ventricular contractions.[18]

Recommendations: Although several studies have pointed out specific instances in which lithium and chlorothiazide are useful (e.g., lithium polyuria and lithium-induced nephrogenic diabetes insipidus) when given concurrently,[19-21] in general they should not be used together. If these drugs must be given simultaneously, the patient should be observed closely for signs and symptoms of lithium-induced neurotoxicity or cardiotoxicity, and a lower dose of lithium may be required. The potassium-sparing diuretics, spironolactone and triamterene, did not affect serum lithium concentrations in a small group of patients[12] and may be safer diuretics to use concurrently with lithium. Amiloride, another potassium-sparing diuretic, may also be considered.

References

1. Thomsen, K., and Shou, M.: Renal lithium excretion in man, Am. J. Physiol. **215:**823, 1968.
2. Petersen, V., and others: Effect of prolonged thiazide treatment on renal lithium clearance, Br. Med. J. **3:**143, 1974.
3. American Medical Association: AMA Drug Evaluations, Chicago, 1980, John Wiley & Sons.
4. Kerry, R.J., and others: Diuretics are dangerous with lithium, Br. Med. J. **281:**371, 1980.
5. Oh, T.E.: Frusemide and lithium toxicity, Anaesth. Intens. Care **5:**60, 1977.
6. Thornton, W.E., and Pray (Thornton), B.J.: Lithium intoxication: a report of two cases, Can. Psychiat. Assoc. J. **20:**281, 1975.
7. Hurtig, H.I., and Dyson, W.L.: Lithium toxicity enhanced by diuresis, N. Engl. J. Med. **290:**748, 1974.
8. Solomon, J.G.: Lithium toxicity precipitated by a diuretic, Psychosomatics **21:**425, 1980.
9. Mehta, B.R., and Robinson, B.H.B.: Lithium toxicity induced by triamterene-hydrochlorothiazide, Postgrad. Med. J. **56:**783, 1980.
10. Macfie, A.C.: Lithium poisoning precipitated by diuretics, Br. Med. J. **1:**516, 1975.
11. Jefferson, J.W., and Kalin, N.H.: Serum lithium levels and long term diuretic use, J.A.M.A. **241:**1134, 1979.
12. Baer, L., and others: Lithium metabolism: its electrolyte actions and relationship to aldosterone. In Williams, T.A., Katz, M.M., and Shield, J.A., editors: Recent advances in the psychobiology of the depressive illnesses, Washington, D.C., 1972, U. S. Government Printing Office.
13. Herrera, F.C.: Inhibition of lithium transport across toad bladder by amiloride, Am. J. Physiol. **222:**499, 1972.
14. Keynes, R.D., and Swan, R.C.: The permeability of frog muscle fibers to lithium ions, J. Physiol. **147:**626, 1959.
15. Demers, R.G., and Heninger, G.R.: Sodium intake and lithium treatment in mania, Am. J. Psychiatry **128:**100, 1971.
16. Singer, I., and Rotenberg, D.: Mechanisms of lithium action, N. Engl. J. Med. **289:**254, 1973.
17. Schou, M., and others: Pharmacological and clinical problems of lithium prophylaxis, Br. J. Psychiatry **116:**615, 1970.
18. Shopsin, B., and Gershon, S.: Pharmacology-toxicology of the lithium ion. In Gershon, S., and Shopsin, B., editors: Lithium its role in psychiatric research and treatment. New York, 1973, Plenum Press.
19. Himmelhoch, J.M., and others: Thiazide-lithium synergy in refractory mood swings, Am. J. Psychiatry **134:**149, 1977.
20. MacNeil, S., and others: Diuretics during lithium therapy, Lancet **1:**1295, 1975.
21. Himmelhoch, J.M., and others: Adjustment of lithium dose during lithium-chlorothiazide therapy, Clin. Pharmacol. Ther. **22:**225, 1977.

Lithium Carbonate–Diazepam

3

Summary: The concurrent use of lithium carbonate and diazepam may result in hypothermia as evidenced by a single case report.[1] When either drug was given alone, hypothermia did not occur.

Related Drugs: There is no documentation regarding a similar interaction between lithium carbonate and the other benzodiazepines (e.g., chlordiazepoxide, flurazepam, triazolam [see Appendix]). There are no drugs related to lithium carbonate.

Mechanism: The mechanism of this interaction is unknown.

Recommendations: Until further studies are done, the concurrent use of these agents need not be avoided. However, if hypothermia occurs, one or both drugs may need to be discontinued.

Reference

1. Naylor, G.J., and others: Profound hypothermia on combined lithium carbonate and diazepam treatment, Br. Med. J. **2**:22, 1977.

Lithium Carbonate–Haloperidol

Summary: Concomitant administration of lithium carbonate and haloperidol has been reported to cause a wide variety of encephalopathic symptoms (lethargy, fever, tremulousness, confusion, and extrapyramidal and cerebellar dysfunction) and in some cases, permanent brain damage or irreversible dyskinesias have resulted.[1-11] Many of the patients who experienced these symptoms had serum lithium levels within the therapeutic range. In other reports it was found that no adverse symptoms developed when both agents were coadministered or that the symptoms were the same when either agent was given alone.[12-16]

Related Drugs: There are no drugs related to lithium carbonate. The interactions between lithium carbonate and other antipsychotics are discussed in other monographs (see Chlorpromazine–Lithium Carbonate, p. 438; and Lithium Carbonate–Thioridazine, p. 467).

Mechanism: The mechanism is not known. Neurologic side effects of lithium or haloperidol are not infrequent. However, the side effects reported in some patients on concomitant therapy suggest a potentiation of the expected additive neurotoxic symptoms seen with either agent alone. It has also been suggested that this interaction is dose related.[1] Other explanations have been offered[17] but not scientifically investigated. Further, the absence of standardized sampling for monitoring lithium serum concentrations may mask what is simply lithium intoxication.[18]

Recommendations: Lithium's onset of action occurs several days after therapy is begun.[12] Therefore, haloperidol is usually added during the acute manic phase and then its dose is tapered and finally discontinued.[13] It is preferable to avoid using these agents together during the acute manic phase since there is a higher risk of combined toxicity at that time.[4,7] If this combination of drugs is to be used during the acute manic symptoms, conservative lithium dosage is recommended.

References

1. Cohen, W.J., and Cohen, N.H.: Lithium carbonate, haloperidol and irreversible brain damage, J.A.M.A. **230:**1283, 1974.
2. Thomas, C., and others: Lithium/haloperidol combinations and brain damage, Lancet **1:**626, 1982.
3. Strayhorn, J.M., and Nash, J.L.: Severe neurotoxicity despite "therapeutic" serum lithium levels, Dis. Nerv. Syst. **38:**107, 1977.
4. Spring, G., and Frankel, M.: New data on lithium and haloperidol, Am. J. Psychiatry **138:**818, 1981.
5. Louden, J.B., and Waring, H.: Toxic reactions to lithium and haloperidol, Lancet **2:**1088, 1976.
6. Coffey, C.E., and Ross, D.R.: Treatment of lithium/neuroleptic neurotoxicity during lithium maintenance, Am. J. Psychiatry **137:**736, 1980.
7. Thornton, W.E., and Pray, B.J.: Lithium intoxication: a report of two cases, Can. Psychiat. Assoc. J. **20:**281, 1975.
8. Prakash, R., and others: Neurotoxicity in patients with schizophrenia during lithium therapy, Compr. Psychiatry **23:**271, 1982.
9. Prakash, R.: Lithium-haloperidol combination and brain damage, Lancet **1:**1468, 1982.

10. Prakash, R., and others: Neurotoxicity with combined administration of lithium and a neuroleptic, Compr. Psychiatry **23:**567, 1982.

11. Kamlana, S.H., and others: Lithium: some drug interactions, Practitioner **224:**1291, 1980.

12. Carman, J.S., and others: Lithium combined with neuroleptics in chronic schizophrenic and schizoaffective patients, J. Clin. Psychiatry **42:**124, 1981.

13. Juhl, R.P., and others: Concomitant administration of haloperidol and lithium carbonate in acute mania, Dis. Nerv. Sys. **38:**675, 1977.

14. Baastrup, P., and others: Adverse reactions in treatment with lithium carbonate and haloperidol, J.A.M.A. **236:**2645, 1976.

15. Biederman, J., and others: Combination of lithium carbonate and haloperidol in schizoaffective disorder, Arch. Gen. Psychiatry **36:**327, 1979.

16. Growe, G.A., and others: Lithium in chronic schizophrenia, Am. J. Psychiatry **136:**454, 1979.

17. Silverman, G.: Lithium/haloperidol combination and brain damage, Lancet **1:**856, 1982.

18. Amdisen, A.: Lithium and drug interactions, Drugs **24:**133, 1982.

Lithium Carbonate–Indomethacin

2

Summary: Increased plasma lithium concentrations have been observed when indomethacin and lithium carbonate are administered simultaneously.[1-5] One study noted an average increase of 59% in plasma lithium concentrations in 3 psychiatric patients and 30% in normal volunteers,[1] whereas a second study reported an increase of 61% in 6 psychiatric patients.[2] Lithium toxicity characterized by polyuria, delirium, muscular weakness, gastrointestinal symptoms, lethargy, and tremor resulting from this combination has been observed.[1,2,5]

Related Drugs: Reports of other nonsteroidal anti-inflammatory agents including ibuprofen,[2,3] diclofenac,[6,7] piroxicam,[8] and phenylbutazone[2,7] show similar elevations in lithium concentrations. Other nonsteroidal anti-inflammatory agents (e.g., naproxen, sulindac, tolmetin [see Appendix]) might be expected to exhibit a similar interaction with lithium carbonate since they may all inhibit prostaglandins to some extent.

Mechanism: Prostaglandins may play an important role in renal lithium clearance.[3-6] Concurrent administration of nonsteroidal anti-inflammatory agents (prostaglandin synthesis inhibitors) with lithium reduces renal lithium clearance,[1,3,5-7] causing an increase in plasma lithium concentration. Enhanced renal reabsorption of lithium induced by indomethacin is another possible explanation for the elevated lithium concentrations.[1]

Recommendations: Careful consideration should precede the decision to use these drugs simultaneously since lithium carbonate has a narrow therapeutic range and symptoms of toxicity may result from the increased plasma lithium concentration. If nonsteroidal anti-inflammatory agents are started in lithium treated patients, careful patient monitoring and possible lithium dosage adjustment should be made to prevent lithium intoxication.

References

1. Frolich, J.C., and others: Indomethacin increases plasma lithium, Br. Med. J. **1:**1115, 1979.
2. Ragheb, M., and others: Interaction of indomethacin and ibuprofen with lithium in manic patients under a steady-state lithium level, J. Clin. Psychiatry **41:**397, 1980.
3. Leftwich, R.B., and others: Inhibition of prostaglandin synthesis increases plasma lithium levels, Clin. Res. **26:**291A, 1978.
4. Reiman, I.W., and others: Indomethacin but not aspirin increases plasma lithium ion levels, Arch. Gen. Psychiatry **40:**283, 1983.
5. Herschberg, S.N., and Sierles, F.S.: Indomethacin-induced lithium toxicity, Am. Fam. Physician **28:**155, 1983.
6. Reimann, I.W.: Risks of nonsteroidal anti-inflammatory drug therapy in lithium treated patients, Naunyn-Schiedeberg's Arch. Pharmacol. **311:**R75, 1980.
7. Reimann, I.W., and Frolich, J.C.: Effects of diclofenac on lithium kinetics, Clin. Pharmacol. Ther. **30:**348, 1981.
8. Kerry, R.J., and others: Possible toxic interaction between lithium and piroxicam, Lancet **1:**418, 1983.

Lithium Carbonate–Mazindol

2

Summary: Apparent lithium intoxication has been observed in 1 case where lithium carbonate and mazindol were administered simultaneously.[1] Signs of intoxication began 3 days after the initiation of mazindol therapy, and the serum lithium concentration rose to 3.2 mmol/L within 9 days after remaining in a therapeutic range of 0.4 to 1.3 mmol/L for 15 months. Complete recovery followed the discontinuation of mazindol and the serum lithium concentration returned to normal.[1]

Related Drugs: Other anorexic agents (e.g., benzphetamine, diethylpropion, phentermine, [see Appendix]) should be used cautiously, since a reduction in caloric/sodium intake may precipitate lithium toxicity. There are no drugs related to lithium carbonate.

Mechanism: The exact mechanism of this interaction is unknown. It is thought that lithium is treated as if it were sodium in the kidney.[2] In the case of negative sodium balance, a compensatory increase in sodium (hence lithium) reabsorption occurs, resulting in decreased lithium clearance.[2] Dieting and the resultant decrease in sodium intake have been shown to induce lithium intoxications in a separate case.[3] It is suggested that the anorexic activity of mazindol was the cause of the rise in serum lithium concentration that lead to symptoms of toxicity.[1]

Recommendations: When an anorexic agent such as mazindol is used concurrently with lithium therapy, care should be taken to assure that sodium intake remains adequate so that increased serum lithium concentrations and possible toxicity are avoided. It may be necessary to lower the dose of lithium during concurrent administration of mazindol.

References

1. Hendy, M.S., and others: Mazindol-induced lithium toxicity, Br. Med. J. **280:**684, 1980.
2. Amdisen, A.: Lithium and drug interaction, Drugs **24:**133, 1982.
3. Furlong, F.W.: Lithium toxicity occurring with a "reducing" diet, Can. Psychiat. Assoc. J. **18:**75, 1973.

Lithium Carbonate–Methyldopa

3

Summary: The concurrent use of lithium carbonate and methyldopa may result in signs of lithium toxicity (sluggishness, hand tremor, etc.) in the presence of therapeutic serum lithium levels as evidenced by several case studies.[1-5]

Related Drugs: There are no drugs related to lithium carbonate or methyldopa.

Mechanism: The mechanism of this interaction is unknown. However, it has been suggested that methyldopa exacerbates the central nervous system response to lithium or perhaps increase the brain uptake of lithium.[1]

Recommendations: Further studies are needed to clarify the interaction between these agents. If symptoms of lithium toxicity occur during concurrent use of these agents, the dose of lithium may need to be decreased or methyldopa may have to be discontinued.

References

1. Osanloo, E., and Deglin, J.H.: Interaction of lithium and methyldopa, Ann. Intern. Med. **92:**433, 1980.
2. Byrd, G.J.: Methyldopa and lithium carbonate: suspected interaction, J.A.M.A. **233:**320, 1975.
3. O'Regan, J.B.: Adverse interaction of lithium carbonate and methyldopa, Can. Med. Assoc. J. **115:**385, 1976.
4. Byrd, G.J.: Lithium carbonate and methyldopa interaction, Clin. Toxicol. **11:**1, 1977.
5. Walker, N., and others: Lithium-methyldopa interaction in normal subjects, Drug Intell. Clin. Pharm. **14:**638, 1980.

Lithium Carbonate–Metoprolol

Summary: In 2 patients with a history of bronchospastic disease, the use of metoprolol produced objective and subjective improvement of lithium carbonate–induced tremors.[1]

Related Drugs: Propranolol has been reported to be effective in reducing lithium tremor,[2,3] but is contraindicated in patients with a history of bronchospastic disease. Another nonselective beta blocking agent, pindolol, has also proved to be useful.[4,5] Although documentation is lacking, a similar interaction may be expected to occur with the other noncardioselective beta-blocking agents (nadolol and timolol); however, these agents would also be contraindicated in bronchospastic patients. The other cardioselective beta-blocking agent (atenolol) would be expected to behave similarly to metoprolol.

Mechanism: The mechanism of this interaction is not fully known, however both $beta_1$ and $beta_2$ receptors have been implicated in essential tremor.[5] Whether both receptors are involved in lithium-induced tremor is not yet known.[1]

Recommendations: Because all beta-blocking agents can improve lithium-induced tremors, it is advisable to use a cardioselective agent such as metoprolol in patients with bronchospastic problems.

References

1. Gaby, N.S., and others: Treatment of lithium tremor with metoprolol, Am. J. Psychiatriy **140:**593, 1938.
2. Kirk, L., and others: Propranolol treatment of lithium induced tremor, Lancet **2:**1086, 1973.
3. LaPierre, Y.D.: Control of lithium tremor with propranolol, Can. Med. Assoc. J. **114:**619, 1976.
4. Floru, L., and others: Die behandlung des lithium tremors mit dem beta-rezeptorenblocker pindolol, Int. Pharmacopsychiatry **14:**149, 1979.
5. Larsen, T.A., and Teravainen, H.: Beta-blockers in essential tremor, Lancet **2:**533, 1981.

Lithium Carbonate–Norepinephrine

3

Summary: Lithium carbonate decreased the pressor response to norepinephrine in 7 of 8 patients in 1 study.[1] In another study, patients showed decreased norepinephrine sensitivity after lithium carbonate treatment.[2]

Related Drugs: A similar interaction may be expected between lithium carbonate and the other direct acting sympathomimetics (e.g., dobutamine, epinephrine, methoxamine [see Appendix]) based on pharmacologic similarity. Patients showed decreased sensitivity to phenylephrine, a mixed acting sympathomimetic, in 1 study.[2] Documentation is lacking regarding a similar interaction with the other mixed acting sympathomimetics (dopamine and metaraminol). The response to tyramine, an indirect acting sympathomimetic, was not altered by lithium carbonate in 2 studies.[1,2] There is no documentation regarding a similar interaction between lithium carbonate and the other indirect acting sympathomimetics (e.g., amphetamine, ephedrine, methylphenidate [see Appendix]). However, these indirect acting sympathomimetics, or anorexic agents, have been reported to increase lithium levels (see Lithium Carbonate–Mazindol, p. 459). There are no drugs related to lithium carbonate.

Mechanism: The mechanism of this interaction is unknown.

Recommendations: If a patient on lithium carbonate is to receive norepinephrine, a higher dose of norepinephrine may be necessary to achieve the desired pressor response.

References

1. Fann, W.E., and others: Effects of lithium on adrenergic function in man, Clin. Pharmacol. Ther. **13:**71, 1972.
2. Ghose, K.: Assessment of peripheral adrenergic activity and its interaction with drugs in man, Eur. J. Clin. Pharmacol. **17:**233, 1980.

Lithium Carbonate–Phenytoin

3

Summary: There have been reports of patients experiencing symptoms of lithium toxicity (e.g., polyuria, polydipsia, tremor, and reduced free thyroxine index) during concomitant therapy with phenytoin. In 1 case[1] lithium toxicity occurred when the serum levels of lithium and phenytoin were within the therapeutic range. The discontinuation of phenytoin and substitution with carbamazepine reversed the clinical signs of lithium toxicity. In another case,[2] a patient stabilized on phenytoin and having lithium carbonate initiated into the regimen (1200 mg/day for 3 days), developed an ataxic gait but no other signs of lithium toxicity. The serum lithium level was reported to be 2.0 mEq/L. After all medications were stopped for 48 hours, the patient was no longer ataxic. Another report stated[3] that the combined therapy resulted in neurologic signs of lithium toxicity despite normal therapeutic levels of lithium. When lithium therapy was discontinued, neurologic symptoms reversed.

Related Drugs: There is a lack of documentation regarding an interaction between lithium and the other hydantoin derivatives (ethotoin and mephenytoin). There are no drugs related to lithium carbonate.

Mechanism: The mechanism of this interaction is unknown.

Recommendations: Until further documentation is available, patients receiving concurrent therapy of lithium and phenytoin should be observed for clinical signs of lithium toxicity. Since toxicity has been reported in the presence of normal therapeutic levels, therapy should be closely supervised and dosing adjustments of lithium may be required.

References

1. MacCallum, W.A.G: Interaction of lithium and phenytoin, Br. Med. J. **280:**610, 1980.
2. Salem, R.B. and others: Ataxia as the primary symptom of lithium toxicity, Drug Intell. Clin. Pharm. **14:**622, 1980.
3. Spiers, J. and Hirsch, S.R.: Lithium toxicity with normal serum concentrations, Br. Med. J. **1:**815, 1978.

Lithium Carbonate–Potassium Iodide

2

Summary: The concurrent administration of lithium carbonate and potassium iodide or other iodine containing compounds may enhance the hypothyroid and goiterogenic effects of either drug.[1-4]

Related Drugs: A possible interaction of lithium carbonate and isopropamide iodide has been reported.[5] Although documentation in the literature is lacking, lithium carbonate could interact with calcium iodate, calcium iodide, hydriodic acid, iodinated glycerol, and sodium iodide. All nonprescription and radiographic products containing iodine may also enhance lithium's antithyroid effects. There are no drugs related to lithium carbonate.

Mechanism: Exogenous iodine given to either animals or humans inhibits thyroid hormone synthesis.[6] Lithium accumulates in the thyroid gland[7,8] and is capable of blocking thyroidal release of liothyronine and thyroxine.[9] Both iodine[10] and lithium[7] have been shown to produce hypothyroidism; therefore, concurrent use of these compounds could have additive or synergistic hypothyroid effects.[11]

Recommendations: Patients receiving lithium carbonate should avoid taking nonprescription or prescription iodine containing preparations. The appearance of goiter or detection of abnormal chemical thyroid tests is not an indication to discontinue lithium therapy. However, it is appropriate to discontinue any iodine-containing drugs and to stabilize thyroid status with appropriate drugs.[12]

References

1. Shopsin, B., and others: Iodine and lithium-induced hypothyrodism, Am. J. Med. **55:**695, 1973.
2. Jorgensen, J.V., and others: Possible synergism between iodine and lithium carbonate, J.A.M.A. **223:**192, 1973.
3. Shopsin, B., and Gershon, S.: Pharmacology-toxicity of the lithium ion. In Gershon, S., and Shopsin, B., editors: Lithium: its role in psychiatric research and treatment. New York, 1973, Plenum Press.
4. Spaulding, S.W., and others: Effect of increased iodide intake on thyroid function in subjects on chronic lithium therapy, Acta Endocrinol. **84:**290, 1977.
5. Luby, E.D., and others: Lithium-carbonate-induced myxedema, J.A.M.A. **218:**1298, 1971.
6. Wolff, J., and Chaikoff, I.L.: Plasma inorganic iodide as a homeostatic regulator of thyroid function, J. Biol. Chem. **174:**555, 1948.
7. Shopsin, B., and others: Lithium-induced thyroid distrubance: case report and review, Compr. Psychiatry **10:**215, 1969.
8. Berens, S.C., and others: Lithium concentration by the thyroid, Endocrinology **87:**1085, 1970.
9. Berens, S.C., and others: Antithyroid effects of lithium, J. Clin. Invest. **49:**1357, 1970.
10. Paris, J., and others: Iodide goiter, J. Clin. Endocrinol. Metab. **20:**57, 1960.
11. Wiener, J.D.: Lithium carbonate-induced myxedema (letter), J.A.M.A. **220:**587, 1972.
12. Shopsin, B., and others: Triiodothyronine and thryoid-stimulating hormone response to thyrotropin-releasing hormone: newer aspects of lithium-induced thryoid disturbances in man. In Prange, A.J., editor: The thyroid axis, drugs, and behavior. New York, 1974, Raven Press.

Lithium Carbonate–Tetracycline

2

Summary: The concurrent administration of lithium carbonate and tetracycline may cause serum concentrations of lithium to increase and may lead to lithium toxicity. A woman stabilized on lithium carbonate demonstrated a significant rise in lithium serum concentrations when tetracycline (long-acting capsules) was added to her regimen. The patient showed slight drowsiness, slurred speech, tremor in both hands, and became very thirsty. Symptoms disappeared when both drugs were discontinued and lithium levels returned to normal.[1]

Related Drugs: Documentation is lacking regarding a similar interaction between lithium carbonate and the other tetracyclines (e.g., doxycycline, minocycline, oxytetracycline [see Appendix]).

Mechanism: The mechanism of this interaction is unknown. Tetracycline has been known to produce anorexia, nausea, vomiting, sodium diuresis, and polyuria in subjects who already have renal insufficiency and this drug may sometimes have a nephrotoxic effect. Lithium may cause diabetes insipidus and negative sodium balance. The fact that the tetracycline was in a sustained release form may also have been important.[1]

Recommendations: Caution should be used when concurrently administering lithium and tetracycline since the possibility of tetracycline-induced nephrotoxicity does exist. Serum lithium concentrations should be determined routinely, since the dose may need to be decreased.

Reference

1. McGennis, A.J.: Lithium carbonate and tetracycline interaction, Br. Med. J. **1:**1183, 1978.

Lithium Carbonate–Theophylline

2

Summary: In a case report, reduced lithium levels as well as worsening of manic symptoms occurred after increasing doses of theophylline were administered.[1]

Related Drugs: It has been shown that aminophylline increases the lithium/creatinine clearance ratio, which may result in decreased serum lithium below the therapeutic level.[2] A similar interaction may be expected between lithium carbonate and the other theophylline derivatives (dyphylline and oxtriphylline) because of pharmacologic similarity. There are no drugs related to lithium carbonate.

Mechanism: The mechanism of this interaction is related to an increase in the renal excretion of lithium by the theophylline derivative.

Recommendations: Patients' lithium levels and therapeutic response should be closely monitored during concurrent theophylline therapy because a higher dose of lithium carbonate may be required.

References

1. Sieles, F.S., and others: Concurrent use of theophylline and lithium in a patient with chronic obstructive lung disease and bipolar disorder, Am. J. Psychiatry **139:**117, 1982.
2. Thomsen, K., and Schou, M.: Renal lithium excretion in man, Am. J. Physiol. **215:**823, 1968.

Lithium Carbonate–Thioridazine

2

Summary: Neurotoxic symptoms (confusion, delirium, seizures, encephalopathy, and abnormal EEG) and somnambulistic episodes have been observed in patients simultaneously receiving lithium carbonate and thioridazine.[1-4] The episodes generally occurred early in combined therapy and with therapeutic doses of each agent. The symptoms were reversible and disappeared when 1 agent was discontinued or the dosage reduced.

Related Drugs: Neurotoxic or somnambulistic episodes have also been reported when lithium was coadministered with thiothixene,[3,4] fluphenazine,[1,4-6] perphenazine,[4,7] and chlorpromazine[4] (see Chlorpromazine–Lithium Carbonate, p. 438). However, it was not clearly established that these symptoms resulted solely from the concomitant use of both agents as compared to either agent alone. Other phenothiazines (e.g., mesoridazine, promazine, trifluoperazine [see Appendix]), the other thioxanthene (chlorprothixene), as well as the dihydroindolone (molindone) and dibenzoxazepine (loxapine), may interact similarly with lithium since they are pharmacologically related, although this has not been specifically documented. Haloperidol, an antipsychotic pharmacologically but not structurally related to the phenothiazines can also interact with lithium carbonate (see Lithium Carbonate–Haloperidol, p. 456). There are no drugs related to lithium carbonate.

Mechanism: The mechanisms responsible for these interactions are not known, yet several have been postulated. The neurotoxicity-type symptoms may be a potentiation[2] or a pharmacologic summation[5] of the antipsychotic agent and lithium. However, it has been argued that the absence of a standardized lithium monitoring schedule may have masked what was simply lithium intoxication.[8]

Recommendations: Plasma level monitoring of either agent is of questionable value since many patients experienced neurotoxic symptoms with plasma concentrations within the therapeutic range. Routine EEG monitoring may aid in the detection or prevention of neurotoxicity; however, it is recommended that therapy be based on the total clinical picture. Conservative use of both agents is warranted, and dosage adjustments of one or both agents may be necessary. If possible, it would be preferable to use only 1 agent.

References

1. Spring, G.K.: EEG observations in confirming neurotoxicity, Am. J. Psychiatry **136:**1099, 1979.
2. Spring, G.K.: Neurotoxicity with combined use of lithium and thioridazine, J. Clin. Psychiatry **40:**135, 1979.
3. Prakash, R., and others: Neurotoxicity in patients with schizophrenia during lithium therapy, Compr. Psychiatry **23:**271, 1982.
4. Charney, D.S., and others: Somnambulistic-like episodes secondary to combined lithium-neuroleptic treatment, Br. J. Psychiatry **135:**418, 1979.
5. Kamlana, S.H., and others: Lithium: some drug interactions, Practitioner **224:**1291, 1980.
6. Singh, S.V.: Lithium carbonate/fluphenazine deconate producing irreversible brain damage, Lancet **2:**278, 1982.
7. Thornton, W.E., and Pray, B.J.: Lithium intoxication: a report of two cases, Can. Psychiat. Assoc. J. **20:**281, 1975.
8. Amdisen, A.: Lithium and drug interactions, Drugs **24:**133, 1982.

Perphenazine–Disulfiram

3

Summary: In a case study, a patient previously maintained on oral perphenazine started therapy with disulfiram. The plasma perphenazine concentration became subtherapeutic and the concentration of the sulfoxide metabolite of perphenazine (pharmacologically inactive) was increased. The dose of perphenazine was increased without improvement of the psychotic symptoms. The route of administration was changed to intramuscular, resulting in a substantial clinical improvement. The plasma perphenazine levels increased and the metabolite concentration fell sharply.[1]

Related Drugs: Documentation is lacking regarding an interaction between disulfiram and the other phenothiazines (e.g., chlorpromazine, thioridazine, triflupromazine [see Appendix]), the thioxanthenes (chlorprothixene and thiothixene), as well as the butyrophenone (haloperidol), dihydroindolone (molindone), and the dibenzoxazepine (loxapine), although based on similar metabolic fates a similar interaction may be expected to occur. There are no drugs related to disulfiram.

Mechanism: It has been suggested that disulfiram activates the liver enzymes to such an extent that oral perphenazine is biotransformed to inactive metabolites. Parenteral administration appears to avoid the first-pass metabolic effect in the liver.[1]

Recommendations: Patients receiving oral perphenazine and disulfiram concurrently should be observed for exacerbated psychotic symptoms. If these symptoms appear, disulfiram may need to be discontinued since increasing the dose of perphenazine failed to control the symptoms.[1] Alternatively, the parenteral use of perphenazine may avoid this interaction.[1]

Reference

1. Hansen, L.B., and Larsen, N.E.: Metabolic interaction between perphenazine and disulfiram, Lancet **2:**1472, 1982.

CHAPTER ELEVEN

Beta–Adrenergic Blocking Agents' Drug Interactions

TABLE 11. Beta-adrenergic Blocking Agents' Drug Interactions

Drug Interaction	Significance Code	Potential Effects	Recommendations	See Page
Atenolol– Ampicillin	3	Some pharmacokinetic parameters of atenolol may be significantly reduced after a single oral dose of ampicillin. Exercise-induced tachycardia may be higher after a single ampicillin dose, although atenolol's antihypertensive effects seem unaffected by 4 weeks of concurrent ampicillin.	Monitor for loss of atenolol's therapeutic effect and increase the dosage if needed.	473
Atenolol– Calcium Carbonate	3	Calcium carbonate may reduce peak plasma concentration and area-under-curve of atenolol, but the elimination half-life may be prolonged. Reduction in beta blockade is shown after 12 hours, but blood pressure response does not significantly change over a 4 week period.	Monitor response to atenolol and adjust the dosage if needed.	474
Metoprolol– Oral Contraceptive Agents	2	Oral contraceptives may increase the effects of metoprolol as indicated by an increased metoprolol area-under-curve.	Reduced metoprolol dosage may be required, or another form of contraception or a noninteracting beta-blocking agent (e.g., atenolol) may be used.	475
Metoprolol– Pentobarbital	2	Pentobarbital reduced oral metoprolol bioavailability approximately 30% in 1 study.	Metoprolol dosage may need to be increased. Alternatively a beta blocker not dependent on hepatic first pass metabolism (e.g., atenolol) may be used.	476
Metoprolol– Rifampin	2	Rifampin reduced metoprolol area-under-curve, which may cause some loss of beta blockade.	Monitor blood pressure carefully and increase the metoprolol dosage if needed.	478
Propranolol– Alcohol, Ethyl	3	Alcohol may increase the elimination and maximum plasma concentration and diminish the antihypertensive effects of propranolol.	As alcohol alone may lead to angina and tachycardia, and concomitant propranolol may potentiate these effects because of decreased levels, patients should be cautioned about ingesting alcohol during therapy.	479
Propranolol– Aluminum Hydroxide	3	Aluminum hydroxide gel decreases propranolol bioavailability. The clinical significance has not been determined.	Advise patients to avoid antacid preparations containing aluminum hydroxide or to separate the dosages by as much time as possible.	480

TABLE 11. Beta-adrenergic Blocking Agents' Drug Interactions—cont'd

Drug Interaction	Significance Code	Potential Effects	Recommendations	See Page
Propranolol– Chlorphenﾂiramﾂine	4	Chlorpheniramine could theoretically antagonize the beta-adrenergic blocking action of propranolol. No data are available to support this possibility.	Concurrent use need not be avoided; however, the possibility of an interaction should be considered.	481
Propranolol– Chlorpromaﾂzine	2	Concurrent use may significantly increase propranolol bioavailability resulting in enhanced pharmacologic activity. Chlorpromazine levels may also increase.	The dose of either agent may need to be lowered.	482
Propranolol– Cimetidine	1	Propranolol plasma concentrations increase 2-fold within 24-28 hours after initiating concomitant cimetidine.	The dosage of either agent may need to be reduced. Ranitidine or a noninteracting beta blocker (e.g., atenolol) may be suitable alternatives.	483
Propranolol– Desipramine	3	The anticholinergic activity of desipramine may theoretically antagonize the myocardial effects of propranolol, although clinical evidence has not been established.	Concurrent use need not be avoided, but precautions appropriate to individual use of these agents should be observed.	485
Propranolol– Epinephrine	1	Propranolol blocks the beta-adrenergic agonist effects of epinephrine and allows unopposed alpha-adrenergic stimulation, causing vasoconstriction that may produce hypertension and bradycardia.	If possible, epinephrine should be avoided in patients receiving nonselective beta blockers, or a cardioselective beta-blocking agent should be used.	486
Propranolol– Ergotamine	3	Concurrent use has resulted in peripheral vasoconstriction, exacerbations of migraine headache, or effective and uneventful use.	The ergotamine dosage may need to be reduced in some patients.	488
Propranolol– Furosemide	2	Furosemide raises propranolol blood levels, which may be accompanied by an increased beta blockade.	Concomitant use need not be avoided. However, monitor patients and adjust dosages of either agent if necessary.	489
Propranolol– Hydralazine	3	Hydralazine significantly increases propranolol bioavailability in normotensive subjects, and the antihypertensive effect of hydralazine is enhanced.	Monitor propranolol levels and decrease the dosage if needed.	490
Propranolol– Indomethacin	2	Indomethacin can reduce the hypotensive effects of propranolol. Blood pressure returns to basal levels after the discontinuation of indomethacin.	Monitor blood pressure closely, and increase propranolol dosage or discontinue indomethacin if needed.	491

471

TABLE 11. Beta-adrenergic Blocking Agents' Drug Interactions—cont'd

Drug Interaction	Significance Code	Potential Effects	Recommendations	See Page
Propranolol–Quinidine	3	Concurrent use may be beneficial in certain patients for converting atrial fibrillation to normal sinus rhythm.	Smaller doses of each drug may be used. This combination may be used for several types of arrhythmias.	492
Propranolol–Thyroid	2	Patients taking thyroid may show a decreased bioavailability of propranolol if the patient is in the hyperthyroid state, although reports are conflicting.	Propranolol dosage may need to be increased, or a noninteracting beta blocker (e.g., atenolol) may be used.	493
Propranolol–Tobacco	2	Propranolol metabolism is significantly induced in smokers, leading to reduced steady-state serum concentrations and increased clearance of propranolol. This effect is greatest in younger patients and diminished in older subjects.	Higher propranolol dosages may be required for smokers. Propranolol dosage may need to be reduced in patients who quit smoking.	494

Atenolol–Ampicillin

3

Summary: In a study involving 6 healthy subjects, some of the pharmacokinetic parameters of atenolol were significantly reduced after a single oral dose of ampicillin, including bioavailability (24% decrease), peak plasma levels (33% decrease), area-under-curve (41% decrease) and steady-state levels (41% decrease). These parameters were further reduced after 6 days of ampicillin treatment. The antihypertensive effects of atenolol seemed unaffected by concurrent ampicillin over a 4 week period in 6 hypertensive patients; however, exercise-induced tachycardia was significantly higher after single doses of each agent in the same 6 patients.[1]

Related Drugs: Documentation is lacking regarding a similar interaction between the other beta-blocking agents (e.g., metoprolol, pindolol, propranolol [see Appendix]) and the other penicillins (e.g., amoxicillin, bacampicillin, hetacillin [see Appendix]).

Mechanism: The mechanism of this interaction is unknown.

Recommendations: Patients should be monitored for a loss of therapeutic effect when atenolol and ampicillin are used concurrently. The dose of atenolol may need to be increased.

Reference

1. Schafer-Korting, M., and others: Atenolol interaction with aspirin, allopurinol, and ampicillin, Clin. Pharmacol. Ther. **33:**283, 1983.

Atenolol–Calcium Carbonate

3

Summary: After the administration of calcium carbonate to 6 patients on atenolol, there was a 51% reduction in the peak plasma concentration of atenolol and a one-third decrease in the atenolol area-under-curve. The elimination half-life, however, was prolonged. A reduction in beta-blockade was demonstrated after 12 hours, but blood pressure response did not significantly change over a 4 week period with atenolol alone or atenolol plus calcium.[1]

Related Drugs: A similar interaction would be expected with the other calcium salts (e.g., gluconate, lactate, phosphate). There is no documentation regarding a similar interaction with the other beta-blocking agents (e.g., nadolol, pindolol, propranolol [see Appendix]).

Mechanism: It has been suggested that the gastrointestinal absorption of atenolol is impaired by calcium salts, although other mechanisms possibly exist.[1]

Recommendations: The patient's response to atenolol should be monitored during administration of concurrent calcium salts, and the atenolol dose may need to be adjusted.

Reference

1. Kirch, W., and others: Interaction of atenolol with furosemide and calcium and aluminum salts, Clin. Pharmacol. Ther. **30:**429, 1981.

Metoprolol–Oral Contraceptive Agents

2

Summary: Metoprolol was administered to 23 female volunteers, 12 of whom were taking oral contraceptive agents. Although there was no difference in the metoprolol elimination half-life between those taking oral contraceptives and those receiving metoprolol only, the area-under-curve for metoprolol was significantly higher in those receiving oral contraceptives concurrently.[1] This finding indicates that the effects of metoprolol may be increased, although this has not been clinically determined.

Related Drugs: Although documentation is lacking, the other beta-blocking agent that undergoes significant first-pass metabolism (propranolol) may be expected to interact similarly with oral contraceptive agents. The other beta-blocking agents that undergo little or no first-pass metabolism (e.g., atenolol, nadolol, pindolol [see Appendix]) would not be expected to interact in a similar manner.

Mechanism: It has been postulated that oral contraceptive agents inhibit hepatic microsomal enzymes, leading to a reduction in first-pass hepatic metabolism of metoprolol and propranolol.

Recommendations: Patients should be monitored for an increased effect of metoprolol and may require a possible dosage adjustment during concurrent oral contraceptive therapy. Alternatively, another form of contraception may be suggested or a noninteracting beta-blocking agent may be used.

Reference

1. Kendall, M. J., and others: Metoprolol pharmacokinetics and the oral contraceptive pill, Br. J. Clin. Pharmacol. **14:**120, 1982.

Summary: Pentobarbital has been reported to reduce the plasma concentration and bioavailability of orally administered metoprolol by 30% in 8 subjects.[1]

Related Drugs: In 1 patient phenobarbital increased the clearance of propranolol.[2] A study performed in dogs reported similar findings as well as an increased plasma protein binding of propranolol and a slight reduction in oral bioavailability.[3,4] Pentobarbital induced sedation has been enhanced with propranolol in mice.[5] Pentobarbital has reduced the plasma concentrations and bioavailability of orally administered alprenolol* and a primary active metabolite by 40% and reduced their efficacy by 20% with no adverse reactions reported.[6,7] Propranolol has been reported to potentiate barbiturate-induced sleeping times, central nervous system toxicity, and reduce the LD_{50} of hexobarbital* in mice.[8-11] Similar adverse effects have not been reported in humans.

Timolol or the beta-blocking agents not dependent on first-pass hepatic metabolism (atenolol, nadolol, and pindolol) have been shown not to interact similarly.[1,2,6,7]

Although no documentation exists, a similar interaction may be expected between metoprolol and other barbiturates (e.g., amobarbital, butabarbital, secobarbital [see Appendix]) since they can also induce hepatic enzymes.

Mechanism: The mechanism of the interaction has not been fully elucidated. However, pentobarbital and phenobarbital have been reported to induce liver microsomal enzymes reducing the bioavailability and plasma concentrations after oral administration of the beta-blocking agents dependent on hepatic metabolism (e.g., alprenolol,* metoprolol, and propranolol).[1,2,6,7]

The enhanced effect of propranolol and hexobarbital in mice appears to be caused by a central rather than peripheral effect.[8] Propranolol is metabolized to naphthyloxylacetic acid among other metabolites,[12] and the naphthyl group of the beta-blocking agents is responsible for the central nervous system (CNS) depressant effect. Animal studies have shown that beta-blocking agents devoid of this group produce stimulation rather than CNS depression.[8,9]

Recommendations: The dosage regimen of orally administered metoprolol may have to be increased if prescribed concomitantly with long-term (longer than 10 days) pentobarbital therapy. The barbiturates do not seem to change the bioavailability of beta-blockers administered intravenously. Patients should be observed for a less than optimal therapeutic effect. Alternatively, timolol or one of the beta-blockers not dependent on hepatic first-pass metabolism (atenolol, nadolol, and pindolol) may be substituted.

*Not available in the U.S.

References

1. Haglund, K., and others: Influence of pentobarbital on metoprolol plasma levels, Clin. Pharmacol. Ther. **26:**326, 1979.
2. Sotaniemi, E.A., and others: Plasma clearance of propranolol and sotalol and hepatic drug-metabolizing enzyme activity, Clin. Pharmacol. Ther. **26:**153, 1979.
3. Vu, V.T., and others: Interactions of phenobarbital with propranolol in the dog. 2. Bioavailability, metabolism, and pharmacokinetics, J. Pharmacol. Exp. Ther. **224:**55, 1983.
4. Bai, S.A., and Abramson, F.: Interactions of phenobarbital with propranolol in the dog. 1. Plasma protein binding, J. Pharmacol. Exp. Ther. **222:**589, 1982.
5. Singh, K.P., and others: Effects of propranolol on some central nervous system parameters, Indian J. Med. Res. **59:**786, 1971.
6. Collste, P., and others: Influence of pentobarbital on effect and plasma levels of alprenolol and 4-hydroxy-alprenolol, Clin. Pharmacol. Ther. **25:**423, 1979.
7. Alvan, G., and others: Effect of pentobarbital on the disposition of alprenolol, Clin. Pharmacol. Ther. **22:**316, 1977.
8. Murmann, W., and others: Effects of hexobarbitone, ether, morphine, and urethane upon the acute toxicity of propranolol and D-(−)INPEA, J. Pharm. Pharmacol. **18:**692, 1966.
9. Murmann, W., and others: Central nervous system effects of four β-adrenergic receptor blocking agents, J. Pharm. Pharmacol. **18:**317, 1966.
10. Hermansen, K.: Effect of different β-adrenergic receptor blocking agents in hexobarbital induced narcosis in mice, Acta Pharmacol. Toxicol. **27:**453, 1969.
11. Davis, W.M., and Hatoum, N.S.: Possible toxic interaction of propranolol and narcotic analgesics, Drug Intell. Clin. Pharm. **15:**290, 1981.
12. Paterson, J.W., and others: The pharmacodynamics and metabolism of propranolol in man, Pharmacologia Clinica **2:**127, 1970.

Metoprolol–Rifampin

2

Summary: Rifampin, when administered concurrently with metoprolol for 15 days in 12 subjects, reduced the area-under-curve of metoprolol by 33%. The elimination rate constant of metoprolol did not change significantly. Some loss of beta-blockade may be expected during concomitant therapy with these agents.[1]

Related Drugs: There are no drugs related to rifampin. Propranolol, the other beta-blocking agent that undergoes extensive first-pass metabolism as does metoprolol, has also been shown to interact with rifampin. In 1 study rifampin caused a large reduction in the steady-state blood level of propranolol and a significant increase in its clearance.[2] Although documentation is lacking, the other beta-blocking agents that are not extensively metabolized by first-pass hepatic metabolism (e.g., atenolol, nadolol, pindolol, and timolol) would not be expected to interact in a similar manner.

Mechanism: Metoprolol is eliminated from the body by hepatic metabolism, and only about 3% of a single oral dose is recovered unchanged in the urine.[3] Since rifampin is a known inducer of hepatic microsomal enzymes, the same mechanism is probably responsible for this interaction.[1,2]

Recommendations: During concurrent use of these agents, blood pressure changes should be carefully monitored as the dose of metoprolol may need to be increased.

References

1. Bennett, P.N., and others: Effect of rifampicin on metoprolol and antipyrine kinetics, Br. J. Clin. Pharmacol. **13:**387, 1982.
2. Herman, R.J., and others: Induction of propranolol metabolism in man by rifampin, Br. J. Clin. Pharmacol. **16:**565, 1983.
3. Regardh, C.G., and others: Comparative bioavailability and effect studies on metoprolol administered as ordinary and slow release tablets in single and multiple doses, Acta Pharmacol. Toxicol. **36:**45, 1975.

Propranolol–Alcohol, Ethyl

Summary: The elimination of propranolol is increased by concomitant administration of alcohol[1,2]; however, alcohol's effect on decreasing propranolol absorption was demonstrated in only 1 of these studies.[1] In 1 crossover study the concomitant ingestion of propranolol and alcohol by 5 volunteers resulted in an increase in maximum plasma concentration and elimination rate of propranolol.[1] In a double-blind crossover study, 8 volunteers received propranolol 12 hours after alcohol ingestion. The elimination rate of propranolol was increased and the blood pressure reducing–effect of propranolol was diminished.[2]

Related Drugs: Although documentation is lacking, the other beta-blocking agent that undergoes extensive hepatic metabolism (metoprolol) may also interact similarly with alcohol. The other beta-blocking agents that are not extensively metabolized by the liver (atenolol, nadolol, pindolol, and timolol) would not be expected to interact similarly with alcohol.

Mechanism: It was suggested that the increased maximum plasma concentration resulted from a decrease in gut motility caused by the alcohol, which prolonged the time propranolol could be absorbed.[1] The increased elimination of propranolol is attributed to an activation of hepatic drug metabolizing enzymes by alcohol, since propranolol is extensively metabolized by the liver.[1,2] Also, blood flow to the liver is increased by alcohol through vascular dilation, thus resulting in an increased amount of propranolol presented to the liver for metabolism.[1,2]

Recommendations: Alcohol alone may lead to incidences of angina and tachycardia. It is possible that the concomitant use of these agents potentiates these adverse reactions as well as other side effects involving neurologic functions.[3] However, it is prudent to caution patients regarding the concurrent use of propranolol and alcohol.

References

1. Grabowski, B.S., and others: Effects of acute alcohol administration on propranolol absorption, Int. J. Clin. Pharmacol. Ther. Toxicol. **18:**317, 1980.
2. Sotaniem, E.A., and others: Propranolol and sotalol after a drinking party, Clin. Pharmacol. Ther. **29:**705, 1981.
3. Noble, E.P., and others: Propranolol-ethanol interaction in man, Fed. Proc. **32:**724, 1973.

Propranolol–Aluminum Hydroxide

3

Summary: Concomitant administration of propranolol and aluminum hydroxide gel resulted in an approximate 60% decrease in propranolol bioavailability in 4 of 5 subjects.[1]

Related Drugs: There is no documentation concerning an interaction between propranolol and other antacid compounds or preparations. Atenolol bioavailability was reduced approximately 35% by an antacid mixture containing aluminum hydroxide, magnesium hydroxide, and magnesium carbonate,[2] and by aluminum hydroxide alone.[3]

When metoprolol was administered with the aluminum hydroxide, magnesium hydroxide, and magnesium carbonate mixture,[2] its bioavailability was increased approximately 25%.

Because of conflicting results it is difficult to determine whether an interaction would occur between aluminum hydroxide and the other beta-blockers (e.g., nadolol, timolol, or pindolol).

Mechanism: The proposed mechanisms involve propranolol being absorbed to or complexing with the antacid compound, therefore inhibiting gastrointestinal absorption. However, 2 reports presented evidence that aluminum hydroxide gel decreases the gastric emptying rate.[4,5] The decreased gastric emptying rate would slow the rate of propranolol absorption, which would decrease the systemic bioavailability because of the extensive first-pass metabolism of propranolol.

The mechanism for the increased metoprolol bioavailability is not known.

Recommendations: The clinical significance of the changes in bioavailability have not been determined for any of the beta-blocking agents. Until such data are available, it would seem prudent to separate the dosages of the antacid and beta-blockers by as much time as possible.

References

1. Dobbs, J.H., and others: Effects of aluminum hydroxide on the absorption of propranolol, Curr. Ther. Res. **21:**887, 1977.
2. Regardh, C.G., and others: The effects of antacid, metoclopramide, and propantheline on the bioavailability of metoprolol and atenolol, Biopharm. Drug Dispos. **2:**79, 1981.
3. Kirch, W., and others: Interaction of atenolol with furosemide and calcium and aluminum salts, Clin. Pharmacol. Ther. **30:**429, 1981.
4. McElnay, J.C., and Temple, D.J.: The use of buccal partitioning as a model to examine the effects of aluminum hydroxide gel on the absorption of propranolol, Br. J. Clin. Pharmacol. **13:**399, 1982.
5. Hurwitz, A., and others: Effects of antacids on gastric emptying, Gastroenterology **71:**268, 1976.

Propranolol–Chlorpheniramine

4

Summary: Chlorpheniramine could theoretically inhibit the beta-adrenergic blocking effect of propranolol and enhance its quinidine-like effect; (i.e., decrease in conduction velocity and increase in effective refractive period); however, this interaction has not been reported in humans or in animals.

Related Drugs: Other beta-adrenergic blocking agents (e.g., metoprolol, nadolol, timolol [see Appendix]) could also theoretically be affected by the antihistamines. Brompheniramine,[1] dexbrompheniramine,[1] dexchlorpheniramine,[1] diphenhydramine,[2] pyrilamine,[3] and tripelennamine[4] have been shown to have effects similar to chlorpheniramine, but there is no documentation regarding an interaction with propranolol.

Mechanism: Propranolol is a competitive antagonist of catecholamines at beta-adrenergic receptor sites. Chlorpheniramine and several other antihistamines have been shown to prevent the uptake of catecholamines at the adrenergic nerve terminal, thereby raising the concentration at the adrenergic receptor sites.[1,2,4] Both propranolol and chlorpheniramine have quinidine-like effects on myocardial conduction (i.e., decrease in conduction velocity and increase in effective refractive period.)[3-5] These effects, however, occur only at doses well above the normal therapeutic levels.

Recommendations: The possibility of an interaction between propranolol and chlorpheniramine is remote but should be considered when these agents are administered concurrently or when large doses of either drug are used. Until more clinical data are available regarding the drug interaction, the concurrent use of these drugs need not be avoided.

References

1. Symchowicz, S., and others: Inhibition of dopamine uptake into synaptosomes of rat corpus striatum by chlorpheniramine and its structural analogs, Life Sci. **10:**35, 1971.
2. Carlsson, A., and Lindquist, M.: Central and peripheral monoaminergic membrane-pump blockade by some addictive analgesics and antihistamines, J. Pharm. Pharmacol. **21:**460, 1969.
3. Osterberg, R.E., and Koppanyi, T.: Effects of chlorpheniramine and pyrilamine on the atrial actions of acetytcholine, tyramine and ephedrine, J. Pharm. Sci. **58:**1313, 1969.
4. Johnson, G.L., and Kahn, J.B.: Cocaine and antihistaminic compounds: comparison of effects of some cardiovascular actions of norepinephrine, tyramine and bretylium, J. Pharmacol. Exp. Ther. **152:**458, 1966.
5. Morales-Aquilera, A., and Vaughn Williams, E.M.: The effects of cardiac muscle of beta-receptor antagonists in relation to their activity as local anaesthetics, Br. J. Pharmacol. **24:**332, 1965.

Propranolol–Chlorpromazine

2

Summary: The concurrent use of propranolol and chlorpromazine may lead to a statistically significant increase in propranolol bioavailability.[1,2] The elevated propranolol plasma levels found in 1 study resulted in enhanced pharmacologic activity. In another study serum chlorpromazine levels increased significantly during concurrent propranolol administration, and the active metabolites of chlorpromazine were increased as well.[3]

Related Drugs: Although documentation is lacking, other phenothiazines (e.g., promazine, thioridazine, trifluoperazine [see Appendix]), the thioxanthenes (chlorprothixene and thiothixene), as well as the butyrophenone (haloperidol), dihydroindolone (molindone), and dibenzoxazepine (loxapine) may interact in a similar manner with propranolol because of pharmacologic similarity. If the mechanism deals with a decreased first-pass hepatic metabolism, the other beta-blocking agent extensively metabolized by the liver (metoprolol) would be expected to interact similarly, although documentation is lacking. Conversely, the beta-blocking agents that do not exhibit extensive first-pass metabolism (atenolol, nadolol, pindolol, and timolol) would not be expected to interact similarly with chlorpromazine.

Mechanism: It has been suggested that the bioavailability of propranolol is increased as a result of a decrease in the first-pass hepatic metabolism by chlorpromazine. It is not known how propranolol may increase chlorpromazine serum levels.

Recommendations: Patients should be closely monitored since a lower dose of propranolol and/or chlorpromazine may be necessary.

References:

1. Wallin, B.A., and others: Propranolol in chronic schizophrenia: a controlled study in neuroleptic treated patients, Ann. Intern. Med. **90:**993, 1979.
2. Vestal, R.E., and others: Inhibition of propranolol metabolism by chlorpromazine, Clin. Pharmacol. Ther. **25:**19, 1979.
3. Peet, M., and others: Pharmacokinetic interaction between propranolol and chlorpromazine in schizophrenic patients, Lancet **2:**978, 1980.

Propranolol–Cimetidine

1

Summary: Concurrent administration of cimetidine and propranolol has resulted in approximately a 2-fold increase in propranolol plasma concentrations after single doses of propranolol[1-6] or multiple propranolol dosing.[7-9] The alterations in propranolol levels were seen within 24 to 48 hours.[7,8,10]

Cimetidine does not influence many pharmacodynamic parameters of propranolol,[8,11] but may significantly lower resting pulse rates compared to propranolol alone.[12]

Related Drugs: Cimetidine produced similar changes in the disposition of metoprolol[5,6,9,13] and labetalol,[14] but not atenolol[5,6,9,13] or pindolol.[13] Opposite results have been published in a poorly designed study.[15] Because of conflicting results it is difficult to determine whether an interaction would occur between cimetidine and the other beta-blocking agents (nadolol and timolol). However, if the mechanism only involves inhibition of hepatic enzymes by cimetidine, then these agents would not be expected to interact since they are not hepatically metabolized.

Ranitidine does not increase propranolol plasma concentrations[4,8,16] although it does reduce hepatic blood flow.[8,17,18] In 2 studies ranitidine with concurrent propranolol did not alter heart rate or blood pressure[9] and did not affect plasma propranolol concentrations,[9] clearance, or area-under-curve.[19] In another study, ranitidine had no significant effect on atenolol kinetics. In the same study when ranitidine was used with metoprolol, it increased metoprolol's peak plasma level, area-under-curve and elimination half-life.[20] However, another report challenges the validity of the previous study, citing deficiencies in the study design.[21] Another study reports an increased half-life and area-under-curve of metoprolol when administered with ranitidine[22]; however, this study has also been challenged.[23]

Mechanism: The mechanism most often cited is that cimetidine reduces hepatic blood flow, thereby decreasing the extraction rate of propranolol. It has also been suggested that cimetidine directly inhibits propranolol metabolism, and the degree of inhibition is related to the cimetidine dosage.[24] An increased gastrointestinal absorption may also be involved.[25]

Recommendations: There is sufficient evidence to show that propranolol levels are increased with concomitant cimetidine. Therefore, patients should be monitored for signs of enhanced beta-blocking activity that might require a reduction of the dosage of either propranolol or cimetidine. Ranitidine may provide a more suitable alternative in combination with propranolol. If cimetidine administration is preferred, other beta-blocking agents that are reported not to interact unfavorably with cimetidine (e.g., atenolol and pindolol) may be a suitable alternative to propranolol.

References

1. Feely, J., and others: Reduction of liver blood flow and propranolol metabolism by cimetidine, N. Engl. J. Med. **304**:692, 1981.
2. Donovan, M.A., and others: Cimetidine and bioavailability of propranolol, Lancet **1**:164, 1981.

3. Heagerty, A.M., and others: Influence of cimetidine on pharmacokinetics of propranolol, Br. Med. J. **282:**1917, 1981.
4. Heagerty, A.M., and others: Failure of ranitidine to interact with propranolol, Br. Med. J. **284:**1304, 1982.
5. Kirch, W., and others: Interaction of cimetidine with metoprolol, propranolol, or atenolol, Lancet **2:**531, 1981.
6. Kirch, W., and others: Interaction of metoprolol, propranolol and atenolol with concurrent administration of cimetidine, Klin. Wochenschr. **60:**1401, 1982.
7. Reimann, I.W., and others: Cimetidine increases steady state plasma levels of propranolol, Br. J. Clin. Pharmacol. **12:**785, 1981.
8. Reimann, I.W., and others: Effects of cimetidine and ranitidine on steady-state propranolol kinetics and dynamics, Clin. Pharmacol. Ther. **32:**749, 1982.
9. Kirch, W., and others: Interaction of metoprolol, propranolol and atenolol with cimetidine, Clin. Sci. **63:**451s, 1982.
10. Cunningham, G.M.: Drug-induced internuclear ophthalmoplegia, Can. Med. Assoc. J. **128:**892, 1983.
11. Warburton, S., and others: Does cimetidine alter the cardiac response to exercise and propranolol? South Afr. Med. J. **55:**1125, 1979.
12. Wood, A.J.J., and Feely, J.: Pharmacokinetic drug interactions with propranolol, Clin. Pharmacokinet. **8:**253, 1983.
13. Spahn, H., and others: The interaction of cimetidine with metoprolol, atenolol, propranolol, pindolol and penbutolol, Br. J. Clin. Pharmacol. **15:**500, 1983.
14. Daneshmend, T.K., and Roberts, C.J.C.: Cimetidine and bioavailability of labetalol, Lancet **1:**565, 1981.
15. Houtzagers, J.J., and others: The effect of pretreatment with cimetidine on the bioavailability and disposition of atenolol and metoprolol, Br. J. Clin. Pharmacol. **14:**67, 1982.
16. Wood, J.R.: H_2 receptor antagonists: cimetidine and ranitidine, Br. Med. J. **286:**1440, 1983.
17. Feeley, J., and Guy, E.: Ranitidine also reduces liver blood flow, Lancet **1:**169, 1982.
18. Kirch, W., and others: Influence of beta-receptor antagonists on pharmacokinetics of cimetidine, Drugs **25**(suppl.2):127, 1983.
19. Patel, L., and Weerasuriya, K.: Effect of cimetidine and ranitidine on propranolol clearance, Br. J. Clin. Pharmacol. **15:**152, 1983.
20. Spahn, H., and others: Influence of ranitidine on plasma metoprolol and atenolol concentrations, Br. Med. J. **286:**1546, 1983.
21. Jack, D., and others: Influence of ranitidine on plasma metoprolol concentration (letter), Br. Med. J. **286:**2064, 1983.
22. Janisch, H.D., and others: Interaction between ranitidine and beta receptor blockers like metoprolol and atenolol, Gastroenterology **84:**1197, 1983.
23. Gaginella, T.S., and Bauman, J.H.: Ranitidine hydrochloride, Drug Intell. Clin. Pharm. **17:**873, 1983.
24. Bauman, J.H.: Influence of cimetidine on pharmacokinetics of propranolol, Br. Med. J. **283:**232, 1981.
25. Kitis, G.: Influence of cimetidine on pharmacokinetics of propranolol, Br. Med. J. **283:**309, 1981.

Propranolol–Desipramine

3

Summary: The anticholinergic activity of desipramine may theoretically antagonize the myocardial effects of propranolol, but clinical evidence of this interaction has not been established.[1] On the other hand, a recent report indicated that although propranolol was able to control cardiac symptoms of mitral valve prolapse in a patient receiving desipramine concomitantly, an exacerbation of depressive symptoms necessitated an increase in dosage of the antidepressant. Therefore, the use of propranolol in patients receiving desipramine requires caution until the report is substantiated.[2]

Related Drugs: Although no documentation exists, other tricyclic antidepressants (e.g., amitriptyline, imipramine, nortriptyline [see Appendix]) and the tetracyclic antidepressant (maprotiline), which are pharmacologically related to desipramine, might be expected to interact with propranolol in a similar manner. Also, other beta-blocking agents (e.g., atenolol, nadolol, pindolol [see Appendix]) may be expected to interact with desipramine in a manner analogous to propranolol because of pharmacologic similarity.

Mechanism: The anticholinergic effects of desipramine may antagonize the beta-blocking effects of propranolol in myocardial tissue[1] and may counteract to some degree the bradycardia and decreased inotropic effects produced by propranolol. No mechanism has been proposed for the increase in depressive symptoms when the 2 drugs are given concurrently.

Recommendations: Since substantial clinical evidence is lacking with respect to specific interactions of desipramine with propranolol, no additional precautions are necessary when these drugs are given concurrently. However, precautions appropriate to the individual use of these drugs should be observed.

References

1. Gibson, D.G.: Pharmacodynamic properties of β-adrenergic receptor blocking drugs in man, Drugs **7:**8, 1974.
2. Pariser, S.F., and others: Arrhythmia induced by a tricyclic antidepressant in a patient with undiagnosed mitral valve prolapse, Am. J. Psychiatry **138:**522, 1981.

Propranolol–Epinephrine

1

Summary: Administration of intravenous epinephrine to a patient being treated with propranolol may result in a considerable increase in systolic and diastolic blood pressure and a marked decrease in heart rate.[1-5] This interaction has been reported to cause a hypertensive episode resulting in stroke[6] and several cases of cardiac arrhythmias.[7,8]

Related Drugs: Timolol has been reported to interact with epinephrine in the same manner.[9,10] Other nonspecific beta-blocking agents (nadolol, pindolol) would be expected to interact similarly with epinephrine although cases have not been reported. Conversely, administration of intravenous epinephrine to subjects receiving beta$_1$ specific blocking drugs (metoprolol[1,2,4,5] and atenolol) has resulted in only minor cardiovascular abnormalities.

Phenylephrine has been reported to cause severe hypertension and fatal intracranial hemorrhage when administered with propranolol.[11] Other sympathomimetics with alpha agonist activity (e.g., metaraminol, methoxamine, norepinephrine [see Appendix]) would be expected to interact similarly with propranolol.

The hemodynamic effects of isoproterenol have been shown to be almost completely blocked by propranolol.[2] However, although isoproterenol has beta agonist activity as does epinephrine, it does not have any alpha agonist activity and therefore would not be expected to result in a hypertensive episode with propranolol. Other sympathomimetics with beta agonist activity (e.g., albuterol, metaproterenol, terbutaline [see Appendix]) would be expected to interact with propranolol similarly to isoproterenol.

Mechanism: Concurrent administration of propranolol and epinephrine results in blocking of the beta agonist activity of epinephrine while the alpha-adrenergic effects are unopposed. Increases in systolic and diastolic blood pressure result from blocked vasodilation and unopposed vasoconstriction. Bradycardia is attributed to beta$_1$ blockade and increased vagal tone mediated by the baroreceptors.[12]

Recommendations: Sympathomimetic drugs with alpha agonist activity should be avoided in patients taking nonselective beta antagonists. Alternatively, a cardioselective beta-blocking agent (metoprolol, atenolol) may be used in place of propranolol.

References

1. Houben, H., and others: Influence of selective and nonselective beta-adrenoreceptor blockade on the haemodynamic effect of adrenaline during antihypertensive drug therapy, Clin. Sci. **57:**3975, 1979.
2. Harris, W.S., and others: Effect of beta adrenergic blockade on the hemodynamic responses to epinephrine in man, Am. J. Cardiol. **17:**484, 1966.
3. Houben, H., and others: Effect of low dose epinephrine infusion on hemodynamics after selective and nonselective beta-blockade in hypertension, Clin. Pharmacol. Ther. **31:**685, 1982.
4. Van Herwaarden, C.L.A., and others: Haemodynamic effects of adrenaline during treatment of hypertensive patients with propranolol and metoprolol, Eur. J. Clin. Pharmacol. **12:**397, 1977.

5. Johnson, G.: Influence of metroprolol and propranolol on hemodynamic effects induced by adrenaline and physical work, Acta Pharmacol. Toxicol. **36**(suppl. 5):59, 1975.

6. Hansbrough, J. F., and Near, A.: Propranolol-epinephrine antagonism with hypertension and stroke, Ann. Intern. Med. **92**:717, 1980.

7. Kram, J., and others: Propranolol, Ann. Intern. Med. **80**:282, 1974.

8. Lampman, R.M., and others: Cardiac arrhythmias during epinephrine-propranolol infusions for measurement of in vivo insulin resistance, Diabetes **30**:618, 1981.

9. Struther, J.L., and others: Beta-adrenoreceptor-linked Na/K ATPase: the effect of cardioselective and nonselective beta-blockade, Drugs **25**:253, 1983.

10. Griffing, G.T., and others: Atenolol and timolol, N. Engl. J. Med. **307**:1344, 1982.

11. Cass, E., and others: Hazards of phenylephrine topical medications in persons taking propranolol, Can. Med. Assoc. J. **120**:1261, 1979.

12. Hollaron, T.J., and Phillips, C.E.: Propranolol intoxication, Arch. Intern. Med. **141**:810, 1981.

Propranolol–Ergotamine

3

Summary: In a study involving a single patient who was receiving a preparation of ergotamine, the addition of propranolol (30 mg daily) to the regimen resulted in peripheral vasoconstriction as evidenced by "purple and painful" feet.[1] In another study, a patient previously controlled on an ergot preparation had exacerbations of migraine headache when propranolol was added to the regimen.[2] The attacks ceased after propranolol was stopped but returned when propranolol was restarted at 30 mg daily. Other evidence indicates that the concurrent use of these agents is effective and uneventful.[3,4]

Related Drugs: Although undocumented, if the mechanism involves the blocking of the vasodilatory effect of beta$_2$-adrenergic receptors in the vessels, then the beta$_1$ cardioselective beta-blocking agents (atenolol and metoprolol) would not be expected to interact similarly. However, the other noncardioselective beta-blocking agents (nadolol, pindolol, and timolol) may be expected to interact similarly with all other ergot alkaloids (e.g., dihydroergotamine, ergoloid mesylates, ergonovine [see Appendix]).

Mechanism: It has been proposed that this interaction occurs because the one natural pathway for vasodilation, which is under beta$_2$ receptor control, is blocked by the noncardioselective beta-adrenergic blocking agents allowing the ergot alkaloid to produce a maximum vasoconstriction.

Recommendation: In certain patients receiving concomitant propranolol and ergot alkaloids, the dose of the ergot alkaloid may need to be adjusted downward.

References

1. Baumrucker, J.F.: Drug interaction-propranolol and cafergot, N. Engl. J. Med. **288**:916, 1973.
2. Blank, N.K., and Rieder, M.J.: Paradoxical response to propranolol in migraine, Lancet **2**:1336, 1973.
3. Diamond, S.: Propranolol and ergotamine tartrate (cont.), N. Engl. J. Med. **289**:159, 1973.
4. Weber, R.B., and Reinmuth, O.M.: The treatment of migraine with propranolol, Neurology **22**:366, 1972.

Propranolol–Furosemide

2

Summary: The concurrent administration of furosemide and propranolol results in higher blood levels of propranolol, and this increase can be accompanied by a simultaneous increase in beta-adrenergic blockade.[1]

Related Drugs: Atenolol kinetics have been shown not to be affected by concurrent furosemide.[2] Documentation is lacking regarding an interaction between furosemide and the other beta-blocking agents (e.g., metoprolol, nadolol, pindolol [see Appendix]). There is also a lack of documentation regarding an interaction between propranolol and the other loop diuretics (bumetanide and ethacrynic acid) although a similar interaction may be expected to occur because of pharmacologic similarity.

Mechanism: The mechanism is unknown, although it has been postulated that a furosemide-induced reduction in extracellular fluid volume is responsible. However, alterations in propranolol absorption or protein binding cannot be ruled out.[1]

Recommendations: The concurrent use of these agents need not be avoided. However, patients should be closely monitored, and a corresponding dosage adjustment of either agent should be made if necessary.

References

1. Chiariello, M., and others: Effect of furosemide on plasma concentration and beta-blockade by propranolol, Clin. Pharmacol. Ther. **26:**433, 1979.
2. Kirch, W., and others: Interaction of atenolol with furosemide and calcium and aluminum salts, Clin. Pharmacol. Ther. **30:**429, 1981.

Propranolol–Hydralazine

3

Summary: Concurrent oral administration of hydralazine and propranolol significantly increased the bioavailability of propranolol in normotensive subjects.[1] Propranolol reportedly enhanced the antihypertensive activity of hydralazine.[2]

Related Drugs: Concomitant hydralazine resulted in similar plasma concentration increases with metoprolol, but not with nadolol or acebutolol*.[3] The other beta-blocking agents (atenolol, pindolol, and timolol) do not undergo significant first-pass metabolism like propranolol and metoprolol, therefore they would not be expected to interact with hydralazine. There are no drugs related to hydralazine.

Mechanism: Although the mechanism is not completely understood, hydralazine may enhance the systemic availability of propranolol by alteration of first-pass clearance. The change in first-pass clearance could result from reduction in extraction by inhibition of metabolism by hydralazine metabolites or from transient changes in splanchnic flow.[1,4] Absorption changes do not appear to be responsible since propranolol is almost completely absorbed, and studies of systemic clearance showed that the increase in systemic bioavailability did not reflect decreased rate of removal from systemic circulation.[1] Metoprolol, like propranolol, has a high liver extraction, whereas acebutolol and nadolol have a moderate or no hepatic extraction, respectively.

    The mechanism by which propranolol prolongs the antihypertensive effect of hydralazine is not known.[5] It has been shown that these 2 agents prolonged the left ventricular ejection time compared to propranolol alone.[6]

Recommendations: The clinical significance of the increased propranolol bioavailability has not been determined in long-term administration studies. Some patients may develop symptoms of propranolol toxicity (e.g., bradycardia, bronchospasm). If such symptoms appear, plasma propranolol should be monitored, and decreasing the propranolol dosage may be indicated.

References

1. McLean, A.J., and others: Interaction between oral propranolol and hydralazine, Clin. Pharmacol. Ther. **27:**726, 1980.
2. Moses, C.: Drug treatment of mild hypertension: adverse consequences, Ann. N.Y. Acad. Sci. **304:**84, 1978.
3. Jack, D.B., and others: The effect of hydralazine on the pharmacokinetics of three different beta adrenoceptor antagonists: metoprolol, nadolol, and acebutolol, Biopharm. Drug Disposition **3:**47, 1982.
4. Jackman, G.P., and others: No stereoselective first-pass hepatic extraction of propranolol, Clin. Pharmacol. Ther. **30:**291, 1981.
5. Schafer-Korting, M., and Mutschler, E.: Pharmacokinetics of bendroflumethiazide alone and in combination with propranolol and hydralazine, Eur. J. Clin. Pharmacol. **21:**315, 1982.
6. Kyle, M.C., and Fries, E.D.: Serial measurements of systolic time intervals: effects of propranolol alone and combined with other agents in hypertensive patients, Hypertension **2:**111, 1980.

*Not available in the U.S.

Propranolol–Indomethacin

2

Summary: Several studies indicate that indomethacin therapy can reduce the hypotensive effects of propranolol.[1-4] One study showed the diastolic blood pressure was 13 mm Hg higher when indomethacin was administered concurrently with a beta-blocking agent (propranolol or pindolol) than when the beta-blocking agent was used alone.[1] Similar results were seen in another study using propranolol. Two weeks after indomethacin was discontinued, blood pressure in these patients returned to basal levels.[3]

Related Drugs: One study suggested that indomethacin did not have an antagonistic action on the negative chronotropic effect of metoprolol.[5] There is a lack of documentation regarding an interaction between indomethacin and the other beta-blocking agents (e.g., atenolol, nadolol, timolol [see Appendix]) although because of pharmacologic similarity, a similar interaction may be expected to occur. Documentation is also lacking regarding a similar interaction with the other nonsteroidal anti-inflammatory agents (e.g., ibuprofen, naproxen, sulindac [see Appendix]). However, since all of these agents inhibit prostaglandin synthesis to some extent, a similar interaction may be expected to occur.

Mechanism: Indomethacin alone has been reported to increase blood pressure.[6-8] It has also been suggested that indomethacin, which inhibits prostaglandin synthesis, inhibits the prostaglandin responsible for vasodilation as well, resulting in an increase in blood pressure.

Recommendations: Patients' blood pressure should be monitored closely during concurrent use of these agents. If a loss of blood pressure control is noted, the dose of propranolol may need to be increased or indomethacin may need to be discontinued.

References

1. Durao, V., and others: Modification of antihypertensive effects of beta-adrenoreceptor-blocking agents by inhibition of endogenous prostaglandin synthesis, Lancet **2:**1005, 1977.
2. Lopez-Ovejero, J.A., and others: Effects of indomethacin alone and during diuretic or beta-adreno-receptor-blockade therapy on blood pressure and the renin system in essential hypertension, Clin. Sci. Molec. Med. **55:**203s, 1978.
3. Watkins, J., and others: Attenuation of hypotensive effect of propranolol and thiazide diuretics by indomethacin, Br. Med. J. **281:**702, 1980.
4. Salvetti, A., and others: Interaction between oxprenolol and indomethacin on blood pressure in essential hypertension patients, Eur. J. Clin. Pharmacol. **22:**197, 1982.
5. Smith, S.R., and others: Failure of indomethacin to modify beta-adrenoceptor blockade, Br. J. Clin. Pharmacol. **15:**267, 1983.
6. Patak, R.V., and others: Antagonism of the effects of furosemide by indomethacin in normal and hypertensive man, Prostaglandins **10:**649, 1975.
7. Mills, E.H., and others: Non-steroidal anti-inflammatory drugs and blood pressure, Aust. N.Z. J. Med. **12:**478, 1982.
8. Barrientos, A., and others: Indomethacin and beta-blockers in hypertension, Lancet **1:**277, 1978.

Summary: Propranolol and quinidine have been found to have a beneficial effect when used together for the treatment of cardiac arrhythmias so that smaller doses of each drug can be used. Concurrent administration of both agents may be therapeutically beneficial in certain patients.[1,2]

Related Drugs: Although not documented, it would seem that other beta-adrenergic blockers (e.g., atenolol, nadolol, pindolol [see Appendix]) would exert the same effect with quinidine because of their pharmacologic similarity to propranolol.

Mechanism: Quinidine and propranolol both depress pacemaker activity, resting membrane potential, and conduction velocity and increase the refractory period.[3] The mechanism of the enhancement by combined drug effects is unclear but probably results from a reduced depolarization rate of the cardiac transmembrane action potential, an effect shared by both drugs. The effect is manifested by a decreased response of the myocardial tissue and a decreased rate of phase 4 diastolic depolarization.

Recommendations: Propranolol and quinidine may be useful in combined therapy in the conversion of atrial fibrillation to normal sinus rhythm.[1] There do not appear to be any pharmacokinetic interactions with these agents.[4,5] This combination of propranolol and quinidine may be advantageous in the therapy of several arrhythmias.

References

1. Stern, S., and Borman, J.B.: Early conversion of atrial fibrillation after open-heart surgery by combined propranolol and quinidine treatment, Isr. J. Med. Sci. **5:**102, 1969.
2. Fors, Jr., W.J., and others: Evaluation of propranolol and quinidine in the treatment of quinidine-resistant arrhythmias, Am. J. Cardiol. **27:**190, 1971.
3. Stern, S.: Synergistic action of propranolol with quinidine, Am. Heart J. **72:**569, 1966.
4. Fenster, P., and others: Kinetic evaluation of the propranolol-quinidine combination, Clin. Pharmacol. Ther. **27:**450, 1980.
5. Kates, R.E., and Blanford, M.F.: Disposition kinetics of oral quinidine when administered concurrently with propranolol, J. Clin. Pharmacol. **19:**378, 1979.

Propranolol–Thyroid

2

Summary: Several studies indicate that patients taking thyroid may show a decreased bioavailability of propranolol if the patient is in the hyperthyroid state.[1-5] However, other studies show conflicting results.[6-8] Although results may vary from patient to patient, plasma levels of propranolol are significantly lower in the hyperthyroid compared to the euthyroid state, and it is important to be aware of this when using concurrent thyroid replacement therapy.

Related Drugs: The other beta-blocking agent that undergoes extensive first-pass metabolism (metoprolol) is also altered in the hyperthyroid state.[4] The beta-blocking agents that do not undergo significant first-pass metabolism (e.g., atenolol, nadolol, pindolol [see Appendix]) do not appear to be affected by hyperthyroidism.[4] A similar interaction may be expected between propranolol and the other thyroid drugs (e.g., levothyroxine, liothyronine, liotrix [see Appendix]). In hypothyroid patients the plasma levels of propranolol and metoprolol appear to be increased, which may explain a possible interaction with the antithyroid thioamine compounds (methimazole and propylthiouracil).

Mechanism: Several studies suggest the decreased bioavailability of propranolol and metoprolol result from an increase in presystemic clearance directly related to the extent of first-pass metabolism.[1-5] Conversely, in the hypothyroid state, the interaction may be produced by a decrease in presystemic clearance.

Recommendations: Although a specific drug interaction has not been determined, it is prudent to be aware of a possible interaction while treating a patient with a thyroid abnormality. Therefore, when using a thyroid drug concurrently with propranolol or metoprolol, the dose of the beta-blocking agent may need to be increased. Alternatively, a noninteracting beta-blocking agent may be used.

References

1. Feely, J., and others: Increased clearance of propranolol in thyrotoxicoses, Ann. Intern. Med. **94:**472, 1981.
2. Feely, J., and others: The influence of age, smoking and hyperthyroidism on plasma propranolol steady state concentration, Br. J. Clin. Pharmacol. **12:**73, 1981.
3. Feely, J., and others: Plasma propranolol steady state concentrations in thyroid disorders, Eur. J. Clin. Pharmacol. **19:**329, 1981.
4. Hallengren, B., and others: Influence of hyperthyroidism on the kinetics of methimazole, propranolol, metoprolol and atenolol, Eur. J. Clin. Pharmacol. **21:**379, 1982.
5. Aro, A., and others: Pharmacokinetics of propranolol and sotalol in hyperthyroidism, Eur. J. Clin. Pharmacol. **21:**373, 1982.
6. Kelly, J.G., and McDevitt, D.G.: Plasma protein binding of propranolol and isoprenaline in hyperthyroidism and hypothyroidism, Br. J. Clin. Pharmacol. **6:**123, 1978.
7. Riddell, J.G., and others: Effects of thyroid dysfunction on propranolol kinetics, Clin. Pharmacol. Ther. **28:**565, 1980.
8. Tawara, K., and others: Pharmacokinetics and pharmacodynamics of propranolol stereoisomers in hyperthyroid patients, Eur. J. Clin. Pharmacol. **19:**197, 1981.

Propranolol–Tobacco

2

Summary: Smoking has resulted in reduced steady-state serum propranolol concentrations and increased propranolol clearance in both patients and normal subjects.[1-3] The affect of smoking was greatest in younger patients but diminished in older patients. Smoking enhanced the hyperthyroid-induced reduction in plasma propranolol concentrations[4] and inhibited the therapeutic effect of propranolol in the treatment of angina pectoris.[5,6]

Related Drugs: Although no documentation exists, the other beta-blocking agent dependent on hepatic metabolism (metoprolol) may be expected to interact similarly with tobacco. The other beta-blocking agents (e.g., atenolol, nadolol, pindolol [see Appendix]), because of nonliver dependent metabolism, would not be expected to interact with tobacco.

Mechanism: Tobacco smoke and some of its components are known to be inducers of hepatic microsomal enzymes, and propranolol is eliminated primarily by hepatic clearance. The evidence also suggests that tobacco's ability to induce microsomal enzymes decreases with age.

Recommendations: Patients beginning propranolol therapy who regularly smoke may require larger doses than nonsmokers to achieve the same therapeutic effect. This should present no specific problem unless the patient quits smoking while continuing with propranolol. In those cases, propranolol serum levels would be expected to increase, necessitating a dosage reduction of propranolol.

References

1. Vestal, R.E., and others: Effect of age and cigarette smoking on the disposition of propranolol in man, Clin. Pharmacol. Ther. **26:**8, 1979.
2. Vestal, R.E., and Wood, A.J.J.: Influence of age and smoking on drug kinetics in man, Clin. Pharmacokinet. **5:**309, 1980.
3. Gardner, S.K., and others: Effect of smoking on the elimination of propranolol hydrochloride, Int. J. Clin. Pharmacol. Ther. Toxicol. **18:**421, 1980.
4. Feely, J., and others: The influence of age, smoking, and hyperthyroidism on plasma propranolol steady-state concentration, Br. J. Clin. Pharmacol. **12:**73, 1981.
5. Fox, K., and others: Interaction between cigarettes and propranolol in treatment of angina pectoris, Br. Med. J. **281:**191, 1980.
6. Deanfield, J., and others: Treatment of angina pectoris with propranolol: the harmful effect of cigarette smoking, Cardiology **68**(suppl.):186, 1981.

CHAPTER TWELVE

Cardiac Glycoside Drug Interactions

TABLE 12. Cardiac Glycoside Drug Interactions

Drug Interaction	Significance Code	Potential Effects	Recommendations	See Page
Digitalis–Calcium Chloride	2	IV calcium salts during digitalis therapy may alter cardiac electrophysiologic activity resulting in tachycardia or arrhythmias.	If IV calcium is necessary, the procedure should be accomplished slowly and cautiously.	499
Digitalis–Phenytoin	2	Although phenytoin is used for treating digitalis glycoside–induced supraventricular arrhythmias, some patients react adversely. It has been shown that long-term phenytoin use may lead to increased digitoxin elimination.	It is important to remember that certain individuals may not respond to co-therapy.	500
Digitalis–Reserpine	3	Concurrent use of these agents may result in enhanced cardiotoxicity.	An alternative to reserpine may be best. If concomitant use is necessary, observe patients carefully for adverse effects.	501
Digitoxin–Cholestyramine	2	Cholestyramine may reduce GI absorption and thus significantly reduce the bioavailability of digitoxin.	Monitor digitoxin serum levels. Giving cholestyramine 1½ hours after digitoxin may avoid a significant interaction.	502
Digitoxin–Phenobarbital	2	Phenobarbital may decrease plasma levels and shorten the half-life of digitoxin.	Monitor for underdigitalization and increase the digitoxin dosage if necessary.	504
Digitoxin–Phenylbutazone	3	Phenylbutazone markedly reduced serum digitoxin levels in 1 patient.	The digitoxin dosage may need to be increased.	505
Digitoxin–Rifampin	1	Rifampin may significantly reduce serum concentrations and half-life of digitoxin, probably by induction of microsomal enzymes, thereby increasing the metabolism of digitoxin.	Monitor for underdigitalization and increase the digitoxin dosage as necessary.	506
Digitoxin–Spironolactone	3	Spironolactone may either reduce the toxicity of digitoxin, reduce its half-life and volume of distribution, or prolong digitoxin elimination. The therapeutic action of digitoxin may be increased or decreased.	Monitor potassium and digitoxin levels frequently.	507
Digoxin–Aluminum Hydroxide, Magnesium Hydroxide, Magnesium Trisilicate	2	Antacids containing these agents may significantly decrease the GI absorption of digoxin. Digoxin capsules may not be affected.	Administer antacids 1-2 hours before or after the digoxin dose.	509

Abbreviations: IV, intravenous; GI, gastrointestinal.

TABLE 12. Cardiac Glycoside Drug Interactions—cont'd

Drug Interaction	Significance Code	Potential Effects	Recommendations	See Page
Digoxin– Aminosalicylic Acid	3	Aminosalicylic acid may reduce the area-under-curve and decrease the excretion of digoxin, possibly from decreased GI absorption. The clinical significance has not been determined.	An increased digoxin dosage may be necessary, or separating the administration of the drugs by as much time as possible may be beneficial.	510
Digoxin– Cyclophosphamide, Prednisone, Procarbazine, Vincristine	2	Chemotherapy with these agents may reduce the digoxin area-under-curve. It is not known whether the individual antineoplastic agents alone will produce the same effect.	Digoxin dosage may need to be increased. Digitoxin may be an alternative to digoxin since it has been shown not to interact.	511
Digoxin– Diazepam	2	Diazepam may moderately increase the half-life and decrease the urinary excretion of digoxin.	Monitor patients for increased digoxin levels and lower the dose if needed.	512
Digoxin– Disopyramide	3	Disopyramide may significantly reduce the volume of distribution and elimination half-life of an IV bolus of digoxin. However, this interaction does not occur with oral digoxin, although mean serum digoxin levels may increase after 1 week of cotherapy.	Concurrent use need not be avoided until further studies determine the clinical significance of this interaction.	513
Digoxin– Erythromycin Base	1	Erythromycin may increase steady-state serum digoxin concentration, thus decreasing urinary and fecal excretion of digoxin reduction products.	Monitor patients closely for overdigitalization.	514
Digoxin– Furosemide	2	Cardiac arrhythmias may develop during concurrent use, primarily because furosemide disturbs the normal potassium gradient across cell membranes.	It may be necessary to add oral potassium to the patients therapy. A potassium-sparing diuretic may be a suitable alternative.	515
Digoxin– Hydroxychloroquine	2	Hydroxychloroquine may increase serum digoxin levels, although digoxin toxicity may not appear.	Monitor patients closely and reduce digoxin dosage if needed.	517
Digoxin– Ibuprofen	2	Ibuprofen may significantly increase serum digoxin levels.	Monitor patients closely and decrease the dosage if digoxin toxicity appears.	518
Digoxin– Kaolin	2	Kaolin-pectin suspension significantly reduces digoxin bioavailability.	Giving kaolin at least 2 hours after digoxin may avoid the interaction, or the soft gelatin capsule or digoxin elixir may be advisable.	519

TABLE 12. Cardiac Glycoside Drug Interactions—cont'd

Drug Interaction	Significance Code	Potential Effects	Recommendations	See Page
Digoxin–Metoclopramide	2	Metoclopramide may reduce steady-state serum digoxin concentrations.	Monitor digoxin serum concentration frequently.	520
Digoxin–Neomycin	2	Neomycin may depress serum digoxin concentration, which may decrease the digoxin area-under-curve.	Monitor patients for a change in digoxin serum concentration.	521
Digoxin–Penicillamine	2	Penicillamine may significantly reduce serum digoxin levels.	The digoxin dosage may need to be increased.	522
Digoxin–Propantheline	1	Propantheline may prolong the intestinal emptying time, which may significantly increase the absorption of digoxin.	Selection of a quickly absorbed digoxin preparation may prevent this interaction.	523
Digoxin–Psyllium	3	Psyllium hydrophilic mucilloid may reduce the bioavailability of digoxin.	Monitor patients for decreasing digoxin serum concentration.	524
Digoxin–Quinidine	1	Increased plasma digoxin concentration, reduced volume of distribution, prolonged half-life, and reduced clearance have been reported with co-therapy.	Monitor for digoxin toxicity and reduce the dosage if needed.	525
Digoxin–Succinylcholine	2	Succinylcholine has caused cardiac arrhythmias in patients stabilized on digoxin.	Succinylcholine should be used with caution in patients receiving digoxin or other digitalis glycosides.	528
Digoxin–Sulfasalazine	2	Sulfasalazine reduces serum digoxin levels. Increasing the digoxin dosage did not increase serum levels.	Monitor digoxin levels carefully and discontinue sulfasalazine if needed.	529
Digoxin–Tetracycline	1	Tetracycline reportedly increases steady-state serum digoxin concentrations, with a decrease in urinary and fecal excretion of digoxin reduction products.	Monitor patients for overdigitalization.	530
Digoxin–Thyroid	2	The therapeutic efficacy of digoxin may be decreased in patients with hyperthyroidism or those treated with thyroid hormones.	Monitor patients stabilized on digoxin closely.	531
Digoxin–Verapamil	1	Verapamil significantly increases serum digoxin concentrations, and both therapeutic and toxic effects of digoxin have been increased.	It is important to monitor digoxin serum levels and cardiac function.	532

Digitalis–Calcium Chloride (intravenous)

Summary: Effects of digitalis glycosides on the heart are increased by elevated extracellular concentrations of ionic calcium. Intravenous administration of calcium salts during digitalis therapy may result in altered cardiac electrophysiologic activity such as tachycardia or arrhythmias.[1,2]

Related Drugs: Because of pharmacologic similarities, the other digitalis glycosides (deslanoside, digitoxin, and digoxin) may be expected to interact in a similar manner with calcium chloride. Multiple forms of calcium compounds (e.g., calcium gluconate, gluceptate, levulinate) are available for parenteral administration and may be expected to interact in a similar manner with the digitalis glycosides. Although antacids may influence oral bioavailability of digitalis, calcium carbonate tablets do not themselves have such an effect.[3]

Mechanism: The mechanism of action of digitalis glycosides appears to be intimately associated with its ability to cause an increase in excitation-contraction coupling mediated through the effects of calcium. Excitable tissues in the heart experience inhibition of sodium/potassium ATPase (the membrane "sodium pump") by digitalis glycosides and so attain relatively higher intracellular Na^+ and lower K^+ concentrations.[4] Higher intracellular Na^+ concentrations facilitate exchange of extracellular Ca^{+2} ions and the inward and internal flux of calcium results in modified transmembrane potentials and stronger contractions of cardiac muscle. Elevated extracellular concentrations of Ca^{+2} after parenteral calcium salts further facilitate these inward calcium fluxes.[5]

Recommendations: If intravenous administration of calcium is necessary in patients receiving digitalis therapy, it is recommended that this procedure be accomplished slowly and with caution. If cardiac toxicity does develop from intravenous calcium administration to a digitalized patient, supportive measures without additional antiarrhythmics may be sufficient, based on studies of massive digitalis intoxication.[6] Calcium chelation with ethylenediaminetetraacetic acid (EDTA) may produce only transient improvement while adding its own toxicity and therefore has been considered unsatisfactory in treating digitalis toxicity in general.[5]

References

1. Bower, J.O., and Mengle, H.A.K.: The additive effects of calcium and digitalis, J.A.M.A. **106**:1151, 1936.
2. Nola, G.T., and others: Assessment of the synergistic relationship between serum calcium and digitalis, Am. Heart J. **79**:499, 1970.
3. Brown, D.D., and Juhl, R.P.: Altered bioavailability of digoxin produced by gastrointestinal medications (abstract), Clin. Res. **27**:610, 1979.
4. Hougen, T.J., and Smith, T.W.: Inhibition of myocardial monovalent cation active transport by subtoxic doses of ouabain in the dog, Circ. Res. **42**:856, 1978.
5. Brown, R.H., and others: The interactions of protons, calcium, and potassium ions on cardiac Purkinje fibers, J. Physiol. (Lond.) **282**:345, 1978.
6. Hansteen, V., and others: Acute, massive poisoning with digitoxin: report of seven cases and discussion of treatment, Clin. Toxicol. **18**:679, 1981.

Digitalis–Phenytoin

Summary: The administration of phenytoin to a patient experiencing supraventricular cardiotoxicity from digitalis has been utilized as a positive interaction with generally beneficial results. Phenytoin has been considered the antiarrhythmic drug of choice in treating digitalis glycoside–induced supraventricular arrhythmias and it has the further advantage of not adding to glycoside-induced atrioventricular block.[1] There are occasional reports of patients reacting adversely to treatment with phenytoin.[2] In addition, it has been observed that long-term phenytoin will lead to increased digitalis (digitoxin) elimination by induction of liver enzymes.[3]

Related Drugs: Since they are pharmacologically related, the other digitalis glycosides (deslanoside, digitoxin, and digoxin) may be expected to interact in a similar manner with phenytoin. There is no documentation regarding the use of the other hydantoin anticonvulsants (ethotoin and mephenytoin) as antiarrhythmic agents for digitalis-induced arrhythmias; however, these drugs may also be expected to act in a similar manner to phenytoin based on pharmacologic similarity.

Mechanism: The effectiveness of phenytoin in antagonizing supraventricular arrhythmias induced by digitalis overdosage appears to result from a pharmacodynamic interaction on the membranes of myocardial pacemaker cells. Local anaesthetic activity,[4] stimulation of Na^+/K^+ ATPase activity, and blockade of calcium ion effects[5] have all been proposed as mechanisms for the rather specific antidotal action of phenytoin in digitalis glycoside intoxication. Phenytoin's kinetic effects on digitoxin metabolism are of uncertain clinical significance but would appear to be of less concern in patients treated with digitalis glycosides that undergo more extensive renal elimination such as digoxin.

Recommendations: With appropriate safeguards, phenytoin appears to be a useful adjunct to management of digitalis-induced superventricular arrhythmias. It must be borne in mind that certain individuals may not respond or may experience a worsening in cardiac function after therapeutic doses of phenytoin. Long-term antiarrhythmic treatment with phenytoin may increase the elimination of digitalis and therefore use of an alternate antiarrhythmic drug may be advantageous. If phenytoin is deleted from combination therapy with digitalis, appropriate adjustment of the cardiac glycoside dosage may be necessary.

References

1. Helfant, R.H., and others: The electrophysiological properties of diphenylhydantoin sodium as compared to procaine amide in the normal and digitalis-intoxicated heart, Circulation **36:**108, 1967.
2. Zoneraich, S., and others: Sudden death following intravenous sodium diphenylhydantoin, Am. Heart J. **91:**375, 1976.
3. Perrier, D., and others: Clinical pharmacokinetics of digoxin, Clin. Pharmacokinet. **2:**292, 1977.
4. Binnion, P.F.: Drug interactions with digitalis glycosides, Drugs **15:**369, 1978.
5. Rahwan, R.G., and others: The role of calcium antagonism in the therapeutic action of drugs, Can. J. Physiol. Pharmacol. **57:**443, 1979.

Digitalis–Reserpine

3

Summary: The clinical literature documents an interaction between cardiac glycosides and reserpine characterized by enhanced cardiotoxicity.[1,2] Patients with atrial fibrillation were at greatest risk to experience enhanced supraventricular arrhythmias and impairment in conduction.

Related Drugs: All the clinically employed digitalis glycosides share similar mechanisms of action and differ primarily in their pharmacokinetic disposition. Therefore, it might be expected that the other digitalis glycosides (deslanoside, digitoxin, and digoxin) may all potentially interact with reserpine. Other rauwolfia alkaloids (e.g., alseroxylon, deserpidine, rescinnamine [see Appendix]) may also be expected to interact with digitalis because of pharmacologic similarity.

Mechanism: Many of the effects of digitalis on the heart are mediated through the autonomic nervous system.[3] Alteration of sympathetic nervous system activity by reserpine in the heart itself has been implicated as significantly contributing to the digitalis interaction in animals.[4] In humans the situation is unclear but the possibilities of adrenergic receptor supersensitivity[5] or differential effects on cardiac sympathetic nerves[6] by reserpine and/or digitalis cannot be ruled out. Other direct or indirect effects of these 2 drugs may actually underlie this interaction.

Recommendations: It may be wise to consider the many alternatives to reserpine for controlling hypertension in patients using digitalis glycosides. If reserpine is necessary in a digitalized individual, it can be successfully used, but careful observation of the patient is in order. If atrial fibrillation preexists, the potential for this adverse drug interaction appears to be greatly enhanced.

References

1. Lown, B., and others: Effect of digitalis in patients receiving reserpine, Circulation **24**:1185, 1961.
2. Dick, H.L.H., and others: Reserpine-digitalis toxicity, Arch. Intern. Med. **109**:503, 1962.
3. Roberts, J., and others: Role of adrenergic influences in digitalis-induced ventricular arrhythmia, Life Sci. **18**:665, 1976.
4. Lathers, C.M., and others: The action of reserpine, 6-hydroxydopamine, and bretylium on digitalis-induced cardiotoxicity, Eur. J. Pharmacol. **76**:371, 1981.
5. Schwartz, P.J., and Stone, H.L.: Left stellectomy and denervation supersensitivity in conscious dogs, Am. J. Cardiol. **49**:1185, 1982.
6. Lathers, C.M., and others: Nonuniform cardiac sympathetic nerve discharge: mechanism for coronary occlusion and digitalis-induced arrhythmia, Circulation **57**:1058, 1978.

Digitoxin–Cholestyramine

2

Summary: Concurrent administration of cholestyramine and orally administered digitoxin can decrease the gastrointestinal absorption of digitoxin and result in a significantly reduced bioavailability.[1,2] The extent of the decreased bioavailability can be directly related to the dose of cholestyramine administered.[3,4] A reduction in the half-life of digitoxin has been reported in 3 studies.[1,5,6]

Related Drugs: In short-term studies in normal volunteers the concurrent administration of cholestyramine and orally administered digoxin resulted in significantly reduced digoxin bioavailability.[3,4] However, in long-term studies the inhibition of digoxin bioavailability was not significantly reduced.[7,8]

Another study has shown increased gastrointestinal absorption of digoxin during administration of cholestyramine in rats.[9] Such data imply that binding of digoxin by cholestyramine is negligible or nonexistent in the gastrointestinal tract. Cholestyramine may be expected to interact with the other digitalis glycosides (deslanoside and digitalis) by a mechanism similar to digoxin or digitoxin. However, the significance of such interactions has not been documented.

Colestipol, another anion exchange resin, reduced digitoxin plasma concentrations in 4 patients with digitoxin intoxication.[2] Interactions between colestipol and the other digitalis glycosides have not been documented.

Mechanism: Cholestyramine has been reported to bind digitoxin in the gastrointestinal tract, inhibiting its absorption and enterohepatic circulation, resulting in reduced reabsorption and increased fecal excretion of digitoxin.[1] The mechanism for an inhibition in the absorption of digoxin as a result of concurrent administration of cholestyramine may be different and has not been fully elucidated.[7,9]

Recommendations: Patients receiving digitalis glycosides, especially digitoxin, should be monitored for appropriate serum levels of the glycoside and observed for clinical signs and symptoms. Administration of the digitalis glycoside at least 1.5 hours before cholestyramine will avoid significant gastrointestinal interference between the 2 drugs.[10]

References

1. Caldwell, J.H., and others: Interruption of the enterohepatic circulation of digitoxin by cholestyramine, J. Clin. Invest. **50:**2638, 1971.
2. Bazzano, G., and Bazzano, G.S.: Digitalis intoxication: treatment with a new steroid-binding resin, J.A.M.A. **220:**828, 1972.
3. Brown, D.D., and others: Decreased bioavailability of digoxin produced by dietary fiber and cholestyramine, Am. J. Cardiol. **39:**297, 1977.
4. Brown, D.D., and others: Decreased bioavailability of digoxin due to hypocholesterolemic intervention, Circulation **58:**164, 1978.
5. Caldwell, J.H., and Greenberger, N.J.: Cholestyramine enhances digitalis excretion and protects against lethal intoxication, J. Clin. Invest. **49:**16a, 1970.
6. Carruthers, S.G., and Dujovne, C.A.: Cholestyramine and spironolactone and their combination in digitoxin elimination, Clin. Pharmacol. Ther. **27:**184, 1980.

7. Hall, W.H., and others: Effect of cholestyramine on digoxin absorption and excretion in man, Am. J. Cardiol. **39**:213, 1977.
8. Bazzano, G., and Bazzano, G.S.: Effect of digitalis binding resins on cardiac glycoside plasma levels, Clin. Res. **20**:24, 1972.
9. Thompson, W.G.: Effect of cholestyramine on absorption of ^{3}H digoxin in rats, Dig. Dis. **18**:851, 1973.
10. Begger, J.T., and Strauss, H.C.: Digitalis toxicity: drug interactions promoting toxicity and the management of toxicity, Sem. Drug Treat. **2**:147, 1972.

Digitoxin–Phenobarbital

2

Summary: Phenobarbital may decrease plasma digitoxin levels and shorten the digitoxin half-life.[1-3] Patients receiving these drugs concurrently may demonstrate increased digitoxin dose requirements.

Related Drugs: Although not documented, digitalis leaf may be expected to interact in a similar manner with phenobarbital because digitalis, like digitoxin, is highly metabolized by liver microsomal enzymes. The other digitalis glycosides (deslanoside and digoxin) are eliminated largely through renal mechanisms and would not be expected to interact significantly with phenobarbital on the basis of the mechanism described below.

Although there is insufficient documentation, other barbiturates (e.g., amobarbital, butabarbital, secobarbital [see Appendix]) would be expected to interact with cardiac glycosides in a similar manner.[1,2]

Mechanism: Phenobarbital has been shown to increase the metabolism of digitoxin to digoxin, probably by inducing hepatic microsomal enzymes.[1,4]

Recommendations: When phenobarbital or another barbiturate is added to the regimen of a patient receiving digitoxin, careful monitoring for underdigitalization should be performed. It may be necessary to increase the digitoxin dose in some patients. Conversely, patients receiving combined therapy should be monitored carefully for digitalis toxicity if the barbiturate is withdrawn from the regimen.

References

1. Jelliffe, R.W., and Blankenhorn, D.H.: Effect of phenobarbital on digitoxin metabolism, Clin. Res. **14:**160, 1966.
2. Solomon, H.M., and Abrams, W.B.: Interactions between digitoxin and other drugs in man, Am. Heart J. **83:**277, 1972.
3. Solomon, H.M., and others: Induction of the metabolism of digitoxin in man by phenobarbital, Clin. Res. **19:**356, 1971.
4. Jelliffe, R.W., and others: A mathematical study of the metabolic conversion of digitoxin to digoxin in man, Math. Biosci. **6:**387, 1970.

Digitoxin–Phenylbutazone

3

Summary: Phenylbutazone markedly reduced serum digitoxin levels in a study involving a single patient. When phenylbutazone was discontinued, the plasma concentration of digitoxin returned to control levels.[1]

Related Drugs: There is no documentation regarding an interaction between digitoxin and oxyphenbutazone, although a similar interaction may be expected to occur since they are pharmacologically related. Documentation is also lacking regarding an interaction between phenylbutazone and the other digitalis glycosides (deslanoside, digitalis, and digoxin). However, since deslanoside and digoxin are excreted renally whereas digitoxin and digitalis undergo hepatic metabolism, a similar interaction would not be expected to occur with deslanoside and digoxin, but may occur with digitalis.

Mechanism: The mechanism is unknown; however, it has been postulated that phenylbutazone may increase the hepatic metabolism of digitoxin.

Recommendations: Patients should be closely monitored during concurrent therapy, and the dose of digitoxin may need to be increased.

Reference

1. Solomon, H.M., and others: Interactions between digitoxin and other drugs in vitro and in vivo, Ann. N.Y. Acad. Sci. **179:**362, 1971.

Digitoxin–Rifampin

1

Summary: Serum digitoxin concentrations can be significantly reduced with concurrent use of rifampin.[1-4] Another study reported that the digitoxin half-life was reduced approximately 50% by rifampin.[5] Most of these alterations were seen within a week of beginning co-therapy.

Related Drugs: Rifampin caused a patient to develop subtherapeutic digoxin serum concentrations.[6] There is no documentation that rifampin alters the disposition of the other digitalis glycosides (deslanoside and digitalis); however, based on pharmacologic similarity an interaction may be expected to occur. There are no drugs related to rifampin.

Mechanism: Rifampin is a known inducer of microsomal enzymes responsible for the metabolism of many drugs. It is therefore suggested that rifampin increases the metabolism of digitoxin. This is further supported by the observation that rifampin caused an increased rate of 12-beta-hydroxylation of digitoxin to digoxin.[5]

Recommendations: Patients should be monitored for underdigitalization during concurrent therapy with rifampin. It would be expected that the dosage of the glycoside will need to be increased within the first week of co-therapy.

References

1. Peters, U., and others: The effects of antituberculosis drugs on the pharmacokinetics of digitoxin, Dtsch. Med. Wochenschr. **99:**2381, 1974.
2. Boman, G., and others: Acute cardiac failure during treatment with digitoxin—an interaction with rifampin, Br. J. Clin. Pharmacol. **10:**89, 1980.
3. Acocella, G., and Conti, R.: Interaction of rifampicin with other drugs, Tubercle **61:**171, 1980.
4. Poor, D.M., and others: Interaction of rifampin and digitoxin, Arch. Intern. Med. **143:**599, 1983.
5. Zilly, W., and others: Pharmacokinetics interactions with rifampicin, Clin. Pharmacokinet. **2:**61, 1977.
6. Novi, C., and others: Rifampin and digoxin: possible drug interaction in a dialysis patient, J.A.M.A. **244:**2521, 1980.

Digitoxin–Spironolactone

3

Summary: Because of conflicting data, whether spironolactone administration increases or reduces the therapeutic action of digitoxin cannot be documented. Animal studies to date show a reduced toxicity of digitoxin,[1,2] and a study in 8 patients who were pretreated with spironolactone for at least 10 days before digitoxin administration showed a reduction in the half-life and volume of distribution of digitoxin.[3] However, another study in healthy volunteers showed prolongation of digitoxin elimination after spironolactone administration. Digitoxin was given for 30 days before spironolactone.[4]

Related Drugs: Digoxin's volume of distribution, plasma clearance, and renal clearance were decreased after spironolactone.[5,6] Correspondingly, the plasma digoxin concentrations increased. In a case study, serum digoxin concentration decreased from 2.4 ng/ml to 1.5 ng/ml after the discontinuation of spironolactone.[7] Conflicting reports make it difficult to predict whether an interaction would occur between spironolactone and the other digitalis glycosides (deslanoside and digitalis).

Other potassium sparing diuretics (amiloride and triamterene) have not been shown to interact with digitoxin; however, amiloride caused an increase in the renal clearance and a decrease in the nonrenal clearance of digoxin, although the total body clearance was only slightly reduced.[8] It appears that the interaction has little or no dependence on the potassium-sparing effects of spironolactone.

Mechanism: The evidence suggests that the reduced effect of digitoxin in animals and the reduced half-life and volume of distribution in humans are caused by spironolactone's ability to act as an enzyme-inducing agent in the liver, resulting in a shorter half-life for digitoxin.[1-3]

The mechanism for spironolactone increasing the half-life of digitoxin in humans is purely speculative. It is possible that spironolactone does not enhance digitoxin elimination in human bile as it does in animals. The data are consistent, but no explanation for this effect can be provided.[3]

The study with digoxin showed a slight increase in steady-state plasma concentrations of digoxin. The effect was attributed to reduced renal tubular clearance of digoxin caused by competitive blocking by spironolactone.[5,7] This may be the mechanism that occurs with digitoxin as well, but again this is not known.[5] It has also been suggested that spironolactone and its metabolites interfere with the commonly used digoxin radioimmunoassay procedure, thereby producing elevated serum digoxin concentrations.[7]

Recommendations: Until more clinical data are published, the combination of spironolactone and digitoxin should be monitored closely if the 2 must be given concurrently. Potassium and digitalis glycoside levels should be monitored frequently to assure therapeutic effectiveness.[9]

References

1. Selye, H., and others: Effect of spironolactone and norbolethone on the toxicity of digitalis compounds in the rat, Br. J. Pharmacol. **37:**485, 1969.
2. Solymoss, B., and others: Protection by spironolactone and oxandrolone against chronic digitoxin or indomethacin intoxication, Toxicol. Appl. Pharmacol. **18:**586, 1971.
3. Wirth, K.E., and others: Metabolism of digitoxin in man and its modification by spironolactone, Eur. J. Clin. Pharmacol. **9:**345, 1976.
4. Carruthers, S.G., and Dujovne, C.A.: Cholestyramine and spironolactone and their combination in digitoxin elimination, Clin. Pharmacol. Ther. **27:**184, 1980.
5. Steiness, E.: Renal tubular secretion of digoxin, Circulation **50:**103, 1974.
6. Waldorff, S., and others: Spironolactone-induced changes in digoxin kinetics, Clin. Pharmacol. Ther. **24:**162, 1978.
7. Paladino, J.A., and others: Influence of spironolactone on serum digoxin concentration, J.A.M.A. **251:**470, 1984.
8. Waldorff, S., and others: Amiloride-induced changes in digoxin dynamics and kinetics: abolition of digoxin-induced inotropism with amiloride, Clin. Pharmacol. Ther. **30:**172, 1981.
9. Doherty, J.E., and Kane, J.J.: Clinical pharmacology and therapeutic use of digitalis glycosides, Drugs **6:**182, 1973.

Digoxin–Aluminum Hydroxide, Magnesium Hydroxide, Magnesium Trisilicate

2

Summary: Simultaneous administration of oral antacids containing magnesium trisilicate, magnesium hydroxide, and aluminum hydroxide may significantly decrease the gastrointestinal absorption of digoxin from oral tablets.[1-3] There is some evidence that digoxin capsules may not be affected by concurrent aluminum/magnesium hydroxide ingestion.[3]

Related Drugs: The absorption of digoxin tablets was not impaired by concurrent administration of oral calcium carbonate in 1 study.[4] The absorption of digitoxin is also reduced by magnesium trisilicate.[5] Although this effect has not been documented, the other digitalis glycosides (deslanoside and digitalis) may interact with antacids to a variable degree.

The extent to which other magnesium or aluminum containing antacids affect digoxin absorption is not known.

Mechanism: In vitro studies indicate that the adsorptive capacity of antacids (especially magnesium trisilicate) may be partially responsible for decreased digoxin absorption.[5,6] It has also been suggested that liquid antacids coat digoxin tablets and thereby interfere with proper dissolution or disintegration of the tablets in the gastrointestinal tract.[7] A reduction in gut transit time is an unlikely explanation, in view of the fact that decreased absorption occurs after both constipating and diarrheal preparations.[1]

Recommendations: Oral digoxin tablets should not be given simultaneously with certain antacids (e.g., aluminum/magnesium hydroxide and magnesium trisilicate). When both digoxin and antacids are indicated, antacid preparations containing magnesium trisilicate, magnesium hydroxide, and aluminum hydroxide should be administered at least 1 to 2 hours before or after the digoxin. Serum digoxin levels and the clinical status of the patient should be monitored carefully for signs of underdigitalization.

References

1. Brown, D.D., and Juhl, R.P.: Decreased bioavailability of digoxin due to antacids and kaolin-pectin, N. Engl. J. Med. **295**:1034, 1976.
2. McElnay, J.C., and others: Interaction of digoxin with antacid constituents, Br. Med. J. **1**:1554, 1978.
3. Allen, M.D., and others: Effect of magnesium-aluminum hydroxide and kaolin-pectin on absorption of digoxin from tablets and capsules, J. Clin. Pharmacol. **21**:26, 1981.
4. Brown, D.D., and Juhl, R.P.: Altered bioavailability of digoxin produced by gastrointestinal medications, Clin. Res. **27**:610a, 1979.
5. Khalil, S.A.H.: The uptake of digoxin by some antacids, J. Pharm. Pharmacol. **26**:961, 1974.
6. Khalil, S.A.H.: Bioavailability of digoxin in presence of antacids, J. Pharm. Sci. **63**:1642, 1974.
7. Brown, D.D., and others: Drug interactions with digoxin, Drugs **20**:198, 1980.

Digoxin–Aminosalicylic Acid

3

Summary: In a study involving 10 healthy volunteers, the concurrent administration of a single digoxin dose and aminosalicylic acid (2 g 4 times a day for 2 weeks) resulted in a reduced digoxin area-under-curve and a decrease in the 6 day cumulative urinary excretion. The half-life of digoxin was not affected.[1] The clinical significance of this interaction was not determined.

Related Drugs: Although documentation is lacking, a similar interaction may be expected between aminosalicylic acid and the other digitalis glycosides (deslanoside, digitalis, and digitoxin) because of pharmacologic similarity. There are no drugs related to aminosalicylic acid.

Mechanism: Aminosalicylic acid is known to induce malabsorption; therefore, decreased gastrointestinal absorption of digoxin is believed to be the mechanism in this interaction. This proposed mechanism was strengthened by in vitro adsorption data.[1]

Recommendations: Patients' digoxin serum levels should be monitored during concomitant use of these agents. An increased digoxin dose may be necessary, or separating the administration of the 2 drugs by as much time as possible may be beneficial.

Reference

1. Brown, P.D., and others: Decreased bioavailability of digoxin due to hypercholesterolemic interventions, Circulation **58**:164, 1978.

Digoxin–Cyclophosphamide, Prednisone, Procarbazine, Vincristine

2

Summary: A single dose of digoxin was administered to 6 patients with malignant lymphoma before and 24 hours after the first dose of treatment with cyclophosphamide, prednisone, procarbazine, and vincristine (COPP therapy) or 24 hours after a 3 to 5 day course of cyclophosphamide, prednisone, and vincristine (COP therapy). The digoxin area-under-curve was reduced by 29% to 30% in all 6 patients. The effects of this interaction continued for several days after discontinuation of the chemotherapeutic agents.[1]

Related Drugs: In another study with 15 patients, digoxin was administered every day before, during, and after treatment with COPP, COP, and COP plus another chemotherapy combination including cytarabine or doxorubicin, bleomycin, and prednisone. The renal excretion and plasma levels of digoxin were reduced by approximately 50%.[1] A similar interaction may be expected with the other vinca alkaloid (vinblastine) when used in combination chemotherapy, although this has not been documented. The extent of digitoxin absorption is not altered by combination chemotherapy, not including bleomycin, as shown in 1 study.[2] There is lack of documentation regarding a similar interaction with the other digitalis glycosides (deslanoside and digitalis). However, if the mechanism involves a decrease in the gastrointestinal absorption of digoxin, it appears that an interaction may occur with these agents as well.

Mechanism: Although the mechanism has not been fully elucidated, it has been suggested that the decreased digoxin levels indicate a reduction in the extent of gastrointestinal absorption of digoxin, possibly resulting from impairment of the intestinal mucosa membrane by the cytotoxic drugs.[1,2]

Recommendations: It is not known whether the individual antineoplastic agents alone will produce the same effect on digoxin therapy, but it may be prudent to be aware of this interaction whether the agents are used in combination or not. Therefore, patients should be closely monitored since a higher dose of digoxin may be necessary. Alternatively, digitoxin may be used in place of digoxin because it was shown to not interact with chemotherapy agents.[2]

References

1. Kuhlman, J., and others: Effects of cytostatic drugs on plasma level and renal excretion of beta-acetyldigoxin, Clin. Pharmacol. Ther. **30:**518, 1981.
2. Kuhlman, J., and others: Cytostatic drugs are without significant effect on digitoxin plasma level and renal excretion, Clin. Pharmacol. Ther. **32:**646, 1982.

Digoxin–Diazepam

2

Summary: During concurrent administration of digoxin and diazepam in 7 subjects, a moderate increase in digoxin half-life was reported in 5 subjects and a substantial decrease in urinary excretion of digoxin was reported in all 7 subjects.[1]

Related Drugs: There appear to be no reports of a similar interaction between the other digitalis glycosides (deslanoside, digitalis, and digitoxin) and diazepam. However, if the interaction is due to a renal mechanism, then deslanoside may interact with diazepam based on a similar metabolic fate. Digitoxin and digitalis are hepatically metabolized and would not be expected to interact similarly. Because of pharmacologic similarity, the other benzodiazepines (e.g., clorazepate, flurazepam, triazolam [see Appendix]) may interact with digoxin, although documentation is lacking.

Mechanism: The mechanism of this interaction is unknown. An increase of about 15% in digoxin binding to plasma proteins was produced by diazepam in vitro. This effect could play a part in the diminished renal excretion of digoxin, although an effect of diazepam on the renal tubular transport of digoxin cannot be excluded.[1]

Recommendations: Patients should be monitored for an increase in digoxin levels, and a lower dose of digoxin may be necessary.

Reference

1. Castillo-Ferando, J.R., and others: Digoxin levels and diazepam, Lancet **1:**368, 1980.

Digoxin–Disopyramide

3

Summary: After an intravenous bolus dose of digoxin (0.8 mg) in 5 healthy subjects, the administration of disopyramide (600 mg/day) significantly reduced the volume of distribution (39% decrease) and elimination half-life (45% decrease) of digoxin. Total clearance and distribution half-life of digoxin did not significantly change.[1] However, in 9 other male subjects the concurrent use of oral digoxin (0.375 mg/day) and disopyramide (300 mg/day) did not alter steady-state digoxin serum concentrations above baseline. However, after the subjects had received disopyramide at 600 mg/day for 1 week, the mean serum digoxin level increased (33%). The clinical significance of this interaction was not determined. In another study involving 10 patients receiving long-term oral digoxin (0.25 to 0.5 mg/day), the concurrent use of disopyramide (300 to 600 mg/day) did not affect serum digoxin levels.[2]

Related Drugs: It is not known whether a similar interaction would occur between disopyramide and the other digitalis glycosides (deslanoside, digitalis, and digitoxin). There are no drugs related to disopyramide.

Mechanism: The mechanism of this interaction is unknown.

Recommendations: Until further studies are done, the concurrent use of these agents need not be avoided, and no special precautions appear necessary.

References

1. Risler, T., and others: On the interaction between digoxin and disopyramide, Clin. Pharmacol. Ther. **34:**176, 1983.
2. Wellens, H.J.J., and others: Effect of oral disopyramide on serum digoxin levels, a prospective study, Am. Heart J. **100:**934, 1980.

Digoxin–Erythromycin Base

1

Summary: Steady-state serum digoxin concentrations were reported to be 2 times higher with a 5-day course of erythromycin base therapy in 2 subjects.[1] There was a corresponding decrease in the urinary and fecal excretion of digoxin reduction products. The effect of erythromycin on the formation of digoxin reduction products may persist for several months after the discontinuation of the antibiotic.

Related Drugs: Other erythromycin salts (estolate, ethylsuccinate, gluceptate, lactobionate, stearate, and sulfate) are expected to undergo a similar interaction with digoxin. There are no reports of the other macrolide antibiotics (oleandomycin and troleandomycin) interacting with digoxin or any of the other digitalis glycosides. However, based on their pharmacologic activity a similar interaction may be expected to occur. It is not known if an interaction will occur between erythromycin and the other digitalis glycosides (deslanoside, digitalis, and digitoxin).

Mechanism: Approximately 10% of the patients who receive digoxin convert a substantial portion of it to digoxin reduction products.[1,2] These products are formed predominantly by the bacteria in the gastrointestinal tract. The antibiotic, by destroying the bacteria, decreases digoxin metabolism, which would account for the increased digoxin serum concentrations.[2]

Recommendations: Digoxin serum concentrations should be monitored when initiating or discontinuing concurrent erythromycin therapy. Patients who are receiving erythromycin and being digitalized should be closely monitored for overdigitalization.

References

1. Lindenbaum, J., and others: Inactivation of digoxin by the gut flora: reversal by antibiotic therapy, N. Engl. J. Med. **305:**789, 1981.
2. Friedman, H.S., and others: Erythromycin-induced digoxin toxicity, Chest **82:**202, 1982.

Digoxin–Furosemide

2

Summary: Six of 12 patients with congestive heart failure receiving maintenance therapy with digoxin and either furosemide or bumetanide developed cardiac arrhythmias compatible with digoxin toxicity in the presence of stable, normal serum digoxin concentrations.[1] In another study, 22% of the patients receiving this combination also developed digoxin toxicity.[2] Perhaps the most significant aspect of this interaction involves the hypokalemia resulting from extracellular fluid potassium losses. However, other potassium depleting diuretic-induced alterations such as hypercalcemia[3] and hypomagnesemia[4] may also contribute to the enhanced digitalis glycoside toxicity. Studies have shown that diuretic induced potassium losses generally involve less than 10% of total body potassium.[5] Losses are derived from extracellular fluid, and over a period of several months' treatment, stabilization of serum potassium levels tends to occur via redistribution from tissues. To circumvent potential hypokalemic digitalis-induced arrhythmias during diuretic therapy, prophylactic potassium supplements may be necessary.

Related Drugs: Other digitalis glycosides that have been reported to interact with diuretics are digitalis and digitoxin.[6,7] Although no documentation exists, the other digitalis glycoside (deslanoside) may be expected to interact in a similar manner based on pharmacologic similarity.

All potassium-depleting diuretics may be expected to interact with digoxin in a similar manner to furosemide. These include the thiazides (e.g., chlorothiazide,[7] hydrochlorothiazide,[2] polythiazide [see Appendix]), the other loop diuretic (ethacrynic acid), the mercurial diuretic (mersalyl),[6,7] and thiazide related diuretics (e.g., chlorthalidone, metolazone, indapamide [see Appendix]).

Mechanism: Digoxin acts on excitable tissues of the myocardium to inhibit sodium/potassium dependent ATPase. In hypokalemia there is less extracellular potassium available to exchange for intracellular sodium through remaining sodium pump activity, and membranes become even more depolarized. Thus furosemide and other diuretics enhance the electrophysiologic effects of digoxin primarily by disturbing the normal potassium gradient across cell membranes.

Recommendations: There is a growing uncertainty about the clinical significance of diuretic-induced hypokalemia.[8] Although it is possible that furosemide will not cause a severe long-term depletion of total body potassium and therefore not significantly or consistently increase digoxin toxicity, it may be prudent to supplement patients with oral potassium chloride preparations when initiating furosemide therapy. Gastrointestinal lesions have been associated with the use of enteric-coated potassium formulations as a result of the high concentrations of the chloride salt that are released after dissolution of the enteric coat. This is seldom a problem with the more modern preparations that have a wax matrix, but remains a possibility.[8] Therefore, these agents should be used with caution. Intact renal function is necessary to minimize the potential of potassium toxicity and careful monitoring of the patient's serum potassium level is necessary.[5] Selection of a potassium-sparing diuretic or combined thiazide/potassium-sparing diuretic therapy may be an alternative approach to managing hypertension and/or edema in a digitalized patient.[9]

References

1. Steiness, E., and Olesen, K.H.: Cardiac arrhythmias induced by hypokalemia and potassium loss during maintenance digoxin therapy, Br. Heart J. **38:**167, 1976.
2. Shapiro, S., and others: The epidemiology of digoxin, a study in three Boston hospitals, J. Chron. Dis. **22:**361, 1969.
3. Mohamadi, M., and others: Effect of thiazides on serum calcium, Clin. Pharmacol. Ther. **26:**390, 1979.
4. Iseri, L.T., and others: Magnesium deficiency and cardiac disorders, Am. J. Med. **58:**837, 1975.
5. Sandor, F.F., and others: Variations of plasma potassium concentrations during long-term treatment of hypertension with diuretics without potassium supplements, Br. Med. J. **284:**710, 1982.
6. Tawakkol, A.A., and others: A prospective study of digitalis toxicity in a large city hospital, Med. Ann. D.C. **36:**402, 1967.
7. Soffer, A.: The changing clinical picture of digitalis intoxication, Arch. Intern. Med. **107:**681, 1961.
8. Lawson, A.R.H.: Potassium replacement: when is it necessary? Drugs **21:**354, 1981.
9. Kohvakka, A., and others: Maintenance of potassium balance during diuretic therapy, Acta Med. Scand. **205:**319, 1979.

Digoxin–Hydroxychloroquine

Summary: Serum digoxin levels exceeded 3.1 nmol/L in 2 patients receiving hydroxychloroquine for rheumatoid arthritis, although digoxin toxicity did not appear in either patient. When hydroxychloroquine was discontinued, digoxin serum levels fell by more than two-thirds.[1]

Related Drugs: Documentation is lacking regarding a similar interaction between the other digitalis glycosides (deslanoside, digitalis, and digitoxin) and the other aminoquinolines (chloroquine and primaquine); however, based on pharmacologic similarity an interaction may be expected to occur.

Mechanism: The mechanism of this interaction is unknown. However, hydroxychloroquine is a semisynthetic cinchona derivative related to quinidine, and the interaction between digoxin and quinidine is well documented (see Digoxin-Quinidine, p. 525). Therefore, a similar mechanism may be involved here as well.[1]

Recommendations: Patients should be closely monitored for signs of digoxin toxicity during concurrent use of these agents, and the dose of digoxin may need to be reduced.

Reference

1. Leden, I.: Digoxin-hydroxychloroquine interaction? Acta Med. Scand. **211:**411, 1982.

Digoxin–Ibuprofen

2

Summary: Serum digoxin levels were significantly increased in 12 patients after concurrent administration of ibuprofen for 7 days. However, there was no significant difference in digoxin levels after 28 days of concomitant therapy.[1]

Related Drugs: There is a lack of documentation regarding an interaction between ibuprofen and the other digitalis glycosides (deslanoside, digitalis, and digitoxin). However, if the mechanism involves decreased renal excretion then deslanoside may interact similarly. Digitalis and digitoxin are hepatically metabolized and would not be expected to interact with ibuprofen. Indomethacin-induced digoxin toxicity in 3 premature infants has been reported in 1 study.[2] Documentation is lacking regarding an interaction with the other nonsteroidal anti-inflammatory agents (e.g., naproxen, piroxicam, sulindac [see Appendix]); however, based on pharmacologic similarity an interaction may be expected to occur.

Mechanism: The mechanism of this interaction is unknown. However, a potential mechanism may be decreased digoxin renal excretion, since nonsteroidal anti-inflammatory agents are known to depress kidney function in patients with underlying renal disease.[1]

Recommendations: Patients should be monitored for digoxin toxicity throughout concurrent therapy with ibuprofen. If toxicity appears, the dose of digoxin may need to be decreased.

References

1. Quattrocchi, F.P., and others: The effect of ibuprofen on serum digoxin concentrations, Drug Intell. Clin. Pharm. **17:**286, 1983.
2. Mayes, L.C., and Boerth, R.C.: Digoxin-indomethacin interaction, Pediatr. Res. **14:**469, 1980.

Digoxin—Kaolin

Summary: Concurrent administration of kaolin-pectin suspension and digoxin tablets resulted in a significant reduction in digoxin bioavailability.[1-3] One steady-state study reported only a slight reduction in digoxin bioavailability.[4] When the kaolin-pectin suspension was given 2 hours before or after digoxin, there was less reduction in digoxin bioavailability.[1,4] The suspension had no effect on digoxin disposition when digoxin was given as the soft gelatin capsule.[3]

Related Drugs: There appear to be no reported studies of the effect of kaolin-pectin suspension on the bioavailability of the other digitalis glycosides (deslanoside, digitalis, and digitoxin), although based on pharmacologic similarity an interaction may be expected to occur. In 1 study, the bioavailability of digoxin was decreased by concurrent diphenoxylate and atropine, an antidiarrheal combination, as measured by the cumulative 6 day urinary excretion.[4]

Mechanism: Although the mechanism is not fully elucidated, part of the interaction may result from the adsorption of digoxin to kaolin preventing the gastrointestinal absorption of digoxin. Another proposed mechanism is that kaolin alters the gastrointestinal motility; however, this has been challenged.[2]

Recommendations: The steady-state study[4] indicates that the interaction is not of major clinical significance, although other studies report a significant decrease in digoxin bioavailability. Administering the kaolin-pectin suspension at least 2 hours after digoxin appears to avoid the interaction. If the agents must be administered simultaneously, then digoxin as the soft gelatin capsule or the elixir is recommended. The patient receiving both digoxin and kaolin-pectin suspension concurrently should be observed for signs and symptoms of underdigitalization.

References

1. Albert, K.S., and others: Influence of kaolin-pectin suspension on digoxin bioavailability, J. Pharm. Sci. **67:**1582, 1978.
2. Brown, D.D., and Juhl, R.P.: Decreased bioavailability of digoxin due to antacids and kaolin-pectin, N. Engl. J. Med. **295:**1034, 1976.
3. Allen, M.D., and others: Effect of mangesium-aluminum hydroxide and kaolin-pectin on absorption of digoxin from tablets and capsules, J. Clin. Pharmacol. **21:**26, 1981.
4. Albert, K.S., and others: Influence of kaolin-pectin suspension on steady state plasma digoxin levels, J. Clin. Pharmacol. **21:**449, 1981.

Digoxin–Metoclopramide

2

Summary: Steady-state serum digoxin concentrations were reduced approximately one-third in a group of elderly female patients receiving metoclopramide.[1] The reduction was attributed to a decreased digoxin bioavailability, although one study disagreed with that conclusion.[2] When metoclopramide was discontinued, digoxin concentrations returned to previous levels. Currently, no information is available concerning whether an interaction will occur with the soft gelatin digoxin capsule.[3]

Related Drugs: There appear to be no reports of a similar interaction with the other digitalis glycosides (deslanoside, digitalis, and digitoxin); however, based on pharmacologic similarity an interaction may be expected to occur. There are no drugs related to metoclopramide.

Mechanism: Metoclopramide stimulates the smooth muscle in the gastrointestinal tract to increase peristalsis. It is suggested this action reduces the time digoxin is at the absorption site, causing less drug to be absorbed since digoxin absorption is dissolution-rate limited.[4-6] One report has proposed that metoclopramide alters digoxin levels by increasing biliary excretion of digoxin.[7]

Recommendations: Metoclopramide will influence digoxin absorption less from fast-dissolving digoxin tablets or liquid preparations than from slow-dissolving tablets. Thus, slow-dissolving preparations may underdigitalize patients currently receiving metoclopramide. Digoxin serum concentrations should therefore be monitored when these agents are used concomitantly.

References

1. Manninen, V., and others: Altered absorption of digoxin in patients given propantheline and metoclopramide, Lancet **1:**398, 1973.
2. Michalopoulos, C.D., and Koutoulidis, C.V.: Altered digoxin bioavailability, Lancet **1:**167, 1974.
3. Personal communication, Burroughs-Wellcome Co., 1983.
4. Manninen, V., and others: Effect of propantheline and metoclopramide on absorption of digoxin, Lancet **1:**1118, 1973.
5. Medin, S., and Nyberg, L.: Effect of propantheline and metoclopramide on absorption of digoxin, Lancet **1:**1391, 1973.
6. Fraser, E.J., and others: Dissolution-rates and bioavailability of digoxin tablets, Lancet **1:**1393, 1973.
7. Thompson, W.G.: Altered absorption of digoxin in patients given propantheline and metoclopramide, Lancet **1:**783, 1973.

Digoxin–Neomycin

2

Summary: Concurrent administration of neomycin sulfate markedly depressed serum digoxin concentrations, which resulted in an average decrease of 41% to 51% in the serum digoxin area-under-curve.[1,2] Urinary recovery data and time to peak concentration data were consistent with a decreased and delayed digoxin absorption. Neomycin did not alter the digoxin half-life. When neomycin was given with maintenance digoxin doses, steady-state digoxin serum concentrations were reduced an average of 28%[2]

Related Drugs: There is no documentation regarding an interaction between neomycin and the other digitalis glycosides (deslanoside, digitalis, and digitoxin) or between digoxin and the other available oral aminoglycosides (kanamycin and paromomycin) although an interaction may be expected to occur due to pharmacologic similarity.

Mechanism: The exact mechanism has not been established. Proposed mechanisms are that neomycin causes a precipitation of digoxin or that neomycin changes the intestinal membrane permeability.

Recommendations: The interaction was seen with neomycin dosages from 1.0 g to 3.0 g with tablets or solutions of both digoxin and neomycin, or when neomycin was given 3 or 6 hours before digoxin.[2] Therefore, if neomycin is added to or discontinued from concurrent digoxin therapy, patients must be monitored for changing digoxin serum concentrations and dosage adjustments should be made.[3] Patients receiving neomycin who are being digitalized should be closely monitored for underdigitalization.

References

1. Lindenbaum, J., and others: Impairment of digoxin absorption by neomycin, Clin. Res. **20:**410, 1972.
2. Lindenbaum, J., and others: Inhibition of digoxin absorption by neomycin, Gastroenterology **71:**399, 1976.
3. Lindenbaum, J., and others: Urinary excretion of reduced metabolites of digoxin, Am. J. Med. **71:**67, 1981.

Digoxin–Penicillamine

Summary: Two reports show that concurrent use of digoxin and penicillamine results in significantly reduced serum digoxin levels, regardless of the route of administration of digoxin.[1,2]

Related Drugs: There is no documentation regarding a similar interaction between penicillamine and the other digitalis glycosides (deslanoside, digitalis, and digitoxin). There are no drugs related to penicillamine.

Mechanism: The exact mechanism is not known. Whether digoxin is eliminated faster or sequestered in the noncirculating part of the body by penicillamine, a chelating agent, is unknown.[1]

Recommendations: Patients should be monitored for decreased digoxin levels. The dose of digoxin may need to be increased.

References

1. Moezzi, B., and others: The effect of penicillamine on serum digoxin levels. Jpn. Heart J. **19:**366, 1978.
2. Moezzi, B., and others: Reversal of digoxin-induced changes in erythrocyte electrolyte concentrations by penicillamine in children, Jpn. Heart J. **21:**335, 1980.

Digoxin–Propantheline

Summary: Absorption of digoxin may be significantly increased by concomitant administration of propantheline. A slowly absorbed tablet will have a greater than expected
bioavailability as a result of the prolonged emptying time induced by propantheline.
The selection of a fast absorption formulation of digoxin or the elixir will circumvent
the risk of inconsistent digoxin blood levels. With liquid or fast-dissolving tablets,
consistent bioavailability will be achieved in spite of prolonged gastrointestinal transit time. The soft gelatin capsule form, which contains a solution of digoxin dissolved
in a mixture of PEG 400, 8% ethyl alcohol, propylene glycol, and purified water is
also absorbed rapidly; therefore, an interaction between propantheline and the gelatin capsule form of digoxin may not prove to be as significant as the effect that
occurs with the slowly absorbed tablet.[1]

Related Drugs: Undocumented risk may be anticipated with all the anticholinergics
(e.g., atropine, dicyclomine, scopolamine [see Appendix]) based on pharmacologic
similarity. It is difficult to determine whether an interaction would occur between
propantheline and the other digitalis glycosides (deslanoside, digitalis, and digitoxin) since the interaction appears to depend on the rate of dissolution of the dosage
form. However, all slowly dissolving digitalis glycoside preparations may be expected to interact similarly.

Mechanism: The medication in a slow-dissolving tablet will be more extensively
absorbed if the time spent in the intestine is increased.[2] The prolonged intestine
emptying time induced by propantheline (i.e., decreased tone, amplitude, and frequency of peristaltic contraction), will facilitate more complete absorption[3-5] than
normally experienced.

Recommendations: The problem presented by a patient who requires propantheline
and digoxin can be circumvented by the selection of quickly absorbed digoxin preparations: either rapidly solubilized tablets or the liquid digoxin. The soft gelatin
capsule form of digoxin might also be considered because of its rapid dissolution.
Should digitalized patients experience symptoms indicative of digitalis glycoside
intoxication with the use of propantheline or similar drugs, it may be from excessive
absorption of digoxin from a slowly disintegrating tablet. Changing to a rapidly
absorbed preparation will give predictable blood levels.

References

1. Personal communication, Burroughs Wellcome Co., Aug., 1983.
2. Hoffman, B.F., and Bigger, J.T., Jr.: Digitalis and allied cardiac glycosides. In Gilman, A.G., Goodman,
   L.S., and Gilman, A., editors: The pharmacological basis of therapeutics, New York, 1980, Macmillan
   Publishing Co.
3. Manninen, V., and others: Altered absorption of digoxin in patients given propantheline and metoclopramide, Lancet **1**:398, 1973.
4. Huffmann, D.H., and Azarnoff, D.L.: Absorption of orally given digoxin preparations, J.A.M.A.
   222:957, 1972.
5. Doherty, J.E.: The clinical pharmacology of digitalis glycosides, a review, Am. J. Med. Sci. **255**:382,
   1968.

Digoxin–Psyllium

3

Summary: In a single dose, crossover study with 10 normal volunteers, coadministration of psyllium hydrophilic mucilloid reduced the bioavailability of digoxin compared to digoxin alone.[1] In the coadministration trial, 7 g of psyllium were given 8 hours before digoxin and an additional 7 g with digoxin.

Related Drugs: There appear to be no other reports that any of the digitalis glycosides (deslanoside, digitalis, and digitoxin) interact similarly with other bulk producing laxatives (e.g., methylcellulose, hemicellulose, barley malt extract [see Appendix]), although an interaction may be expected to occur based on the mechanism.

Mechanism: Possible physical binding of digoxin to psyllium or other absorptive hindrance may explain this interaction.

Recommendations: Although information is limited, the interaction seems to produce some degree of reduced digoxin absorption. If long-term psyllium and digoxin cotherapy is undertaken, patients should be monitored for decreasing digoxin serum concentrations. A 2 hour interval between dosage with these drugs may prevent any problem.

Reference

1. Brown, D.D., and Juhl, R.P.: Altered bioavailability of digoxin produced by gastrointestinal medications, Clin. Res. **27:**610A, 1979.

Digoxin–Quinidine

Summary: It is well documented that quinidine alters digoxin pharmacokinetics when administered simultaneously. A roughly 2-fold increase in plasma digoxin concentration has been observed when quinidine is coadministered.[1-30] Reduced digoxin volume of distribution, prolonged digoxin elimination half-life, and reduced total digoxin clearance have been reported with combined digoxin-quinidine therapy. There is some indication that the rise in digoxin concentration depends on the dosage of quinidine.[14,16,18] Significant changes in serum digoxin levels may appear within the first day of combined therapy[16,18,19] and persist as long as combination therapy is continued.[7,13,16]

Related Drugs: Similar effects have been seen when quinidine and digitoxin are combined, since digitoxin serum concentration increased, clearance was decreased, and its elimination half-life prolonged by oral quinidine administration.[29,31-33] However, 1 study found that quinidine had no statistically significant effect on the distribution or clearance of intravenous digitoxin.[34] The other cinchona alkaloid, quinine, was found to increase digoxin plasma concentration when used concurrently.[35,36] Conflicting results make it difficult to determine whether a similar interaction would occur between quinidine and the other digitalis glycosides (deslanoside and digitalis).

Mechanism: Reduction in digoxin renal clearance and displacement from tissue digoxin binding sites, leading to a reduced volume of distribution, appear to be the predominant mechanisms involved in this interaction. It has been suggested that quinidine inhibits the renal secretion of digoxin, reducing total renal digoxin clearance.[8,23] Digoxin absorption and bioavailability do not appear to be altered by quinidine.[5] It has been suggested that the reduction in digitoxin clearance by quinidine results from a reduction in hepatic metabolism or biliary excretion or that quinidine interferes with the urinary excretion of the unchanged drug or its cardioactive metabolites.[32]

Recommendations: Because of the well-documented occurrence of this interaction, it is suggested that the digoxin dosage be reduced when quinidine is to be given concurrently.[2,8,19,20,23,37] Some reports suggest reducing the digoxin dosage by 30% to 50%[11,13,23] when quinidine is to be coadministered. Digoxin toxicity (anorexia, nausea, vomiting) may be enhanced by quinidine.[8,13,38] Therefore, patients receiving both drugs should be monitored carefully for these symptoms. To avoid this interaction, an alternative antiarrhythmic drug such as disopyramide or procainamide may be considered for use instead of quinidine.[10,13,21] However, digoxin may also interact with disopyramide (see Digoxin-Disopyramide, p. 513). A fall in serum digoxin levels should be expected when the quinidine-digoxin combination is discontinued and appropriate digoxin dosage adjustments made to counteract this decrease.

References

1. Ejvinsson, G.: Effect of quinidine on plasma concentrations of digoxin, Br. Med. J. **1:**279, 1978.
2. Reiffel, J.A., and others: A digoxin/quinidine adverse drug interaction, Am. J. Cardiol. **41:**368, 1978.
3. Leahey, E.B., and others: Interaction between quinidine and digoxin, J.A.M.A. **240:**533, 1978.
4. Hooymans, P.M., and Merkus, F.W.H.M.: Effect of quinidine on plasma concentration of digoxin, Br. Med. J. **2:**1022, 1978.
5. Hager, W.D., and others: Digoxin bioavailability during quinidine administration, Clin. Pharmacol. Ther. **30:**594, 1981.
6. Schenck-Gustafsson, K., and others: Effect of quinidine on digoxin concentration in skeletal muscle and serum in patients with atrial fibrillation, Med. Intell. **305:**209, 1981.
7. Leahey, E.B., and others: Enhanced cardiac effect of digoxin during quinidine treatment, Arch. Intern. Med. **139:**519, 1979.
8. Hager, W.D., and others: Digoxin-quinidine interaction: pharmacokinetic evaluation, N. Engl. J. Med. **300:**1238, 1979.
9. Ochs, H.R., and others: Impairment of digoxin clearance by coadministration of quinidine, J. Clin. Pharmacol. **21:**396, 1981.
10. Burkle, W.S., and Matzke, G.R.: Effect of quinidine on serum digoxin concentrations, Am. J. Hosp. Pharm. **36:**968, 1979.
11. Doering, W.: Quinidine-digoxin interaction, pharmacokinetics, underlying mechanism and clinical implications, N. Engl. J. Med. **301:**400, 1979.
12. Holt, D.W., and others: Clinically significant interaction between digoxin and quinidine, Br. Med. J. **2:**1401, 1979.
13. Lopez, L.M., and Mehta, J.: Digoxin-quinidine interaction, U.S. Pharmacist **6:**50, 1981.
14. Risler, T., and others: Quinidine-digoxin interaction, N. Engl. J. Med. **302:**175, 1980.
15. Powell, J.R., and others: Letter to the editor, N. Engl. J. Med. **302:**176, 1980.
16. Fenster, P.E., and others: Onset and dose dependence of the digoxin-quinidine interaction, Am. J. Cardiol. **45:**413, 1980.
17. Pedersen, K.E., and Hvidt, S.: Digoxin-quinidine interaction (letter), N. Engl. J. Med. **302:**176, 1980.
18. Powell, R., and others: Quinidine-digoxin interaction: multiple dose pharmacokinetics, Clin. Pharmacol. Ther. **27:**279, 1980.
19. Dahlqvist, R., and others: Effect of quinidine on plasma concentration and renal clearance of digoxin. A clinically important drug interaction, Br. J. Clin. Pharmacol. **9:**413, 1980.
20. Moench, T.R.: The quinidine-digoxin interaction (letter), N. Engl. J. Med. **302:**864, 1980.
21. Leahey, E.B., and others: The effect of quinidine and other oral antiarrhythmic drugs on serum digoxin, Ann. Intern. Med. **92:**605, 1980.
22. Steiness, E., and others: Reduction of digoxin-induced inotropism during quinidine administration, Clin. Pharmacol. Ther. **27:**791, 1980.
23. Pedersen, K.E., and others: The effect of quinidine on digoxin kinetics in cardiac patients, Acta Med. Scand. **207:**291, 1980.
24. Chen, T.S., and Friedman, H.S.: Alteration of digoxin pharmacokinetics by a single dose of quinidine, J.A.M.A. **244:**669, 1980.
25. Schenck-Gustafsson, K.: Digitalis and quinidine, Lancet **1:**105, 1981.
26. Fenster, P.E., and others: Digoxin-quinidine interaction in patients with chronic renal failure, Circulation **66:**1277, 1982.
27. Bigger, J.T., and Leakey, E.B.: Quinidine and digoxin: an important interaction, Drugs **24:**229, 1982.
28. Pieroni, R.E., and Marshall, J.: Fatal digoxin-quinidine interaction in an elderly woman, J. Am. Geriatr. Soc. **29:**422, 1981.
29. Woodcock, B.G., and Rietbrock, N.: Digitalis-quinidine interactions, Trends Pharm. Sci. **3:**118, 1982.
30. Fichtl, B., and Doering, W.: The quinidine-digoxin interaction in perspective, Clin. Pharmacokinet. **8:**137, 1983.
31. Fenster, P.E., and others: Combined digitoxin-quinidine administration: pharmacokinetic evaluation, Clin. Res. **28:**235A, 1980.

32. Garty, M., and others: Digitoxin elimination reduced during quinidine therapy, Ann. Intern. Med. **94:**35, 1981.
33. Peters, U., and others: Interaction of quinidine and digitoxin in the human, Dtsch. Med. Wochenschr. **105:**438, 1980.
34. Ochs, H.R., and others: Noninteraction of digitoxin and quinine, N. Engl. J. Med. **303:**672, 1980.
35. Wandell, M., and others: Effect of quinine on digoxin kinetics, Clin. Pharmacol. Ther. **28:**425, 1980.
36. Aronson, J.K., and Carver, J.G.: Interaction of digoxin with quinidine, Lancet **1:**1418, 1981.
37. Friedman, H.S., and Chen, T.: Use of control steady-state serum digoxin levels for predicting serum digoxin concentrations after quinidine administration, Am. Heart J. **104:**72, 1982.
38. Walker, A.M., and others: Drug toxicity in patients receiving digoxin and quinidine, Am. Heart J. **105:**1025, 1983.

Digoxin–Succinylcholine

2

Summary: There have been reports of cardiac arrhythmias occurring after the administration of succinylcholine to patients stabilized on digoxin.[1]

Related Drugs: In 1 study, the nondepolarizing neuromuscular blocking agents (e.g., atracurium, pancuronium, tubocurarine [see Appendix]) have not been shown to be involved in the interaction and have been used to abolish the arrhythmias.[2] However, in a conflicting report, 6 of 18 patients developed sinus tachycardia and 2 developed atrial flutter after concurrent administration of digoxin and pancuronium,[3] although deficiencies in study design make it difficult to make any firm conclusions from either study.

The other digitalis glycosides (deslanoside, digitalis, and digitoxin) may also be expected to interact with succinylcholine similarly since they are pharmacologically related.

Mechanism: The mechanism through which this interaction occurs is unclear, but may be related to a loss of intracellular potassium that results from the depolarizing neuromuscular blocking agents shifting potassium from inside the muscle cell to the outside. Other postulated mechanisms include sympathetic postganglionic stimulation and a direct effect on the myocardium by succinylcholine.[4]

Recommendations: Succinylcholine should be used with caution in patients receiving digoxin or other digitalis glycosides.

References

1. Smith, R.B., and Petrusack, J.: Succinylcholine, digitalis and hypercalcemia: a case report, Anesth. Analg. (Cleve.) **51:**202, 1972.
2. Dowdy, E.G., and Fabian, L.W.: Ventricular arrhythmias induced by succinylcholine in digitalized patients: a preliminary report, Anesth. Anal. (Cleve.) **42:**501, 1963.
3. Bartolone, R.S., and others: Dysrhythmia following muscle relaxant administration in patients receiving digitalis, Anesthesiology **58:**567, 1983.
4. Perez, H.R.: Cardiac arrhythmias after succinylcholine anesthesia and analgesia, Curr. Res. **49:**36, 1970.

Digoxin–Sulfasalazine

Summary: The serum levels of digoxin were reduced after 6 days of sulfasalazine therapy in 10 normal subjects. The finding was initially observed in 1 patient receiving 8 g of sulfasalazine daily, and subsequently confirmed in normal volunteers.[1]

Related Drugs: No documentation is available that indicates that sulfasalazine interacts similarly with the other digitalis glycosides (deslanoside, digitalis, and digitoxin). Also, there appears to be no evidence that other sulfonamides (e.g., sulfadiazine, sulfisoxazole, sulfamethoxazole [see Appendix]) interact with digoxin.

Mechanism: The mechanism of this interaction if unknown, although it is known that physical adsorption of digoxin to sulfasalazine is not the mechanism.

Recommendations: Careful monitoring of digoxin serum levels is recommended to detect subtherapeutic levels when digoxin is taken concurrently with sulfasalazine. Increasing the digoxin dosage or switching to the elixir form did not increase digoxin levels, nor did separating the times of administration,[1] results suggesting that sulfasalazine may need to be discontinued. In an acute situation, parenteral digoxin may be indicated.[1] No literature is available at this time regarding the interaction of sulfasalazine and the soft gelatin capsule form of digoxin.[2]

References

1. Juhl, R.P., and others: Effect of sulfasalazine on digoxin bioavailability, Clin. Pharmacol. Ther. **20:**387, 1976.
2. Professional information, Lanoxin®, Burroughs-Wellcome, Research Triangle Park, N.C., 1983.

Digoxin–Tetracycline

1

Summary: Steady-state serum digoxin concentrations were reported to be 30% higher after a 5 day course of concurrent tetracycline hydrochloride therapy in 1 subject.[1] There was a corresponding decrease in the urinary and fecal excretion of digoxin reduction products. The effect of tetracycline on the formation of digoxin reduction products may persist for several months after the discontinuation of the antibiotic.

Related Drugs: Although no documentation exists, the tetracycline derivatives (e.g., doxycycline, minocycline, oxytetracycline [see Appendix]) may be expected to undergo a similar interaction with digoxin based on pharmacologic similarity. There is no documentation that tetracycline undergoes a similar reaction with the other digitalis glycosides (deslanoside, digitalis, and digitoxin).

Mechanism: Approximately 10% of the patients who receive digoxin convert a substantial portion of it to digoxin reduction products.[1,2] These products are formed predominantly by the bacteria in the gastrointestinal tract. The antibiotic, by destroying the bacteria, decreases digoxin metabolism, which would account for the increased digoxin serum concentrations.

Recommendations: Digoxin serum concentrations should be monitored when initiating or discontinuing concurrent tetracycline therapy. Patients who are receiving tetracycline and being digitalized should be closely monitored for overdigitalization.

References

1. Lindenbaum, J., and others: Inactivation of digoxin by the gut flora: reversal by antibiotic therapy, N. Engl. J. Med. **305:**789, 1981.
2. Lindenbaum, J., and others: Urinary excretion of reduced metabolites of digoxin, Am. J. Med. **71:**67, 1981.

Digoxin–Thyroid

2

Summary: The therapeutic efficacy of digoxin may be decreased in patients with hyperthyroidism or in patients being treated with thyroid hormones.[1-6] Larger digoxin doses may be required to prevent relapse of cardiac arrhythmias or congestive heart failure. Conversely, hypothyroid patients or those on antithyroid drug therapy (methimazole or propylthiouracil) may require smaller doses of digoxin because the therapeutic and toxic effects of digoxin may be increased.

Related Drugs: Digitoxin has been shown to be similarly affected by hyperthyroidism.[7-9] Although not documented, the other digitalis glycosides (deslanoside and digitalis) may be expected to interact in a similar manner since they are pharmacologically related.

　　　　The interaction with thyroid hormones may occur primarily with liothyronine (triiodothyronine),[1] but all other thyroid preparations (e.g., levothyroxine, liotrix, thyroglobulin [see Appendix]) may be expected to interact similarly based on pharmacologic similarity.

Mechanism: Hyperthyroidism results in lower serum levels of digoxin and other digitalis glycosides.[2,3,7,8] Decreased serum levels and half-lives have been correlated with increases in the renal excretion of the cardiac glycosides.[3,7] Altered tissue distribution[2] and malabsorption[10] may also contribute to lowered serum digoxin levels in patients with hyperthyroidism.

Recommendations: Patients stabilized on digoxin should be monitored closely when concurrent thyroid therapy is initiated to avoid a decrease in the therapeutic effect of the digoxin. Conversely, increased digoxin sensitivity may result from withdrawal of thyroid preparations in patients maintained on the digitalis glycoside.

References

1. Frye, R.L., and Braunwald, E.: Studies on digitalis. III. The influence of triiodothyronine on digitalis requirements, Circulation **23**:376, 1961.
2. Doherty, J.E., and Perkins, W.H.: Digoxin metabolism in hypo- and hyperthyroidism, Ann. Intern. Med. **64**:469, 1966.
3. Croxsen, M.S., and Ibbertson, H.K.: Serum digoxin in patients with thyroid disease, Br. Med. J. **3**:566, 1975.
4. Nielson, T.P., and others: Serum digoxin and thyroid hormones, Ann. Intern. Med. **81**:126, 1974.
5. Lawrence, J.R., and others: Digoxin kinetics in patients with thyroid dysfunction, Clin. Pharmacol. Ther. **22**:7, 1977.
6. Huffman, D.H., and others: Digoxin in hyperthyroidism, Clin. Pharmacol. Ther. **22**:533, 1977.
7. Eickenbusch, W., and others: Serum concentrations and urinary excretion of ^{3}H-ouabain and ^{3}H-digitoxin in patients suffering from hyperthyroidism and hypothyroidism, Klin. Wochenschr. **48**:270, 1970.
8. Morrow, D.H., and others: Studies on digitalis. VII. Influence of hyper- and hypothyroidism on the myocardial response to ouabain, J. Pharmacol. Exp. Ther. **140**:324, 1963.
9. Rosen, A., and Moran, N.C.: Comparison of the action of ouabain on the heart in hypothyroid, euthyroid, and hyperthyroid dogs, Circ. Res. **12**:479, 1963.
10. Watters, K., and Tomkin, G.H.: Serum digoxin in patients with thyroid disease, Br. Med. J. **4**:102, 1975.

Digoxin–Verapamil

1

Summary: Serum digoxin concentrations are increased 50% to 70% with concurrent verapamil therapy. The increased digoxin concentrations occur within 7 days after initial verapamil therapy,[1-5] and the digoxin parameters significantly affected are total body clearance and half-life.[6] Both the therapeutic and toxic effects of digoxin have been increased as a result of increased digoxin levels.[7-9] Also, digoxin has been reported to increase the half-life of verapamil in 1 study.[10]

Related Drugs: Two reports state that digoxin serum concentrations were increased 45% with coadministration of nifedipine,[2,8] but one study showed that nifedipine significantly changed only the extrarenal clearance of digoxin.[11] The increase in serum digoxin levels have been reported to be similar with both verapamil and nifedipine.[4] Diltiazem, like verapamil, prolongs atrioventricular (AV) node refractory periods without significantly prolonging sinus node recovery time. It has been suggested that concurrent use of diltiazem and digoxin may result in additive effects on cardiac conduction; however, domestic studies without controls suggest that concurrent use is usually well tolerated. Available controlled study data are not sufficient to predict the effects of concomitant treatment. The effect of diltiazem on serum digoxin levels has not been examined.[12]

There is a lack of information concerning the effects of an interaction between verapamil and the other digitalis glycosides (deslanoside, digitalis, and digitoxin).

Mechanism: Verapamil impairs both the renal and extrarenal clearance of digoxin,[4,7,10,13] but it is not known how this inhibition occurs. The reduction in renal clearance may result from inhibition of tubular secretion, as shown in an in vitro animal study.[14] This is also supported by the fact that digoxin renal clearance is decreased by verapamil without altering glomerular filtration or changing creatinine clearance.[7,15] It has been shown that inhibition of digoxin renal elimination is transient, but the inhibition of extrarenal clearance continues.[13] One study reports that verapamil-induced elevation of digoxin levels may be dose-dependent.[16] Nifedipine slightly increases the extrarenal clearance of digoxin, but the renal clearance is reduced more than the total body clearance.[8,11]

Recommendations: Patients receiving concomitant verapamil and digoxin need close monitoring of digoxin serum levels. It is also important to monitor cardiac function. Since both verapamil and digoxin slow AV conduction, patients should be monitored for AV block and excessive bradycardia. This interaction is clinically significant, and although verapamil can serve as an adjunct to digoxin in certain cases, the dosage of digoxin may have to be lowered with concomitant verapamil therapy.

References

1. Klein, H.O., and others: Verapamil-digoxin interaction, N. Engl. J. Med. **303:**160, 1980.
2. Belz, G.G., and others: Digoxin plasma concentrations and nifedipine, Lancet **1:**844, 1981.
3. Doering, W.: Quinidine-digoxin interaction: pharmacokinetics, underlying mechanism and clinical implications, N. Engl. J. Med. **301:**400, 1979.

4. Pedersen, K.E., and others: Digoxin-verapamil interaction, Clin. Pharmacol. Ther. **30:**311, 1981.

5. Schwartz, J.B., and others: Acute and chronic pharmacodynamic interaction of verapamil and digoxin in atrial fibrillation, Circulation **65:**1163, 1982.

6. Pedersen, K.E., and others: Verapamil-induced changes in digoxin kinetics and intraerythrocytic sodium concentration, Clin. Pharmacol. Ther. **34:**8, 1983.

7. Klein, H.O., and others: The influence of verapamil on serum digoxin concentration, Circulation **65:**998, 1982.

8. Belz, G.G., and others: Interaction between digoxin and calcium antagonists and antiarrhythmic drugs, Clin. Pharmacol. Ther. **33:**410, 1983.

9. Kounis, N.G.: Asystole after verapamil and digoxin, Br. J. Clin. Pract. **34:**57, 1980.

10. Koren, G.: Digoxin-verapamil interaction: is it mutual? Circulation **67:**707, 1983.

11. Pedersen, K.E., and others: Effect of nifedipine on digoxin kinetics in healthy subjects, Clin. Pharmacol. Ther. **32:**562, 1982.

12. Professional production information, Diltiazem®, Marion Labs Inc., Nov. 1982.

13. Pedersen, K.E., and others: The long term effect of verapamil on plasma digoxin concentration and renal digoxin clearance in healthy subjects, Eur. J. Clin. Pharmacol. **22:**123, 1982.

14. Koren, G., and others: Digoxin-verapamil interaction: in vitro studies in rat tissue, J. Cardiovasc. Pharmacol. **5:**443, 1983.

15. Belz, G.G., and others: Digoxin-antiarrhythmics: pharmacodynamic and pharmacokinetic studies with quinidine, propafenon, and verapamil, Clin. Pharmacol. Ther. **31:**202, 1982.

16. Long, R., and others: Effect of verapamil on blood level and renal clearance of digoxin, Circulation **62:** (suppl. 3):3, 1980.

CHAPTER THIRTEEN

Diuretic Drug Interactions

TABLE 13. Diuretic Drug Interactions

Drug Interaction	Significance Code	Potential Effects	Recommendations	See Page
Bendroflume-thiazide–Indo-methacin	2	Indomethacin can reduce the hypotensive effects of bendro-flumethiazide. Indomethacin alone may increase blood pressure, inhibit the prostaglandin responsible for vasodilation, and reduce sodium and water excretion.	Monitor blood pressure closely and increase the bendroflume-thiazide dosage if needed.	537
Chlorothiazide–Colestipol	3	Concurrent use of a single dose of chlorothiazide and colestipol may significantly reduce the 24 hour cumulative urinary excretion of chlorothiazide.	Separate the administration of these drugs by as much time as possible. Increased chloro-thiazide dosage may be necessary.	539
Chlorothiazide–Probenecid	3	Probenecid may increase the diuretic effect of chlorothia-zide, whereas chlorothiazide may diminish the uricosuric effect of probenecid and elevate the uric acid concentrations.	If serum uric acid levels increase, an increased probenecid dosage and/or a decreased chlorothiazide dose may be necessary.	540
Ethacrynic Acid–Cisplatin	2	Concurrent use in animals produced prolonged and permanent ototoxicity. This has not been studied in humans, although it may theoretically occur.	Monitor eighth cranial nerve function. Lower doses of etha-crynic acid may avoid or lessen the potential for this interaction.	542
Furosemide–Aspirin	3	Aspirin may suppress the renal hemodynamic effects of furose-mide and markedly reduce diuresis, although data are conflicting.	If the diuretic effect of furose-mide decreases, adjust the fu-rosemide dosage.	543
Furosemide–Chloral Hydrate	3	Concurrent IV furosemide and chloral hydrate may cause uneasiness, diaphoresis, hot flashes, and blood pressure changes including hypertension. It is unknown whether oral furosemide results in a similar interaction.	Discontinuing chloral hydrate will reverse symptoms. A benzodiazepine may be considered for a nocturnal sedative.	544
Furosemide–Indomethacin	3	Indomethacin antagonizes several pharmacologic effects of furosemide including diuresis and natriuresis.	Discontinue indomethacin if a failure in co-therapy occurs since there appears to be no dose dependency of the antagonism.	545
Hydrochlorothi-azide–Fenflur-amine	3	Concurrent use reduces blood pressure in obese patients previously unresponsive to hydro-chlorothiazide.	Use cautiously in normotensive patients because hypotension is a possibility; however, it may be useful in the hypertensive obese patient.	547

Abbreviations: IV, intravenous.

535

TABLE 13. Diuretic Drug Interactions—cont'd

Drug Interaction	Significance Code	Potential Effects	Recommendations	See Page
Hydrochlorothiazide, Triamterene–Amantadine	3	One or both agents of the combination drug containing hydrochlorothiazide and triamterene may reduce clearance, raise plasma levels, and produce toxic effects of amantadine.	Use these agents concurrently with caution. Amantadine dosage may need to be decreased.	548
Spironolactone–Aspirin	3	Aspirin reduced the natriuretic effects of spironolactone in normal subjects, but this has not been reported in clinical practice.	Concurrent use need not be avoided at this time.	549
Spironolactone–Potassium Chloride	1	Serious hyperkalemic effects such as cardiac failure and arrest may result from using a potassium-sparing diuretic and a potassium supplement together.	A potassium supplement should not be used concurrently with spironolactone.	550
Triamterene–Indomethacin	2	Concurrent use of these agents may lead to reversible acute renal failure.	Concomitant use requires caution. Discontinue 1 or both drugs if renal function deteriorates.	551

Bendroflumethiazide–Indomethacin

Summary: Indomethacin can reduce the hypotensive effects of concurrent bendroflumethiazide. In 1 study involving patients with mild essential hypertension, mean supine blood pressure increased by 13/9 mm Hg after addition of indomethacin. Two weeks after indomethacin was discontinued, blood pressure returned to basal levels.[1]

Related Drugs: In 1 study involving 10 healthy volunteers, indomethacin had no affect on the diuretic activity or pharmacokinetic parameters of a single dose of hydrochlorothiazide.[2] Similar results were shown in 2 other studies.[3,4] However, 1 study reported a decrease in natriuresis when indomethacin and hydrochlorothiazide were used concurrently.[5] Another study reported that indomethacin blunted the antihypertensive effect of chlorthalidone.[6] Because of conflicting results it is difficult to determine whether an interaction would occur between indomethacin and the other thiazide diuretics (e.g., chlorothiazide, methyclothiazide, polythiazide [see Appendix]) or the other thiazide related diuretics (indapamide, metolazone, and quinethazone). In a study involving 10 patients with essential hypertension, sulindac significantly enhanced the antihypertensive effect of either bendroflumethiazide, hydrochlorothiazide, or amiloride.[7] Documentation is lacking regarding an interaction between thiazide-type diuretics with the other nonsteroidal anti-inflammatory agents (e.g., ibuprofen, naproxen, piroxicam [see Appendix]); however, based on pharmacologic similarity an interaction may be expected to occur.

Mechanism: Indomethacin alone has been reported to increase blood pressure.[1,8] It has been suggested that indomethacin, which inhibits prostaglandin synthesis, inhibits the prostaglandin responsible for vasodilation as well, causing an increase in blood pressure. Also, indomethacin has been shown to acutely reduce sodium and water excretion. Sodium retention, which itself may depend on inhibition of prostaglandin synthesis in the kidney, may represent another mechanism by which indomethacin antagonizes the hypotensive action of thiazides.[1] Regarding the effect of sulindac on blood pressure, it has been shown that sulindac inhibits exclusively the extrarenal prostaglandin synthesis and does not affect the renal excretion of PGE_2. Therefore, this inhibition of the extrarenal synthesis decreases blood pressure.[7]

Recommendations: Patient's blood pressure should be closely monitored during concurrent therapy of these agents. The dose of the thiazide diuretics may need to be increased.

References

1. Watkins, J., and others: Attenuation of hypotensive effect of propranolol and thiazide diuretics by indomethacin, Br. Med. J. **281:**702, 1980.
2. Williams, R.L., and others: Hydrochlorothiazide pharmacokinetics and pharmacologic effect: the influence of indomethacin, J. Clin. Pharmacol. **22:**32, 1982.
3. Davis, R.O., and others: Lack of effect of indomethacin on diuretic effects and plasma levels of hydrochlorothiazide, Clin. Pharmacol. Ther. **25:**220, 1979.

4. Favre, L., and others: Interaction of diuretics and non-steroidal anti-inflammatory drugs in man, Clin. Sci. **64:**407, 1983.
5. Kramer, H.J., and others: Interaction of conventional and antikaliuretic diuretics with the renal prostaglandin system, Clin. Sci. **59:**67, 1980.
6. Lopez-Ovejero, J.A., and others: Effects of indomethacin alone and during diuretic or beta-adrenoreceptor-blockade therapy on blood pressure and the renin system in essential hypertension, Clin. Sci. **55:**2035, 1978.
7. Steiness, E., and Waldorff, S.: Different interactions of indomethacin and sulindac with thiazides in hypertension, Br. Med. J. **285:**1703, 1982.
8. Salvetti, A., and others: Interaction between oxprenolol and indomethacin on blood pressure in essential hypertensive patients, Eur. J. Clin. Pharmacol. **22:**197, 1982.

Chlorothiazide–Colestipol

3

Summary: In a study involving 10 patients, the concurrent use of a single dose of chlorothiazide and colestipol resulted in a significant reduction in the 24 hour cumulative urinary excretion of chlorothiazide.[1] The response to the change in chlorothiazide's decreased excretion was not measured in these studies.

Related Drugs: In a study involving 6 healthy subjects, both cholestyramine and colestipol were administered 2 minutes before and 6 and 12 hours after a single dose of hydrochlorothiazide. The 24 hour urinary excretion of hydrochlorothiazide was reduced by both of these agents, although to a greater extent by cholestyramine. The plasma levels of hydrochlorothiazide were also lower, especially after cholestyramine.[2] Documentation is lacking regarding an interaction between chlorothiazide and cholestyramine, although a similar interaction may be expected to occur since they are pharmacologically related. Similar results may be expected between colestipol and the other thiazide diuretics (e.g., bendroflumethiazide, methyclothiazide, polythiazide [see Appendix]), and thiazide related diuretics (e.g., chlorthalidone, indapamide, metolazone [see Appendix]) based on the proposed mechanism.

Mechanism: Colestipol and cholestyramine (anion exchange resins) have both been shown to bind chlorothiazide and hydrochlorothiazide in vitro.[1,3] A similar mechanism may be expected in vivo, although this is not documented.

Recommendations: If concurrent use of colestipol and chlorothiazide is necessary, it may be advisable to separate their administration by as much time as possible. However, patients should still be closely monitored since an increased dose of the thiazide diuretic may be necessary.

References

1. Kauffman, R., and Azarnoff, D.L.: Effect of colestipol on gastrointestinal absorption of chlorothiazide in man, Clin. Pharmacol. Ther. **14:**886, 1973.
2. Hanninghake, D.B., and others: The effect of cholestyramine and colestipol on the absorption of hydrochlorothiazide, Int. J. Clin. Pharmacol. **20:**151, 1982.
3. Phillips, W.A., and others: Effect of colestipol hydrochloride on drug absorption in the rat. II, J. Pharm. Sci. **65:**1285, 1976.

Chlorothiazide–Probenecid

Summary: Probenecid may increase the diuretic effect of chlorothiazide.[1,2] Chlorothiazide has the potential to elevate serum uric acid concentrations and diminish the uricosuric effect of probenecid.

Related Drugs: Probenecid blocks the secretion of furosemide[3,4] and bumetanide[5] at the proximal renal tubule. The diuretic effect of furosemide was not altered,[4] and for bumetanide the diuretic effect was diminished or not affected.[5,6] Bendroflumethiazide,[7] hydrochlorothiazide,[8-11] and methyclothiazide[12] cause serum uric acid retention and may be expected to antagonize the uricosuric effect of probenecid. Other thiazide diuretics (e.g., benzthiazide, cyclothiazide, polythiazide [see Appendix]) may be expected to interact similarly, although no documentation on such interactions exists. The loop diuretics bumetanide,[13] ethacrynic acid,[14] and furosemide[2,14]; the thiazide related diuretics chlorthalidone,[9,10] metolazone,[15] quinethazone,[16,17] and indapamide; possibly triamterene[10]; and the antidiuretic thiazide diazoxide[18] may also increase uric acid concentrations.

Mechanism: Probenecid blocks the secretion of chlorothiazide at the proximal renal tubule, resulting in enhancement, through prolongation, of the diuretic effect of chlorothiazide.[1,2] Hyperuricemia from the thiazide diuretics is attributed to either competitive inhibition of uric acid secretion within the kidney[8,19] or to indirect enhancement of renal reabsorption of uric acid through redistribution of blood flow.[13,20] Since probenecid acts by blocking the reabsorption of uric acid in the proximal renal tubules,[21,22] the thiazide diuretics may decrease the uricosuric effect of probenecid.

Recommendations: The use of chlorothiazide with probenecid usually causes only a small increase in serum uric acid concentrations. More frequent monitoring of uric acid concentrations is unnecessary. However, if feasible, baseline serum uric acid concentrations should be obtained when concurrent administration of these drugs is initiated. If serum uric acid concentrations become elevated from baseline values, an increase in the dosage of probenecid should be considered. Similarly a decreased dosage of chlorothiazide may be considered, because of the increased diuretic effect of chlorothiazide caused by probenicid.

References

1. Brater, D.C.: Increase in diuretic effect of chlorothiazide by probenecid, Clin. Pharmacol. Ther. **23**:259, 1978.
2. Steele, T.H., and Oppenheimer, S.: Factors affecting urate excretion following diuretic administration in man, Am. J. Med. **47**:564, 1969.
3. Honari, J., and others: Effects of probenecid on furosemide kinetics and natriuresis in man, Clin. Pharmacol. Ther. **22**:395, 1977.
4. Homeida, M., and others: Influence of probenecid and spironolactone on furosemide kinetics and dynamics in man, Clin. Pharmacol. Ther. **22**:402, 1977.
5. Brater, D., and Che-navasin, P.: Effects of probenecid and indomethacin on the response to bumetanide, Clin. Pharmacol. Ther. **27**:246, 1980.

6. Brater, D.C., and others: Interaction studies with bumetanide and furosemide: effects of probenecid and of indomethacin on response to bumetanide in man, J. Clin. Pharmacol. **21:**647, 1981.

7. Feldman, L.H.: A new antihypertensive preparation combining rauwolfia, bendroflumethiazide and potassium, N.C. Med. J. **23:**248, 1962.

8. Freis, E.D., and Sappington, R.F.: Long-term effect of probenecid on diuretic-induced hyperuricemia, J.A.M.A. **198:**127, 1966.

9. Bryant, J.M., and others: Hyperuricemia induced by the administration of chlorthalidone and other sulfonamide diuretics, Am. J. Med. **33:**408, 1962.

10. Spilkerman, R.F., and others: Potassium sparing effects of triamterene in the treatment of hypertension, Circulation **34:**524, 1966.

11. Aronoff, A., and Barkum, H.: Hyperuricemia and acute gouty arthritis precipitated by thiazide derivatives, Can. Med. Assoc. J. **84:**1181, 1961.

12. Stern, F.H.: The use of methyclothiazide (Enduron) in geriatric patients, J. Am. Geriatr. Soc. **10:**256, 1962.

13. Cuthbert, M.F.: Reports of adverse reactions with bumetanide, Postgrad. Med. J. **51**(suppl. 6):51, 1975.

14. McSherry, J.: Acute gout complicating frusemide therapy, Practitioner **201:**809, 1968.

15. Searle Laboratories: Diulo® product information. In Angel. J.E., publisher: Physician's desk reference, 37 edition, Oradell, N.J., 1983. Medical Economics Co.

16. Brest, A.N., and others: Drug control of diuretic-induced hyperuricemia, J.A.M.A. **195:**42, 1966.

17. Parkes, W.E., and others: Treatment of hypertension with quinethazone alone or in combination with reserpine, Practitioner **203:**194, 1969.

18. Schering Corporation: Proglycem® product information. In Angel, J.E., publisher: Physician's desk reference, 37 edition, Oradell, N.J., 1983, Medical Economics Co.

19. Demartini, F.E., and others: Effect of chlorothiazide on the renal excretion of uric acic, Am. J. Med. **32:**572, 1962.

20. Suki, W.N., and others: Mechanism of the effect of thiazide diuretics on calcium and uric acid (abstract), J. Clin. Invest. **46:**1121, 1967.

21. Fanelli, G.M., and Weiner, I.M.: Pyrozinoate excretion in the chimpanzee. Relation to urate disposition and the action of uricosuric drugs, J. Clin. Invest. **52:**1946, 1973.

22. Steele, T.H., and Boner, G.: Origins of the uricosuric response, J. Clin. Invest. **52:**1368, 1973.

Ethacrynic Acid–Cisplatin

2

Summary: The concurrent use of ethacrynic acid and cisplatin, although not studied in human subjects, has been shown in experimental animals to produce prolonged and permanent ototoxic effects when given at doses that produce reversible ototoxic effects when administered alone.[1] Both drugs have been documented to cause ototoxicity in humans when used alone; therefore, the interaction seen in animals can theoretically occur in humans as well.

Related Drugs: There are no drugs related to cisplatin. There is no documentation regarding an interaction between cisplatin and the other loop diuretics (bumetanide and furosemide); however, they also have the potential to cause ototoxicity and therefore may interact in a similar manner.

Mechanism: The mechanism appears to be related to the synergistic toxicity of each agent.

Recommendations: Although this interaction is based on animal studies only, the ototoxicity of each agent is well documented. Therefore, it is important to monitor eighth cranial nerve function during and after concurrent therapy. The use of lower doses of ethacrynic acid may also avoid or lessen the potential for an interaction.

Reference

1. Komune, S., and others: Potentiating effects of cisplatin and ethacrynic acid in ototoxicity, Arch. Otolaryngol. **107:**594, 1981.

Furosemide–Aspirin

Summary: In 6 of 8 nonazotemic cirrhotic patients, the concurrent use of aspirin and furosemide suppressed the renal hemodynamic effects of furosemide and markedly reduced the diuretic effect, and the signs of renal insufficiency that developed with aspirin alone were abolished when furosemide was added.[1] In another study in patients with chronic renal insufficiency, a single dose of aspirin reduced the diuretic effect of furosemide.[2] However, 2 other studies in normal subjects failed to show any effect of aspirin on furosemide's diuretic action.[3,4]

Related Drugs: One study found that diflunisal, a salicylate derivative, had no effect on furosemide.[5] Because of conflicting results it is difficult to determine whether a similar interaction would occur between the other loop diuretics (bumetanide and ethacrynic acid) and the other salicylates (e.g., choline salicylate, salicylamide, sodium salicylate [see Appendix]).

Mechanism: It has been suggested that aspirin and furosemide have opposing effects on renal prostaglandin synthesis.[1]

Recommendations: During concurrent administration of these agents, the dose of furosemide may need to be adjusted if the diuretic effect decreases. However, whether this interaction occurs in all patients or only those with renal insufficiency remains to be determined.

References

1. Planas, R., and others: Acetylsalicylic acid suppresses the renal hemodynamics effect and reduces the diuretic action of furosemide in cirrhosis with ascites, Gastroenterology **84:**247, 1983.
2. Berg, K.J., and others: Acute effects of acetylsalicylic acid in patients with chronic renal insufficiency, Eur. J. Clin. Pharmacol. **11:**110, 1977.
3. Berg, K.J., and others: Acute effects of acetylsalicylic acid in patients with chronic renal insufficiency, Eur. J. Clin. Pharmacol. **11:**117, 1977.
4. Bartoli, E., and others: Blunting of furosemide diuresis by aspirin in man, J. Clin. Pharmacol. **20:**452, 1980.
5. Tolert, J.A., and others: Diflunisal-furosemide interaction, Clin. Pharmacol. Ther. **27:**289, 1980.

Furosemide–Chloral Hydrate

3

Summary: In 6 patients with acute coronary disease, an intravenous bolus of furosemide (40 to 120 mg) injected within 24 hours after administration of chloral hydrate resulted in uneasiness, diaphoresis, hot flashes, and blood pressure changes (including hypertension). There was no apparent adverse effect or reaction during a 3 day period in which furosemide was continued without chloral hydrate. The use of flurazepam as a nocturnal sedative did not result in a similar interaction, a finding that suggests a drug interaction between the previous agents did occur.[1] In a retrospective study of 43 patients receiving intravenous furosemide and chloral hydrate, 1 patient exhibited similar symptoms and 2 patients were identified as having possible reactions.[2] It is not known whether oral furosemide will result in a similar interaction with chloral hydrate.

Related Drugs: Documentation is lacking regarding a similar interaction between the other loop diuretics (bumetanide and ethacrynic acid) and the other chloral derivative (triclofos). However, based on pharmacologic similarity an interaction may be expected to occur with triclofos.

Mechanism: A proposed mechanism suggests that furosemide displaces bound trichloroacetic acid (a metabolite of chloral hydrate) from plasma protein binding sites which in turn displaces thyroxine. The increase in free thyroxine levels can result in a hypermetabolic state. The rapid excretion of free thyroxine would explain the brief duration of effects (generally less than 24 hours).[1]

Recommendations: In patients with acute coronary disease, the concurrent use of these agents may need to be avoided. However, since this interaction does not occur in all patients, concomitant administration should at least be used with caution. If the interaction does occur, the discontinuation of chloral hydrate has been shown to lead to a reversal of the symptoms.[1] Alternatively, the use of flurazepam or another benzodiapine may be considered as a nocturnal sedative.

References

1. Malach, M., and Berman, N.: Furosemide and chloral hydrate. Adverse drug interaction, J.A.M.A. **232:**638, 1975.
2. Pevonka, M.P., and others: Interaction of chloral hydrate and furosemide, Drug Intell. Clin. Pharm. **11:**332, 1977.

Furosemide–Indomethacin

Summary: Indomethacin decreased the diuretic and natriuretic effects of furosemide when given 12 hours before furosemide.[1-10] Indomethacin also blocked the acute audiologic effect[11] and the rise in plasma renin activity associated with furosemide therapy.[11-13] Furosemide has also been reported to reduce indomethacin plasma concentrations when both agents were orally administered.[14]

Related Drugs: Indomethacin has reportedly produced a similar attenuation of the effects of ethacrynic acid[9] and bumetanide.[15-18] The pharmacologic action of furosemide has also been reduced by naproxen[19,20] and ibuprofen.[20] Diflunisal has been reported not to cause a deleterious effect on the action of furosemide.[21] There is no documentation of a similar interaction with the other nonsteroidal anti-inflammatory agents (e.g., mefenamic acid, piroxicam, sulindac [see Appendix]), although based on pharmacologic similarity an interaction may be expected to occur.

Mechanism: Indomethacin and other nonsteroidal anti-inflammatory agents are inhibitors of prostaglandin synthesis; they have been shown to decrease the levels of prostaglandins that cause sodium diuresis.[22,23] This effect varies with the individual nonsteroidal anti-inflammatory agent used with furosemide.

Recommendations: This interaction may not occur or be clinically significant in all patients; however, it is still important to be aware of potential problems. Increasing furosemide dosage in an attempt to overcome the interaction was not successful in 1 report, although patients had preexisting renal failure.[20] Discontinuation of the nonsteroidal anti-inflammatory agent may be indicated since there is no indication that the blockade of furosemide's activity is dose-dependent.

References

1. Brater, D.C.: Analysis of the effect of indomethacin on the response to furosemide in man: effect of dose on furosemide, J. Pharmacol. Exp. Ther. **210:**386, 1979.
2. Chennavasin, P., and others: Pharmacokinetic-dynamic analysis of the indomethacin-furosemide interaction in man, J. Pharmacol. Exp. Ther. **215:**77, 1980.
3. Smith, D.E., and others: Attenuation of furosemide's diuretic effect by indomethacin: pharmacokinetic evaluation, J. Pharmacokinet. Biopharm. **7:**265, 1979.
4. Patak, R.V., and others: Antagonism of the effects of furosemide by indomethacin in normal and hypertensive man, Prostaglandins **10:**649, 1975.
5. Benet, L.Z.: Pharmacokinetics/pharmacodynamics of furosemide in man: a review, J. Pharmacokinet. Biopharm. **7:**1, 1979.
6. Brater, D.C., and others: Effects of indomethacin on furosemide-stimulated urinary PGE$_2$ excretion in man, Eur. J. Pharmacol. **65:**231, 1980.
7. Kramer, H.J., and others: Interaction of conventional and antikaliuretic diuretics with the renal prostaglandin system, Clin. Sci. **59:**67, 1980.
8. Favre, L., and others: Interaction of diuretics and nonsteroidal anti-inflammatory drugs in man, Clin. Sci. **64:**407, 1983.
9. Williams, R.L., and others: Hydrochlorothiazide pharmacokinetics and pharmacologic effect: the influence of indomethacin, J. Clin. Pharmacol. **22:**32: 1982.
10. Allan, S.G., and others: Interaction between diuretics and indomethacin, Br. Med. J. **283:**1611, 1981.

11. Arenberg, I.K., and Goodfriend, T.L.: Indomethacin blocks acute audiologic effects of furosemide in Meniere's disease, Arch. Otolaryngol. **106:**383, 1980.
12. Tan, S.Y., and Mulrow, P.J.: Inhibition of the renin-aldosterone response to furosemide by indomethacin, J. Clin. Endocrinol. Metab. **45:**174, 1977.
13. Frolich, J.C., and others: Suppression of plasma renin activity by indomethacin in man, Circ. Res. **39:**447, 1976.
14. Brooks, P.M., and others: The effect of frusemide on indomethacin plasma levels, Br. J. Clin. Pharmacol. **1:**485, 1974.
15. Brater, D.C., and others: Interaction studies with bumetanide and furosemide. Effects of probenecid and of indomethacin on response to bumetanide in man, J. Clin. Pharmacol. **21:**647, 1981.
16. Kaufman, J., and others: Bumetanide-induced diuresis and natriuresis: effect of prostaglandin synthetase inhibition, J. Clin. Pharmacol. **21:**663, 1981.
17. Pedrinelli, R., and others: Influence of indomethacin on the natriuretic and renin-stimulating effect of bumetanide in essential hypertension, Clin. Pharmacol. Ther. **28:**722, 1980.
18. Brater, C., and Chennavasin, P.: Indomethacin and the response to bumetanide, Clin. Pharmacol. Ther. **27:**421, 1980.
19. Faunch, R.: Nonsteroidal anti-inflammatory drugs and frusemide-induced diuresis, Br. Med. J. **283:**989, 1981.
20. Yeung-Laiwah, A.C., and Mactier, R.A.: Antagonistic effect of nonsteroidal anti-inflammatory drugs on frusemide-induced diuresis in cardiac failure, Br. Med. J. **283:**714, 1981.
21. Poe, T.E., and others: Interaction of indomethacin with furosemide, J. Fam. Pract. **16:**610, 1983.
22. Brater, D.C.: Effect of indomethacin on salt and water homeostasis, Clin. Pharmacol. Ther. **25:**322, 1974.
23. Lee, J.B., and others: Renal prostaglandins and the regulation of blood pressure and sodium and water homeostasis, Am. J. Med. **60:**798, 1976.

Hydrochlorothiazide–Fenfluramine

Summary: Fenfluramine in combination with hydrochlorothiazide has been shown to reduce blood pressure in obese patients who were previously unresponsive to hydrochlorothiazide.[1] After 2 weeks of combined therapy in 9 obese patients, both systolic and diastolic pressures fell by 16 ± 3 mm Hg and 12 ± 3 mm Hg, respectively, and plasma norepinephrine levels decreased to below control values after being elevated by hydrochlorothiazide alone. Both blood pressure and norepinephrine levels remained reduced over the remainder of the study.

Related Drugs: Based on pharmacologic similarity, it is anticipated that an interaction would occur between fenfluramine and the other thiazide diuretics (e.g., chlorothiazide, methyclothiazide, polythiazide [see Appendix]) and thiazide related diuretics (e.g., chlorthalidone, indapamide, metolazone [see Appendix]) as well as between hydrochlorothiazide and the other anorexic agents (e.g., benzphetamine, mazindol, phentermine [see Appendix]), although documentation is lacking.

Mechanism: The mechanism of action of fenfluramine in lowering plasma norepinephrine levels and in enhancing the hypotensive effects of hydrochlorothiazide is not clear. Thiazide diuretics deplete plasma volume, thus reducing blood pressure and eliciting compensatory sympathetic nervous system activation, as was shown by the increased plasma norepinephrine. Both basal and reflex induced levels of norepinephrine were reduced by the addition of fenfluramine. Fenfluramine appears to interfere with the reflex activation of the sympathetic nervous system induced by hydrochlorothiazide, therefore allowing blood pressure to fall.[1]

Recommendations: Because of the combined anorectic and hypotensive effects of fenfluramine, it may be useful in combination with a thiazide diuretic in the hypertensive obese patient. Caution should be used when prescribing fenfluramine and a thiazide diuretic in a normotensive patient because of the possibility of hypotension.[1]

Reference

1. Lake, R.C., and others: Fenfluramine potentiation of antihypertensive effects of thiazides, Clin. Pharmacol. Ther. **28:**22, 1980.

Hydrochlorothiazide / Triamterene ⟩ Amantadine

3

Summary: Under controlled conditions, a patient was given amantadine alone for 1 week followed by amantadine plus a combination of hydrochlorothiazide and triamterene for 1 week. Amantadine's urinary excretion decreased and the plasma concentration increased. It was concluded that 1 or both agents of the combination drug (hydrochlorothiazide and triamterene) reduced the clearance and produced higher plasma levels and toxic effects (ataxia, slurred speech, auditory and visual hallucinations, and, rarely, seizures) of amantadine.[1]

Related Drugs: Because it is not known which agent was responsible for the interaction, it is also not certain whether other thiazide diuretics (e.g., chlorothiazide, bendroflumethiazide, polythiazide [see Appendix]), thiazide related diuretics (e.g., chlorthalidone, indapamide, metolazone [see Appendix]), or the other potassium-sparing diuretics (amiloride and spironolactone), either alone or in combination, would cause a similar interaction with amantadine. There are no drugs related to amantadine.

Mechanism: Ninety percent of the amantadine a patient absorbs is excreted unchanged in the urine. The renal clearance of amantadine is usually greater than the creatinine clearance, suggesting a net tubular secretion of the drug.[2] It has been postulated that 1 or both of the components of the combination diuretic reduces the tubular secretion of amantadine.[1]

Recommendations: The concurrent use of these agents should be used with caution. If symptoms of amantadine toxicity occur, the dose of amantadine may need to be decreased.

References

1. Wilson, T.W., and Rajput, A.H.: Amantadine-Dyazide interaction, Can. Med. Assoc. J. **129:**974, 1983.
2. Horadam, V.W., and others: Pharmacokinetics of amantadine hydrochloride in subjects with normal and impaired renal function, Ann. Intern. Med. **94:**454, 1981.

Spironolactone–Aspirin

3

Summary: Concurrent usage of aspirin and spironolactone showed a decrease in the natriuretic effect of spironolactone[1,2] in a small group of normal subjects. However, this drug interaction has not been reported in clinical practice.

Related Drugs: Although no clinical reports of this interaction have been noted in the biomedical literature, such a potential may exist. Further studies are needed to determine any possible effects caused by other salicylates (e.g., choline salicylate, salicylamide, sodium salicylate [see Appendix]). There is also a lack of documentation regarding a similar interaction between aspirin and the other potassium-sparing diuretics (amiloride and triamterene).

Mechanism: The mechanism by which aspirin decreases the natriuresis of spironolactone is controversial and unclear at this point. One theory is that aspirin may block the renal tubular secretion of the active metabolite (canrenone) of spironolactone.[3]

Recommendations: The concurrent usage of spironolactone and aspirin need not be avoided, unless additional study establishes a clinically significant effect.

References

1. Elliott, H.C.: Reduced adrenocortical steroid excretion rates in man following aspirin administration, Metabolism **11:**1015, 1962.
2. Tweeddale, M.G., and Ogilvie, R.I.: Antagonism of spironolactone-induced natriuresis by aspirin in man, N. Engl. J. Med. **289:**198, 1973.
3. Ramsay, L.E., and others: Influence of acetylsalicylic acid on the renal handling of spironolactone metabolite in healthy subjects, Eur. J. Clin. Pharmacol. **10:**43, 1976.

Spironolactone–Potassium Chloride

1

Summary: In the presence of a potassium sparing diuretic, an added source of potassium can result in serious symptoms of hyperkalemia, which may lead to cardiac failure and arrest. The risk of hyperkalemia is further enhanced in the presence of patients with impaired renal function.

Related Drugs: Other potassium-sparing diuretics (amiloride and triamterene) may be expected to interact in a similar manner with all absorbable forms of potassium (e.g., potassium acetate, bicarbonate, chloride, citrate, gluconate, iodide, and, to a lesser extent, potassium in fruit juices and salt substitutes).

Mechanism: Spironolactone effectively competes with endogenous mineralocorticoids and produces retention of potassium ions while enhancing sodium ion excretion.[1,2] The hyperkalemia resulting from simultaneous use of a potassium-sparing diuretic and a potassium supplement is a consequence of the accumulation of potassium resulting from decreased renal excretion and additional intake.[3,4]

Recommendations: A potassium supplement may not be needed and should not be used concurrently with spironolactone. If spironolactone is prescribed, evaluation of serum potassium levels is mandatory, especially if kidney failure exists, congestive heart failure is evident, or development of prerenal azotemia is shown.

References

1. Kagawa, C.M., and others: Action of new steroids in blocking effects of aldosterone and deoxycorticosterone on salt, Science **126:**1015, 1957.
2. Mashford, W.L., and Robertson, M.B.: Spironolactone and ammonium and potassium chloride, Br. Med. J. **4:**298, 1972.
3. Edmonds, C.S., and Jasani, B.: Total body potassium in hypertensive patients during prolonged diuretic therapy, Lancet **2:**8, 1972.
4. Greenblatt, D.J., and Koch-Weser, J.: Adverse reactions to spironolactone, J.A.M.A. **225:**40, 1973.

Triamterene–Indomethacin

Summary: The concurrent use of triamterene and indomethacin may lead to reversible acute renal failure. In 1 study involving 4 healthy subjects with normal renal function, 2 subjects showed a marked decrease in creatinine clearance (62% and 72%) after concomitant administration of the 2 drugs. Renal function was restored to normal after 4 weeks. When triamterene or indomethacin was given alone, renal function remained normal.[1] Similar results were shown in another study.[2]

Related Drugs: The same experimental method of comparing the effects of 3 other diuretics (furosemide, hydrochlorothiazide, and spironolactone) that act at different sites in the renal tubule, was performed in 18 healthy volunteers pretreated with indomethacin. Only a slight decrease in creatinine clearance which did not exceed 16% was found.[1] It is not known whether the other potassium-sparing diuretic (amiloride) would result in renal failure when used concurrently with indomethacin. However, 1 study showed that hyperkalemia resulted in 1 patient when indomethacin was administered concomitantly with a combination product containing amiloride and hydrochlorothiazide. The hyperkalemia was not seen when either agent was used alone.[3] There is a lack of documentation regarding a similar interaction between triamterene and the other nonsteroidal anti-inflammatory agents (e.g., ibuprofen, naproxen, sulindac [see Appendix]). In the study cited the authors believed that this interaction is limited to a particular nonsteroidal anti-inflammatory agent and a particular diuretic.[1]

Mechanism: Urinary prostaglandin E_2 was stimulated by triamterene and inhibited by indomethacin in all 4 subjects in the study; however, both changes were more marked in the 2 sensitive subjects. Therefore, prostaglandin inhibition by indomethacin may unmask triamterene toxicity and contribute to the pathogenesis of the renal failure observed.[1] The hyperkalemia in the patient receiving indomethacin and the combination product containing amiloride and hydrochlorothiazide may result from a decreased uptake of potassium by the cells secondary to the coadministration of these drugs.[3]

Recommendations: The concurrent use of these agents requires caution. If renal function deteriorates during concomitant therapy, one or both agents may need to be discontinued.

References

1. Favre, L., and others: Reversible acute renal failure from combined triamterene and indomethacin, Ann. Intern. Med. **96:**317, 1982.
2. Favre, L., and others: Interaction of diuretics and non-steroidal anti-inflammatory drugs in man, Clin. Sci. **64:**407, 1983.
3. Mor, R., and others: Indomethacin- and moduretic-induced hyperkalemia, Isr. J. Med. Sci. **19:**535, 1983.

CHAPTER FOURTEEN

Hypoglycemic Drug Interactions

TABLE 14. Hypoglycemic Drug Interactions

Drug Interaction	Significance Code	Potential Effects	Recommendations	See Page
Chlorpropamide–Alcohol, Ethyl	1	Concurrent use can result in unpredictable and varied reactions, ranging from mild flushing to severe hypoglycemic reactions. Chlorpropamide has produced a disulfiram-like reaction to alcohol.	Reduced alcohol intake or abstinence is recommended for patients on antidiabetic therapy.	556
Chlorpropamide–Allopurinol	3	Allopurinol may increase the serum half-life of chlorpropamide. However, the clinical significance of this is unknown.	Monitor patients for an increased effect of chlorpropamide.	558
Chlorpropamide–Aspirin	2	Aspirin may potentiate the hypoglycemic effect of chlorpropamide.	The chlorpropamide dosage may need to be reduced.	559
Chlorpropamide–Clofibrate	2	Clofibrate may enhance the activity of chlorpropamide, possibly because of decreased chlorpropamide excretion.	Blood glucose levels should be closely monitored and the chlorpropamide dosage reduced if needed.	561
Chlorpropamide–Cortisone	2	The intrinsic hyperglycemic activity of cortisone may decrease the hypoglycemic effects of chlorpropamide.	Monitor patients for decreased hypoglycemic action.	563
Chlorpropamide–Hydrochlorothiazide	2	Impaired diabetic control may result from current therapy. Hypokalemia may be a contributing factor in this interaction.	Monitor patients for hyperglycemia. The interaction may be reversed by discontinuing the diuretic, increasing the sulfonylurea dosage, or using a potassium supplement.	565
Chlorpropamide–Probenecid	3	Probenecid reportedly increases chlorpropamide's half-life.	Monitor patients for excessive hypoglycemic effects, but concurrent use need not be avoided.	567
Insulin–Aspirin	3	Aspirin may potentiate the hypoglycemic activity of insulin.	Monitor blood glucose levels and lower the insulin dosage if needed.	568
Insulin–Chlorpromazine	3	Chlorpromazine may produce a dose- and duration-dependent increase in plasma glucose concentrations that may lead to loss of diabetic control.	Monitor patients for loss of diabetic control during concurrent therapy.	570
Insulin–Clofibrate	2	Clofibrate may lower blood glucose levels and improve glucose tolerance in insulin-dependent diabetics, although another study showed no effect.	It is important to monitor blood glucose levels and adjust the insulin dosage if necessary.	572

TABLE 14. Hypoglycemic Drug Interactions—cont'd

Drug Interaction	Significance Code	Potential Effects	Recommendations	See Page
Insulin–Epinephrine	3	Epinephrine raises blood glucose levels and may increase insulin requirements.	Monitor patients stabilized on insulin when administering a sympathomimetic.	573
Insulin–Fenfluramine	2	The intrinsic hypoglycemic effect of fenfluramine may increase the effects of insulin resulting in hypoglycemia.	Although this interaction may be beneficial in some diabetics, patients should be closely monitored.	574
Insulin–Guanethidine	2	Long-term guanethidine therapy may improve glucose tolerance in diabetics, necessitating a reduction in insulin dose.	Monitor diabetics closely when guanethidine is added to or withdrawn from the drug regimen.	575
Insulin–Isoniazid	3	Isoniazid antagonizes the hypoglycemic action of insulin by elevating blood sugar levels.	Monitor patients for increases in blood glucose levels. This interaction may be of greater significance in patients with hepatic dysfunction or in slow acetylators.	576
Insulin–Oxytetracycline	2	Concurrent use of these agents may cause hypoglycemia.	Monitor patients closely as a decreased insulin dosage or increased carbohydrate intake may be necessary.	577
Insulin–Phenelzine	2	Phenelzine may potentiate the action of insulin, resulting in enhanced hypoglycemia.	Monitor patients for excessive hypoglycemia. A reduction in the insulin dosage may be required.	578
Insulin–Phenytoin	3	High doses of phenytoin have produced hyperglycemia and glycosuria, with convulsions, coma, and other neurologic effects, in patients receiving antidiabetic treatment.	Dosage reduction of phenytoin may prevent or alleviate the symptoms.	580
Insulin–Propranolol	1	Propranolol can delay recovery from hypoglycemia and modify normal cardiovascular response to insulin-induced hypoglycemia. Hypertensive responses may also occur.	A cardioselective beta blocker, (e.g., atenolol) may be a suitable alternative to propranolol. Patients on concurrent therapy should be advised of the diaphoretic response that occurs with hypoglycemia.	582
Insulin–Thyroid	2	Initiation of thyroid replacement therapy may increase insulin or oral hypoglycemic requirements. Insulin may affect thyroid hormone binding and disrupt thyroid function.	It is important to monitor both diabetic control and thyroid function.	584

TABLE 14. Hypoglycemic Drug Interactions—cont'd

Drug Interaction	Significance Code	Potential Effects	Recommendations	See Page
Tolbutamide–Chloramphenicol	2	Chloramphenicol may increase tolbutamide half-life, causing a prolonged hypoglycemic response.	The tolbutamide dose may need to be reduced.	585
Tolbutamide–Diazoxide	3	One report suggests that diazoxide may enhance tolbutamide-induced insulin release when given before the sulfonylurea. The hyperglycemia that may occur may be caused by diazoxide alone.	If hyperglycemia occurs, adjust dosages of 1 or both drugs as needed.	586
Tolbutamide–Dicumarol	2	Dicumarol may significantly increase the serum half-life of tolbutamide.	Monitor serum glucose concentrations and adjust the tolbutamide dose accordingly.	587
Tolbutamide–Phenylbutazone	1	Concurrent use of these agents can result in severe hypoglycemic reactions.	Avoid concurrent use. If co-therapy is necessary, intense monitoring of serum glucose levels is required.	589
Tolbutamide–Sulfamethizole	2	Sulfamethizole may prolong tolbutamide half-life and enhance hypoglycemic effects.	Adverse reactions occur less often after patients are stabilized on co-therapy for a few weeks. The extent of caution indicated is dependent on several factors (agents used, renal and hepatic function, etc.).	591

Chlorpropamide—Alcohol, Ethyl

1

Summary: The combination of alcohol and antidiabetic agents can result in unpredictable and varied reactions, ranging from mild flushing to severe hypoglycemic reactions. Clinical significance is dependent on the hypoglycemic agent involved, amount and type of alcohol ingested, pattern of alcohol use and dietary intake, and state of hepatic function.

Chlorpropamide has frequently been reported to induce facial flushing after alcohol ingestion in some individuals, particularly noninsulin-dependent diabetics.[1-11] A disulfiram-type reaction to alcohol has been produced by chlorpropamide.[1,2,10,12,13]

Related Drugs: Cases of profound hypoglycemic coma have been reported in chronic alcoholics who were also insulin-dependent[14] diabetics. Ample documentation exists of an interaction between tolbutamide and alcohol in nonalcoholic diabetic patients, alcoholics, and normal subjects.[8,9,15-19] There is 1 report of reduced tolerance for alcohol in a patient on tolazamide therapy.[20] There is no documentation regarding an interaction between alcohol and the other first generation sulfonylurea hypoglycemic agent (acetohexamide); however, based on pharmacologic similarity an interaction may be expected to occur. Glipizide and glyburide have been reported to have a very low incidence of disulfiram-like reactions with concurrent alcohol; however, in 1 study 5 of 11 patients taking glyburide developed a flush after a test dose of alcohol.[10]

Mechanism: Alcohol, by means of its intrinsic hypoglycemic activity, can induce hypoglycemia and interfere with gluconeogenesis in the liver.[14,17,18] Conversely, use of some alcoholic beverages may increase serum glucose levels because of high carbohydrate content.[12] Chronic alcohol intake has been shown to greatly reduce the half-life of tolbutamide, probably through an increase in tolbutamide metabolism in the liver.[11,14-16,19]

Recommendations: Although abstinence from alcohol would be ideal for patients receiving antidiabetic therapy, practical management will more often involve recommendation for reduced alcohol intake and cautioning the patient regarding potential effects of alcohol while taking antidiabetic agents, as well as the importance of adequate dietary intake to minimize the potential for adverse effects.

References

1. Medbak, S., and others: Chlorpropamide alcohol flush and circulating metenkephalin: a positive link, Br. Med. J. **283:**937, 1981.
2. Leslie, R.D., and Pyke, D.A.: Chlorpropamide alcohol flushing: a dominantly inherited trait associated with diabetes, Br. Med. J. **2:**1519, 1978.
3. Kobberling, J., and others: The chlorpropamide alcohol flush, Diabetalogia **19:**359, 1980.
4. DeSilva, N.E., and others: Low incidence of chlorpropamide alcohol flushing in diet-treated non-insulin dependent diabetics, Lancet **1:**128, 1981.
5. Strakosch, C.R., and others: Blockade of chlorpropamide alcohol flush by aspirin, Lancet **1:**394, 1980.

6. Leslie, R., and others: Asthma induced by enkephalin, Br. Med. J. **280:**16, 1980.
7. Barnett, A.H., and Pyke, D.A.: Chlorpropamide-alcohol flushing and large-vessel disease in non-insulin dependent diabetes, Br. Med. J. **281:**261, 1980.
8. Harris, E.L.: Adverse reactions to oral antidiabetic agents, Br. Med. J. **3:**29, 1971.
9. Capretti, L., and others: Chlorpropamide- and tolbutamide-alcohol flushing in non-insulin-dependent diabetes, Br. Med. J. **283:**1361, 1981.
10. Wardle, E.N., and Richardson, G.O.: Alcohol and glibenclamide, Br. Med. J. **3:**309, 1971.
11. Barnett, A.H., and others: Blood concentrations of acetaldehyde during chlorpropamide-alcohol flush, Br. Med. J. **283:**939, 1981.
12. Walsh, C.H., and others: Effect of moderate alcohol intake on control of diabetes, Diabetes **23:**440, 1974.
13. Fitzgerald, M.G., and others: Alcohol sensitivity in diabetics receiving chlorpropamide, Diabetes **11:**40, 1962.
14. Arky, R.A., and others: Irreversible hypoglycemia, a complication of alcohol and insulin, J.A.M.A. **206:**575, 1968.
15. Shah, M.N., and others: Comparison of blood clearance of ethanol and tolbutamide and the activity of hepatic ethanol-oxidizing and drug metabolizing enzymes in chronic alcoholic subjects, Am. J. Clin. Nutr. **25:**135, 1972.
16. Iber, F.L.: Drug metabolism in heavy consumers of alcohol, Clin. Pharmacol. Ther. **22:**735, 1977.
17. Dornhorst, A., and Ouyang, A.: Effect of alcohol on glucose tolerance, Lancet **3:**957, 1971.
18. Jackson, J.E., and Bressler, R.: Clinical pharmacology of sulphonylurea hypoglycemic agents: part 2, Drugs **22:**295, 1981.
19. Kater, R.M.H., and others: Increased rate of tolbutamide metabolism in alcoholic patients, J.A.M.A. **207:**363, 1969.
20. McKendry, J.B., and Gfeller, K.F.: Clinical experience with the oral antidiabetic compound, tolazamide, Can. Med. Assoc. J. **96:**531, 1967.

Chlorpropamide–Allopurinol

3

Summary: Serum half-life of chlorpropamide may be significantly increased by concurrent administration of allopurinol, although supporting clinical data are scarce and inconclusive.

Related Drugs: There have been no reports of other sulfonylurea hypoglycemic drugs (e.g., acetohexamide, tolazamide, tolbutamide [see Appendix]) interacting with allopurinol; however, a similar interaction may be expected to occur based on pharmacologic similarity. Glyburide and glipizide may not interact to the same extent as the other sulfonylureas since they are excreted as less active metabolites by both renal and biliary routes. There are no drugs related to allopurinol.

Mechanism: Both chlorpropamide and allopurinol are excreted slowly, with the half-life of allopurinol increasing in proportion to the degree of renal impairment.[1-3] Although documentation is lacking, the suggested mechanism of interaction between chlorpropamide and allopurinol is a competition for renal tubular secretion.[3] In the only clinical report of this interaction,[4] long term allopurinol therapy increased the half-life of chlorpropamide in patients with renal dysfunction and in 1 patient with normal renal function; a shorter length of allopurinol administration (1 to 2 days) did not produce this response in 3 other patients.

Recommendations: Because of the extremely limited evidence of this drug interaction, the clinical significance must be considered minimal. It would be prudent to monitor patients on oral hypoglycemic agents for increases in pharmacologic effect or serum half-life if allopurinol is administered concurrently.

References

1. Larner, J.: Insulin and oral hypoglycemic drugs; glucagon. In Gilman, A.G., Goodman, L.S., and Gilman, A., editors: The pharmacological basis of therapeutics. New York, 1980, MacMillan Publishing.
2. Flower, R.J., and others: Analgesic-antipyretics and anti-inflammatory agents; drugs employed in the treatment of gout. In Gilman, A.G., Goodman, L.S., and Gilman, A., editors: The pharmacological basis of therapeutics, New York, 1980, MacMillan Publishing.
3. Jackson, J.E., and Bressler, R.: Clinical pharmacology of sulphonylurea hypoglycaemic agents: part 2, Drugs **22:**295, 1981.
4. Petitpierre, B., and others: Behavior of chlorpropamide in renal insufficiency and under the effect of associated drug therapy, Int. J. Clin. Pharmacol. Ther. Toxicol. **62:**120, 1972.

Chlorpropamide–Aspirin

2

Summary: There appears to be an increased risk of chlorpropamide toxicity when aspirin is added to a therapeutic regimen with this sulfonylurea oral hypoglycemic drug. Specifically, the most prominent feature of such an interaction is a prolonged and possibly severe hypoglycemia.[1] Because chlorpropamide possesses significant intrinsic toxicity and a rather long elimination half-life and because this effect can occur with analgesic doses of aspirin,[2,3] this interaction is moderately hazardous and necessitates appropriate clinical action.

Related Drugs: Other sulfonylurea hypoglycemic agents (acetohexamide, tolbutamide, and tolazamide) may also interact with aspirin based on pharmacologic similarity. It appears that chlorpropamide may represent the greatest potential for such an interaction since it possesses the longest elimination half-life of this group and it is most dependent on renal mechanisms of excretion.[4] Glyburide and glipizide are less susceptible to protein displacement by anionic substances such as aspirin and may not interact to the same degree as other sulfonylureas.[5,6]

Although no documentation exists, other salicylates (e.g., choline salicylate, salicylamide, sodium salicylate [see Appendix]) share many pharmacologic activities with aspirin and may also interact with chlorpropamide.

Mechanism: Sulfonylureas tend to bind extensively to plasma protein where aspirin may cause a displacement and increased concentrations of free drug.[7] In addition, aspirin has very complex effects upon glucose metabolism, partly because of its ability to uncouple oxidative phosphorylation, which can further alter glucose homeostasis in the diabetic individual receiving oral hypoglycemic drugs.[4]

Recommendations: An individual receiving both chlorpropamide and aspirin therapy should have the chlorpropamide dose adjusted downward. The patient should be carefully monitored. Serum or urinary glucose levels will facilitate proper management of such patients. Upon discontinuation of aspirin administration, the requirement for chlorpropamide will increase. It may be beneficial to consider switching to insulin or dietary control in patients requiring aspirin therapy, particularly those who exhibit poor response with the oral hypoglycemic drug. Cases of hypoglycemia can be treated by traditional methods or by the use of glucose plus diazoxide.[8]

References

1. Schulz, E.: Severe hypoglycemic reactions after tolbutamide, carbutamide, and chlorpropamide, Arch. Klin. Med. **214:**125, 1968.
2. vonEickstedt, K.W.: Insulin, glucagon and oral hypoglycemic drugs. In Dukes, M.N.G., editor: Meyler's side effects of drugs, ed. 9, Amsterdam, 1980, Excerpta Medica.
3. Hays, A.H.: Therapeutic implications of drug interactions with acetaminophen and aspirin, Arch. Intern. Med. **141:**301, 1981.
4. Larner, J.: Insulin and oral hypoglycemic drugs: glucagon. In Gilman, A.G., Goodman, L.S., and Gilman, A., editors: The pharmacological basis of therapeutics, New York, 1980, Macmillan Publishing.

5. Brown, K.F., and Crooks, M.J.: Displacement of tolbutamide, glibenclamide and chlorpropamide from serum albumin by anionic drugs, Biochem. Pharmacol. **25:**1175, 1976.

6. Shuman, C.R.: Glipizide: an overview, Am. J. Med. **11:**15, 1983.

7. Wishinsky, H., and others: Protein interactions of sulfonylurea compounds, Diabetes **2**(suppl.):18, 1962.

8. Johnson, S.F., and others: Chlorpropamide induced hypoglycemia. Successful treatment with diazoxide, Am. J. Med. **16:**799, 1977.

Chlorpropamide–Clofibrate

Summary: The hypoglycemic activity of chlorpropamide may be enhanced by concurrent administration of clofibrate.[1-5] A reduction in the dose of the hypoglycemic agent may be necessary in some patients to prevent the development of symptomatic hypoglycemia.

Related Drugs: Other sulfonylureas, including acetohexamide,[4] tolazamide,[1] and tolbutamide,[6] have demonstrated a similar interaction with clofibrate. Glyburide and glipizide may interact in a similar manner because of pharmacologic similarity if the mechanism relates to decreased insulin resistance by clofibrate or if clofibrate has intrinsic hypoglycemic activity.

Halofenate,* an antilipidemic agent, reportedly enhances the hypoglycemic effect of the sulfonylureas to a greater degree than clofibrate.[1,2,7]

Mechanism: Clofibrate has been postulated to increase the half-life of chlorpropamide by competing for renal tubular secretion sites and thereby decreasing chlorpropamide's excretion.[4] Clofibrate also has greater affinity for plasma protein binding sites and may displace chlorpropamide and other sulfonylureas from these sites.[1,2] A decrease in insulin resistance by clofibrate has also been suggested as a possible mechanism for the enhanced hypoglycemia.[6]

Recent studies have demonstrated that clofibrate has hypoglycemic activity in itself.[8-10] Although the mechanism whereby clofibrate produces hypoglycemia is not established, results of 1 study indicate that the effect may result from increased insulin sensitivity.[10]

Recommendations: When clofibrate is added to the regimen of diabetic patients receiving chlorpropamide or other sulfonylureas, blood glucose levels should be monitored closely for hypoglycemia; it may be necessary to decrease the dose of the sulfonylurea in some patients. Conversely, when clofibrate is discontinued in patients receiving chlorpropamide concurrently, blood glucose levels should be monitored closely for deterioration in diabetic control.

References

1. Jain, A.K., and others: Potentiation of hypoglycemic effect of sulfonylureas by halofenate, N. Engl. J. Med. **293**:1283, 1975.
2. Ryan, J.R.: The metabolic spectrum of halofenate, J. Clin. Pharmacol. Biopharm. **12**:239, 1975.
3. Daubresse, J., and others: Potentiation of hypoglycemic effect of sulfonylureas by clofibrate, N. Engl. J. Med. **294**:613, 1976.
4. Petitpierre, B., and others: Behavior of chlorpropamide in renal insufficiency and under the effect of associated drug therapy, Int. J. Clin. Pharmacol. Ther. Toxicol. **6**:120, 1972.
5. Daubresse, J., and others: Clofibrate and diabetes control in patients treated with oral hypoglycemic agents, Br. J. Clin. Pharmacol. **7**:599, 1979.
6. Ferrari, C., and others: Potentiation of hypoglycemic response to intravenous tolbutamide by clofibrate, N. Engl. J. Med. **294**:1184, 1976.
7. Kudzma, D.J., and Friedberg, S.J.: Potentiation of hypoglycemic effect of chlorpropamide and phenformin by halofenate, Diabetes **26**:291, 1977.

*Not available in the U.S.

8. Calvert, G.D., and others: The effects of clofibrate on plasma glucose, lipoproteins, fibrinogen, and other biochemical and haematological variables in patients with mature onset diabetes mellitus, Eur. J. Clin. Pharmacol. **17:**355, 1980.

9. Barnett, D., and others: Effect of clofibrate on glucose tolerance in maturity onset diabetes, Br. J. Clin. Pharmacol. **4:**455, 1977.

10. Ferrari, C., and others: Effects of short-term clofibrate administration on glucose tolerance and insulin secretion in patients with chemical diabetes or hypertriglyceridemia, Metabolism **26:**129, 1977.

Chlorpropamide–Cortisone

Summary: The intrinsic hyperglycemic activity of cortisone may decrease the hypoglycemic effects of concurrently administered chlorpropamide, resulting in a moderately clinically significant interaction.[1,2]

Related Drugs: Short-term prednisone treatment did not significantly influence tolbutamide disposition in 2 studies of healthy individuals.[3,4] Since prolonged treatment with glucocorticoids has been found to elevate plasma glucagon,[2,5] the other sulfonylurea hypoglycemics (e.g., acetohexamide, glyburide, tolazamide [see Appendix]) and other corticosteroids (e.g., betamethasone, hydrocortisone, triamcinolone [see Appendix]) may be expected to interact similarly.

Mechanism: Glucocorticoids promote gluconeogenesis by both peripheral and hepatic actions. Peripherally they act to mobilize amino acids from a number of tissues. In the liver, they produce enzyme induction after a matter of hours.[1] Prolonged, but not acute, treatment with glucocorticoids has been found to elevate plasma glucagon, contributing to the enhanced synthesis of glucose.[1,2,5] The deposition of glycogen in the liver found after treatment with glucocorticoids is believed to be at least in part secondary to the rise in plasma insulin concentration elicited by the elevated plasma glucose.[3] Chlorpropamide and other sulfonylureas acutely increase beta cell sensitivity to glucose as a stimulus to insulin release in both normal and diabetic subjects.[6] In vitro studies[7,8] suggest that chlorpropamide inhibits glucagon-stimulated hepatic gluconeogenesis and augments insulin-mediated suppression of hepatic glucose release.

Recommendations: Occurrence of glycosuria should not be an important factor in the decision to discontinue corticosteroid therapy or to initiate it in diabetic patients. However, patients on antidiabetic therapy should be monitored for decreased hypoglycemic action while on concurrent glucocorticoid treatment. To maintain diabetic control during high dose or long-term corticosteroid treatment, increased dosage of chlorpropamide may be required.

References

1. Haynes, R.C., and Murad, F.: Adrenocorticotropic hormone; adrenocortical steroids and their synthetic analogs; inhibitors of adrenocortical steroid biosynthesis. In Gilman, A.G., Goodman, L.S., and Gilman, A., editors: The pharmacological basis of therapeutics. New York, 1980, Macmillan Publishing.
2. Wise, J.K., and others: Influence of glucocorticoids on glucagon secretion and plasma amino acid concentrations in man, J. Clin. Invest. **52:**2774, 1973.
3. Kreutner, W., and Goldberg, N.D.: Dependence on insulin of the apparent hydrocortisone activation of hepatic glycogen synthetase, Proc. Nat. Acad. Sci. U.S.A. **58:**1515, 1967.
4. Breimer, D.D., and others: Influence of corticosteroid on hexobarbital and tolbutamide disposition, Clin. Pharmacol. Ther. **24:**208, 1978.
5. Marco, J., and others: Hyperglucagonism induced by glucocorticoid treatment in man, N. Engl. J. Med. **288:**128, 1973.
6. Jackson, J.E., and Bressler, R.: Clinical pharmacology of sulphonylurea hypoglycaemic agents, part 2, Drugs **22:**295, 1981.

7. Blumenthal, S.A.: Potentiation of hepatic action of insulin by chlorpropamide, Diabetes **26:**485, 1977.

8. Blumethal, S.A., and Whitmer, K.R.: Hepatic effects of chlorpropamide, inhibition of glucagon-stimulated gluconeogenesis in perfused livers of fasted rats, Diabetes **28:**646, 1979.

Chlorpropamide–Hydrochlorothiazide

Summary: Diabetic patients regulated by chlorpropamide may exhibit impaired diabetic control when hydrochlorothiazide is added to the drug regimen.[1-6] This effect is usually reversible when the diuretic is discontinued, a larger dose of the hypoglycemic agent is used, or increased potassium supplementation is provided.

Related Drugs: This drug interaction may also occur with the other sulfonylurea hypoglycemics (e.g., acetohexamide, glyburide, tolbutamide [see Appendix]).[1] All thiazide diuretics (e.g., cyclothiazide, methyclothiazide, polythiazide [see Appendix]) have the potential of producing hypokalemia,[7] which is probably a factor in the etiology of the interaction. Chlorothiazide,[1] trichlormethiazide,[1] bendroflumethiazide,[6] benzthiazide,[2] and dihydroflumethiazide[8*] have been documented to interact with antidiabetic agents. Chlorthalidone[6,9] and the other thiazide related diuretics, metolazone, quinethazone, and indapamide, may also cause hyperglycemia. Most studies have shown that furosemide has little effect on the glucose tolerance of diabetic and nondiabetic patients.[3,4,10,11] Ethacrynic acid also is less likely to affect glucose tolerance.[3,4] The other loop diuretic (bumetanide) may be expected to interact similarly. There is no evidence to suggest that the thiazides inhibit the hypoglycemic effect of exogenously administered insulin.

Mechanism: The mechanism of this interaction is not fully understood. It has been suggested that thiazides inhibit the release of insulin by the pancreas.[10-11] However, in vitro studies using rat pancreatic tissue have failed to demonstrate this effect.[12,13] Hypokalemia is believed to be a contributing factor in the pathogenesis of the interaction.[5,14]

Recommendations: Diabetic patients controlled by diet, with oral hypoglycemic agents, or by insulin should be monitored closely for hyperglycemia before and after thiazide or thiazide-like diuretics are initiated. Also, patients who have been maintained on such combination therapy should be observed for symptoms of hypoglycemia when the diuretic is withdrawn from the regimen. Since the development of hypokalemia may be responsible for the pathogenesis of the interaction, therapy should be directed toward preventing abnormal potassium loss. Additionally, the dose of the hypoglycemic drug may be increased or insulin therapy may be substituted in sufficient dosage to control the diabetic state.

References

1. Kansel, P.C., and others: Thiazide diuretics and control of diabetes mellitus, South. Med. J. **62:**1374, 1969.
2. Runyan, J.W., Jr.: Influence of thiazide diuretics on carbohydrate metabolism in patients with mild diabetes, N. Engl. J. Med. **267:**541, 1962.
3. Kohner, E.M., and others: Effect of diuretic therapy on glucose tolerance in hypertensive patients, Lancet. **1:**1986, 1971.
4. Breckenridge, A.: Glucose tolerance in hypertensive patients on long-term diuretic therapy, Lancet **1:**61, 1967.

*Not available in the U.S.

5. Amery, A., and others: Glucose tolerance during diuretic therapy, Lancet **1:**681, 1978.

6. Lewis, P.J., and others: Deterioration of glucose tolerance in hypertensive patients on prolonged diuretic treatment, Lancet. **1:**564, 1976.

7. Mudge, G.H.: Diuretics and other agents employed in the mobilization of edema fluid. In Gilman, A.G., Goodman, L.S., and Gilman, A., editors: The pharmacologic basis of therapeutics, New York, 1980, MacMillan Publishing.

8. Goldner, M.G., and others: Hyperglycemia and glycosuria due to thiazide derivatives administered in diabetes mellitus, N. Engl. J. Med. **262:**403, 1960.

9. Caliner, N.H., and others: Thiazide- and phthalimidine-induced hyperglycemia in hypertensive patients, J.A.M.A. **191:**535, 1965.

10. Jackson, W.P.U., and Nellen, M.: Effect of frusemide on carbohydrate metabolism, blood-pressure and other modalities: a comparison with chlorothiazide, Br. Med. J. **2:**333, 1966.

11. Fajans, S.S., and others: Benzothiadiazine suppression of insulin release from normal and abnormal islet tissue in man, J. Clin. Invest. **45:**481, 1966.

12. Malaisse, W., and Malaisse-Lagae, F.: Effect of thiazide upon insulin secretion in vitro, Arch. Int. Pharmacodyn. Ther. **171:**235, 1968.

13. Kaldor, A., and others: Diabetogenic effect of oral diuretics in asymptomatic diabetes, Int. J. Clin. Pharmacol. **11:**232, 1975.

14. Conn, J.W.: Hypotension, the potassium ion and impaired carbohydrate tolerance, N. Engl. J. Med. **273:**1135, 1965.

Chlorpropamide–Probenecid

3

Summary: Probenecid was reported to increase the half-life of chlorpropamide in 6 patients from approximately 36 to 50 hours.[1] This report has not been confirmed or refuted by subsequent clinical study and is of dubious clinical significance.

Related Drugs: Probenecid was reported to prolong the half-life of tolbutamide[2]; however, this finding was not confirmed by a second well-controlled study.[3] It is not known whether the other sulfonylurea hypoglycemic agents (e.g., acetohexamide, glyburide, tolazamide [see Appendix]) would interact with probenecid in a similar manner. In 6 normal subjects on sulfinpyrazone therapy (800 mg/day), the half-life of tolbutamide approximately doubled and clearance was reduced 10% following parenteral tolbutamide administration.[4] In 1 study involving 19 diabetics, the concurrent use of glyburide and sulfinpyrazone (200 mg 4 times a day) had no significant effect on blood and urine glucose concentration or blood cholesterol or triglyceride concentrations, as compared to glyburide and concomitant placebo.[5]

Mechanism: The purported mechanism of this interaction is that probenecid inhibits the renal excretion of chlorpropamide.[1] This interaction was reported before it was generally known that chlorpropamide is widely metabolized by the liver to metabolites of unknown activity.[6] The metabolic fate of chlorpropamide may account for the lack of reports of clinical hypoglycemia in patients receiving the combination. Sulfinpyrazone is thought to depress the metabolism of tolbutamide resulting in decreased elimination.[4]

Recommendations: No changes are necessary during combined therapy; however, patients should be observed for excessive hypoglycemic effects. Neither chlorpropamide nor probenecid should be used in patients with impaired renal function.

References

1. Petitpierre, B., and others: Behaviour of chlorpropamide in renal insufficiency and under the effect of associated drug therapy, Int. J. Clin. Pharmacol. Ther. Toxicol. **6**:120, 1972.
2. Stowers, J.M., and others: Pharmacology and mode of action of the sulphonylureas in man, Lancet **1:**278, 1958.
3. Brook, R., and others: Failure of probenecid to inhibit the rate of metabolism of tolbutamide in man, Clin. Pharmacol. Ther. **9**:314, 1968.
4. Stockley, I.H.: Drug interactions with sulphinpyrazone, Pharmacol. J. **230**:163, 1983.
5. Kritz, H., and others: Sulfinpyrazone and glibenclamide study of interaction in diabetics of type II, Wien. Med. Wochenschr. **133**:237, 1983.
6. Taylor, J.A.: Pharmacokinetics and biotransformation of chlorpropamide in man, Clin. Pharmacol. Ther. **13**:710, 1972.

Insulin—Aspirin

Summary: The hypoglycemic activity of insulin may be potentiated by concurrent use of aspirin or other salicylates. Three studies have shown that moderate doses of aspirin (3.0 to 3.2 g/day) when administered to normal subjects,[1-3] adult-onset diabetics,[2] and insulin-requiring diabetics[1] significantly increased early insulin release and decreased plasma glucose in response to intravenous glucose in the normal subjects. Basal plasma glucose levels were lower[1-3] and basal insulin also rose.[3]

Related Drugs: Four studies in which moderate doses of intravenous sodium salicylate were used in normal subjects,[4-7] adult-onset diabetics,[4-5] or insulin-dependent diabetics[6,7] showed similar results, including an improvement in glucose tolerance and an augmented plasma-insulin response. Also, the oral administration of 3-methyl salicylic acid (0.9 to 1.8 g/day) to diabetic and nondiabetic patients produced a significant increase in plasma insulin levels.[8] Although documentation is lacking, a similar interaction may be expected to occur with the other salicylates (e.g., choline salicylate, salicylamide, salsalate [see Appendix]) since they are pharmacologically related.

Mechanism: The reduction of plasma glucose by aspirin is dependent on continuing beta cell function. In the absence of beta cell function the stimulatory effect of aspirin on glucagon production becomes the major determinant of aspirin's effect on plasma glucose. The effects of aspirin on pancreatic islet cell function appear to be the major determinant of its effect on glucose handling.[1] Other explanations have been suggested, including a change in hepatic glucose production, an inhibition of intestinal glucose production, or an increase in peripheral glucose uptake and oxidation.[2-4] Also, because prostaglandins (specifically PGE_1 and PGE_2) significantly decrease the early insulin response, it has been suggested that aspirin, a prostaglandin inhibitor, exerts its effect by inhibiting PGE_1 and PGE_2.[2,5]

Recommendations: Patients should be monitored for a change in their blood glucose levels during concurrent use of these agents. If necessary, a lower dose of insulin may be administered.

References

1. Prince, R.L., and others: The effect of acetylsalicylic acid on plasma glucose and the response of glucose regulatory hormones to intravenous glucose and arginine in insulin treated diabetics and normal subjects, Metabolism **30:**293, 1981.
2. Micossi, P., and others: Aspirin stimulates insulin and glucagon secretion and increases glucose tolerance in normal and diabetic subjects, Diabetes **27:**1196, 1978.
3. Giugliano, P., and others: The effect of acetylsalicylic acid on insulin response to glucose and argenine in normal man, Diabetologia **14:**359, 1978.
4. Chen, M.C., and others: Restoration of the acute insulin response by sodium salicylate: a glucose dose-related phenomenon, Diabetes **27:**750, 1978.
5. Robertson, R.P., and Chen, M.: A role for prostaglandin E in defective insulin secretion and carbohydrate intolerance in diabetes mellitus, J. Clin. Invest. **60:**747, 1977.

6. Field, J.B., and others: Effect of salicylate infusion on plasma-insulin and glucose tolerance in healthy persons and mild diabetics, Lancet **1**:1191, 1967.
7. Gilgore, S.G., and Rupp, J.J.: Response of blood glucose to intravenous salicylate, Metabolism **10**:419, 1961.
8. Hyams, D.E., and others: The effect of 3-methyl salicylic (0-cresotinic) acid on plasma insulin and glucose tolerance in diabetic and non-diabetic subjects, Diabetologia **7**:94, 1971.

Insulin–Chlorpromazine

3

Summary: Chlorpromazine may produce a dose- and duration-dependent increase in plasma glucose concentrations that may lead to loss of diabetic control in predisposed individuals. This effect of chlorpromazine has been confirmed by numerous reports in both diabetics and nondiabetics.[1-12] Chlorpromazine has also been used to treat hyperinsulinemic hypoglycemia.[13]

Related Drugs: Animal and human studies have demonstrated that fluphenazine, perphenazine, thioridazine, and trifluoperazine may also increase blood glucose levels.[9,14] Although documentation is lacking, other phenothiazines (e.g., carphenazine, mesoridazine, promazine [see Appendix]), thioxanthenes (chlorprothixene and thiothixene), as well as the butyrophenone (haloperidol), dihydroindolone (molindone), and dibenzoxazepine (loxapine) may be expected to interact with insulin in a similar manner because of pharmacologic similarity.

Because of the mechanism of this interaction, sulfonylurea hypoglycemic agents (e.g., acetohexamide, chlorpropamide, glyburide [see Appendix]) may also be affected by chlorpromazine administration.

Mechanism: Animal studies have established that this interaction is a result of the inhibition of insulin release from the pancreas,[14-17] although chlorpromazine probably also stimulates epinephrine release from the adrenal medulla, which will raise blood sugar levels.[18] Evidence of the dose/duration dependency of this reaction comes from several different studies demonstrating (1) a higher incidence of this effect at higher dosages (more than 100 mg/day) or longer duration (more than 1 year)[9]; (2) no effect of chlorpromazine on blood sugar levels with short duration of therapy (less than 2 weeks)[19]; or (3) no effect of chlorpromazine with small doses.[12]

Recommendations: Patients receiving hypoglycemic therapy with insulin or sulfonylureas should be observed for loss of diabetic control if high doses of phenothiazines are added to their medication regimen.

References

1. Hiles, B.H.: Hyperglycaemia and glycosuria following chlorpromazine therapy, J.A.M.A. **162:**1651, 1956.
2. Dobkin, A., and others: Some studies with largactil, Can. Med. Assoc. J. **70:**626, 1954.
3. Mayer, J., and others: Chlorpromazine as a therapeutic agent in clinical medicine, Arch. Intern. Med. **95:**202, 1955.
4. Lancaster, N.P., and Jones, D.H.: Chlorpromazine and insulin in psychiatry, Br. Med. J. **2:**565, 1954.
5. Charatan, F., and Bartlett, N.: The effect of chlorpromazine (largactil) on glucose tolerance, J. Ment. Sci. **101:**351, 1955.
6. Cooperberg, A.A., and Eidlow, S.: Haemolytic anaemia, jaundice and diabetes mellitus following chlorpromazine therapy, Can. Med. Assoc. J. **75:**746, 1956.
7. Arneson, G.: Phenothiazine derivatives and metabolism, J. Neuropsychiatry **5:**181, 1964.
8. Amdisen, A.: Diabetes mellitus as a side effect of treatment with tricyclic neuroleptics, Acta Psychiatry Scand. **40**(suppl.):411, 1964.

9. Thonnard-Neumann, E.: Phenothiazines and diabetes in hospitalized women, Am. J. Psychiatry **124:**978, 1968.
10. Korenyi, C., and Lowenstein, B.: Chlorpromazine induced diabetes, Dis. Nerv. Syst. **29:**327, 1968.
11. Marmow, A.: Diabetes in chronic schizophrenia, Dis. Nerv. Syst. **32:**777, 1971.
12. Erle, G., and others: Effect of chlorpromazine on blood glucose and plasma insulin in man, Eur. J. Clin. Pharmacol. **11:**15, 1977.
13. Federspil, G., and others: Chlorpromazine in the treatment of endogenous organic hyperinsulinism, Diabetologia **10:**189, 1974.
14. Proakis, A.G., and Borowitz, J.L.: Blockage of insulin release by certain phenothiazines, Biochem. Pharmacol. **23:**1693, 1974.
15. Jori, A., and Carrara, M.C.: On the mechanism of the hyperglycemic effect of chlorpromazine, J. Pharm. Pharmacol. **18:**623, 1966.
16. Susten, A.S., and others: Effect of chlorpromazine on glucose and tolbutamide-stimulated insulin release in the adrenalectomized rat, Toxicol. Appl. Pharmacol. **24:**364, 1973.
17. Ammon, H.P., and others: Effect of chlorpromazine (CPZ) on insulin release in vivo and in vitro in the rat, J. Pharmacol. Exp. Ther. **187:**423, 1973.
18. Bonaccurosi, A., and others: Studies on the hyperglycemia induced by chlorpromazine in rats, Br. J. Pharmacol. **23:**93, 1964.
19. Schwarz, L., and Munoz, R.: Blood sugar levels in patients treated with chlorpromazine, Am. J. Psychiatry **125:**253, 1968.

Insulin–Clofibrate

2

Summary: Clofibrate has been shown to lower blood glucose levels in insulin-dependent diabetics in 2 controlled studies[1,2] and to improve glucose tolerance in a study without controls.[3] These beneficial effects were observed without demonstrable changes in circulating concentrations of insulin and glucagon.[1] Similar results were described in another report.[4] However, a controlled study involving 18 juvenile-onset diabetics failed to show any affect of clofibrate on fasting blood glucose, glucose tolerance, or insulin requirements.[5]

Related Drugs: There are no drugs related to clofibrate. An interaction involving clofibrate and the oral sulfonylureas is discussed in another monograph (see Chlorpropamide–Clofibrate, p. 561).

Mechanism: The mechanism of this interaction is unknown. However, it has been suggested that clofibrate causes a change in tissue sensitivity to insulin and/or glucose, and therefore mediates this interaction.[4]

Recommendations: It is important to monitor blood glucose levels during concurrent therapy with these agents. The dose of insulin may need to be adjusted.

References

1. Schade, D.S., and others: Metabolic effects of clofibrate in insulin-dependent ketosis-prone diabetic man, Metabolism **27:**461, 1978.
2. Twomey, C., and Bloom, A.: Clofibrate in insulin-dependent diabetes, Ir. J. Med. Sci. **148:**31, 1979.
3. Miller, R.D.: Atromid in the treatment of post-climacteric diabetes, J. Atherosclerosis Res. **3:**694, 1963.
4. Ferrari, C., and others: Effect of short-term clofibrate administration on glucose tolerance and insulin secretion in patients with chemical diabetes or hypertriglyceridaemia, Metabolism **26:**129, 1977.
5. Danowski, T.S., and others: Ethyl chlorophenoxyisobutyate (CPIB) effects in juvenile-onset diabetes mellitus, Clin. Pharmacol. Ther. **6:**716, 1965.

Insulin–Epinephrine

3

Summary: Epinephrine raises blood glucose levels and may increase insulin requirements.

Related Drugs: Other sympathomimetic agents[1] such as dopamine,[2] dobutamine,[3] norepinephrine,[4] and salbutamol (albuterol),[5-7] may have the same hyperglycemic effect with insulin. Similar precautions should be observed with the other sympathomimetic agents (e.g., indirect: amphetamine; direct: methoxamine; mixed: metaraminol [see Appendix]).

Mechanism: Epinephrine stimulates glycogenolysis, gluconeogenesis, and lipolysis and inhibits insulin secretion.[8] In both normal and diabetic subjects, epinephrine increases blood glucose levels and glucose production while decreasing glucose clearance.[9-11] It may act synergistically with glucagon to antagonize the effects of insulin; however, the interrelationship between the glucose-regulating hormones (including cortisol) has not been fully elucidated.[12]

Recommendations: Patients stabilized on insulin should be monitored for possible increases in blood glucose levels with sympathomimetic administration. Since the parenteral administration of sympathomimetics usually occurs in emergency clinical situations, the elevation of blood glucose may not be of clinical importance. There is no evidence, however, that supports an interaction between epinephrine and exogenously administered insulin.

References

1. Robertson, R.P., and Porte, D.: Adrenergic modulation of basal insulin secretions in man, Diabetes **22:**1; 1973.
2. Leblanc, H., and others: The effect of dopamine infusion on insulin and glucagon secretion in man, J. Clin. Endocrinol. Metab. **44:**196, 1977.
3. Wood, S.M., and others: Effect of dobutamine on insulin requirements in diabetic ketoacidosis, Br. Med. J. **282:**946, 1981.
4. Passwell, J., and others: The metabolic effects of excess noradrenaline secretion from a pheochromocytoma, Am. J. Dis. Child. **131:**1011, 1977.
5. Thomas, D.J.B., and others: Salbutamol-induced diabetic ketoacidosis, Br. Med. J. **2:**438, 1977.
6. Leslie, D., and Coats, P.M.: Salbutamol induced diabetic ketoacidosis, Br. Med. J. **2:**768, 1977.
7. Goldberg, R., and others: Metabolic responses to selective beta adrenergic stimulation in man, Postgrad. Med. J. **51:**53, 1975.
8. Mayer, S.E.: Neurohumoral transmission and the autonomic nervous system. In Gilman, A.G., Goodman, L.S., and Gilman, A., editors: The pharmacological basis of therapeutics, New York, 1980, Macmillan Publishing.
9. Rizza, R.A., and others: Effect of alpha adrenergic stimulation and its blockade on glucose turnover in man, Am. J. Physiol. **238:**E467, 1980.
10. Muller-Hess, R., and others: Interactions of insulin and epinephrine in human metabolism: their influence on carbohydrate and lipid oxidation rate, Diabetes Metab. **1:**151, 1975.
11. Shamoon, H., and others: Altered responsiveness to cortisol, epinephrine, and glucagon in insulin-infused juvenile-onset diabetes, Diabetes **29:**284, 1980.
12. Sacca, L., and others: Insulin antagonistic effects of epinephrine and glucagon in the dog, Am. J. Physiol. **239:**E487, 1979.

Insulin–Fenfluramine

Summary: The intrinsic hypoglycemic effect of fenfluramine may increase the effects of insulin and result in hypoglycemia when used concurrently. In 1 study, this effect was assessed in maturity-onset and insulin-requiring diabetics. When administered before a meal, fenfluramine consistently lowered blood glucose levels in maturity-onset diabetics for at least 2 hours. A similar but less marked action was seen in insulin-requiring diabetics.[1] In a study involving 6 overweight nondiabetic subjects without dietary restrictions and another 6 subjects on a low-calorie diet, the addition of fenfluramine brought about an improvement in glucose tolerance and a decrease in insulin secretion.[2]

Related Drugs: There is lack of documentation regarding an interaction between insulin and the other anorexic agents (e.g., phentermine, benzphetamine, mazindol [see Appendix]). However, because the other anorexic agents lower glucose levels by increasing glucose uptake into skeletal muscle as does fenfluramine, a similar interaction may be expected to occur. In diabetics maintained on diet alone or diet plus tolbutamide, fenfluramine lowered blood glucose levels without any direct effect on insulin secretion.[1] Although this effect is undocumented, a similar interaction may be expected with the other sulfonylureas (e.g., acetohexamide, chlorpropamide, glyburide [see Appendix]) because of pharmacologic similarity.

Mechanism: Fenfluramine lowers blood sugar levels as a result of the increased uptake of glucose into skeletal muscle.[2,3] This hypoglycemic effect is additive in combination with insulin.

Recommendations: This interaction may be beneficial in certain diabetic patients, and this effect is most marked when fenfluramine is administered immediately before a meal.[1] However, patients must be closely monitored when fenfluramine is added to or withdrawn from diabetic therapy.

References

1. Turtle, J.R., and Burgess, J.A.: Hypoglycemic effect of fenfluramine in diabetes mellitus, Diabetes **22:**858, 1973.
2. Dykes, J.R.W.: The effect of a low-calorie diet with and without fenfluramine, and fenfluramine alone on the glucose tolerance and insulin secretion of overweight non-diabetics, Postgrad. Med. J. **49:**314, 1973.
3. Kirby, M.J. and Turner, P.: Effect of amphetamine, fenfluramine and norfenfluramine on glucose uptake into human isolated skeletal muscle, Br. J. Clin. Pharmacol. **1:**340, 1974.

Insulin–Guanethidine

2

Summary: Long-term guanethidine therapy may improve glucose tolerance in diabetic patients necessitating a reduction in insulin dose.[1-3] Guanethidine also improves glucose tolerance in thyrotoxicosis patients[4] and in normal subjects.[5]

Related Drugs: There is no documentation regarding an interaction between insulin and the other drugs pharmacologically related to guanethidine (bethanidine,* debrisoquin,* and guanadrel) although a similar interaction may be expected to occur. Also, no documentation exists regarding a similar interaction between guanethidine and the sulfonylurea hypoglycemics (e.g., acetohexamide, chlorpropamide, tolbutamide [see Appendix]).

Mechanism: The exact mechanism is unknown. The antihypertensive effect of guanethidine is primarily the result of its ability to block the release of norepinephrine from the sympathetic nerve endings. This blockade is apparently dependent on its active transport into the nerve terminal. Long-term guanethidine also depletes tissue catecholamines involved with raising blood sugar levels, and therefore guanethidine decreases blood glucose levels and improves glucose tolerance.[1-5] It has been postulated that guanethidine may exert its hypoglycemic response by increasing the sensitivity of tissues to endogenous insulin.[5]

Recommendations: Diabetic patients should be closely observed when guanethidine is added to or deleted from the drug regimen. A decrease in insulin dose may be required when guanethidine is added, or an increase in insulin dose may be necessitated when guanethidine is withdrawn.[3]

References

1. Gupta, K.K., and Lillicrap, C.A.: Guanethidine and diabetes, Br. Med. J. **2:**697, 1968.
2. Gupta, K.K.: Guanethidine and glucose tolerance in diabetics, Br. Med. J. **3:**679, 1968.
3. Gupta, K.K.: The antidiabetic action of guanethidine, Postgrad. Med. J. **45:**455, 1969.
4. Woeber, K.A., and others: Reversal by guanethidine of abnormal glucose tolerance in thyrotoxicosis, Lancet **1:**895, 1966.
5. Kansal, P.C., and others: Effect of guanethidine and reserpine on glucose tolerance, Curr. Ther. Res. **13:**517, 1971.

*Not available in the U.S.

Insulin–Isoniazid

3

Summary: Isoniazid (250 to 400 mg/day) antagonizes the hypoglycemic action of insulin by elevating blood sugar levels.[1,2] Although administration of isoniazid to diabetic patients has resulted in increased insulin requirements,[3,4] blood glucose levels have not been found to be affected by the commonly used tuberculostatic agents at usual therapeutic dosage ranges.[5]

Related Drugs: Tolbutamide has been found to have no interaction with isoniazid in some studies[4,6] and reportedly resulted in hypoglycemia in another.[7] Because of conflicting results, it is difficult to determine whether an interaction occurs between isoniazid and the other sulfonylurea hypoglycemics (e.g., acetohexamide, chlorpropamide, glyburide [see Appendix]). There are no drugs related to isoniazid.

Mechanism: Insulin and many polypeptides reportedly greatly enhance the membrane transport of isoniazid,[8] normally considered to cross cell membranes by passive diffusion. Thus the intestinal uptake of isoniazid is enhanced by insulin.[8] By causing disturbances in carbohydrate metabolism,[3] isoniazid may increase blood glucose levels[1,2] and impair glucose tolerance, although potentiations of the hypoglycemic effect has also been noted.[7] In contrast to rifampin, isoniazid is not reported to be an enzyme-inducing agent.[6]

Recommendations: Patients on concurrent therapy with antidiabetic agents and isoniazid should be monitored for possible increases in blood glucose levels. This may be of greater clinical significance in patients with hepatic dysfunction or those who are slow acetylators of isoniazid.

References

1. Brown, C.V.: Acute isoniazid poisoning, Am. Rev. Resp. Dis. **105:**206, 1972.
2. Terman, D.S., and Teitelbaum, D.T.: Isoniazid self-poisoning, Neurology **20:**299, 1970.
3. Luntz, G.R., and Smith, S.G.: Effect of isoniazid on carbohydrate metabolism in controls and diabetics, Br. Med. J. **1:**296, 1953.
4. Dickson, I.: Glycosuria and diabetes mellitus following I.N.A.H. therapy, Med. J. Aust. **49:**325, 1962.
5. Syvalahti, E., and others: Effect of tuberculostatic agents on the response of serum growth hormone and immunoreactive insulin to intravenous tolbutamide and on the half-life of tolbutamide, Int. J. Clin. Pharmacol. **13:**83, 1976.
6. Danysz, A., and Wisniewski, K.: Control of drug transport through cell membranes, Mater. Med. Pol. **2:**35, 1970.
7. Segarra, F.O., and others: Experiences with tolbutamide and chlorpropamide in tuberculous diabetic patients, Ann. N.Y. Acad. Sci. **74:**656, 1959.
8. Conney, A.H.: Pharmacological implications of microsomal enzyme induction, Pharmacol. Rev. **19:**317, 1967.

Insulin–Oxytetracycline

2

Summary: Several cases have been reported in which the administration of oxytetracycline to diabetic patients receiving insulin caused hypoglycemia, necessitating a decrease in insulin dosage or an increase in carbohydrate intake.[1,2]

Related Drugs: Hypoglycemia has been reported when oxytetracycline and tolbutamide were used concurrently.[3] Because of pharmacologic similarity the other sulfonylurea hypoglycemics (e.g., acetohexamide, chlorpropamide, glyburide [see Appendix]) may also interact with oxytetracycline; however, documentation of this effect is lacking. There is no information regarding other tetracyclines (e.g., doxycycline, minocycline, tetracycline [see Appendix]) causing a similar drug interaction; however, this possibility may exist based on similar pharmacologic activity.

Mechanism: It is hypothesized that oxytetracycline exerts this hypoglycemic effect by increasing the half-life of insulin or by interfering with the action of epinephrine.[3]

Recommendations: Patients whose diabetes is controlled on insulin therapy who receive oxytetracycline should be monitored closely because of the possibility of hypoglycemia.

References

1. Miller, J.B.: Hypoglycaemic effect of oxytetracycline, Br. Med. J. **2:**1007, 1966.
2. Sen, S., and Murkerjee, A.B.: Hypoglycaemic action of oxytetracycline. A preliminary study, J. Indian. Med. Assoc. **52:**366, 1969.
3. Hiatt, N., and Bonoriss, G.: Insulin response in pancreatectomized dogs treated with oxytetracycline, Diabetes **19:**307, 1970.

Insulin–Phenelzine

Summary: Phenelzine can potentiate the action of insulin, resulting in an enhanced hypoglycemic state. Monoamine oxidase (MAO) inhibitors have an effect on carbohydrate metabolism,[1-3] and subsequent enhancement of the hypoglycemic action of insulin is documented in animal[3-10] and human studies.[1,2,11-13]

Related Drugs: Tranylcypromine[6] has produced a rapid and significant stimulation of insulin secretion in animals; pargyline[6] did not produce similar effects in this study, although it was shown to enhance hypoglycemic activity of insulin in other animal studies.[7,8] In another report long-term administration of tranylcypromine potentiated insulin- and tolbutamide-induced hypoglycemia in animal studies.[4] Furazolidone and procarbazine, which possess monoamine oxidase inhibitor activity, may interact similarly with insulin.

There are no reports regarding a similar interaction with other sulfonylurea hypoglycemics (e.g., acetohexamide, chlorpropamide, glyburide [see Appendix]), although an interaction may be expected to occur based on pharmacologic similarity.

Mechanism: The exact mechanism by which MAO inhibitors affect carbohydrate metabolism is not clear; however, a diminution in the epinephrine response following insulin-induced hypoglycemia has been proposed.[4,14] In vitro studies have shown that MAO inhibitors are capable of both potentiating and inhibiting insulin release, depending on their concentrations.[3,9,10] Stimulation of glucose-mediated insulin secretion is believed to be related to the MAO inhibitory effects of the drugs.

Recommendations: Concurrent MAO inhibitor therapy for depression in a diabetic patient will often require reduction in dosage of the hypoglycemic agent because of enhanced hypoglycemic effects. Since the extent of the reaction is highly unpredictable, any diabetic patients receiving MAO inhibitors should be monitored for possible excessive hypoglycemia.

References

1. VanPraag, H.M., and Leijnsef, B.: The influence of some antidepressives of the hydrazine type on the glucose metabolism in depressed patients, Clin. Chim. Acta **8:**466, 1963.
2. Weiss, J., and others: Effects of iproniazid and similar compounds on the gastrointestinal tract, Ann. N.Y. Acad. Sci. **80:**854, 1959.
3. Aleyassine, H., and Gardiner, R.J.: Dual action of antidepressant drugs (MAO inhibitors) on insulin release, Endocrinology **96:**702, 1975.
4. Cooper, A.J., and Ashcroft, G.: Potentiation of insulin hypoglycaemia by M.A.O.I. antidepressant drugs, Lancet **1:**407, 1966.
5. Barrett, A.M.: Modification of the hypoglycaemic response to tolbutamide and insulin by mebanazine. An inhibitor of monoamine oxidase, J. Pharm. Pharmacol. **17:**19, 1965.
6. Adnitt, P.I.: Hypoglycemic action of monoamine oxidase inhibitors (MAOI's) and mebanazine, Diabetes **17:**628, 1968.
7. Frohman, L.A.: Stimulation of insulin secretion in rats by pargyline and mebanazine, Diabetes **20:**266, 1971.

8. Potter, W.Z., and others: Possible role of hydrazine group in hypoglycemia associated with the use of certain monoamine oxidase inhibitors (MAOI's), Diabetes **18:**538, 1969.

9. Aleyassine, H., and Lee, S.H.: Inhibition of insulin release by substrates and inhibitors of monoamine oxidase, Am. J. Physiol. **222:**565, 1972.

10. Aleyassine, H., and Lee, S.H.: Inhibition by hydrazine, phenelzine and pargyline of insulin release from rat pancreas, Endocrinology **89:**125, 1971.

11. Cooper, A.J., and Keddie, K.M.: Hypotensive collapse and hypoglycaemia after mebanazine, a monoamine oxidase inhibitor, Lancet **1:**1133, 1964.

12. Patrignani, A., and Miele, V.: The influence of MAOI on the glycemic balance: the potentiation of insulin hypoglycemia by beta-phenylethylhydrazine (Nardil), G. Psychiat. Neuropat. **96:**29, 1968.

13. Adnitt, P.I., and others: The hypoglycaemic action of monoamine oxidase inhibitors (MAOI's), Diabetologia **4:**379, 1968.

14. Cooper, A.J., and Ashcroft, G.: Modification of insulin and sulfonylurea hypoglycemia by monoamine oxidase inhibitor drugs, Diabetes **16:**272, 1967.

Insulin–Phenytoin

3

Summary: Phenytoin alone may inhibit endogenous insulin secretion, resulting in clinically significant symptoms of hyperglycemia (e.g., ataxia, coma, drowsiness, lethargy, hypotension, polydipsia, and polyuria), as evidenced by several reports using oral and parenteral phenytoin.[1-11] There is no evidence that phenytoin antagonizes exogenously administered insulin; however, based on the mechanism and 1 case report,[2] an interaction may theoretically occur. In this report, a patient developed hyperglycemia 3 hours after phenytoin administration, and subsequent insulin did not lower serum glucose levels to normal.[2] However, the lack of response to insulin may have resulted from concomitant renal failure, since the hyperglycemic response of phenytoin may be more pronounced in patients with renal failure or uremia.[2,3]

Related Drugs: Mephenytoin has been shown through in vitro studies to be equivalent to phenytoin in inhibition of insulin secretion.[12] Although it is not documented, the other hydantoin anticonvulsant (ethotoin) may be expected to produce the same hyperglycemic effect as phenytoin because of pharmacologic similarity.

Since oral sulfonylurea hypoglycemic agents (e.g., chlorpropamide, glyburide, tolbutamide [see Appendix]) act by stimulation of the pancreatic beta cells to release insulin, their action may theoretically be affected by phenytoin as well. It has also been shown that tolbutamide,[13] acetohexamide, chlorpropamide, and tolazamide[14] may displace phenytoin from plasma protein binding sites, leading to high phenytoin plasma levels; however, the significance of this effect is not known. It is unknown if glyburide or glipizide will displace phenytoin from binding sites.

Mechanism: Phenytoin can induce hyperglycemia in humans[1-11] and animals[15-18] through inhibition of endogenous insulin secretion, possibly by decreasing intracellular sodium via stimulation of the sodium-potassium ATPase pump in the islet cell membrane.[12,19,20]

Recommendations: Diabetic patients receiving phenytoin should be closely monitored for elevation of serum glucose levels and symptoms of hyperglycemia. Dosage reduction of phenytoin may prevent or alleviate the symptoms, since some adverse reactions have occurred at high phenytoin dosages.[3,11] Also, adjusting the sulfonylurea dose whenever phenytoin is added to or withdrawn from therapy may be advisable.

References

1. Goldberg, E.M., and Sanbar, S.S.: Hyperglycemic hyperosmolar coma following administration of Dilantin (diphenylhydantoin), Diabetes **20**:177, 1971.
2. Goldberg, E.M., and Sanbar, S.S.: Hyperglycemic, nonketotic coma following administration of Dilantin (diphenylhydantoin), Diabetes **18**:101, 1969.
3. Klein, J.P.: Diphenylhydantoin intoxication associated with hyperglycemia, J. Pediatr. **69**:463, 1966.
4. Dahl, J.R.: Diphenylhydantoin toxic psychosis with associated hyperglycemia, Calif. Med. **107**:345, 1967.

5. Said, D.M., and others: Hyperglycemia associated with diphenylhydantoin (Dilantin) intoxication, Med. Ann. D. C. **37:**170, 1968.

6. Peters, B.H., and Samaan, N.A.: Hyperglycemia with relative hypoinsulinemia in diphenylhydantoin toxicity, N. Engl. J. Med. **281:**91, 1969.

7. Fariss, B.L., and Lutcher, C.L.: Diphenylhydantoin-induced hyperglycemia and impaired insulin release. Effect of dosage, Diabetes **20:**177, 1971.

8. Gerich, J.E., and others: Clinical and metabolic characteristics of hyperosmolar nonketotic coma, Diabetes **20:**228, 1971.

9. Treasure, T., and Toseland, P.A.: Hyperglycaemia due to phenytoin toxicity, Arch. Dis. Child. **46:**563, 1971.

10. Hofeldt, F.D., and others: Effects of diphenylhydantoin upon glucose-induced insulin secretion in three patients with insulinoma, Diabetes **83:**192, 1974.

11. Stambough, J.E., and others: Effect of diphenylhydantoin on glucose tolerance in patients with hypoglycemia, Diabetes **23:**679, 1974.

12. Kizer, J.S., and others: The in vitro inhibition of insulin secretion by diphenylhydantoin, J. Clin. Invest. **49:**1942, 1970.

13. Wesseling, H., and Mols-Thurkow, I.: Interaction of diphenylhydantoin (DPH) and tolbutamide in man, Eur. J. Clin. Pharmacol. **8:**75, 1975.

14. Wesseling, H., and others: Effect of sylphonylureas (tolazamide, tolbutamide and chlorpropamide) on the metabolism of diphenylhydantoin in the rat, Biochem. Pharmacol. **22:**3033, 1973.

15. Levin, S.R., and others: Inhibition of insulin secretion by diphenylhydantoin in the isolated perfused pancreas, J. Clin. Endocrinol. Metab. **30:**400, 1970.

16. Belton, N.R., and others: Effects of convulsions and anticonvulsants on blood sugar in rabbits, Epilepsia **6:**243, 1965.

17. Sanbar, S., and others: Diabetogenic effect of Dilantin (diphenylhydantoin), Diabetes **16:**533, 1967.

19. Malherbe, C., and others: Effect of diphenylhydantoin on insulin secretion in man, N. Engl. J. Med. **286:**339, 1972.

20. Pace, C.S., and Livingston, E.: Ionic basis of phenytoin sodium inhibition of insulin secretion in pancreatic islets, Diabetes **28:**1077, 1979.

Insulin—Propranolol

Summary: Propranolol can delay recovery from hypoglycemia (blood glucose rebound) in diabetics as well as in normal subjects. Propranolol also modifies the normal cardiovascular response to insulin-induced hypoglycemia, thereby possibly decreasing patient awareness of the hypoglycemic condition. This combination of effects is of considerable significance for diabetic patients, particularly those inclined toward hypoglycemic attacks. Also, patients taking propranolol may have clinically important hypertensive responses to hypoglycemia.

Related Drugs: According to most reports, neither atenolol[1-3] nor metoprolol[1,4-6] produces the prolonging effect on insulin-induced hypoglycemia. In the only conflicting study, metoprolol potentiated the initial hypoglycemic effect of insulin in normal individuals; however, metoprolol significantly delayed the return to normoglycemia.[7] There is no documentation regarding an interaction between insulin and the other noncardioselective beta-blockers (nadolol, pindolol, and timolol); however, they may be expected to interact similarly to propranolol. Effects of beta-adrenergic blockers on long-term sulfonylurea therapy have not been determined, although hyperglycemia has been reported in a patient on chlorpropamide and propranolol.[8] One study involving hypertensive diabetics and nondiabetics indicated that tolbutamide-stimulated insulin secretion is unaffected by beta-blocking agents (metoprolol or propranolol).[9] In a study involving 8 diabetics, the concurrent use of glyburide and propranolol or acebutolol* (a noncardioselective beta-blocking agent) resulted in an increased blood glucose area-under-curve when compared to the use of glyburide alone. The difference between the propranolol and acebutolol groups was not significant.[10] Because of conflicting reports, it is difficult to determine whether an interaction would occur with the other sulfonylurea hypoglycemics (acetohexamide, glipizide, and tolazamide).

Mechanism: The mechanism is complicated and unclear. Beta-adrenergic blocking agents are known to considerably modify carbohydrate metabolism.[11] D, L-Propranolol exerts a blocking effect on insulin release through blockage of beta-adrenergic receptors at the level of the pancreatic beta cell.[12] D-Propranolol also inhibits insulin release, probably by a mechanism of membrane stabilization.[3,9] Alteration of peripheral insulin receptor affinity has also been suggested.[13] Propranolol does not affect plasma glucose or insulin concentrations in normal individuals or the rate or magnitude of the fall of plasma glucose after insulin, but it does slow the subsequent recovery of glucose concentration and prevents the usual rebound of plasma glycerol.[1,3,9,14,15]

Recommendations: When use of a beta-blocking agent is indicated in a diabetic patient, particularly one prone to hypoglycemic attacks, one of the cardioselective agents rather than propranolol should be used, both to decrease the risk of hyper-

*Not available in the U.S.

tensive attacks and to permit more rapid recovery from low blood glucose levels. The danger of unrecognized hypoglycemia in the insulin-dependent diabetic taking propranolol can be reduced if the patient is aware of the associated diaphoretic response.

References

1. Anon: Beta blockers for diabetics, Lancet **1:**843, 1977.
2. Deacon, S.P., and others: Acebutol, atenolol and propranolol and metabolic responses to acute hypoglycaemia in diabetics, Br. Med. J. **2:**1255, 1977.
3. Deacon, S.P., and Barnett, D.: Comparison of atenolol and propranolol during insulin-induced hypoglycaemia, Br. Med. J. **2:**272, 1976.
4. Linton, S.P., and others: Blood sugar and beta blockers, Br. Med. J. **2:**877, 1976.
5. Waal-Manning, H.J.: Metabolic effects of β-adrenoreceptor blockers, Drugs **2**(suppl. 1):121, 1976.
6. Leslie, R.D., and others: Sensitivity to enkephalin as a cause of non-insulin dependent diabetes, Lancet **1:**341, 1979.
7. Newman, R.J.: Comparison of propranolol, metoprolol, and acebutolol on insulin-induced hypoglycaemia, Br. Med. J. **2:**447, 1976.
8. Holt, R.J., and Gaskins, J.D.: Hyperglycemia associated with propranolol and chlorpropamide coadministration, Drug Intell. Clin. Pharm. **15:**599, 1981.
9. Potterman, K.J., and Groop, L.G.: No effect of propranolol and metoprolol on tolbutamide-stimulated insulin-secretion in hypertensive diabetic and non-diabetic patients, Ann. Clin. Res. **14:**190, 1982.
10. Zaman, R., and others: The effect of acebutolol and propranolol on the hypoglycemic action of glibenclamide, Br. J. Clin. Pharmacol. **13:**507, 1982.
11. Weiner, N.: Drugs that inhibit adrenergic nerves and block adrenergic receptors. In Gilman, A.G., Goodman, L.S., and Gilman, A., editors: The pharmacological basis of therapeutics, New York, 1980, Macmillan Publishing.
12. Cerasi, E., and others: Effect of adrenergic blocking agents on insulin response to glucose infusion in man, Acta Endocrinol. **69:**335, 1972.
13. Blum, I., and others: Suppression of hypoglycemia by DL-propranolol in malignant insulinoma, N. Engl. J. Med. **299:**487, 1978.
14. Abramson, E.A., and others: Effects of propranolol on the hormonal and metabolic responses to insulin-induced hypoglycaemia, Lancet **2:**1386, 1966.
15. Davidson, N., and others: Observations in man of hypoglycaemia during selective and non-selective beta-blockade, Scott. Med. J. **22:**69, 1977.

Insulin–Thyroid

Summary: Although clinical data are lacking, the initiation of thyroid replacement therapy may cause an increase in insulin or oral hypoglycemic requirements.[1] Insulin administration may also affect thyroid hormone binding and may disrupt thyroid function.[2]

Related Drugs: There have been no published reports of an interaction between hypoglycemic therapy and thyroid replacement therapy in human patients. The effects of insulin administration on serum thyroid hormone have been examined in healthy subjects.[2] The interactions of liothyronine (T_3), thyroxine (T_4), and insulin have been investigated in several animal models.[3-6] Based on the available evidence and mechanism, it would seem that any thyroid hormone (e.g., levothyroxine, liotrix, thyroglobulin, etc. [see Appendix]) can interact with any hypoglycemic therapy, including insulin and the oral sulfonylurea hypoglycemics (e.g., acetohexamide, chlorpropamide, glyburide [see Appendix]).

Mechanism: Although the reasons for this effect are poorly understood, animal studies have established that levothyroxine increases the rate of carbohydrate absorption from the gastrointestinal tract and both liothyronine and thyroxine suppress insulin secretion from the pancreas.[3-7] Insulin administration in humans increases serum thyroxine levels and may increase its metabolic rate.[2]

Recommendations: The management of patients on this combination requires attention to both diabetic control and thyroid function, especially at initiation of therapy.

References

1. Refetoff, S.: Thyroid hormone therapy, Med. Clin. North Am. **59**:1147, 1975.
2. Blum, C., and others: Effect of insulin administration on plasma thyroxine in euthyroid subjects, Isr. Med. Sci. **8**:767, 1972.
3. Lenzen, S.: Proceedings: studies on the inhibitory effect of thyroxine on insulin secretion from the perfused rat pancreas, Naunyn-Schmiedeberg's Arch. Pharmacol. **287**(suppl.):R58, 1975.
4. Lenzen, S., and others: Thyroxine treatment and insulin secretion in the rat, Diabetologia **11**:49, 1975.
5. Lenzen, S., and Hasselblatt, A.: The effect of thyroxine treatment on the dynamics of insulin release from the isolated perfused rat pancreas, Naunyn-Schmiedeberg's Arch. Pharmacol. **282**:317, 1974.
6. Mueller, M.K., and others: Interaction of gastric inhibitory polypeptide and arginine with glucose in the perfused pancreas of rats treated with triiodothyronine, Can. J. Physiol. Pharmacol. **60**:297, 1982.
7. Shah, J.H.: Hypoinsulinemia of hypothyroidism, Arch. Intern. Med. **132**:657, 1973.

Tolbutamide–Chloramphenicol

2

Summary: There are published reports of prolonged hypoglycemic response after chloramphenicol administration in diabetic patients on tolbutamide therapy because of an increased tolbutamide half-life.[1,2] Reactions have varied from mild[3] symptoms to collapse.[1] Patients with renal insufficiency may be at greater risk for this interaction.

Related Drugs: Chlorpropamide half-life has also been considerably increased by administration of chloramphenicol.[4,5] No studies have been reported with tolazamide or acetohexamide; however, their half-lives may be expected to be similarly affected. Based on the proposed mechanism, glyburide and glipizide may also interact with chloramphenicol since they are excreted by both renal and biliary routes. There are no drugs related to chloramphenicol.

Mechanism: Interference with renal elimination has been proposed as a mechanism for the increased half-life and elevated serum levels of the sulfonylurea.[5,6] Potentiation of tolbutamide through microsomal enzyme inhibition by chloramphenicol is also considered to be a factor.[6]

Recommendations: Reduction in the sulfonylurea dose may be necessary if concurrent chloramphenicol administration is indicated. Frequent monitoring of serum glucose levels may enable control during this time. Temporary use of insulin may be required if serum glucose levels cannot be controlled with the oral agent. Since some studies have shown higher serum tolbutamide levels in morning measurements compared to those later in the day, patients can be monitored for symptoms and cautioned accordingly.[3]

References

1. Skovsted, L., and others: Inhibition of drug metabolism in man. In Morselli, P.L. and others, editors: Drug interactions. New York, 1974, Raven Press.
2. Soelder, J.S., and Steinke, J.: Hypoglycemia in tolbutamide-treated diabetics, J.A.M.A. **193:**398, 1965.
3. Brunova, E., and others: Interaction of tolbutamide and chloramphenicol in diabetic patients, Int. J. Clin. Pharmacol. **15:**7, 1977.
4. Petitpierre, B., and others: Behavior of chlorpropamide in renal insufficiency and under the effect of associated drug therapy, Int. J. Clin. Pharmacol. Ther. Toxicol. **6:**120, 1972.
5. Petitpierre, B., and Fabre, J.: Chlorpropamide and chloramphenicol, Lancet **1:**789, 1970.
6. Christensen, L.K., and Skovsted, L.: Inhibition of drug metabolism by chloramphenicol, Lancet **2:**1397, 1969.

Tolbutamide–Diazoxide

Summary: Hyperglycemia has occurred in patients receiving short-term intravenous diazoxide for treatment of severe hypertension, or after long-term oral administration in the treatment of hypoglycemia.[1-5] However, there are no clinical reports indicating that diazoxide interferes with the hypoglycemic effectiveness of tolbutamide therapy in diabetes. One report suggests that it enhances tolbutamide-induced insulin release when administered before the sulfonylurea.[6] However, until more clinical data are available, increased blood glucose levels in diabetic patients receiving diazoxide may be viewed as being caused by this agent.

Related Drugs: Although no documentation exists, the other sulfonylurea hypoglycemics (e.g., acetohexamide, chlorpropamide, glyburide [see Appendix]) may interact similarly with diazoxide based on pharmacologic similarity. There are no drugs related to diazoxide.

Mechanism: Diazoxide, related structurally to tolbutamide, has been shown to inhibit the release of insulin in vitro by a direct effect on the pancreatic beta cells.[7,8] Although this accounts for at least part of its hyperglycemic effect, the underlying cellular mechanism including an effect on cell-membrane calcium flux has not been elucidated.

Recommendations: Diabetic patients receiving diazoxide should be monitored for an increase in blood glucose levels. Should hyperglycemia occur, an appropriate adjustment in dosage of one or both drugs is necessary. Treatment with insulin should be considered in patients with severe hyperglycemia resulting from diazoxide administration.

References

1. Graber, A.L., and others: Clinical use of diazoxide and mechanism for its hyperglycemic effects, Diabetes **15:**143, 1966.
2. Fajans, S.S., and others: Further studies on diazoxide suppression of insulin release from abnormal and normal islet tissue in man, Ann. N.Y. Acad. Sci. **150:**261, 1968.
3. Porte, D. Jr.: Inhibition of insulin release by diazoxide and its relation to catecholamine effects in man, Ann. N.Y. Acad. Sci. **150:**281, 1968.
4. Field, J.B., and others: Clinical and physiological studies using diazoxide in the treatment of hypoglycemia, Ann. N.Y. Acad. Sci. **150:**415, 1968.
5. Seltzer, H.S., and Allen, E.W.: Hyperglycemia and inhibition of insulin secretions during administration of diazoxide and trichlormethiazide in man, Diabetes **18:**19, 1969.
6. Greenwood, R.H., and others: Improvement in insulin secretion in diabetes after diazoxide, Lancet **1:**444, 1976.
7. Frerichs, H., and others: Insulin secretion in vitro. II. Inhibition of glucose-induced insulin release by diazoxide [German with an English summary], Diabetologia **2:**269, 1966.
8. Howell, S.L., and Taylor, K.W.: Effects of diazoxide on insulin secretion in vitro, Lancet **1:**128, 1966.

Tolbutamide–Dicumarol

2

Summary: Dicumarol may significantly increase the serum half-life of tolbutamide.[1-3] The effect usually begins within 4 days after initiation of dicumarol therapy and may result in acute hypoglycemic episodes.[1,2] Sulfonylurea hypoglycemics do not appear to have a significant overall effect on the pharmacokinetics or hypoprothrombinemic activity of coumarin anticoagulants.[4,5] One study describes a prolonged prothrombin time in 2 patients on concurrent dicumarol and tolbutamide; however, no effect was noted in 3 other patients.[6]

Related Drugs: The serum half-life of chlorpropamide is also increased by concurrent dicumarol administration.[7] Although there is a lack of documentation, dicumarol may similarly interact with the other sulfonylurea hypoglycemics (e.g., acetohexamide, glyburide, tolazamide [see Appendix]) based on pharmacologic similarity.

The other coumarin anticoagulants (warfarin and phenprocoumon) and the indandione derivatives (anisindione and phenindione) apparently do not interact with tolbutamide.[4,8-10] Warfarin had a minimal effect on glyburide binding to human serum albumin in vitro.[11] In 1 study, glyburide had no significant effect on the pharmacokinetics or efficacy of phenprocoumon.[12]

Mechanism: On the basis of indirect evidence it has been suggested that dicumarol inhibits the hepatic metabolism of tolbutamide[1,2] and chlorpropamide.[7] In addition, there is in vitro evidence that dicumarol displaces the sulfonylureas from their plasma protein binding sites.[13]

Recommendations: If dicumarol and a sulfonylurea must be given concurrently, serum glucose concentrations should be closely monitored and the sulfonylurea dose adjusted accordingly when dicumarol is added to or withdrawn from the drug regimen. Also, it is prudent to closely monitor prothrombin times since the dose of dicumarol may need to be adjusted.

References

1. Kristensen, M., and Hansen, J.M.: Potentiation of the tolbutamide effect by dicumarol, Diabetes **16:**211, 1967.
2. Solomon, H.M., and Schrogie, J.J.: Effect of phenyramidol and bishydroxycoumarin on the metabolism of tolbutamide in human subjects, Metabolism **16:**1029, 1967.
3. Skovsted, L., and others: The effect of different oral anticoagulants on diphenylhydantoin (DPH) and tolbutamide metabolism, Acta Med. Scand. **199:**513, 1976.
4. Poucher, R.L., and Vecchio, T.J.: Absence of tolbutamide effect on anticoagulant therapy, J.A.M.A. **197:**1069, 1966.
5. Jahnchen, E., and others: Pharmacokinetic analysis of the interaction between dicumarol and tolbutamide in man, Eur. J. Clin. Pharmacol. **10:**349, 1976.
6. Chaplin, H., and Cassell, M.: Studies on the possible relationship of tolbutamide to dicumarol in anticoagulant therapy, Am. J. Med. Sci. **235:**706, 1958.
7. Kristensen, M., and Hansen, J.M.: Accumulation of chlorpropamide caused by dicoumarol, Acta Med. Scand. **183:**83, 1968.
8. Petitpierre, B., and others: Behavior of chlorpropamide in renal insufficiency and under the effect of associated drug therapy, Int. J. Clin. Pharmacol. Toxicol. **6:**120, 1972.

9. Kolenda, K.D., and others: Drug interaction during therapy with tolbutamide, Med. Clin. **74:**1914, 1979.

10. Heine, P., and others: The influence of hypoglycaemic sulphonylureas on elimination and efficacy of phenprocoumon following a single dose in diabetic patients, Eur. J. Clin. Pharmacol. **10:**31, 1976.

11. Brown, K.F., and Crooks, M.J.: Displacement of tolbutamide, glibenclamide and chlorpropamide from serum albumin by anionic drugs, Biochem. Pharmacol. **25:**1175, 1976.

12. Heine, P., and others: The influence of hypoglycemic sulfonylureas on elimination and efficacy of phenprocoumon following a single oral dose in diabetic patients, Eur. J. Clin. Pharmacol. **10:**31, 1976.

13. Judis, J.: Displacement of sulfonylureas from human serum proteins by coumarin derivatives and cortical steroids, J. Pharm. Sci. **62:**232, 1973.

Tolbutamide–Phenylbutazone

1

Summary: Documentation exists concerning several cases of severe hypoglycemic reactions after phenylbutazone administration to patients on long-term tolbutamide therapy.[1-11] This has occurred with the use of the drugs within usual recommended dosage ranges, and enhanced hypoglycemic response can be expected whenever these drugs are given concurrently. In a study involving 9 patients, not only did the tolbutamide half-life increase but the half-life of phenylbutazone was reduced significantly when these agents were used concurrently. It was suggested that the therapeutic effect of phenylbutazone is reduced.[12]

Related Drugs: Two cases have been reported of hypoglycemic collapse after phenylbutazone administration in chlorpropamide-treated patients.[8] In a case study involving a single patient, phenylbutazone potentiated the hypoglycemic action of acetohexamide.[13] Phenylbutazone has been shown to slow the excretion of hydroxyhexamide, an active metabolite of acetohexamide.[5,14-16] Tolbutamide half-life has been increased in chronic administration of oxyphenbutazone[7,17] in normal subjects. In animal studies the rate of elimination of a constant dose of tolazamide[18] was reduced by various intravenous doses of oxyphenbutazone. Sulfinpyrazone reduced tolbutamide clearance by 40%.[19] In 1 study, phenylbutazone had no significant effect on glyburide plasma levels, rate of elimination, or metabolism after the administration of ^{14}C-labeled intravenous glyburide; however, significantly less glyburide metabolite was renally excreted.[20] Phenylbutazone also had a minimal effect on glyburide binding in vitro.[21] Glipizide may interact with phenylbutazone in a manner similar to glyburide since they both are bound to albumin by nonionic forces and exhibit a similar metabolic fate. In a study involving 40 diabetics receiving tolmetin and glyburide, blood and urine glucose concentrations were not significantly different as compared to glyburide and placebo.[22]

In a study of 12 tolbutamide-treated maturity-onset diabetics with stable glycemic control, sulindac[20] did not significantly affect tolbutamide serum concentration or blood sugar. A study of 10 maturity-onset diabetics showed no effects of naproxen[21] on glucose metabolism or tolbutamide pharmacokinetics. There is no documentation regarding an interaction between tolbutamide and the other nonsteroidal anti-inflammatory agents (e.g., indomethacin, mefenamic acid, piroxicam [see Appendix]); however, they may be expected to interact in a manner similar to sulindac and naproxen.

Mechanism: Tolbutamide is significantly bound to plasma proteins and presumably tissue proteins. Phenylbutazone is also highly bound to plasma and tissue proteins and is capable of displacing tolbutamide, acetohexamide, and chlorpropamide from albumin in vitro.[1,5,7,9,13,18] Phenylbutazone prolongs the half-life of tolbutamide by inhibiting its oxidation,[5-7,16] and this appears to increase with repeated dosing.[8,18] The delayed inhibition of tolbutamide metabolism by phenylbutazone may be the result of the induction of a form of cytochrome P-450 that has low affinity for tolbutamide hydroxylation.[18] It has also been suggested that phenylbutazone may inhibit the excretion of tolbutamide.[11] It is not known how tolbutamide reduced the half-life of phenylbutazone.

Recommendations: Because of the possibility of a severe or even fatal hypoglycemic reaction that can result, use of this combination requires intense monitoring of serum glucose levels and probable dosage reduction of the sulfonylurea. If concurrent long-term therapy is necessary, agents other than phenylbutazone or oxyphenbutazone should be used whenever possible (e.g., sulindac).

References

1. Dent, L.A., and Jue, S.G.: Tolbutamide-phenylbutazone interaction, Drug Intell. Clin. Pharm. **10:**711, 1976.
2. Macgregor, H.G., and others: Drug interaction, Br. Med. J. **1:**389, 1971.
3. Slade, I.H., and Iosefra, R.N.: Fatal hypoglycemic coma from the use of tolbutamide in elderly patients: report of two cases, J. Am. Geriat. Soc. **15:**948, 1967.
4. Avery, G.S.: Drug interactions that really matter: a guide to major importance drug interactions, Drugs **14:**132, 1977.
5. Jodis, J.: Binding of sulfonylurea to serum protein, J. Pharm. Sci. **61:**89, 1972.
6. Christensen, L.K., and others: Sulphaphenazole-induced hypoglycaemic attacks in tolbutamide-treated diabetes, Lancet **2:**1298, 1963.
7. Rowland, M., and others: Kinetics of tolbutamide interactions. In Morselli, P.L., Garattini, S., and Cohen, S.N., editors: Drug interactions, New York, 1974, Raven Press.
8. Jackson, J.E., and Bressler, R.: Clinical pharmacology of sulphonylurea hypoglycemic agents: part 2, Drugs **22:**295, 1981.
9. Harris, E.L.: Adverse reactions to oral antidiabetic agents, Br. Med. J. **3:**29, 1971.
10. Tannenbaum, H., and others: Phenylbutazone-tolbutamide drug interaction, N. Engl. J. Med. **290:**344, 1974.
11. Ober, K.F.: Mechanism of interaction of tolbutamide and phenylbutazone in diabetic patients, Eur. J. Clin. Pharmacol. **7:**291, 1974.
12. Szita, M., and others: Interaction of phenylbutazone and tolbutamide in man, Int. J. Clin. Pharmacol. **18:**378, 1980.
13. Healey, L.A.: Phenylbutazone: drug potentiator, Med. Times **109:**52, 1981.
14. Field, J.B., and others: Potentiation of acetohexamide hypoglycemia by phenylbutazone, N. Engl. J. Med. **277:**889, 1967.
15. Shen, S-W., and Bressler, R.: Clinical pharmacology of oral antidiabetic agents, N. Engl. J. Med. **296:**493, 1977.
16. Metz, R.: Case notes, Bull. Mason Clin. **30:**38, 1976.
17. Pond, S.M., and others: Mechanisms of inhibition of tolbutamide metabolism: phenylbutazone, oxyphenbutazone, sulfaphenazole, Clin. Pharmacol. Ther. **22:**573, 1977.
18. Abidi, S.E., and Kebbe, A.H.: Pharmacokinetic interaction of tolazamide and oxyphenbutazone in dogs, J. Pharm. Sci. **71:**29, 1982.
19. Miners, J.O., and others: The effect of sulphinpyrazone on oxidative drug metabolism in man: inhibition of tolbutamide elimination, Eur. J. Clin. Pharmacol. **22:**321, 1982.
20. Schulz, E., and others: Ursachen der potenzierung der hypoglykamischen wirkung von sulfonylharnstoff-derivaten durch medikamente: II. Pharmacokokinetik und metabolismus von glibenclamid (HB419) in gegenwart von phenylbutazon, Eur. J. Clin. Pharmacol. **4:**32, 1971.
21. Brown, K.F., and Crooks, M.J.: Displacement of tolbutamide, glibenclamide and chlorpropamide from serum albumin by anionic drugs, Biochem. Pharmacol. **25:**1175, 1976.
22. Chlud, K., and Kaik, B.: Clinical studies of the interaction between tolmetin and glibenclamide, Int. J. Clin. Pharmacol. **15:**409, 1977.
23. Ryan, J.R., and others: On the question of an interaction between sulindac and tolbutamide in the control of diabetes, Clin. Pharmacol. Ther. **21:**231, 1977.
24. Whiting, B., and others: Effect of naproxen on glucose metabolism and tolbutamide kinetics and dynamics in maturity onset diabetes, Br. J. Pharmacol. **11:**295, 1981.

Tolbutamide–Sulfamethizole

2

Summary: Tolbutamide-treated patients have developed enhanced hypoglycemic effects after administration of sulfamethizole.[1] Administration of tolbutamide to patients on sulfamethizole therapy also produced prolonged tolbutamide half-life.[1,2] Although this is the most predictable combination of the interacting sulfonamides, documentation for this specific interaction is limited.

Related Drugs: There are contradictory reports regarding the effect of concomitant sulfisoxazole[3-5] or sulfadiazine[6,7] on serum glucose or serum tolbutamide levels in diabetics. Sulfadimethoxine* has been shown to displace tolbutamide from plasma protein binding sites in vitro[8,9] but did not produce hypoglycemic episodes similar to sulfaphenazole.*[6] The best documented interaction between sulfonylureas and sulfonamides is that between tolbutamide and sulfaphenazole.[6,10-13] There appears to be no interaction with sulfamethoxypyridazine,[5,6] sulfamethoxine,*[5,6] and sulfamethoxazole.[5,6] There are no reports regarding the other sulfonamides (sulfacytine and sulfasalazine), and because of conflicting results it is difficult to determine whether an interaction would occur with tolbutamide.

Sulfisoxazole[4] along with sulfamethazine[14] produced hypoglycemic coma in diabetic patients maintained on chlorpropamide. There is no documentation regarding alteration of the half-life of other sulfonylurea hypoglycemics (e.g., acetohexamide, glyburide, tolazamide [see Appendix]) by concurrent sulfonamides, but they may interact similarly to tolbutamide due to pharmacologic similarity.

Mechanism: Sulfamethizole can prolong the serum half-life of tolbutamide by inhibiting its hepatic oxidation. Inhibition of carboxylation has been proposed as the specific mechanism.[2] Because onset of action of the metabolic inhibition of tolbutamide by sulfamethizole was rapid, it has been suggested that the latter acts as an inhibitor of the aromatic ring-hydroxylating enzyme system.[1] Results from 1 study also suggested that the enhanced hypoglycemic response results from displacement of the sulfonylurea from plasma protein binding sites by the sulfonamide.[4,6,14]

Recommendations: The extent of caution indicated with concurrent sulfonylurea-sulfonamide therapy is dependent on the specific agents used, with tolbutamide and sulfaphenazole being most likely to result in enhanced hypoglycemic effects. Increased risk is associated with concurrent renal or hepatic dysfunction or restricted food intake in the elderly. Adverse reactions occur less often after the patient has been stabilized on the combination for a few weeks.[13]

References

1. Lumholtz, B., and others: Sulfamethizole-induced inhibition of diphenylhydantoin, tolbutamide, and warfarin metabolism, Clin. Pharmacol. Ther. **17:**731, 1975.
2. Siersbaek-Nielsen, K., and others: Sulfamethizole-induced inhibition of diphenylhydantoin and tolbutamide metabolism in man, Clin. Pharmacol. Ther. **14:**148, 1973.

*Not available in the U.S.

3. Dubach, U.C., and others: Einflus von sulfonamiden auf die blutzuckersenkende wirkung oraler antidiabetica, Schweiz Med. Wochenschr **96:**1483, 1966.

4. St. George Tucker, H., and Hirsch, J.I.: Sulfonamide-sulfonylurea interaction, N. Engl. J. Med. **286:**110, 1972.

5. Soeldner, J.S., and Steinke, J.: Hypoglycemia in tolbutamide-treated diabetics: report of two cases with measurement of serum insulin, J.A.M.A. **193:**398, 1965.

6. Christensen, L.K., and others: Sulphaphenazole-induced hypoglycaemic attacks in tolbutamide-treated diabetics, Lancet **2:**1298, 1963.

7. Kristensen, M., and Christensen, L.K.: Drug induced changes of the blood glucose lowering effect of oral hypoglycemic agents, Acta Diabetol. Lat. **6**(suppl. 1):116, 1969.

8. Thiessen, J.J., and Rowland, M.: Kinetics of drug-drug interactions in sheep: tolbutamide and sulfa-dimethoxine, J. Pharm. Sci. **66:**1063, 1977.

9. Jodis, J.: Binding of sulfonylurea to serum protein, J. Pharm. Sci. **61:**89, 1972.

10. Shen, S-W, and Bressler, R.: Clinical pharmacology of oral antidiabetic agents, N. Engl. J. Med. **296:**493, 1977.

11. Prescott, L.F.: Pharmacokinetic drug interactions, Lancet **2:**1239, 1969.

12. Pond, S.M., and others: Mechanisms of inhibition of tolbutamide metabolism: phenylbutazone, oxy-phenbutazone, sulfaphenazole, Clin. Pharmacol. Ther. **22:**573, 1977.

13. Jackson, J.E., and Bressler, R.: Clinical pharmacology of sulphonylurea hypoglycaemic agents: part 2. Drugs **22:**295, 1981.

14. Dall, J.L., and others: Hypoglycaemia due to chlorpropamide, Scott. Med. J. **12:**403, 1967.

Sedative-Hypnotic Drug Interactions

*Not available in the U.S.

TABLE 15. Sedative-Hypnotic Drug Interactions

Drug Interaction	Significance Code	Potential Effects	Recommendations	See Page
Alcohol, Ethyl– Amitriptyline	2	Studies have variously reported that amitriptyline enhances, antagonizes, or has no effect on the CNS depressant effects of alcohol.	Warn patients about possible impairment that may result from concurrent use.	596
Alcohol, Ethyl– Cimetidine	3	Cimetidine may increase the peak plasma level and area-under-curve of alcohol.	Advise patients that an increased level of intoxication may occur with concomitant use.	598
Alcohol, Ethyl– Diphenhydra-mine	2	Concurrent use of these agents may cause greater impairment of motor and mental performance than either drug alone.	Advise patients that ability to drive or operate dangerous equipment may be impaired.	599
Alcohol, Ethyl– Disulfiram	1	Alcohol ingestion while taking disulfiram results in throbbing in the head and neck, palpitations, tachycardia, hypotension, sweating, nausea, and vomiting. Disulfiram is used in the treatment of alcoholism.	Concurrent use should be avoided as even small doses (e.g., 15 ml) of alcohol lead to this interaction.	600
Alcohol, Ethyl– Glutethimide	2	Concurrent use of these agents may cause greater CNS depression that when either agent is taken alone.	Warn patients of possible impairment from concurrent use.	601
Alcohol, Ethyl– Metoclopra-mide	3	Metoclopramide may increase the rate of alcohol absorption and sedation.	Avoid concurrent use of these agents, although the clinical significance is not completely documented.	602
Alcohol, Ethyl– Metronidazole	2	Concurrent use of these agents has been associated with disulfiram-like reactions with symptoms of nausea, facial flushing, headache, and sweating. Other studies failed to show this.	Advise patients of the possible effects that may occur.	603
Amobarbital– Tranylcypro-mine	3	Pretreatment with tranylcypromine may prolong the CNS depressant effect of amobarbital.	Lengthen the dosage interval of amobarbital if concurrent use cannot be avoided.	604
Chloral Hy-drate–Alcohol, Ethyl	2	Concurrent use of these agents results in greater CNS depression than when either agent is taken alone. A vasodilation reaction may also occur.	Warn patients of possible effects that may occur.	605

Abbreviations: CNS, central nervous system; MAO, monoamine oxidase.

TABLE 15. Sedative-Hypnotic Drug Interactions—cont'd

Drug Interaction	Significance Code	Potential Effects	Recommendations	See Page
Chloral Hydrate–Furazolidone	4	Furazolidone inhibits MAO and can theoretically inhibit chloral hydrate metabolism, thus enhancing CNS depression. However, no reports have been made of this interaction.	Since the clinical significance is unsubstantiated and the interaction is based on theory, no special precautions are advised with concurrent use.	606
Hexobarbital*– Rifampin	3	Rifampin may increase the metabolism and clearance of hexobarbital.	Increased hexobarbital dosage may be required.	607
Meprobamate– Alcohol, Ethyl	2	Acute ingestion of alcohol with meprobamate may cause additive or synergistic CNS depression and increase the half-life of meprobamate. Conversely, in long-term alcohol use, enhanced drug metabolism can result in tolerance to pharmacologic effects of meprobamate.	Warn patients of these possible effects. Concurrent use of these agents should be avoided.	608
Meprobamate– Imipramine	3	Imipramine may enhance the CNS effect of meprobamate.	Advise patients that enhanced drowsiness and dizziness may occur with concomitant use.	609
Phenobarbital– Alcohol, Ethyl	2	Acute alcohol ingestion may increase the action and half-life of phenobarbital. Conversely, results of studies with long-term alcohol ingestion are inconsistent.	Since the effects appear to be dose-related, large amounts of alcohol should be avoided.	610
Phenobarbital– Chlorcyclizine	3	Concurrent use of these agents may result in enhanced CNS depression.	Caution patients about this possible interaction.	611
Phenobarbital– Dexamethasone	2	Large doses of phenobarbital may decrease systemic effects of dexamethasone.	A benzodiazepine may be a suitable alternative to phenobarbital. If concurrent use is unavoidable, the dexamethasone dosage may need to be increased.	612
Phenobarbital– Oral Contraceptive Agents	2	Concurrent use of these agents may cause failure of the contraceptive. Phenobarbital also decreases unbound serum concentration of the steroid.	An alternative form of contraception may be advisable, or increasing the ethinyl estradiol content may be necessary.	614

*Not available in the U.S.

Summary: The effects of the concurrent use of amitriptyline and alcohol are unpredictable. Various studies have reported that amitriptyline can enhance (within the first week of therapy),[1-3] antagonize,[4,5] or have no effect on the central nervous system depressant effects of alcohol[6] and may also impair gastrointestinal activity.[7] The combination has been associated with overdose deaths.[8] One study reported that alcohol increased the area-under-curve of free amitriptyline by 48% and the area-under-curve of total amitriptyline by 44.4%, and this resulted in psychomotor impairment in 5 healthy volunteers.[9]

Related Drugs: Doxepin has been reported to both minimize[1] and enhance[4] the psychomotor impairment produced by alcohol. Nortriptyline was observed to have a slight antagonistic effect on the central nervous system depressant effect of alcohol in 1 study.[5] However, another study concluded that nortriptyline and clomipramine* had minimal effects on the psychomotor impairment produced by alcohol.[1] Other tricylic antidepressants (e.g., desipramine, imipramine, protriptyline [see Appendix]) and the tetracyclic antidepressant (maprotiline) may be expected to interact similarly with alcohol based on pharmacologic similarity.

Mechanism: Amitriptyline is an antidepressant that also has sedative effects. Since alcohol is a central nervous system depressant, the enhanced sedation seen with the combination of amitriptyline and alcohol probably results from the additive effect of the 2 agents.[1] Theories that amitriptyline alters the pharmacokinetics of alcohol have not been substantiated.[8,10] There is no established mechanism for the interaction that suggests amitriptyline antagonizes the effect of alcohol.[4]

Recommendations: The most hazardous of the possible interactions is the enhanced central nervous system depression of alcohol while the patient is on amitriptyline. Patients receiving amitriptyline should be informed that concurrent ingestion of alcohol may produce a greater than expected impairment of the ability to drive an automobile or operate dangerous machinery.[1] The impairment in psychomotor skills caused by the combination of alcohol and amitriptyline may become less harmful with continued amitriptyline administration.[1,3]

References

1. Seppala, T., and others: Effect of tricyclic antidepressants and alcohol on psychomotor skills related to driving, Clin. Pharmacol. Ther. **17:**515, 1975.
2. Landauer, A.A., and others: Alcohol and amitriptyline effects on skills related to driving behavior, Science **163:**1467, 1969.
3. Seppala, T.: Psychomotor skills during acute and two week treatment with mianserin and amitriptyline and their combined effects with alcohol, Am. Clin. Res. **9:**66, 1977.
4. Milner, G., and others: The effects of doxepin, alone and together with alcohol, in relation to driving safety, Med. J. Aust. **1:**837, 1973.
5. Hughes, F.W., and others: Delayed audiofeedback for induction of anxiety: effect of nortriptyline,

*Not available in the U.S.

ethanol, or nortriptyline-ethanol combinations on performance with delayed audiofeedback, J.A.M.A. **185:**556, 1963.

6. Patman, J., and others: The combined effect of alcohol and amitriptyline on skills similar to motor-car driving, Med. J. Aust. **2:**946, 1969.

7. Lockett, M.F., and others: Combining the antidepressant drugs, Br. Med. J. **1:**921, 1965.

8. Scott, D.B., and others: Amitriptyline and zimelidine in combination with ethanol, Psychopharmacology **76:**209, 1982.

9. Dorian, P., and others: Amitriptyline and ethanol: pharmacokinetic and pharmacodynamic interaction, Eur. J. Clin. Pharmacol. **25:**325, 1983.

10. Cott, J.M., and others: Antidepressant drugs and ethanol behavior and pharmacokinetic interactions in mice, J. Neural. Transm. **48:**223, 1980.

Summary: In 1 study, 8 volunteers received either cimetidine or placebo for 7 days and then were given a 20% alcohol solution. In those who received cimetidine the peak plasma alcohol level and the area-under-curve were significantly increased.[1] In another study 6 healthy subjects received the same therapy. The subjects who received cimetidine had peak alcohol concentrations that were 10% higher and occurred earlier than those in a comparative placebo subject.[2]

Related Drugs: There are no drugs related to alcohol. In the study cited,[1] the subjects who received ranitidine and alcohol showed neither an increased alcohol area-under-curve nor an increased peak plasma alcohol level.

Mechanism: Because the elimination rate of alcohol was not changed by either cimetidine or ranitidine, the mechanism does not appear to be related to inhibition of hepatic metabolism. It has been suggested that alcohol absorption may be increased with concurrent cimetidine.[1]

Recommendations: Patients should be aware that alcohol blood levels may be increased during concurrent cimetidine, and an increased level of intoxication can result.

References

1. Seitz, H.K., and others: Increased blood ethanol levels following cimetidine but not ranitidine, Lancet **1:**760, 1983.
2. Feely, J., and others: Effect of cimetidine on the elimination and actions of ethanol, J.A.M.A. **247:**2819, 1982.

Summary: Concurrent administration of diphenhydramine and alcohol may result in a greater impairment of motor and mental performance than the ingestion of either drug alone.[1-5] There appears to be a wide variation among individuals in the effect of this combination.[3]

Related Drugs: Evidence indicates that tripelennamine also interacts with alcohol.[5] Although not reported, other antihistamines (e.g., brompheniramine, chlorpheniramine, pyrilamine [see Appendix]) may also interact with alcohol.

Mechanism: The mechanism of the interaction between diphenhydramine and alcohol is unknown.

Recommendations: Patients receiving diphenhydramine or other antihistamines should be advised that the concurrent use of alcohol may result in increased mental and motor impairment and may impair their ability to drive an automobile or operate dangerous equipment.

References

1. Baugh, R., and Calvert, R.T.: The effect of diphenhydramine alone and in combination with ethanol on histamine skin response and mental performance, Eur. J. Clin. Pharmacol. **12:**201, 1977.
2. Linnoila, M.: Effects of drugs and alcohol on psychomotor skills related to driving, Ann. Clin. Res. **6:**7, 1974.
3. Linnoila, M.: Effects of antihistamines, chlormezanone and alcohol on psychomotor skills related to driving, Eur. J. Clin. Pharmacol. **5:**247, 1973.
4. Forney, R.B.: International seminar research on alcohol, drugs and driving, Pharmakopsychiatr. Neuropsychopharmakol. **6:**104, 1973.
5. Hughes, R.W., and Fortney, R.B.: Comparative effects of three antihistamines and ethanol on mental and motor performances, Clin. Pharmacol. Ther. **5:**414, 1964.

Alcohol, Ethyl–Disulfiram

Summary: Extensive documentation shows that patients ingesting alcohol or using topical preparations that contain alcohol while taking disulfiram will experience throbbing in the head and neck, palpitations, tachycardia, hypotension, sweating, nausea, and vomiting.[1] The duration of the interaction varies from 30 to 60 minutes to several hours depending on the amount of alcohol consumed.[2] Disulfiram is therapeutically utilized in the treatment of alcoholism.

Related Drugs: There are no drugs related to alcohol or disulfiram.

Mechanism: Disulfiram alters the intermediary metabolism of alcohol. Acetaldehyde is produced as a result of an initial alcohol dehydrogenase oxidation in the liver. Acetaldehyde is normally further oxidized by aldehyde dehydrogenase but this step is slowed by disulfiram. Acetaldehyde blood levels accumulate leading to the undesired responses. Other biochemical mechanisms may be responsible for some of the reaction symptoms since not all of the symptoms can be produced by administering acetaldehyde.

Recommendations: Consumption of even small doses (e.g., 15 ml) of alcohol lead to this interaction; therefore, concomitant administration should be avoided. Patients have suffered this interaction from taking cough mixtures[3] and using topical preparations such as aftershave lotions[4] and antipsoriatic preparations[5] that contained alcohol.

References

1. Kwentus, J., and Major, L.F.: Disulfiram in the treatment of alcoholism: a review, J. Stud. Alcohol **40:**428, 1979.
2. Hald, J., and others: The sensitizing effects of tetraethylthiuram disulphide (Antabuse) to ethyl alcohol, Acta Pharmacol. **4:**285, 1948.
3. Koff, R.S., and others: Alcohol in cough medicines: hazards to the disulfiram user, J.A.M.A. **215:**1988, 1971.
4. Mercurio, F.: Antabuse-alcohol reaction following the use of after-shave lotion, J.A.M.A. **149:**82, 1952.
5. Ellis, C.N., and others: Tar gel interaction with disulfiram, Arch. Dermatol. **115:**1367, 1979.

Alcohol, Ethyl–Glutethimide

2

Summary: Concurrent ingestion of alcohol and glutethimide may result in a greater central nervous system depression than when either agent is taken alone.[1-3]

Related Drugs: Methyprylon may be expected to interact with alcohol in a manner similar to glutethimide, but documentation is not available. Other drugs that possess central nervous system (CNS) depressant activity such as ethchlorvynol and possibly methaqualone* may also interact with alcohol.[4,5]

Mechanism: The mechanism of this interaction is not documented. However, it is postulated that the CNS depressant effects result from synergism.

Recommendations: Concurrent ingestion of alcohol and glutethimide or other central nervous system depressants previously mentioned may result in an increased depressant activity. Patients should be warned of this possible enhancement of the depressant effects and also that this combination may produce a greater impairment of their ability to drive or operate hazardous machinery.

References

1. Mould, G.P., and others: Interaction of glutethimide and phenobarbitone with ethanol in man, J. Pharm. Pharmacol. **24:**894, 1972.
2. Maher, J.F., and others: Acute glutethimide intoxication. I. Clinical experience (22 patients) compared to acute barbiturates intoxication (63 patients), Am. J. Med. **33:**70, 1962.
3. Saario, I., and Linnoila, M.: Effects of subacute treatment with hypnotics alone or in combination with alcohol, on psychomotor skills related to driving, Acta Pharmacol. Toxicol. **38:**382, 1976.
4. Flemenbaum, A., and Gunby, B.: Ethchlorvynol (Placidyl) abuse and withdrawal, Dis. Nerv. Syst. **32:**188, 1971.
5. Inaba, D.S., and others: Methaqualone abuse. Luding out, J.A.M.A. **224:**1505, 1973.

*Not available in the U.S.

Alcohol, Ethyl–Metoclopramide

3

Summary: Concurrent administration of metoclopramide and alcohol resulted in significant increases in the rate of alcohol absorption and sedation in fasting normal volunteers.[1-3] Alcohol plasma concentrations were significantly higher and the peak concentration occurred earlier. The effect of metoclopramide could be seen when alcohol was administered 3 hours later.

Related Drugs: There are no drugs related to metoclopramide.

Mechanism: The mechanism for the enhanced alcohol absorption is not fully known. Metoclopramide hastens gastric emptying, probably through prolactin inhibiting factor by increasing endogenous prolactin serum concentrations. The more rapid gastric emptying results in a quicker absorption onset.

Recommendations: The clinical significance of the interaction is not completely documented. However, administration of these agents together led to an enhanced alcohol sedation,[2] suggesting that concurrent use should be avoided.

References

1. Gibbons, D.O., and Lant, A.F.: Effects of intravenous and oral propantheline and metoclopramide on ethanol absorption, Clin. Pharmacol. Ther. **17:**578, 1975.
2. Bateman, D.N., and others: Pharmacokinetic and concentration effect studies with intravenous metoclopramide, Br. J. Clin. Pharmacol. **6:**401, 1978.
3. Finch, J.E., and others: An assessment of gastric emptying by breathalyser, Br. J. Clin. Pharmacol. **1:**233, 1974.

Alcohol, Ethyl–Metronidazole

2

Summary: Concurrent use of metronidazole with alcohol has been associated with a disulfiram-type reaction resulting in symptoms of nausea, facial flushing, headache, and sweating.[1-3] Other studies have failed to observe such an effect.[4-10]

Related Drugs: There are no drugs related to metronidazole.

Mechanism: In vitro studies[11-15] showed that metronidazole produces an inhibition of aldehyde dehydrogenase and other alcohol-oxidizing enzymes. This results in the accumulation of acetaldehyde, which is responsible for the reaction symptoms.

Recommendations: Although adverse effects from concurrent ingestion of metronidazole and alcohol are infrequent, the possibility exists. Therefore, the patient should be advised that facial flushing, headache, sweating, and nausea may result if alcohol is ingested during metronidazole therapy.

References

1. Penick, S., and others: Metronidazole in the treatment of alcoholism, Am. J. Psychiatry **125**:1063, 1969.
2. Taylor, J.T.: Metronidazole. A new agent combined somatic and psychic therapy of alcoholism, Bull. Los Angeles Neurol. Soc. **29**:158, 1964.
3. Lehmann, H.E., and others: Metronidazole in the treatment of the alcoholic, Psychiat. Neurol. **152**:395, 1966.
4. Gelder, M.C., and Edwards, G.: Metronidazole in the treatment of alcohol addiction: a controlled trial, Br. J. Psychiatry **1134**:473, 1968.
5. Goodwin, D.W.: Metronidazole in the treatment of alcoholism: a negative report, Am. J. Psychiatry **123**:1276, 1967.
6. Eagan, W.P., and Goetz, R.: Effect of metronidazole on drinking by alcoholics, Q. J. Stud. Alcohol **29**:899, 1968.
7. Dallant, D.M., and others: A six-month controlled evaluation of metronidazole in chronic alcoholic patients, Curr. Ther. Res. **10**:82, 1968.
8. Platz, A., and others: Metronidazole and alcoholism. An evaluation of specific and nonspecific factors in drug treatment, Dis. Nerv. Syst. **31**:631, 1970.
9. Strassman, H.D., and others: Metronidazole effect on social drinkers, Q. J. Stud. Alcohol **31**:394, 1970.
10. Lowenstein, I.: Metronidazole and placebo in the treatment of chronic alcoholism, Psychosomatics **10**:43, 1970.
11. Gupta, N., and others: Effect of metronidazole on liver alcohol dehydrogenase, Biochem. Pharmacol. **19**:2805, 1970.
12. Kitson, T.M.: The disulfiram-ethanol reaction, J. Stud. Alcohol **38**:96, 1977.
13. Edwards, J.A., and Price, J.: Metronidazole and atypical human alcohol dehydrogenase, Biochem. Pharmacol. **16**:2026, 1967.
14. Fried, R., and Fried, L.W.: The effect of Flagyl on xanthine oxidase and alcohol dehydrogenase, Biochem. Pharmacol. **15**:1890, 1966.
15. Paltrinieri, E.: Inhibitory action on alcohol-dehydrogenase by hydroxy-2'-ethyl-1-methyl-2-nitro-5-imidazole, Farmaco. (Sci.) **22**:1054, 1967.

Amobarbital–Tranylcypromine

3

Summary: Pretreatment with tranylcypromine may prolong the central nervous system (CNS) depressant effect of amobarbital.[1]

Related Drugs: It is probable that other monoamine oxidase inhibitors (isocarboxazid, pargyline, and phenelzine) prolong the CNS depressant effects of the other barbiturates (e.g., butabarbital, phenobarbital, secobarbital [see Appendix]) based on a similar effect on the metabolism of barbiturates, although documentation is lacking.

Mechanism: Monoamine oxidase inhibitors produce this effect by interference with the metabolism of the barbiturates rather than through the effect on monoamine oxidase.[1-3]

Recommendations: Amobarbital and possibly other barbiturates should be used with caution in patients receiving tranylcypromine or other monoamine oxidase inhibitors or other drugs that possess monoamine oxidase inhibitor activity such as furazolidone or procarbazine. If concurrent administration is required, the dosage interval of the barbiturate may need to be lengthened because of the prolongation of CNS depression.

References

1. Domino, E.F., and others: Barbiturate intoxication in a patient treated with a MAO inhibitor, Am. J. Psychiatry **118**:941, 1962.
2. Laroche, M., and Brodie, B.B.: Lack of relationship between inhibition of monamine oxidase and potentiation of hexobarbital hypnosis, J. Pharmacol. Exp. Ther. **130**:143, 1960.
3. Fouts, J.R., and Brodie, B.B.: On the mechanism of drug potentiation by iproniazid (2-isopropyl-1-isonicotinyl hydrazine), J. Pharmacol. Exp. Ther. **116**:480, 1956.

Chloral Hydrate–Alcohol, Ethyl

2

Summary: Concurrent ingestion of chloral hydrate and alcohol results in greater central nervous system (CNS) depression than that occurring when either agent is taken alone.[1,2] In addition, a disulfiram-like reaction characterized by vasodilation, flushing, tachycardia, hypotension, or headache occasionally occurs when alcohol is ingested by a patient who has been receiving chloral hydrate for several days.[1,3]

Related Drugs: Although there is no clinical documentation, based on the mechanism triclofos and other products metabolized to yield trichloroethanol may be expected to interact in a similar manner with alcohol.

Mechanism: After concurrent ingestion of these agents, enhanced CNS depression occurs because of an altered production of active metabolites of both chloral hydrate and alcohol. Alcohol stimulates the reduction of chloral hydrate to trichloroethanol, which is a longer-acting hypnotic than the parent compound.[3] Trichloroethanol in turn inhibits the oxidation of alcohol to acetaldehyde by alcohol dehydrogenase.

  The mechanism for the development of the vasodilation reaction is not established, but it is not related to increased acetaldehyde levels such as those seen after concurrent alcohol-disulfiram ingestion.[1,3,4]

Recommendations: All patients taking chloral hydrate should be warned that the CNS depressant effects of both chloral hydrate and alcohol are increased by concurrent ingestion. Patients with cardiovascular disease who receive chloral hydrate long-term should be especially careful about ingesting alcohol in view of the tachycardia and hypotension that can result from the vasodilation reaction.

References:

1. Sellers, E.M., and others: Interaction of chloral hydrate and ethanol in man. II. Hemodynamics and performance, Clin. Pharmacol. Ther. **13:**50, 1972.
2. Gessner, P.K., and Cabana, B.E.: Chloral alcoholate: reevaluation of its role in the interaction between hypnotic effects of chloral hydrate and ethanol, J. Pharmacol. Exp. Ther. **156:**602, 1967.
3. Sellers, E.M., and others: Interaction of chloral hydrate and ethanol in man. I. Metabolism, Clin. Pharmacol. Ther. **13:**37, 1967.
4. Asmussen, E.M., and others: The pharmacological action of acetaldehyde on the human organism, Acta Pharmacol. Toxicol. **4:**311, 1948.

Chloral Hydrate–Furazolidone

Summary: Furazolidone is a broad-spectrum antimicrobial agent effective against the majority of gastrointestinal tract pathogens.[1] Because furazolidone or its metabolite has been shown to inhibit monoamine oxidase and presumably other enzyme systems as well, it can theoretically inhibit the metabolism of chloral hydrate, thereby enhancing the central nervous system (CNS) depressant effect of the latter.[2] However, there are no reports of this interaction.

Related Drugs: Although no documentation exists, other monoamine oxidase inhibitors (e.g., isocarboxazid, phenelzine, tranylcypromine [see Appendix]) or procarbazine, an antineoplastic with monoamine oxidase inhibitor activity, might be expected to interact with chloral hydrate in a manner analogous to furazolidone.

Mechanism: Inhibition of monoamine oxidase by furazolidone has been demonstrated experimentally in humans by the enhancement of tyramine and amphetamine sensitivity and by directly measuring monoamine oxidase inhibition.[3,4] The monoamine oxidase inhibitors inhibit many liver enzymes responsible for drug metabolism.[5] Since chloral hydrate is normally metabolized by the liver enzyme systems, it could show exaggerated effects in the presence of monoamine oxidase inhibitors, primarily CNS depression.

Recommendations: Since the drug interaction between chloral hydrate and furazolidone is based on theoretic considerations and has not been documented in humans, the clinical significance of this drug interaction is unsubstantiated, and no special precautions are advised with concurrent use.

References

1. Chamberlain, R.E.: Chemotherapeutic properties of prominent nitrofurans, J. Antimicrob. Chemother. **2:**325, 1976.
2. Stern, I.J., and others: The anti-monoamine oxidase effects of furazolidone, J. Pharmacol. Exp. Ther. **156:**492, 1967.
3. Pettinger, W.A., and others: Monoamine oxidase inhibition by furazolidone in man, Clin. Res. **14:**258, 1966.
4. Pettinger, W.A., and others: Inhibition of monoamine oxidase in man by furazolidone, Clin. Pharmacol. Ther. **9:**442, 1968.
5. Ghoneim, M.M.: Drug interaction in anesthesia, a review, Can. Anaesth. Soc. J. **18:**353, 1971.

Hexobarbital*–Rifampin

Summary: Eight days of rifampin therapy increased hexobarbital metabolism approximately 3-fold and reduced the effectiveness of hexobarbital.[1] Similar reports further indicated that hexobarbital clearance was increased even in patients with chronic liver disease[2] and returned to pre-rifampin levels within 14 days after discontinuation of rifampin.[3]

Related Drugs: Concomitant rifampin and phenobarbital lowered plasma rifampin concentrations and reduced the rifampin half-life but such changes were judged to be of little clinical significance.[4] Because of conflicting results, it is difficult to determine whether an interaction would occur between rifampin and the other barbiturates (e.g., amobarbital, butabarbital, secobarbital [see Appendix]). There are no drugs related to rifampin.

Mechanism: Rifampin is a known inducer of hepatic microsomal enzymes responsible for the metabolism of many drugs. Rifampin appears to significantly stimulate the metabolism of hexobarbital, reducing its effectiveness.

Recommendations: A reduction in the effectiveness of hexobarbital may be expected with concurrent rifampin and may necessitate an increased hexobarbital dosage. Whether this occurs with other barbiturates is unknown at this time.

References

1. Zilly, W., and others: Induction of drug metabolism in man after rifampin treatment measured by increased hexobarbital and tolbutamide clearance, Eur. J. Clin. Pharmacol. **9:**219, 1975.
2. Zilly, W., and others: Stimulation of drug metabolism by rifampicin in patients with cirrhosis or cholestasis measured by increased hexobarbital and tolbutamide clearance, Eur. J. Clin. Pharmacol. **11:**287, 1977.
3. Breimer, D.D., and others: Influence of rifampicin on drug metabolism: differences between hexobarbital and antipyrine, Clin. Pharmacol. Ther. **21:**470, 1977.
4. Zilly, W., and others: Pharmacokinetic interaction with rifampicin, Clin. Pharmacokinet. **2:**61, 1977.

*Not available in the U.S.

Meprobamate–Alcohol, Ethyl

Summary: Acute alcohol intoxication in patients receiving meprobamate can lead to additive or synergistic central nervous system (CNS) depression as well as an increase in the half-life of meprobamate.[1] The CNS depression is usually mild or insignificant if alcohol intake does not exceed 1 or 2 drinks (90 to 120 ml of 100-proof whiskey) and meprobamate is taken in a single dose of 200 to 400 mg. However, with long-term use of alcohol, enhanced drug metabolism can result in tolerance to the pharmacologic effects of meprobamate.[2]

Related Drugs: Propanediol derivatives (e.g., carisoprodol, chlorphenesin, methocarbamol [see Appendix]) are chemically and pharmacologically related to meprobamate and may be expected to interact with alcohol in a similar manner.

Mechanism: The effects of this interaction may be described as enhanced CNS depression produced by 2 agents having sedative-hypnotic properties. Acutely, alcohol has been shown to increase the half-life of meprobamate, presumably by competitive inhibition of the meprobamate-oxidizing enzyme system.[1,3] More recently it has been reported that acute alcohol administration inhibits absorption of meprobamate orally and decreases the peak blood meprobamate concentration by approximately 20% 4 hours after a dose.[4] Long-term alcohol ingestion, on the other hand, results in the acceleration of the rate of disappearance of meprobamate from the blood consistent with a stimulation of the hepatic microsomal drug metabolizing enzymes responsible for meprobamate biotransformation.[3]

Recommendations: Patients receiving meprobamate should be cautioned regarding the enhancement of the CNS depressant effects of this drug when alcohol is ingested concurrently, because more pronounced and possibly dangerous effects (impairment of driving ability) have been observed when meprobamate was administered to some patients on a long-term basis. If either drug is taken in large doses, these agents can enhance CNS depression, resulting in death.[5] Habitual use of alcohol while taking meprobamate should likewise be avoided.

References

1. Rubin, E., and others: Inhibition of drug metabolism by acute ethanol intoxication: a hepatic microsomal mechanism, Am. J. Med. **49:**801, 1970.
2. Rubin, E., and Gang, C.S.: Alcoholism, alcohol, and drugs, Science **172:**1097, 1971.
3. Misra, P.S., and others: Increase of ethanol, meprobamate and pentobarbital metabolism after chronic ethanol administration in man and in rats, Am. J. Med. **51:**346-351, 1971.
4. Cobby, J.M., and Ashford, J.R.: Drug interactions: the effects of alcohol and meprobamate applied singly and jointly in human subjects. IV. The concentrations of alcohol and meprobamate in the blood, J. Stud. Alcohol **7**(suppl.):162, 1975.
5. Felby, S.: Concentrations of meprobamate in the blood and liver following fatal meprobamate poisoning, Acta Pharmacol. Toxicol. **28:**334, 1970.

Summary: Imipramine has been shown to enhance the central nervous system effect of meprobamate in animals.[1] The clinical significance of this effect has not been established in humans.

Related Drugs: Propanediol derivatives (e.g., carisoprodol, chlorphenesin, methocarbamol [see Appendix]) are chemically and pharamcologically related to meprobamate and may be expected to interact with imipramine in a similar manner. Other tricyclic antidepressants (e.g., desipramine, nortriptyline, protriptyline [see Appendix]) and the tetracyclic antidepressant (maprotiline) may also be expected to interact with meprobamate based on pharmacologic similarity.

Mechanism: Imipramine enhanced the sedative effects of meprobamate and carisoprodol in rats and inhibited the in vitro metabolism of these drugs in rat liver microsomal enzyme preparations.[1] This evidence suggests the enhanced sedative effects of meprobamate in rats is mediated by hepatic microsomal enzyme inhibition rather than additive central depression.

Recommendations: Although 1 study[2] suggested drowsiness and dizziness in humans were enhanced by the combination of meprobamate and a tricyclic antidepressant, it appears that this interaction is of minor clinical significance. However, patients should be aware that the combination of these drugs may result in enhanced drowsiness and dizziness.

References

1. Kato, R., and others: Mechanism of potentiation of barbiturates and meprobamate actions by imipramine, Biochem. Pharmacol. **12:**357, 1963.
2. Rickels, K., and others: Drug treatment in depression: antidepressant or tranquilizer? J.A.M.A. **201:**105, 1967.

Phenobarbital–Alcohol, Ethyl

Summary: Concurrent use of alcohol and barbiturates may result in enhanced central nervous system (CNS) depressant effects.[1] With acute alcohol ingestion, the action and half-life of phenobarbital increase.[2-4] Conversely, chronic alcohol ingestion results in lack of consistency and great variability in humans.

Related Drugs: With chronic ingestion of alcohol, pentobarbital has been shown to have a decreased half-life and action.[4] Other barbiturates (e.g., amobarbital, butabarbital, secobarbital [see Appendix]) may be expected to interact with acute alcohol consumption similarly to phenobarbital since they are pharmacologically related.

Mechanism: The CNS depression of this interaction is caused by a synergistic effect of phenobarbital and alcohol and the results are similar to the effects of either agent alone, except more intense. After acute alcohol ingestion, inhibition of hepatic microsomal enzyme activity has been demonstrated, which increases barbiturate activity and half-life.[2-4] In chronic alcohol consumption, although the effect is variable, alcohol seems to stimulate hepatic microsomal enzymes that accelerate the metabolism of phenobarbital, resulting in decreased activity and half-life.[4]

Recommendations: The effects of this interaction are dose-related. Relatively moderate amounts of alcohol (90 to 120 ml of 100-proof whiskey ingested during 1 hour) may impair a patient's ability to drive or operate machinery, and this danger is increased when barbiturates are taken concurrently. Large amounts of alcohol (150 to 200 ml of 100-proof whiskey) should be avoided while the patient is receiving barbiturates. Although benzodiazepines also interact with alcohol, they may be preferred over barbiturates for treatment of alcohol withdrawal since they result in less respiratory depression and do not disturb sleep patterns.[5,6]

References

1. Curry, S.H., and Scales, A.H.: Interaction of phenobarbitone and ethanol in mice studied from dose-response curves and drug concentration in blood, J. Pharm. Pharmacol. **26:**771, 1974.
2. Thomas, B.H., and others: Effect of ethanol on the fate of pentobarbital in the rat, Biochem. Pharmacol. **21:**2605, 1972.
3. Rubin, E., and others: Inhibition of drug metabolism by acute ethanol intoxication, Am. J. Med. **49:**801, 1970.
4. Sellers, E.M., and Holloway, M.R.: Drug kinetics and alcohol ingestion, Clin. Pharmacokinet. **3:**440, 1978.
5. Greenblatt, D.J., and Greenblatt, M.: Which drug for alcohol withdrawal? J. Clin. Pharmacol. **12:**429, 1972.
6. Rothstein, E.: Prevention of alcohol withdrawal seizures: the roles of diphenylhydantoin and chlordiazepoxide, Am. J. Psychol. **130:**1381, 1973.

Summary: Concurrent administration of the antihistamine chlorcyclizine and the barbiturate phenobarbital may result in an enhanced central nervous system (CNS) depression. There are no clinical data on the interaction between chlorcyclizine and phenobarbital, but the CNS depressant effect of either agent alone is well documented.[1,2]

Related Drugs: Although this effect is undocumented, other antihistamines (e.g., chlorpheniramine, diphenhydramine, pyrilamine [see Appendix]) and other barbiturates (e.g., amobarbital, butabarbital, secobarbital [see Appendix]) may cause similar additive depressant action when given together.

Mechanism: The hepatic microsomal enzyme-inducing properties of both drugs are noted[3,4]; however, this particular metabolic degradation of drug activity is not believed to be of clinical importance in acute concurrent administration. The probable mechanism for this interaction is the additive synergistic CNS depressant effect of each agent.

Recommendations: Patients receiving both antihistamines and barbiturates should be cautioned about the combined CNS depressant effects particularly when driving or operating hazardous machinery. Patients should be reminded that antihistamines occur widely in nonprescription formulas, especially cough and cold remedies.

References

1. Harvey, S.C.: Hypnotics and sedatives. In Gilman, A.G., Goodman, L.S., Gilman, A., editors: The pharmacological basis of therapeutics. New York, 1980, MacMillan Publishing.
2. Douglas, W.W.: Histamine and 5-hydroytriptamine (serotonin) and their antagonists. In Gilman, A.G., Goodman, L.S., Gilman, A., editors: The pharmacological basis of therapeutics. New York, 1980, MacMillan Publishing.
3. Conney, A.H., and others: Stimulatory effect of chlorcyclizine on barbiturate metabolism, J. Pharmacol. Exp. Ther. **132:**202, 1961.
4. Conney, A.H.: Pharmacological implications of microsomal enzyme induction, Pharmacol. Rev. **19:**317, 1967.

Phenobarbital–Dexamethasone

Summary: Large doses of barbiturates, such as phenobarbital, may act to decrease the systemic effects of corticosteroids such as dexamethasone.[1] This effect may persist for several days after the barbiturate has been discontinued.

Related Drugs: In addition to decreasing the effects of dexamethasone, phenobarbital and other barbiturates may decrease the efficacy of prednisone,[1] prednisolone,[2] methylprednisolone,[3] and hydrocortisone.[4] Other corticosteroids (e.g., betamethasone, fludrocortisone, triamcinolone [see Appendix]) may also interact with barbiturates because of a similar metabolic fate, but clinical evidence of this interaction has not appeared in the literature.

Several other barbiturates have been noted to affect the metabolism of the corticosteroids. These include pentobarbital[5-7] and primidone,[8] which is metabolized to phenobarbital. Note should be made of the metabolites of primidone, which include phenethylmalonic acid (PEMA) and phenobarbital,[9] a fact that explains the role of primidone in this potential interaction. Other barbiturates (e.g., amobarbital, mephobarbital, secobarbital [see Appendix]) have not been documented in the literature to interact with corticosteroids, but because of similar effects on hepatic microsomes responsible for drug metabolism,[10,11] they may be expected to affect the clinical efficacy of the corticosteroids.

Mechanism: The concurrent administration of barbiturates can induce the activity of hepatic microsomes responsible for drug metabolism in rats and guinea pigs and has also been shown to influence the metabolism of testosterone and cortisol in humans.[12]

Recommendations: Current evidence reveals that if barbiturates, such as phenobarbital, are taken in high doses (i.e., 120 mg/day or more) by patients dependent on steroid therapy, these patients should be observed for clinical evidence of decreased corticosteroid effectiveness.[1,13,14] Alternative therapy should be considered in these patients, or a higher dose of the corticosteroid during concomitant therapy may be necessary.

For treatment of anxiety and sedation, a benzodiazepine such as diazepam could be utilized. This agent has not been shown to significantly interact with steroids.[3,15]

Patients requiring physiologic replacement doses of steroids should be assessed for adrenal function and pharmacologic response to steroid treatment after initiation of barbiturate therapy. Barbiturates should be given with care to patients with borderline hypoadrenal function, whether of pituitary or adrenal origin.

References

1. Brooks, S.M., and others: Adverse effects of pentobarbital on corticosteroid metabolism in patients with bronchial asthma, N. Engl. J. Med. **286:**1125, 1972.
2. Brooks, P.M., and others: Effects of enzyme induction on metabolism of prednisolone, Ann. Rheum. Dis. **35:**339, 1976.

3. Stjiernholm, M.R., and Katz, F.H.: Effects of diphenylhydantoin, phenobarbital, and diazepam on the metabolism of methylprednisolone and its sodium succinate, J. Clin. Endocrinol. Metab. **41:**887, 1975.

4. Bernstein, S., and Klaiber, E.L.: Phenobarbital-induced increase in 6-beta-hydroxycortisol excretion: clue to its significance in human urine, J. Clin. Endocrinol. **25:**293, 1965.

5. Rerup, C., and Hedner, P.: The effect of pentobarbital (Nembutal, Membual NFN) on corticotrophin release in the rat, Acta Endocrinol. **39:**518, 1962.

6. Berman, M.L., and Green, O.C.: Acute stimulation of cortisol metabolism by pentobarbital in man, Anesthesiology **34:**365, 1971.

7. Oyama, T., and others: Objective evaluation of pentobarbital as a preanesthetic medication: effects on adrenal cortical function, Curr. Res. Anesth. Analg. **48:**367, 1969.

8. Hancock, K.W., and Levell, M.J.: Primidone-dexamethasone interaction, Lancet **2:**97, 1978.

9. Hollister, L.E.: Neurologic Disorders. In Melmon, K.L., and Morrelli, H.F., editors: Clinical pharmacology: basic principles in therapeutics, ed. 2, New York, Macmillan Publishing Co., pp. 874-912.

10. Conney, A.H.: Pharmacological implications of microsomal enzyme induction, Pharmacol. Rev. **19:**317, 1967.

11. Fouts, J.R.: Factors influencing metabolism of drugs by liver microsomes, Ann. N.Y. Acad. Sci. **104:**875, 1964.

12. Southern, A.L., and others: Stimulatory effect of N-phenylbarbital (Phentharbital) on the metabolism of testosterone and cortisol in man, J. Clin. Endocrinol. **29:**251, 1969.

13. Falliers, C.J.: Corticosteroids and phenobarbital in asthma, N. Engl. J. Med. **287:**201, 1972.

14. Wassner, S.J., and others: The adverse effects of anticonvulsant therapy on renal allograft survival, J. Pediatr. **88:**134, 1976.

15. Cryer, P.E., and Sode, J.: Drug interference with measurement of adrenal hormones in urine: analgesics and tranquilizer-sedatives, Ann. Intern. Med. **75:**697, 1971.

Phenobarbital–Oral Contraceptive Agents

2

Summary: Pretreatment with or the concurrent administration of phenobarbital may result in the failure of oral contraceptive agents, which may persist for days beyond the discontinuation of the barbiturate.[1-4] A disturbance of seizure control has also been reported with concurrent use of these agents when phenobarbital is used as an anticonvulsant.[5,6]

Related Drugs: Animal[7,8] and human studies[9,10] demonstrated that phenobarbital treatment enhanced the metabolism of estrone, progesterone, estradiol, ethinyl estradiol, testosterone, and androsterone.

Other barbiturates (e.g., amobarbital, butabarbital, secobarbital [see Appendix]) also induce hepatic enzymes and may be expected to interact similarly with oral contraceptive agents, but documentation is lacking.

Mechanism: Phenobarbital is known to be a potent inducer of microsomal enzyme systems, which are responsible for the metabolism of a variety of compounds. Therefore, the hormonal steroids apparently have their metabolism increased by this mechanism. Phenobarbital also increases progestogen binding to sex-hormone binding globulin, thereby decreasing the unbound serum concentration of the steroid.[11]

Changes in seizure control have been attributed to fluid retention changes that can influence seizure frequency.[5,12]

Recommendations: Although the incidence of oral contraceptive failure is not known, a sign of developing failure is intermediate breakthrough bleeding or spotting. Two courses of action have been suggested.[11] The first is to increase the ethinyl estradiol content of the oral contraceptive to 50 µg, or to 80 µg if bleeding persists. The second is to use a mechanical form of contraception.

Patients receiving phenobarbital as an anticonvulsant should be monitored for changes in seizure control when oral contraceptive agents are added to or withdrawn from therapy.

References

1. Janz, D., and Schmidt, D.: Anti-epileptic drugs and failure of oral contraceptives, Lancet **1:**1113, 1974.
2. Robertson, Y.R., and Johnson, E.S.: Interactions between oral contraceptives and other drugs: a review, Curr. Med. Res. Opin. **3:**647, 1976.
3. Hemper, E., and Klinger, W.: Drug stimulated biotransformation of hormonal steroid contraceptives: clinical implications, Drugs **12:**442, 1976.
4. Coulam, C.B., and Annegers, J.F.: Do anticonvulsants reduce the efficacy of oral contraceptives? Epilepsia **20:**519, 1979.
5. McArthur, J.: Oral contraceptives and epilepsy, Br. Med. J. **3:**162, 1967.
6. Copeman, H.: Oral contraceptives, Med. J. Aust. **2:**969, 1963.
7. Levin, W., and others: Effect of phenobarbital and other drugs on the metabolism and uterotropic action of estradiol-17B and estrone, J. Pharmacol. Exp. Ther. **159:**362, 1968.
8. Welch, R.M., and others: Stimulatory effect of phenobarbital on the metabolism in vivo of estradiol-17B and estrone in the rat, J. Pharmacol. Exp. Ther. **160:**171, 1968.

9. Conne, A.H.: Pharmacological implications of microsomal enzyme induction, Pharmacol. Rev. **19:**317, 1967.
10. Back, D.J., and others: The interaction of phenobarbital and other anticonvulsants with oral contraceptive steroid therapy, Contraception **22:**495, 1980.
11. Anon: Drug interactions with oral contraceptive steroids, Br. Med. J. **281:**93, 1980.
12. Espir, M., and others: Epilepsy and oral contraception, Br. Med. J. **1:**294, 1969.

CHAPTER SIXTEEN

Vitamin Drug Interactions

TABLE 16. Vitamin Drug Interactions

Drug Interaction	Significance Code	Potential Effects	Recommendations	See Page
Ascorbic Acid– Aspirin	4	Large doses of ascorbic acid had been previously thought to decrease the renal excretion of aspirin, but evidence is inconclusive. Also, it has been reported that aspirin increases the urinary excretion of ascorbic acid, reduces uptake into leukocytes in healthy subjects, and increases uptake in patients with colds.	Concurrent use of these agents need not be avoided. However, monitor for signs of ascorbic acid deficiency.	619
Ascorbic Acid– Ethinyl Estradiol	3	Ascorbic acid may increase plasma ethinyl estradiol concentrations.	Advise patients that starting and stopping ascorbic acid may lead to contraceptive failure.	621
Ergocalciferol– Phenytoin	2	Phenytoin may increase the metabolic inactivation and decrease the half-life of ergocalciferol, possibly resulting in hypocalcemia, osteomalacia, or rickets.	Monitor for decreased serum calcium levels and evidence of bone demineralization.	622
Ferrous Sulfate–Allopurinol	4	Studies in humans do not support animal studies indicating that concurrent use of these agents may increase hepatic iron storage.	Concurrent use of these agents need not be avoided.	624
Ferrous Sulfate–Aluminum Hydroxide, Magnesium Carbonate, Magnesium Hydroxide	2	Ferrous ion absorption is markedly reduced by concurrent administration with an antacid containing these agents, apparently from increased gastric pH.	Administer ferrous salts and antacids several hours apart.	625
Ferrous Sulfate–Ascorbic Acid	3	Ascorbic acid reportedly facilitates the absorption of ferrous ions.	Since absorption of ferrous salts alone is adequate, there is little justifcation for cotherapy.	626
Folic Acid– Sulfasalazine	2	Folate absorption (after oral folic acid administration) may be further reduced in patients with inflammatory bowel disease who are taking sulfasalazine.	Folic acid given by the parenteral route may avoid this interaction.	627
Niacin– Aspirin	3	Aspirin administered before niacin may reduce the flushing response common to niacin use.	Concurrent use may be beneficial to patients who are bothered by the flushing response from niacin.	628

TABLE 16. Vitamin Drug Interactions—cont'd

Drug Interaction	Significance Code	Potential Effects	Recommendations	See Page
Pyridoxine– Levodopa	1	Pyridoxine may reduce or abolish the beneficial effects of levodopa in parkinsonism.	Concurrent use of these agents should be avoided, but if this is not possible the concomitant use of carbidopa may prevent this interaction.	629
Vitamin A– Neomycin	3	Concurrent use of the oral forms of both agents may cause decreased plasma vitamin A levels. These plasma levels may take as long as 5 days to increase after neomycin is withdrawn.	Increased vitamin A doses may be necessary.	630

618

Ascorbic Acid–Aspirin

4

Summary: There is no conclusive evidence that large doses of ascorbic acid (4 to 6 g) will reduce the excretion of aspirin since ascorbic acid does not consistently acidify the urine.[1,2]

However, it has been previously reported that aspirin, administered in doses of 600 mg every 6 hours, resulted in increased urinary excretion of ascorbic acid, reduced uptake of ascorbic acid into the leukocytes of healthy individuals, and increased uptake into the leukocytes of patients suffering from a cold.[3-6]

Related Drugs: The administration of sodium salicylate appears to cause effects similar to aspirin when used concurrently with ascorbic acid.[1-7] The administration of other salicylates (e.g., choline salicylate, salicylamide, salsalate [see Appendix]) either alone or in combination products may produce a similar interaction based on pharmacologic similarity but clinical data are lacking.

Both indomethacin and aspirin have been reported to inhibit the rise in platelet cyclic GMP caused by ascorbic acid.[8] Indomethacin may have decreased the leukocyte levels of ascorbic acid in 2 patients.[6]

The ability of other nonsteroidal anti-inflammatory agents (e.g., ibuprofen, naproxen, sulindac [see Appendix]) to alter ascorbic acid leukocyte levels has not been sufficiently determined.

Mechanism: The mechanism by which aspirin was reported to alter the uptake of ascorbic acid into the leukocytes is not known. The interaction may be significant only in healthy persons.[3-5] Aspirin does not produce the reaction by damaging the cell membrane with subsequent leakage of ascorbic acid from the leukocyte.[5]

Aspirin may displace ascorbic acid from albumin binding sites, but the effect of this displacement is not clear.[9]

Ascorbic acid in doses greater than 4 g causes a significant uricosuric effect, which is inhibited by aspirin, suggesting the site of interaction is the renal tubule.[10]

Recommendations: Since there is no conclusive evidence that large doses of ascorbic acid will reduce the excretion of aspirin, or that aspirin causes a deficiency of ascorbic acid, the concurrent use of these agents need not be avoided.

References

1. Nakata, M.C., and others: Effect of ascorbic acid on urine pH in man, Am. J. Hosp. Pharm. **32:**1234, 1977.
2. Hansten, P.D., and Hayton, W.L.: Effect of antacids and ascorbic acid on sodium salicylate concentration in humans, J. Clin. Pharmacol. **20:**326, 1980.
3. Loh, J.S., and others: The effects of aspirin on the metabolic activity of ascorbic acid in human beings, J. Clin. Pharmacol. **13:**480, 1973.
4. Wilson, C.W.M., and Greene, M.: The relationship of aspirin to ascorbic acid metabolism during the common cold, J. Clin. Pharmacol. **18:**21, 1978.
5. Wilson, C.W.M.: Clinical pharmacological aspects of ascorbic acid, Ann. N.Y. Acad. Sci. **258:**355, 1975.

6. Sahud, M.A., and Cohen, R.J.: Effect of aspirin ingestion on ascorbic acid levels in rheumatoid arthritis, Lancet 1:937, 1971.
7. Williams, R.S., and Hughes, R.E.: Dietary protein, growth and retention of ascorbic acid in guinea pigs, Br. J. Nutr. 28:167, 1972.
8. Pickett, W.C., and others: Inhibition by nonsteroidal anti-inflammatory agents of the ascorbate-induced elevations of platelet cyclic GMP levels, J. Cyclic Nucleotide Res. 3:355, 1977.
9. Lambert, M.B.T., and others: The effect of aspirin on the protein binding of ascorbic acid, Br. J. Pharmacol. 60:300, 1977.
10. Stein, H.B., and others: Ascorbic acid-induced uricosuria. A consequence of megavitamin therapy, Ann. Intern. Med. 84:385, 1976.

Ascorbic Acid–Ethinyl Estradiol

3

Summary: In 1 study 4 of 6 women showed an increase in plasma ethinyl estradiol concentration when a single dose of ethinyl estradiol was administered with ascorbic acid.[1] The same results were noted in another study involving 5 volunteers.[1]

Related Drugs: A patient on an oral contraceptive containing ethinyl estradiol and levonorgestrel had normal withdrawal bleeding after the first 2 courses. During the next 3 courses, the patient took ascorbic acid (1 g/day) intermittently and suffered breakthrough bleeding each time she stopped the ascorbic acid.[2] Several studies indicate that the use of oral contraceptives lower concurrent ascorbic acid levels in both leukocytes and platelets.[3-7] Documentation is lacking regarding an interaction between ascorbic acid and the other estrogenic substances (e.g., chlorotrianisene, conjugated estrogens, estradiol [see Appendix]), although since they are pharmacologically related a similar interaction may be expected. There are no drugs related to ascorbic acid.

Mechanism: It has been suggested that the interaction results from competition for sulfate in the gut wall. This would reduce the first-pass effect of ethinyl estradiol, therefore increasing its systemic bioavailability and plasma concentration.[1] The breakthrough bleeding may be a withdrawal effect of the ascorbic acid causing sudden falls in the ethinyl estradiol levels each time the vitamin was stopped.[2] The lower ascorbic acid levels in contraceptive users may be the result of an increase in the breakdown of ascorbic acid by the oral contraceptives.[3-7] This may occur by their stimulant action on liver release of ceruloplasmin, a copper-containing protein with ascorbate oxidase activity.[3,4]

Recommendations: Patients should be advised that starting and stopping ascorbic acid may lead to contraceptive failure. It has been suggested that the increase in plasma ethinyl estradiol during treatment with ascorbic acid might be of some benefit in permitting wider use of the very-low-dose ethinyl estradiol preparations.[1,2]

References

1. Back, D.J., and others: Interaction of ethinyloestradiol with ascorbic acid in man, Br. Med. J. **282:**1516, 1981.
2. Morris, J.C., and others: Interaction of ethinyloestradiol with ascorbic acid in man, Br. Med. J. **283:**503, 1981.
3. Briggs, M., and Briggs, M.: Vitamin C requirements and oral contraceptives, Nature **4:**238, 1972.
4. Wynn, V.: Vitamins and oral contraceptive use, Lancet **1:**561, 1975.
5. Briggs, M., and Briggs, M.: Oral contraceptives and vitamin requirements, Med. J. Aust. **1:**407, 1975.
6. Harris, A.B., and others: Vitamin and oral contraceptives, Lancet **1:**82, 1975.
7. Larsson-Cohn, U.: Oral contraceptives and vitamins: a review, Am. J. Obstet. Gynecol. **121:**84, 1975.

Ergocalciferol–Phenytoin

2

Summary: Phenytoin may increase the metabolic inactivation of ergocalciferol (vitamin D) and decrease the half-life of the vitamin in the body, possibly resulting in hypocalcemia and, in debilitated patients, clinical osteomalacia or rickets. These effects have been more severe when phenytoin was used in combination with other anticonvulsants.[1,2]

Related Drugs: It may be expected that other hydantoin derivatives (ethotoin and mephenytoin) would have a similar potential to interact with ergocalciferol, since other anticonvulsants, particularly phenobarbital, have been implicated in producing osteomalacia as well.[1,3]

Mechanism: Phenytoin may affect ergocalciferol activity by the following mechanisms: (1) induction of the hepatic microsomal oxidative enzyme system, causing an increase in the hydroxylation of cholecalciferol and 25-hydroxycholecalciferol to more polar inactive metabolites,[4,5] although decreases in serum 25-hydroxycholecalciferol have not been consistently reported,[6,7] or (2) an increase in hepatic glucuronidation of cholecalciferol, which is then excreted as an inactive glucuronide.[8,9] As a result, phenytoin can decrease serum calcium levels and increase serum alkaline phosphatase levels (from both liver and bone),[1,2,10] with changes in these levels noted approximately 1 month after drug initiation.[11] Ergocalciferol independent factors may also play a role in phenytoin-induced hypocalcemia and metabolic bone disease, since phenytoin has inhibited parathyroid-induced mobilization of bone calcium in vitro.[12] The effect of phenytoin on intestinal calcium absorption has been inconsistent, with increases and decreases in calcium absorption being reported.[1,7,13]

Recommendations: Patients receiving phenytoin with risk factors for the development of osteomalacia (e.g., inadequate dietary vitamin D intake, limited sunlight exposure, relative inactivity) should be monitored periodically for decreased serum calcium levels and evidence of bone demineralization. Adequate nutrition, with the ingestion of foods rich in vitamin D such as milk, fish, and eggs, and sufficient sunlight exposure are necessary for patients receiving phenytoin and other anticonvulsants. Ergocalciferol therapy, at an individualized dosage, may be required in certain high-risk patients to prevent development of osteomalacia and rickets, and in patients with evidence of impaired bone and mineral metabolism.

References

1. Hahn, T.J., and Avioli, L.V.: Anticonvulsant osteomalacia, Arch. Intern. Med. **135:**997, 1975.
2. Mosekilde, L., and Melsen, F.: Anticonvulsant osteomalacia determined by quantitative analysis of bone changes, Acta Med. Scand. **199:**349, 1976.
3. Pierides, A.M., and others: Barbiturate and anticonvulsant treatment in relation to osteomalacia with haemodialysis and renal transplantation, Br. Med. J. **1:**190, 1976.
4. Hahn, T.J., and others: Effect of chronic anticonvulsant therapy on serum 25-hydroxycalciferon levels in adults, N. Engl. J. Med. **287:**900, 1972.
5. Hahn, T.J.: Anticonvulsant therapy and vitamin D, Ann. Intern. Med. **78:**308, 1973.

6. Mosekilde, L., and others: The interrelationships between serum 25-hydroxycholecalciferol, serum parathyroid hormone and bone changes in anticonvulsant osteomalacia, Acta Endocrinol. **84:**559, 1977.
7. Wark, J.D., and others: Chronic diphenylhydantoin therapy does not reduce plasma 25-hydroxyvitamin D, Clin. Endocrinol. **11:**267, 1979.
8. Sotaniemi, E., and others: Radiologic bone changes and hypocalcemia with anticonvulsant therapy in epilepsy, Ann. Intern. Med. **77:**389, 1972.
9. Hunter, J., and others: Altered calcium metabolism in epileptic children on anticonvulsants, Br. Med. J. **4:**202, 1971.
10. Tjellesen, L., and Christiansen, C.: Serum vitamin D metabolites in epileptic patients treated with 2 different anticonvulsants, Acta Neurol. Scand. **66:**335, 1982.
11. Reunanen, M.I., and others: Serum calcium balance during early phase of diphenylhydantoin therapy, Int. J. Clin. Pharmacol. **14:**15, 1976.
12. Jenkins, M.V., and others: The effect of anticonvulsant drugs in vitro on bone calcium mobilization by parathyroid hormone, Clin. Sci. Mol. Med. **45:**1p, 1973.
13. Bell, R.D., and others: Effect of phenytoin on bone and vitamin D metabolism, Ann. Neurol. **5:**374, 1979.

Ferrous Sulfate–Allopurinol

4

Summary: Studies in humans[1-4] do not support earlier animal data[1,5] indicating that allopurinol and ferrous ion preparations interact.[6] Information about this interaction was removed from package literature of the original manufacturer of allopurinol before 1981.[6]

Related Drugs: Various ferrous salts are available (e.g., ferrous fumarate, ferrous gluconate, ferrous lactate) and may also be expected to not interact with allopurinol. There are no drugs related to allopurinol.

Mechanism: According to this hypothesis, iron is stored in the liver in the oxidized or ferric state and is tightly bound to protein as ferric ferritin. Xanthine oxidase appears to be involved in the conversion of ferric ferritin to ferrous ferritin. The reduced form of iron is less tightly bound to ferritin and thus is more easily released for utilization. Therefore, a possible inverse relationship between hepatic xanthine oxidase activity and hepatic iron storage exists. Theoretically, the xanthine oxidase inhibitor allopurinol should decrease the activity of xanthine oxidase and increase hepatic iron storage.[1,7]

Recommendations: Clinical studies do not support the existence of this interaction; therefore, no additional precautions are required when these drugs are given together.

References

1. Green, R., and others: The effect of allopurinol on iron metabolism, South Afr. Med. J. **42:**776, 1968.
2. Rundles, R.W.: Allopurinol in the treatment of gout, Ann. Intern. Med. **64:**229, 1966.
3. Emmerson, B.T.: Effects of allopurinol on iron metabolism in man, Ann. Rheum. Dis. **25:**700, 1966.
4. Davis, V., and Deller, D.J.: Effect of a xanthine oxidase inhibitor (allopurinol) on radioiron absorption in man, Lancet **2:**470, 1966.
5. Udall, V., and Deller, D.J.: Allopurinol symposium, 1966, Ann. Rheum. Dis. **25:**704, 1966.
6. Personal communication, Burroughs-Wellcome Company, Research Triangle Park, N.C., 1983.
7. Powell, L.W.: Effects of allopurinol on iron storage in the rat, Ann. Rheum. Dis. **25:**697, 1966.

Ferrous Sulfate–Aluminum Hydroxide, Magnesium Carbonate, Magnesium Hydroxide

2

Summary: Ferrous ion absorption was markedly reduced when ferrous sulfate was coadministered with a suspension containing aluminium hydroxide, magnesium hydroxide, and magnesium carbonate.[1] Such co-therapy may reduce the hematologic response expected with oral ferrous sulfate iron therapy. The effect of these 3 antacids individually on ferrous ion absorption has not been studied.

Related Drugs: The suspension also interfered with ferrous ion absorption when ferrous fumarate and ferrous carbonate were used.[1] In a separate report magnesium trisilicate inhibited the ferrous ion absorption in all 9 subjects given ferrous sulfate.[2]

Mechanism: Ferrous salts are readily dissolved at low pH, but only slightly dissolved at higher pHs. Therefore, the main mechanism seems to be an increase in the gastric pH elicited by the antacid, reducing the solubility and dissolution of the ferrous salt. In addition, the formation of poorly absorbed macromolecular ferrous complexes may also be occurring.

Recommendations: It is not known whether the individual agents (aluminum hydroxide, magnesium carbonate, and magnesium hydroxide) alone affect ferrous ion absorption; however the documentation indicates the combination of the 3 ingredients reduced ferrous ion absorption. Therefore, until further clinical evidence is available, the administration of ferrous salts should be separated by several hours from antacids containing a combination of aluminum hydroxide, magnesium carbonate, and magnesium hydroxide or from those containing magnesium trisilicate.

References

1. Ekenved, G., and others: Influence of a liquid antacid on the absorption of different iron salts, Scand. J. Haematol. **28**(suppl.):65, 1976.
2. Hall, G.J.L., and Davis, A.E.: Inhibition of iron absorption by magnesium trisilicate, Med. J. Aust. **2**:95, 1969.

Ferrous Sulfate–Ascorbic Acid

3

Summary: It has been reported that ferrous ion absorption is facilitated by concurrent administration of ascorbic acid (greater than 200 mg orally).[1,2] However, this enhanced absorption of ferrous ion is not usually required in routine treatment of uncomplicated iron deficiency states.

Related Drugs: The absorption of other iron salts (e.g., ferrous fumarate, ferrous gluconate, ferrous lactate) may also be enhanced in the presence of appropriate amounts of ascorbic acid (greater than 200 mg).

Mechanism: Ascorbic acid is thought to increase the absorption of ferrous ion by virtue of its ability to lower pH (and thus increase the solubility of the ferrous ion) and to reduce the ferric ion to the more soluble ferrous ion, which aids in releasing the metal to the gut wall for absorption.[3]

Recommendations: Since the absorption of ferrous salts alone has been shown to be adequate in most humans, there is little justification for concurrent use of ascorbic acid in the treatment of uncomplicated iron deficiency states.[4]

References

1. Lee, P.C., and others: Large and small doses of ascorbic acid in the absorption of ferrous iron, Can. Med. Assoc. J. **97:**181, 1967.
2. Gorten, M.K., and Bradley, J.E.: The treatment of nutritional anemia in infancy and childhood with oral iron and ascorbic acid, J. Pediatr. **45:**1, 1954.
3. Forth, W., and Rummel, W.: Iron absorption, Physiol. Rev. **53:**724, 1973.
4. Cochrane, W.A.: Overnutrition in prenatal and neonatal life: a problem? Can. Med. Assoc. J. **93:**893, 1965.

Folic Acid–Sulfasalazine

3

Summary: One study demonstrated that folate absorption (after oral folic acid administration) was further reduced in patients with inflammatory bowel disease who were taking sulfasalazine.[1]

Related Drugs: Documentation is lacking regarding a similar interaction between folic acid and the other sulfonamides (e.g., sulfadiazine, sulfisoxazole, sulfamethoxazole [see Appendix]); however, based on pharmacologic similarity an interaction may be expected to occur. There are no drugs related to folic acid.

Mechanism: Low serum folate concentration is often observed in patients with ulcerative colitis and Crohn's disease because of impaired absorption, inadequate dietary intake, and increased tissue utilization.[1] However, it is not known how the use of sulfasalazine may further decrease the absorption of folic acid.

Recommendations: In patients with inflammatory bowel disease who require sulfasalazine and folic acid, the administration of folic acid by the parenteral route may avoid this interaction.[1]

Reference

1. Franklin, J.L., and Rosenberg, I.H.: Impaired folic acid absorption in inflammatory bowel disease: effect of salicylazosulfapyridine (Azulfidine), Gastroenterology **64**:517, 1973.

Niacin—Aspirin

3

Summary: The administration of aspirin (975 mg) before niacin administration (2.86 and 5.71 mg/kg) was effective in reducing the flushing response, a common reaction with the use of niacin, especially at high doses. The flushing response was minimal when lower doses of niacin were used alone, and the concurrent effects of aspirin were not considered significant.

Related Drugs: Documentation is lacking regarding a similar interaction with the other salicylates (e.g., choline salicylate, salicylamide, sodium salicylate [see Appendix]). However, if the mechanism is related to prostaglandin synthesis inhibition, then the other salicylates would be expected to interact similarly with niacin since all can inhibit prostaglandins to some extent. There are no drugs related to niacin.

Mechanism: It has been postulated that the flushing response seen with niacin administration is related to prostaglandin liberation rather than a direct effect.[1] If this hypothesis is correct, then aspirin, a known inhibitor of prostaglandin synthesis, would be expected to antagonize this effect of niacin.

Recommendations: Because the niacin-induced flushing may be bothersome to some patients, the concurrent use of aspirin may be beneficial.

Reference

1. Wilkin, J.K., and others: Aspirin blocks nicotinic acid-induced flushing, Clin. Pharmacol. Ther. **31:**478, 1982.

Pyridoxine–Levodopa

Summary: Pyridoxine (vitamin B_6), in doses of 5 mg or more daily, may reduce or abolish the beneficial effects of levodopa in parkinsonism.[1,2]

Related Drugs: There are no drugs related to pyridoxine and levodopa.

Mechanism: Pyridoxine may alter levodopa's metabolism by Schiff-base formation,[3] increased transamination of levodopa,[4] or acceleration of peripheral nonenzymatic conversion of levodopa to dopamine.[1,5] The favored mechanism is acceleration of the peripheral decarboxylation of levodopa by pyridoxine, probably in the gastrointestinal tract.[6,7]

Recommendations: Patients receiving levodopa therapy should avoid products containing more than the pyridoxine dietary allowance (2 mg per day). Patients with conditions causing pyridoxine deficiency (i.e., diabetes mellitus, chronic alcoholism, malnutrition, and malignancy) may be exceptions to this recommendation. Also included as possible exceptions are patients requiring pyridoxine supplementation because of other drug therapy (i.e., those taking isoniazid or cycloserine, penicillamine, and those with cystinuria or heavy metal poisoning). Concurrent use of carbidopa (a peripheral decarboxylase inhibitor) prevents the inhibitory effect of pyridoxine on levodopa[6,8] and is recommended for use in patients receiving pyridoxine supplementation.

References

1. Duvoisin, R.C., and others: Pyridoxine reversal of L-dopa effects in parkinsonism, Trans. Am. Neurol. Assoc. **94:**81, 1969.
2. Calesia, G.G., and Barr, A.N.: Psychosis and other psychiatric manifestations of levodopa therapy, Arch. Neurol. **23:**193, 1970.
3. Evereo, D.F.: L-dopa as a vitamin B_6 antagonist, Lancet **1:**914, 1971.
4. Sourkes, T.L., and Murphy, G.F.: Determination of catecholamines and catecholamino acids by differential spectrophotofluorimetry, Methods Med. Res. **9:**147, 1961.
5. Cotzias, G.C.: Metabolic modification of some neurologic disorders, J.A.M.A. **210:**1255, 1969.
6. Mars, H.: Levodopa, carbidopa and pyridoxine in Parkinsons disease, Arch. Neurol. **30:**44, 1974.
7. Leon, A.S., and others: Pyridoxine antagonism of levodopa in parkinsonism, J.A.M.A. **218:**1924, 1971.
8. Yahr, M.D., and Duvoisin, R.C.: Pyridoxine levodopa and 1-alpha-methyldopa hydrazine regimen in parkinsonism, J.A.M.A. **216:**2141, 1971.

Vitamin A–Neomycin

Summary: One study noted decreased plasma vitamin A levels when oral neomycin was administered concurrently with oral vitamin A.[1] In another study 6 patients showed a decrease in plasma carotene (a provitamin converted to vitamin A in vivo) concentration during the concurrent administration of oral neomycin.[2] After the cessation of oral neomycin, a lapse of up to 5 days may occur before the plasma level of vitamin A increases. A reversible depression of the serum vitamin A concentration in 7 healthy volunteers receiving 2 g neomycin daily for 1 week was demonstrated in another study.[3]

Related Drugs: Isotretinoin, which is chemically related to vitamin A,[4] may also have decreased levels with concurrent neomycin, although no documentation exists. Documentation is also lacking regarding an interaction between vitamin A and the other oral aminoglycosides (kanamycin and paromomycin), although since they are pharmacologically related a similar interaction may be expected.

Mechanism: Neomycin is thought to interfere with the physiologic activity of the bile acids, thereby reducing the uptake of vitamin A. Neomycin can also inhibit pancreatic lipase and can cause morphologic changes in the mucosa of the small intestine, which may interfere with vitamin A absorption.

Recommendations: It may be advisable to monitor patients on concurrent vitamin A and oral neomycin therapy for a decrease in vitamin A levels. An increased vitamin A dose may be necessary.

References

1. Barrowman, J.G., and others: A single dose of neomycin impairs absorption of vitamin A (retenol) in man, Eur. J. Clin. Pharmacol. **5:**199, 1973.
2. Jacobson, E.D., and others: An experimental malabsorption syndrome induced by neomycin, Am. J. Med. **28:**524, 1960.
3. Levine, R.A.: Effect of dietary gluten upon neomycin-induced malabsorption, Gastroenterology **52:**685, 1967.
4. Product Information, Accutane® (isotretinoin), p. 1643, 1983, Physicians Desk Reference.

CHAPTER SEVENTEEN

Xanthine Drug Interactions

TABLE 17. Xanthine Drug Interactions

Drug Interaction	Significance Code	Potential Effects	Recommendations	See Page
Aminophylline–Halothane	1	Concurrent use of these agents may cause cardiac arrhythmias including multiform ventricular tachycardia.	Aminophylline given after halothane appears to reduce the incidence of this interaction. Enflurane may be substituted for halothane since it does not interact with aminophylline.	635
Aminophylline–Ketamine	3	Concurrent use of these agents may precipitate convulsive seizures. The mechanism is unknown since neither drug alone significantly lowers seizure threshold.	Although concurrent use need not be avoided, caution should be observed. Succinylcholine has been successful in resolving this interaction.	637
Aminophylline–Oral Contraceptive Agents	3	Elimination half-life of aminophylline may increase and plasma clearance may decrease in patients receiving oral contraceptives.	Monitor plasma theophylline levels and decrease the aminophylline dosage if necessary.	638
Aminophylline–Thiabendazole	2	Thiabendazole may increase theophylline plasma levels, producing signs of toxicity including nausea, lethargy, and general malaise.	Aminophylline dosage may need to be decreased or another antihelmintic may be considered.	639
Caffeine–Oral Contraceptive Agents	3	Total plasma clearance of a single caffeine dose may be reduced and elimination half-life prolonged in oral contraceptive users.	Concurrent use need not be avoided, but caffeine may need to be reduced if CNS stimulation occurs.	640
Dyphylline–Probenecid	2	Probenecid increases the half-life and decreases the elimination rate constant and total body clearance of dyphylline.	Monitor dyphylline levels and decrease the dosage if necessary.	641
Theophylline–Allopurinol	2	Large doses of allopurinol may decrease theophylline clearance and increase the risk of toxicity. This apparently does not occur with short courses and smaller daily doses of allopurinol.	Monitor theophylline levels and decrease the dose if necessary.	642
Theophylline–Carbamazepine	3	Carbamazepine may decrease theophylline half-life, resulting in subtherapeutic levels and possible worsening of clinical condition.	Monitor patients and increase the theophylline dose if necessary.	643

Abbreviations: CNS, central nervous system; GI, gastrointestinal.

TABLE 17. Xanthine Drug Interactions—cont'd

Drug Interaction	Significance Code	Potential Effects	Recommendations	See Page
Theophylline–Charcoal	2	Activated charcoal limits the absorption of both uncoated and slow release oral theophylline preparations.	Theophylline overdose can be treated with 5:1 charcoal:theophylline within 1 hour of drug ingestion. If charcoal is not to be used in this situation, increase the theophylline dose or separate the administration of these agents by as much time as possible.	644
Theophylline–Cimetidine	1	Cimetidine impairs the elimination of theophylline, increasing the plasma concentration, and elimination half-life, and decreasing clearance.	Monitor theophylline blood levels closely and consider reducing the theophylline dosage. Ranitidine may be a more judicious choice instead of cimetidine since it does not influence theophylline disposition.	645
Theophylline–Erythromycin	1	Concurrent use of these agents for at least 5 days may increase serum theophylline concentrations and reduce erythromycin concentrations after the 5th day of cotherapy. Conflicting reports may be due to patient status.	Monitor theophylline levels throughout cotherapy.	647
Theophylline–Furosemide	3	Furosemide increased serum theophylline level in adults, whereas levels decreased by the same magnitude in premature neonates.	Monitor theophylline levels. Separate the dosing of these agents by as much time as possible.	650
Theophylline–Hydrocortisone	3	Hydrocortisone may increase theophylline levels, although some studies failed to show any effect.	A reduced theophylline dose may be necessary.	651
Theophylline–Influenza Virus Vaccine	2	The administration of influenza vaccine may increase theophylline half-life and decrease its clearance, although other reports are conflicting and report no effect.	Monitor patients for signs of theophylline toxicity and temporarily decrease the dosage if needed.	652
Theophylline–Phenobarbital	2	Phenobarbital may increase the clearance of theophylline and thus reduce theophylline serum levels.	Monitor theophylline plasma levels closely and increase the dosage if needed.	654
Theophylline–Phenytoin	2	Phenytoin may decrease the half-life and increase clearance of theophylline. Phenytoin levels may also be decreased.	It is important to monitor levels of both drugs and adjust the dosages as needed.	655

633

TABLE 17. Xanthine Drug Interactions—cont'd

Drug Interaction	Significance Code	Potential Effects	Recommendations	See Page
Theophylline–Propranolol	2	Propranolol may significantly reduce the clearance and elimination half-life of theophylline. It antagonizes the pharmacologic action of theophylline on bronchial musculature and increases bronchial resistance.	Monitor theophylline levels closely and adjust the dosage if needed.	656
Theophylline–Tetracycline	3	Increased incidence of side effects were reported in 1 study after concurrent use of these agents, although other studies report no effect. Both agents may cause GI complaints, which may be a summation rather than a kinetic interaction. Theophylline half-life may increase and body clearance may decrease, but this may not be statistically significant with respect to kinetic variables.	These agents need not be avoided; however, theophylline levels should be monitored during concurrent therapy.	657
Theophylline–Tobacco	1	Smoking enhances theophylline elimination, which reduces serum concentrations, shortens half-life, and increases total body clearance of theophylline.	Theophylline dosage may need to be adjusted in smokers or those who quit smoking during therapy.	658
Theophylline–Verapamil	3	Verapamil initiated in a patient stabilized on theophylline caused doubling of theophylline serum concentrations and clinical manifestations of toxicity.	Monitor patients for increased theophylline levels and decrease the dosage if needed.	660

Aminophylline–Halothane

1

Summary: The concurrent use of halothane and aminophylline may lead to cardiac arrhythmias. This was shown to occur in 2 asthmatic patients who developed multiform ventricular tachycardia after concomitant use of these agents.[1] Similar results have been shown to occur in several animal studies.[2-6] However, these studies suggest that the incidence of arrhythmias may be affected by the order that these drugs are administered. Even with nontoxic theophylline levels, the incidence of arrhythmias increases when aminophylline is administered before halothane.[2] Conversely, when aminophylline is administered during halothane anesthesia, the chance of arrhythmias is unlikely unless toxic levels of theophylline are present.[3,4]

Related Drugs: Documentation is lacking regarding an interaction between halothane and the other theophylline derivatives (dyphylline, oxtriphylline, and theophylline), although since they are pharmacologically related, a similar interaction may be expected to occur. An animal study showed that aminophylline administered before enflurane anesthesia did not induce cardiac arrhythmias.[7,8] Documentation is lacking regarding an interaction between aminophylline and the other halogenated inhalation anesthetics (isoflurane and methoxyflurane).

Mechanism: The exact mechanism of this interaction is unknown. However, aminophylline exerts its effect on cardiac muscle partly by its release of cardiac catecholamines and in part by inhibition of phosphodiesterase and enhancement of the cyclic AMP system. Halothane has been reported to cause effects compatible with the activation of adenyl cyclase and cyclic AMP. Therefore, it has been postulated that halothane potentiates the arrhythmogenic effects of aminophylline by the same metabolic pathway.[1,3]

Recommendations: Although some believe there is a wide margin of safety associated with the concurrent use of these agents,[9] caution should be observed since arrhythmias have been reported. It appears that the use of aminophylline after halothane anesthesia reduces the incidence of this interaction.[3,4] Alternatively, the use of a noninteracting anesthetic agent such as enflurane may be considered.[7]

References

1. Roizen, M.F., and Stevens, W.C.: Multiform ventricular tachycardia due to the interaction of aminophylline and halothane, Anesth. Analg. (Cleve.) **57:**738, 1978.
2. Stirt, J.A., and others: Halothane-induced cardiac arrhythmias following administration of aminophylline in experimental animals, Anesth. Analg. (Cleve.) **60:**517, 1981.
3. Stirt, J.A., and others: Arrhythmogenic effects of aminophylline during halothane anesthesia in experimental animals, Anesth. Analg. (Cleve.) **59:**410, 1980.
4. Stirt, J.A., and others: Aminophylline pharmacokinetics and cardiorespiratory effects during halothane anesthesia in experimental animals, Anesth. Analg. (Cleve.) **59:**186, 1980.
5. Takaori, M., and Loehning, R.W.: Ventricular arrhythmias induced by aminophylline during halothane anaesthesia in dogs, Can. Anaesth. Soc. J. **14:**79, 1967.
6. Takaori, M., and Loehning, R.W.: Ventricular arrhythmias during halothane anaesthesia: effect of isoproterenol, aminophylline, and ephedrine, Can. Anaesth. Soc. J. **12:**275, 1965.

7. Stirt, J.A., and others: Safety of enflurane following administration of aminophylline in experimental animals, Anesth. Analg. (Cleve.) **60:**871, 1981.

8. Berger, J.M., and others: Enflurane, halothane and aminophylline uptake and pharmacokinetics, Anesth. Analg. (Cleve.) **67:**733, 1983.

9. Zimmerman, B.L.: Arrhythmogenicity of theophylline and halothane used in combination, Anesth. Analg. (Cleve.) **58:**259, 1979.

Aminophylline–Ketamine

3

Summary: Four cases were reported that implied that maintenance aminophylline administration and ketamine given before surgery could precipitate convulsive seizures.[1] However, all patients were receiving other anesthetics, making a clear cause and effect relationship difficult to determine. In animals, it was shown that combined administration of these agents did reduce the minimal electroshock seizure threshold.[1]

Related Drugs: There are no drugs related to ketamine. Documentation is lacking regarding a similar interaction with the other theophylline derivatives (dyphylline, oxtriphylline, and theophylline).

Mechanism: The mechanism of this interaction is unknown. However, neither drug used alone significantly lowers seizure threshold.[1]

Recommendations: The concurrent use of these agents need not be avoided; however, caution should be used. The administration of succinylcholine was successful in resolving the interaction.[1]

Reference

1. Hirshman, C.A., and others: Ketamine-aminophylline-induced decrease in seizure threshold, Anesthesiology **56:**464, 1982.

Aminophylline–Oral Contraceptive Agents

Summary: In a controlled study involving 16 females, the aminophylline plasma clearance decreased and the elimination half-life increased in the 8 women taking oral contraceptives as compared to the 8 nonusers after the administration of a single dose of aminophylline.[1]

Related Drugs: In 1 study involving 100 patients, a reduced theophylline clearance was associated with oral contraceptive use in smokers. However, since this was a prospective study, no direct cause and effect could be established.[2] The other theophylline derivative metabolized by the liver (oxtriphylline) may be expected to interact similarly, although no documentation exists. Dyphylline, a theophylline derivative that is not converted to theophylline in vivo, is not metabolized by the liver and is rapidly removed from the blood by glomerular filtration or active secretion, or both, and approximately 82% is excreted unchanged in the urine.[3,4] This is in contrast to theophylline, which is extensively metabolized by the liver. Therefore, dyphylline would not be expected to interact with oral contraceptive agents.

Mechansim: It has been suggested that oral contraceptive agents inhibit the metabolism of aminophylline.

Recommendations: Plasma theophylline levels should be monitored during concurrent use of aminophylline and oral contraceptive agents. If theophylline levels are increased, a lower dose of aminophylline may be necessary.

References

1. Tornatore, K.M., and others: Effect of chronic oral contraceptive steroids on theophylline disposition, Eur. J. Clin. Pharmacol. **23:**129, 1982.
2. Jusko, W.J., and others: Factors effecting theophylline clearance: age, tobacco, marijuana, cirrhosis, congestive heart failure, obesity, oral contraceptives, benzodiazepines, barbiturates, and ethanol, J. Pharm. Sci. **68:**1358, 1979.
3. Gisclon, L.G., et al.: Pharmacokinetics of orally administered dyphylline, Am. J. Hosp. Pharm. **36:**1179, 1979.
4. Simons, K.J., and Simons, F.E.K.: Urinary excretion of dyphylline in humans, J. Pharm. Sci. **68:**1327, 1979.

Aminophylline–Thiabendazole

2

Summary: In a single case report, a patient maintained on aminophylline received thiabendazole for *Strongyloides*. During the second course of thiabendazole, the patient suffered severe nausea, lethargy, and general malaise, and his theophylline levels rose from 21 μg/ml to 46 μg/ml (while receiving aminophylline infusion). The aminophylline infusion was stopped, but 18 hours later theophylline levels were still 36 μg/ml. When thiabendazole was discontinued, oral aminophylline resulted in serum levels of 16 μg/ml. Although the patient was receiving other maintenance drugs as well, theophylline levels increased only after the introduction of thiabendazole.[1]

Related Drugs: A similar interaction may be expected between thiabendazole and the other theophylline derivatives (oxtriphylline and theophylline) based on a similar metabolic fate, although documentation is lacking. Dyphylline, in contrast to the other theophylline derivatives, is not converted to theophylline in vivo, is not metabolized by the liver, and is rapidly removed from the blood by glomerular filtration, active secretion, or both, and approximately 82% is excreted unchanged in the urine.[2,3] Therefore, if the mechanism involves hepatic inhibition by thiabendazole, dyphylline would not be expected to interact similarly. There are no drugs related to thiabendazole.

Mechanism: It has been suggested that thiabendazole inhibits the hepatic microsomal enzymes responsible for aminophylline's metabolism.[1]

Recommendations: Theophylline levels should be closely monitored during concomitant use of these agents. The dose of aminophylline may need to be decreased or another anthelmintic may be considered.

References

1. Sugar, A.M., and others: Possible thiabendazole-induced theophylline toxicity? Am. Rev. Resp. Dis. **122:**501, 1980.
2. Gisclon, L.G., and others: Pharmacokinetics of orally administered dyphylline, Am. J. Hosp. Pharm. **36:**1179, 1979.
3. Simons, K.J., and Simons, F.E.K.: Urinary excretion of dyphylline in humans, J. Pharm. Sci. **68:**1327, 1979.

Caffeine–Oral Contraceptive Agents

Summary: The total plasma clearance of a single dose of caffeine was reduced and its elimination half-life prolonged in 9 women taking oral contraceptive agents as compared to 9 women not taking oral contraceptives.[1] The clinical significance of this interaction was not determined.

Related Drugs: There are no drugs related to caffeine.

Mechanism: The mechanism of this interaction is unknown; however, it has been suggested that oral contraceptive agents may inhibit the hepatic metabolism of caffeine.

Recommendations: The concurrent use of these agents need not be avoided. However, if central nervous system stimulation appears, the dose of caffeine may need to be decreased.

Reference

1. Pativardhan, R.V., and others: Impaired elimination of caffeine by oral contraceptive steroids, J. Lab. Clin. Med. **95:**603, 1980.

Dyphylline–Probenecid

2

Summary: The concurrent administration of probenecid and dyphylline has been shown in 2 studies to result in an increase in the half-life of dyphylline, a decrease in the elimination rate constant, a decrease in total body clearance, and no significant change in volume of distribution.[1,2]

Related Drugs: One study with aminophylline showed that concurrent use of probenecid had no significant effect on any of the pharmacokinetic parameters measured (half-life, total body clearance, volume of distribution, etc.).[3] Although documentation is lacking, the same results may be expected when probenecid is used with theophylline and the other theophylline derivative, oxtriphylline, since, like aminophylline, they are also hepatically metabolized. In a study involving 6 subjects the concurrent use of sulfinpyrazone and theophylline resulted in a 22% increase in total plasma theophylline clearance.[4]

Mechanism: Dyphylline is rapidly removed from the blood by glomerular filtration or active secretion, or both, and approximately 82% is excreted unchanged in the urine.[1] It has been suggested that probenecid, which inhibits the renal transport of some compounds, also inhibits the renal elimination of dyphylline.[1,2] In addition to renal transport inhibition, probenecid has also been shown to inhibit the uptake of certain compounds by the liver.[3] Aminophylline, in contrast to dyphylline, is extensively metabolized by the liver, and probenecid has little or no influence on the metabolism of aminophylline.[3]

Recommendations: Dyphylline, although not as potent as some other theophylline salts, also has less incidence of toxic side effects.[1-3] Therefore, this interaction may be of greater clinical importance in aminophylline-sensitive patients. If a patient is currently on dyphylline therapy and probenecid is added, the patient should be monitored for increased dyphylline levels (not detectable by theophylline assays) and a decrease in the dosage of dyphylline may be necessary.

References

1. May, D.C., and Jarboe, C.H.: Effect of probenecid on dyphylline elimination, Clin. Pharmacol. Ther. **33:**822, 1983.
2. May, D.C., and Jarboe, C.H.: Inhibition of clearance of dyphylline by probenecid, N. Engl. J. Med. **304:**791, 1981.
3. Chen, T.W.D., and Patton, T.F.: Effect of probenecid on the pharmacokinetics of aminophylline, Drug Intell. Clin. Pharm. **17:**465, 1983.
4. Birkett, D.J., and others: Evidence for a dual action of sulphinpyrazone on drug metabolism in man: theophylline-sulfinpyrazone interaction, Br. J. Clin. Pharmacol. **15:**567, 1983.

Theophylline–Allopurinol

Summary: Allopurinol may decrease theophylline clearance and increase the risk of toxocity.[1] Decreased metabolism of theophylline has been noted only with large doses of allopurinol (600 mg per day) given over at least 2 weeks. Shorter courses and smaller daily doses of allopurinol have not decreased theophylline clearances.[2,3]

Related Drugs: No interaction has been described between allopurinol and other theophylline derivatives (aminophylline and oxtriphylline). However, because of similar metabolic pathways, a similar interaction may be expected. Dyphylline, a theophylline derivative that is not converted to theophylline in vivo, is not metabolized by the liver and is rapidly removed from the blood by glomerular filtration, active secretion, or both, and approximately 82% is excreted unchanged in the urine.[4,5] This is in contrast to theophylline, which is extensively metabolized by the liver. Therefore, dyphylline would not be expected to interact with allopurinol. There are no drugs related to allopurinol.

Mechanism: It is speculated that allopurinol inhibits hepatic drug metabolizing enzymes.[1] Specific mechanisms are yet to be elucidated.

Recommendations: Large daily doses of allopurinol may decrease theophylline clearance when both drugs are used for longer than 2 weeks. Since increases in serum theophylline concentrations of 25% have been reported, some patients may require monitoring for signs of possible theophylline toxicity and may need lower doses during concurrent allopurinol therapy.

References

1. Manfredi, R.L., and Vesell, E.S.: Inhibition of theophylline metabolism by long-term allopurinol administration, Clin. Pharmacol. Ther. **29:**224, 1981.
2. Grygiel, J.J., and others: Effects of allopurinol on theophylline metabolism and clearance, Clin. Pharmacol. Ther. **26:**660, 1979.
3. Vozeh, S., and others: Influence of allopurinol on theophylline disposition in adults, Clin. Pharmacol. Ther. **27:**194, 1980.
4. Gisclon, L.G., and others: Pharmacokinetics of orally administered dyphylline, Am. J. Hosp. Pharm. **36:**1179, 1979.
5. Simons, K.J., and Simons, F.E.K.: Urinary excretion of dyphylline in humans, J. Pharm. Sci. **68:**1327, 1979.

Theophylline–Carbamazepine

3

Summary: In a case report an asthmatic child was maintained on theophylline and phenobarbital. When the phenobarbital was replaced with carbamazepine, the theophylline levels became subtherapeutic and the half-life was markedly decreased after 3 weeks of concurrent therapy, resulting in worsening of the patient's clinical condition. When carbamazepine was changed to ethotoin, within 3 weeks the patient's asthma was controlled and the half-life of theophylline increased.[1]

Related Drugs: There are no drugs related to carbamazepine. A similar interaction may be expected between carbamazepine and the other theophylline derivatives that are hepatically metabolized (aminophylline and oxtriphylline). Dyphylline, a theophylline derivative that is not converted to theophylline in vivo, is not metabolized by the liver and is rapidly removed from the blood by glomerular filtration, active secretion, or both, and approximately 82% is excreted unchanged in the urine.[2,3] This is in contrast to theophylline, which is extensively metabolized by the liver. Therefore, if the mechanism of this interaction results from increased hepatic metabolism of theophylline, dyphylline would not be expected to interact with carbamazepine.

Mechanism: The mechanism of this interaction remains to be defined. However, it has been suggested that the hepatic metabolism of theophylline is increased by carbamazepine.

Recommendations: Patients should be monitored for subtherapeutic theophylline levels when theophylline and carbamazepine are used concurrently. A higher dose of theophylline may be necessary, or a noninteracting anticonvulsant may be considered.

References

1. Rosenberry, K.R., and others: Reduced theophylline half-life induced by carbamazepine therapy, J. Pediatr. **102:**472, 1983.
2. Gisclon, L.G., et al.: Pharmacokinetics of orally administered dyphylline, Am. J. Hosp. Pharm. **36:**1179, 1979.
3. Simons, K.J., and Simons, F.E.K.: Urinary excretion of dyphylline in humans, J. Pharm. Sci. **68:**1327, 1979.

Theophylline–Charcoal

Summary: Activated charcoal has been shown to limit the absorption of both uncoated and slow-release oral theophylline preparations.[1,2] In a study involving 5 patients, activated charcoal was administered 30 minutes after ingestion of uncoated oral theophylline tablets, and only 40% of the administered dose of theophylline was absorbed.[1] In a similar study 6 volunteers were administered activated charcoal 1 hour after ingestion of a slow-release theophylline, and the mean plasma level of theophylline was reduced 39%.[2]

Related Drugs: Other oral theophylline derivatives (aminophylline, dyphylline, and oxtriphylline) may also be adsorbed by activated charcoal; however, documentation is lacking.

Mechanism: Activated charcoal adsorbs oral theophylline, thereby limiting its absorption from the gastrointestinal tract.[2]

Recommendations: It has been suggested that a dose of 5 : 1 charcoal : theophylline can be used in the treatment of theophylline overdose. The activated charcoal should be given within 1 hour of theophylline administration, if possible, to effectively limit theophylline absorption.[2] However, if charcoal is not to be used to treat theophylline overdose, a higher dose of theophylline or separating the administration of theophylline and charcoal by as much time as possible is necessary.

References

1. Sintek, C., and others: Inhibition of theophylline absorption by activated charcoal, J. Pediatr. **94:**314, 1979.
2. Helliwell, M., and Berry, D.: Theophylline absorption by effervescent activated charcoal, J. Int. Med. Res. **9:**222, 1981.

Theophylline–Cimetidine

Summary: It is well documented that cimetidine impairs the elimination of theophylline when the 2 agents are co-administered to patients.[1-20] Reports indicate theophylline plasma concentrations increase as the elimination half-life of theophylline is prolonged from 36.2% to 73%[1-6,10,13,14] and theophylline clearance is decreased by 18.5% to 40%.[2-4,6,10,13,14,17] Significant changes can be seen within 24 hours[6,8] and may progress as co-therapy continues.[6] One report found no interaction in elderly female patients,[21] but several concerns about that report have been published.[22-26]

Related Drugs: A study involving 10 healthy patients demonstrated that concomitant administration of cimetidine significantly decreased the plasma clearance of oxtriphylline.[26] Since aminophylline exhibits the same pathway of metabolism as theophylline (hepatic metabolism), it may also be involved in a similar interaction. On the other hand, dyphylline, a theophylline derivative that is not converted to theophylline in vivo and is not involved in hepatic metabolism would therefore not be expected to interact with cimetidine. In 1 report cimetidine also decreased the clearance and prolonged the half-life of caffeine.[27] Two reports state that ranitidine does not influence theophylline disposition[14,28]; however, 1 case study reported serum theophylline levels in the toxic range in a patient after concurrent ranitidine. Tachycardia, mild confusion, and anxiety developed within 36 hours of concomitant therapy, and symptoms resolved when the theophylline dosage was decreased from 600 mg every 8 hours to 450 mg every 8 hours.[29]

Mechanism: It is believed that cimetidine or one of its metabolites inhibits the hepatic microsomal mono-oxygenase system involving both the P-450 and P-448 systems.[2,4, 6-11,14,19] This inhibition may result from the binding of cimetidine either to the enzyme systems or to theophylline, which forms a complex that interrupts metabolism.[8] The duration of cimetidine's inhibitory action is uncertain. It appears to reverse rapidly after cimetidine discontinuation in short-term therapy[4] but may persist in prolonged therapy.

Recommendations: Since this seems to be an established interaction, theophylline blood levels should be very closely monitored if cimetidine therapy is to be initiated, changed, or discontinued. Since theophylline has a narrow therapeutic range, dosage reductions up to 30% to 50%[7] should be considered to prevent intoxication when cimetidine therapy is started. Antacids or ranitidine might be more judicious choices than cimetidine in patients receiving theophylline.

References

1. Jackson, J.E., and others: Cimetidine-theophylline interaction, Pharmacologist **22:**231, 1980.
2. Roberts, R.K., and others: Cimetidine impairs the elimination of theophylline and antipyrine, Gastroenterology **81:**19, 1981.
3. Wood, L., and others: Effects of cimetidine on the disposition of theophylline, Aust. N. Z. J. Med. **10:**586, 1980.

4. Campbell, M.A., and others: Cimetidine decreases theophylline clearance, Ann. Intern. Med. **95:**68, 1981.
5. Weinberger, M.M., and others: Decreased theophylline clearance due to cimetidine, N. Engl. J. Med. **304:**672, 1981.
6. Reitberg, D.P., and others: Alteration of theophylline clearance and half-life by cimetidine in normal volunteers, Ann. Intern. Med. **95:**582, 1981.
7. Bauman, J.H., and others: Cimetidine-theophylline interaction: report of four patients, Ann. Allergy **48:**100, 1982.
8. Cluxton, R.J., and others: Cimetidine-theophylline interaction, Ann. Intern. Med. **96:**684, 1982.
9. Fenje, P.C., and others: Interaction of cimetidine and theophylline in two infants, Can. Med. Assoc. J. **126:**1178, 1982.
10. Jackson, J.E., and others: Cimetidine decreases theophylline clearance, Am. Rev. Resp. Dis. **123:**615, 1981.
11. Lalonde, R.L., and others: The effects of cimetidine on theophylline pharmacokinetics at steady state, Chest **83:**221, 1983.
12. Lofgren, R.P., and Gilhertson, R.A.: Cimetidine and theophylline, Ann. Intern. Med. **96:**378, 1982.
13. Lalonde, R.L., and others: Influence of cimetidine on theophylline pharmacokinetics at steady-state, Clin. Pharmacol. Ther. **31:**241, 1982.
14. Powell, J.R., and others: The influence of cimetidine vs. ranitidine on theophylline pharmacokinetics, Clin. Pharmacol. Ther. **31:**261, 1982.
15. Kelly, J.F., and others: The effect of cimetidine on theophylline metabolism in the elderly, Clin. Pharmacol. Ther. **31:**238, 1982.
16. Bauman, J.H., and Fuentes, R.J.: Cimetidine impairs the elimination of theophylline and antipyrine, Gastroenterology **82:**601, 1982.
17. Roberts, R., and others: Cimetidine impairs the elimination of theophylline and antipyrine (reply), Gastroenterology **82:**602, 1982.
18. Anderson, J.R., and others: A fatal case of theophylline intoxication, Arch. Intern. Med. **143:**559, 1983.
19. Schwartz, J.I., and others: Impact of cimetidine on the pharmacokinetics of theophylline, Clin. Pharm. **1:**534, 1982.
20. Roberts, R.K., and others: Cimetidine-theophylline interaction with chronic obstructive airways disease, Med. J. Aust. **140:**279, 1984.
21. Ambrose, P.J., and Harralson, A.F.: Lack of effect of cimetidine on theophylline clearance, Drug Intell. Clin. Pharm. **15:**389, 1981.
22. Bauman, J.H., and Kimelblatt, B.J.: Comment on effect of cimetidine on theophylline clearance, Drug Intell. Clin. Pharm. **15:**808, 1981.
23. Hendeles, L., and others: The interaction of cimetidine and theophylline, Drug Intell. Clin. Pharm. **15:**808, 1981.
24. Jackson, J.E., and Plachetka, J.R.: More on cimetidine-theophylline interaction, Drug Intell. Clin. Pharm. **15:**809, 1981.
25. Ambrose, P.J., and Harralson, A.F.: More on cimetidine-theophylline interaction (reply), Drug Intell. Clin. Pharm. **15:**810, 1981.
26. DeAngelis, C., and others: Effect of low-dose cimetidine on theophylline metabolism, Clin. Pharm. **2:**563, 1983.
27. Broughton, L.J., and Rogers, H.J.: Decreased systemic clearance of caffeine due to cimetidine, Br. J. Clin. Pharmacol. **12:**155, 1981.
28. Breen, K.J., and others: Effects of cimetidine and ranitidine on hepatic drug metabolism, Clin. Pharmacol. Ther. **31:**297, 1982.
29. Fernandes, E., and Melewicz, F.M.: Ranitidine and theophylline, Ann. Intern. Med. **100:**459, 1984.

Theophylline–Erythromycin

1

Summary: Concurrent administration of erythromycin and theophylline for at least 5 days has increased serum theophylline concentrations approximately 2-fold, which required a reduction in theophylline dosage.[1-22]

There are conflicting reports regarding this interaction[23-29]; it may result from a short duration of erythromycin administration, the bioavailability of the erythromycin salt used, smoking habits, age, or disease state of the study population.

The concurrent use of these agents has been reported to have led to a 63% reduction in the mean steady-state serum erythromycin concentrations on the fifth day of co-therapy.[7]

Related Drugs: The interaction has been shown to occur with erythromycin base, ethylsuccinate, and stearate.[1,3,9] Troleandomycin, another macrolide antibiotic, produced a 2-fold increase in serum theophylline concentrations.[30-32] Other theophylline derivatives, aminophylline[8,22,23] and oxitryphylline,[3] have also been shown to interact with erythromycin. Dyphylline, a theophylline derivative that is not converted to theophylline in vivo, is not metabolized by the liver and is rapidly removed from the blood by glomerular filtration or active secretion, or both, and approximately 82% is excreted unchanged in the urine.[33,34] This is in contrast to theophylline, which is extensively metabolized by the liver. Therefore, dyphylline would not be expected to interact with erythromycin.

Mechanism: The mechanism is not clearly established. Theophylline is metabolized to a significant degree, and the evidence would be consistent with erythromycin blocking one or more of the metabolic pathways of theophylline. This has been found to be the case in animal studies.[35,36]

The mechanism by which theophylline lowers erythromycin levels is not known.

Recommendations: Patients receiving theophylline should be closely monitored for theophylline toxicity when concomitant erythromycin is initiated. Some practitioners have suggested that theophylline dosage be lowered by 25% when beginning concurrent erythromycin; however, this may lead to subtherapeutic theophylline levels in patients who have low theophylline plasma levels. It would also be expected that theophylline levels would fall if erythromycin therapy is discontinued.

The clinical significance of the decreased erythromycin bioavailability has not been established. Clinicians should be aware that erythromycin may fail therapeutically when these agents are used together.

References

1. Zarowitz, B.J.M., and others: Effect of erythromycin base on theophylline kinetics, Clin. Pharmacol. Ther. **29:**601, 1981.
2. Renton, K.W., and others: Depression of human theophylline metabolism by erythromycin, Pharmacologist **23:**194, 1981.

3. Renton, K.W., and others: Depression of theophylline elimination by erythromycin, Clin. Pharmacol. Ther. **30:**422, 1981.
4. Walker, J., and Hendeles, L.: The interaction of erythromycin and theophylline in the asthmatic dental patient, J. Am. Dent. Assoc. **99:**995, 1979.
5. Prince, R.A., and others: Effect of erythromycin on theophylline kinetics, J. Allergy Clin. Immunol. **68:**427, 1981.
6. Prince, R.A., and others: The effect of erythromycin on theophylline kinetics, Drug Intell. Clin. Pharm. **14:**637, 1980.
7. Iliopoulou, A., and others: Pharmacokinetic interaction between theophylline and erythromycin, Br. J. Clin. Pharmacol. **14:**495, 1982.
8. Branigan, T.A., and others: The effects of erythromycin on the absorption and disposition kinetics of theophylline, Eur. J. Clin. Pharmacol. **21:**115, 1981.
9. LaForce, C.F., and others: Effect of erythromycin on theophylline clearance in asthmatic children, J. Pediatr. **99:**153, 1981.
10. Pfeifer, H.J., and others: Effect of antibiotics on theophylline kinetics in humans, Clin. Pharmacol. Ther. **23:**124, 1978.
11. May, D.C., and others: The effects of erythromycin on theophylline elimination in normal males, J. Clin. Pharmacol. **22:**125, 1982.
12. Reisz, G.R., and others: Erythromycin induced changes in theophylline kinetics in chronic bronchitis, Am. Rev. Resp. Dis. **125**(suppl.):95, 1982.
13. Richer, C., and others: Theophylline kinetics and ventilatory flow in bronchial asthma and chronic airflow obstruction: influence of erythromycin, Clin. Pharmacol. Ther. **31:**579, 1982.
14. Kozak, P.P., and others: Administration of erythromycin to patients on theophylline, J. Allergy Clin. Immunol. **60:**149, 1977.
15. Kozak, P.P., and others: Interaction between erythromycin and theophylline, Pediatrics **61:**325, 1978.
16. Cummins, L.H., and others: Erythromycin's effect on theophylline blood level, Pediatrics **59:**144, 1977.
17. Cummins, L.H., and others: Theophylline determinations, Ann. Allergy **37:**450, 1976.
18. Murray, M.D., and Brown, B.K.: Theophylline-erythromycin interaction in an infant, Clin. Pharm. **1:**107, 1982.
19. Stults, B.M., and others: Effect of erythromycin stearate on serum theophylline concentration in patients with chronic obstructive lung disease, South. Med. J. **76:**714, 1983.
20. Stratton, M.A.: Theophylline-erythromycin base interaction: case report and kinetic profile, Clin. Pharm. **2:**183, 1983.
21. Parish, R.A., and others: Interaction of theophylline with erythromycin base in a patient with seizure activity, Pediatrics **72:**828, 1983.
22. Green, J.A., and Clementi, W.A.: Decrease in theophylline clearance after the administration of erythromycin to a patient with obstructive lung disease, Drug Intell. Clin. Pharm. **17:**370, 1983.
23. Pfeifer, H.J., and others: Effects of three antibiotics on theophylline kinetics, Clin. Pharmacol. Ther. **26:**36, 1979.
24. Stults, B.M., and others: The effect of oral erythromycin on serum levels of theophylline in patients with chronic obstructive pulmonary disease, Am. Rev. Resp. Dis. **123**(suppl.):105, 1981.
25. Pingleton, S.K., and others: Lack of effect of erythromycin on theophylline serum levels, Chest **78:**352, 1980.
26. Kimelblatt, B.J., and Slaughter, R.L.: Lack of effect of intravenous erythromycin lactobionate on theophylline clearance, J. Allergy Clin. Immunol. **65:**313, 1980.
27. Maddux, M., and others: Erythromycin alteration of theophylline pharmacokinetics: lack of effect at steady state, Am. Rev. Resp. Dis. **123**(suppl.):60, 1981.
28. Maddux, M., and others: Effect of erythromycin on theophylline pharmacokinetics at steady state, Chest **81:**563, 1982.
29. Melethel, S., and others: Steady state urinary excretion of theophylline and its metabolites in the presence of erythromycin, Res. Commun. Chem. Pathol. Pharmacol. **35:**341, 1982.
30. Weinberger, M., and others: Troleandomycin (TAO): an inhibitor of theophylline metabolism, J. Allergy Clin. Immunol. **57:**262, 1976.

31. Weinberger, M., and others: Effect of triacetyloleandomycin (TAO) on the metabolism of theophylline, Clin. Pharmacol. Ther. **19:**118, 1976.
32. Weinberger, M., and others: Inhibition of theophylline clearance by troleandomycin, J. Allergy Clin. Immunol. **59:**228, 1977.
33. Gisclon, L.G., and others: Pharmacokinetics of orally administered dyphylline, Am. J. Hosp. Pharm. **36:**1179, 1979.
34. Simons, K.J., and Simons, F.E.K.: Urinary excretion of dyphylline in humans, J. Pharm. Sci. **68:**1327, 1979.
35. Hemsworth, T.C., and Renton, K.W.: Depression of theophylline metabolism and elimination by troleandomycin and erythromycin, Biochem. Pharmacol. **30:**1299, 1981.
36. Reisz, G., and others: The effect of erythromycin on theophylline pharmacokinetics in chronic bronchitis, Am. Rev. Respir. Dis. **127:**581, 1983.

Theophylline–Furosemide

3

Summary: Two reports have shown opposite effects of furosemide on the steady-state serum concentrations of theophylline.[1,2] In 10 adult patients, serum theophylline levels (from aminophylline) increased approximately 3 μg/ml within 4 hours of intravenous furosemide.[1] Theophylline levels fell 2 to 3 μg/ml in 4 premature neonates receiving either oral or intravenous furosemide when administered within 30 minutes of theophylline.[2]

Related Drugs: No reports are available of an interaction between furosemide and the theophylline derivative oxtriphylline, although a similar effect may be expected. Dyphylline, a theophylline derivative that is not converted to theophylline in vivo and does not undergo hepatic metabolism, has not been shown to interact with furosemide. There is no documentation regarding an interaction between theophylline and the other loop diuretics (bumetanide and ethacrynic acid); however, based on pharmacologic similarity an interaction may be expected to occur.

Mechanism: The mechanism is not known, but several factors may be involved. Furosemide may decrease theophylline's volume of distribution associated with diuresis in adults,[1] or it may decrease hepatic congestion,[3] thereby increasing theophylline clearance in neonates.[2] In addition, furosemide can displace theophylline from serum proteins in vitro.[4]

The opposite effect of furosemide on theophylline disposition is most likely the result of the many physiologic parameters (protein binding, binding affinity, body water distribution) that are different in adults and premature infants. It is well established that theophylline clearance is age dependent.

Recommendations: The data suggest that age-graded studies are required to fully elucidate the specificity of this interaction. The limited reports do show a clinically significant change in serum theophylline concentrations, and patients may need to be monitored during chronic co-therapy with furosemide. Separating the dosing of these agents as much as possible may be useful, since no interaction occurred when they were administered at least 2 hours apart.[2]

References

1. Conlon, P.F., and others: Effect of intravenous furosemide on serum theophylline concentration, Am. J. Hosp. Pharm. **38:**1345, 1981.
2. Toback, J.W., and Gilman, M.E.: Theophylline-furosemide inactivation, Pediatrics **71:**140, 1983.
3. Nakagawa, R.S.: Theophylline-furosemide interaction, Am. J. Hosp. Pharm. **39:**242, 1982.
4. Shaw, L.M., and others: Factors influencing theophylline serum protein binding, Clin. Pharmacol. Ther. **32:**490, 1982.

Theophylline–Hydrocortisone

3

Summary: In a study involving 3 patients with status asthmaticus maintained on theophylline, the concurrent administration of hydrocortisone resulted in increased theophylline levels, which elevated to between 40 and 50 μg/ml. Two of these patients complained of nausea and headache. No change in serum theophylline concentrations was observed in the control patient who received saline in place of hydrocortisone.[1] Two other studies, however, failed to show any effect of hydrocortisone on theophylline levels.[2,3] In 1 of these studies, theophylline clearance was 21% higher after a hydrocortisone injection.[3]

Related Drugs: In a study involving 7 healthy volunteers, an intravenous injection of methylprednisolone had no significant effect on theophylline serum levels.[3] Theophylline has also been reported not to interact with dexamethasone.[4] The mean relative bioavailability of theophylline (from aminophylline) was not significantly affected by concomitant oral prednisone administration in 6 healthy subjects. However, mean plasma concentrations for both theophylline and prednisone were lower.[5] Because of lack of consistent data, it is not known whether theophylline would interact with other corticosteroids (e.g., betamethasone, fluprednisolone, triamcinolone [see Appendix]). Documentation is also lacking regarding an interaction between hydrocortisone and the other theophylline derivatives (aminophylline, dyphylline, and oxtriphylline). If the mechanism for the interaction proves to be related to an inhibition of theophylline metabolism by hydrocortisone, then dyphylline, which is not metabolized by the liver like the other theophylline derivatives, would not be expected to interact with hydrocortisone, whereas aminophylline and oxtriphylline would probably interact similarly.

Mechanism: The mechanism of this interaction is unknown. Subsequent studies failed to determine whether the interaction leading to increased theophylline levels was the result of an alteration in theophylline distribution or the inhibition of theophylline metabolism by hydrocortisone.[1]

Recommendations: Theophylline levels should be monitored if concurrent corticosteroids are indicated. A lower dose of theophylline may be necessary.

References

1. Buchanan, N., and others: Asthma—a possible interaction between hydrocortisone and theophylline, South Afr. Med. J. **56:**1147, 1979.
2. Jusko, W.J., and others: Factors affecting theophylline clearances: age, tobacco, marijuana, cirrhosis, congestive heart failure, obesity, oral contraceptives, benzodiazepines, barbiturates, and ethanol, J. Pharm. Sci. **68:**1358, 1979.
3. Leavengood, D.C., and others: The effect of corticosteroids on theophylline metabolism, Ann. Allergy **50:**24, 1983.
4. Brooks, S.M., and others: The effects of ephedrine and theophylline on dexamethasone metabolism on bronchial asthma, J. Clin. Pharmacol. **17:**308, 1977.
5. Anderson, J.L., and others: Potential pharmacokinetic interaction between theophylline and prednisone, Clin. Pharm. **3:**187, 1984.

Theophylline–Influenza Virus Vaccine

Summary: In 1 study the elimination of theophylline was assessed in 4 healthy volunteers both before and after influenza vaccination. The mean theophylline half-life before vaccination was 3.3 hours and increased to 7.3 hours 24 hours after vaccination. Theophylline clearance decreased, although the apparent volume of distribution was unchanged.[1] Another report confirms this interaction since theophylline levels rose to levels exceeding 32 µg/ml.[2] However, 4 other studies showed conflicting results and failed to show any significant influence of influenza vaccine on theophylline levels.[3-6] These studies involved 20 asthmatics and 16 patients with chronic airway obstruction. One of these patients needed a reduction in the theophylline dosage as toxic theophylline levels developed.[4]

Related Drugs: In a study involving 3 patients who had been receiving oxtriphylline, 2 of 3 patients showed toxic signs characteristic of theophylline within 12 to 24 hours after vaccination. The serum theophylline concentrations increased 219%, 89%, and 85%.[1] Seven patients were given a constant intravenous infusion of aminophylline, and also received an intramuscular vaccination with 0.5 ml inactivated subvirion trivalent influenza vaccine. There was no significant difference in the mean total theophylline clearance rate before and after vaccination.[7] Dyphylline, a theophylline derivative not converted to theophylline in vivo, is not metabolized by the liver and is rapidly removed from the blood by glomerular filtration or active secretion, or both, and approximately 82% is excreted unchanged in the urine.[8,9] This is in contrast to theophylline, which is extensively metabolized by the liver. Therefore, if the mechanism involves inhibition of hepatic metabolism, dyphylline would not be expected to interact with influenza virus vaccine.

Mechanism: Theophylline is partially metabolized by hepatic cytochrome P-450, and alterations in the rate of metabolism can alter the rate of theophylline elimination. It is postulated that influenza virus vaccine inhibits the hepatic metabolism of theophylline.[9] Also, it has been demonstrated in animals that the stimulation of host defense mechanisms by a variety of biologic agents results in a decreased theophylline biotransformation. It has been suggested that influenza vaccine may be such an agent.[1] Stults and Hashisaki suggested that different vaccine preparations have maximal effect on hepatic metabolism at different times and that only certain preparations may depress hepatic metabolism, or different groups of patients may react differently.[7]

Recommendations: After an influenza vaccination, patients should be monitored for signs of theophylline toxicity. The dose of theophylline may need to be decreased temporarily.

References

1. Renton, K.W., and others: Decreased elimination of theophylline after influenza vaccination, Can. Med. Assoc. J. **123:**288, 1980.

2. Walker, S., and others: Serum theophylline levels after influenza vaccination, Can. Med. Assoc. J. **125:**243, 1981.
3. Goldstein, R.S., and others: Decreased elimination of theophylline after influenza vaccination, Can. Med. Assoc. J. **126:**470, 1982.
4. Fischer, R.G., and others: Altered theophylline clearance during an influenza B outbreak, Can. Med. Assoc. J. **126:**1312, 1982.
5. San Joaquin, V.H., and others: Influenza vaccination in asthmatic children on maintenance theophylline therapy, Clin. Pediatr. **21:**724, 1982.
6. Patriarca, P.A., and others: Influenza vaccination and warfarin or theophylline toxicity in nursing-home residents, N. Engl. J. Med. **308:**1601, 1983.
7. Stults, B.M., and Hashisaki, P.A.: Influenza vaccination and theophylline pharmacokinetics in patients with chronic obstructive lung disease, West. J. Med. **139:**651, 1983.
8. Gisclon, L.G., and others: Pharmacokinetics of orally administered dyphylline, Am. J. Hosp. Pharm. **36:**1179, 1979.
9. Simons, K.J., and Simons, F.E.K.: Urinary excretion of dyphylline in humans, J. Pharm. Sci. **68:**1327, 1979.
10. Kraemer, M.J., and others: Influence of trivalent influenza vaccine on serum theophylline levels, Pediatrics **69:**476, 1982.

Theophylline–Phenobarbital

2

Summary: The concurrent use of phenobarbital and theophylline may reduce theophylline serum levels. One study showed that a 34% increase in serum theophylline clearance occurred after phenobarbital pretreatment.[1] Another study demonstrated an insignificant increase in theophylline plasma clearance.[2] However, it was theorized that in this study phenobarbital was not administered for a long enough period.[1]

Related Drugs: One report demonstrated the induction of theophylline clearance by secobarbital in the presence of phenobarbital. The decrease in theophylline clearance occurred while phenobarbital dosage remained stable. During this time it was necessary to administer theophylline at a dosage 4 times above that usually recommended.[3] Although documentation is lacking, a similar interaction may be expected between theophylline and the other barbiturates (e.g., amobarbital, butabarbital, pentobarbital [see Appendix]) since they also induce hepatic enzymes. Documentation is also lacking regarding a similar interaction with the other theophylline derivatives (aminophylline and oxtriphylline), although based on their similar metabolic fate an interaction with phenobarbital would be likely. Dyphylline, a theophylline derivative that is not converted to theophylline in vivo, is not metabolized by the liver and is rapidly removed from the blood by glomerular filtration or active secretion, or both, and approximately 82% is excreted unchanged in the urine.[4,5] This is in contrast to theophylline, which is extensively metabolized by the liver. Therefore, dyphylline would not be expected to interact with phenobarbital.

Mechanism: The mechanism of this interaction is thought to be related to barbiturate induction of hepatic microsomal enzyme activity, since theophylline is metabolized by the cytochrome P-450 system.[1,4]

Recommendations: Theophylline plasma levels should be closely monitored during concurrent barbiturate therapy. The dose of theophylline may need to be increased.

References

1. Landay, R.A., and others: Effect of phenobarbital on theophylline disposition, J. Allergy Clin. Immunol. **62:**271, 1978.
2. Piafsky, K.M., and others: Effect of phenobarbital on the disposition of intravenous theophylline, Clin. Pharmacol. Ther. **22:**336, 1977.
3. Paladino, J.A., and others: Effect of secobarbital on theophylline clearance, Ther. Drug. Monit. **5:**135, 1983.
4. Gisclon, L.G., and others: Pharmacokinetics of orally administered dyphylline, Am. J. Hosp. Pharm. **36:**1179, 1979.
5. Simons, K.J., and Simons, F.E.K.: Urinary excretion of dyphylline in humans, J. Pharm. Sci. **68:**1327, 1979.

Theophylline–Phenytoin

Summary: In a study involving 10 healthy volunteers, the half-life of theophylline decreased and its clearance increased approximately 2-fold when phenytoin was administered for 10 to 15 days in doses that produced plasma concentrations in the usual therapeutic range.[1] Two other studies reported similar results.[2,3] In another study, withdrawal of theophylline resulted in a 40% rise in the mean serum phenytoin level in 5 of 14 subjects. The phenytoin levels were decreased during concurrent therapy.[4]

Related Drugs: There is a lack of documentation regarding an interaction between theophylline and the other hydantoin anticonvulsants (ethotoin and mephenytoin), although since they are pharmacologically related, a similar interaction may be expected to occur. In a study involving 5 healthy subjects the concurrent use of aminophylline and phenytoin resulted in an increased clearance of aminophylline.[5] The other theophylline derivative (oxtriphylline) would be expected to interact with phenytoin based on a similar metabolic fate. Dyphylline, a theophylline derivative not converted to theophylline in vivo is not metabolized by the liver and is rapidly removed from the blood by glomerular filtration, active secretion, or both, and approximately 82% is excreted unchanged in the urine.[6,7] This is in contrast to theophylline, which is extensively metabolized by the liver. Therefore, if the mechanism of this interaction involves hepatic enzyme induction, dyphylline would not be expected to interact with phenytoin.

Mechanism: Although the mechanism is not fully known, it has been suggested that phenytoin increases the metabolism of theophylline by inducing hepatic microsomal enzymes.[1,5] Regarding the decreased phenytoin levels, it has been postulated that theophylline induces the metabolism of phenytoin or interferes with its absorption.[4,8]

Recommendations: It is important to monitor the levels of both phenytoin and theophylline during concurrent therapy. If necessary, the dose of theophylline or phenytoin may need to be increased.

References

1. Marquis, J.F., and others: Phenytoin-theophylline interaction, N. Engl. J. Med. **307**:1189, 1982.
2. Rosenberg, K.R., and others: Reduced theophylline half-life induced by carbamazepine therapy, J. Pediatr. **102**:472, 1983.
3. Reed, R.C., and others: An interaction between theophylline and phenytoin, N. Engl. J. Med. **308**:724, 1983.
4. Taylor, J.W., and others: The interaction of phenytoin and theophylline, Drug Intell. Clin. Pharm. **14**:638, 1980.
5. Miller, M.E., and others: The effect of Dilantin on theophylline elimination, Clin. Res. **31**:104A, 1983.
6. Gisclon, L.G., and others: Pharmacokinetics of orally administered dyphylline, Am. J. Hosp. Pharm. **36**:1179, 1979.
7. Simons, K.J., and Simons, F.E.K.: Urinary excretion of dyphylline in humans, J. Pharm. Sci. **68**:1327, 1979.
8. Fincham, R.W., and others: Advances in epileptology. New York, 1978, Raven Press, p. 505.

Theophylline–Propranolol

2

Summary: In a study involving 8 healthy subjects, theophylline clearance was significantly reduced by concurrent propranolol. The apparent volume of distribution of theophylline did not change significantly; however, the elimination rate constant was reduced by propranolol in both smokers and nonsmokers.[1] However, propranolol and the other noncardioselective beta-blocking agents (nadolol, pindolol, and timolol) increase bronchial resistance and are pharmacologic antagonists of the xanthines.

Related Drugs: In the same study, metoprolol did not reduce theophylline clearance in all subjects but had some effect in those who smoked and who had a high theophylline clearance initially.[1] Documentation is lacking regarding an interaction between the other theophylline derivatives (aminophylline, dyphylline, and oxtriphylline) and the other noncardioselective beta-blocking agents (nadolol, pindolol, and timolol), although one would expect some degree of a similar interaction. Atenolol, which is noncardioselective and is not involved in hepatic metabolism, would be less likely, if at all, to interact with theophylline.

Mechanism: Beta-blocking agents antagonize the pharmacologic action of theophylline on the bronchial musculature and also increase bronchial resistance (particularly noncardioselective beta-blocking agents).[2,3] The inhibition of phosphodiesterase by theophylline derivatives causes beta-adrenergic stimulation;[4] therefore, it may be expected that propranolol and theophylline would have some antagonistic effects. It is also known that theophylline is metabolized by the hepatic mixed-function oxidase system, and propranolol has been shown to reduce the clearance of drugs metabolized by the liver. It has been postulated that propranolol interferes with the N-demethylation metabolism of theophylline by blocking cyclic AMP in the cytochrome system.[1] If this is true, dyphylline would not be expected to interact with propranolol since it is not metabolized by the liver like theophylline and its other derivatives.

Recommendations: Patients' theophylline levels should be monitored during concurrent therapy with propranolol. The dose of theophylline may need to be adjusted.

References

1. Conrad, K.A., and Nyman, D.W.: Effects of metoprolol and propranolol on theophylline elimination, Clin. Pharmacol. Ther. **28:**463, 1980.
2. Horvath, J.S., and others: A comparison of metoprolol and propranolol on blood pressure and respiratory function in patients with hypertension, Aust. N.Z. J. Med. **8:**1, 1978.
3. Mue, S., and others: Clinical pharmacokinetics of theophylline and propranolol, Int. J. Clin. Pharmacol. Biopharm. **17:**346, 1979.
4. Ensinck, J.W., and others: Effect of aminophylline on the secretion of insulin, glucagon, leutinizing hormone and growth hormone in humans, J. Clin. Endocrinol. Metab. **31:**153, 1970.

Theophylline–Tetracycline

3

Summary: An increased incidence of side effects (mainly gastrointestinal complaints) was noted in patients after concurrent use of tetracycline and theophylline in 1 study.[1] However, 2 other studies conflict with this report and find no interaction during concomitant therapy.[2,3] In 1 of these reports, 6 of 9 subjects demonstrated an increased theophylline elimination half-life and a decrease in body clearance, although no statistically significant difference between kinetic variables and control values could be shown.[2]

Related Drugs: Documentation is lacking regarding a similar interaction between the other theophylline derivatives (aminophylline, dyphylline, and oxtriphylline) and the other tetracyclines (e.g., chlortetracycline, doxycycline, oxytetracycline [see Appendix]).

Mechanism: Because of conflicting reports, the mechanism of this interaction is unknown. Gastrointestinal complaints may occur with both agents, and the increased frequency of adverse effects previously reported from the combination[1] may simply have been a summation and not necessarily caused by a kinetic drug interaction.[3]

Recommendations: The concurrent use of these agents need not be avoided. However, it is prudent to monitor theophylline levels and adjust the dose accordingly if necessary.

References

1. Pfeifer, H., and Greenblatt, D.: Clinical toxicity of theophylline in relation to cigarette smoking: a report from the Boston collaborative drug surveillance program, Chest **73**:455, 1978.
2. Pfeifer, H., and others: Effects of three antibiotics on theophylline kinetics, Clin. Pharmacol. Ther. **26**:36, 1979.
3. Mathis, J., and others: Effect of tetracycline hydrochloride on theophylline kinetics, Clin. Pharm. **1**:446, 1982.

Theophylline–Tobacco

1

Summary: Numerous studies have demonstrated that theophylline elimination is enhanced by tobacco smoking.[1-14] Reduced serum theophylline concentrations, shortened theophylline half-life, and a 42% increase in total body clearance were all observed in smokers.[4] Smokers also exhibited fewer adverse reactions to theophylline than nonsmokers,[1] a finding consistent with smoking-induced reductions in serum theophylline concentrations.

Related Drugs: Several reports have shown that theophylline from aminophylline undergoes the same interaction.[1,2,4,5,11,14] Smoking may be expected to interact similarly with the other theophylline derivative that is hepatically metabolized (oxtriphylline). Dyphylline, a theophylline derivative not converted to theophylline in vivo, is not metabolized by the liver and is rapidly removed from the blood by glomerular filtration, active secretion, or both, and approximately 82% is excreted unchanged in the urine.[15,16] This is in contrast to theophylline, which is extensively metabolized by the liver. Therefore, dyphylline would not be expected to interact with tobacco. Chronic users of marijuana also exhibited a 42% increase in total theophylline clearance, whereas users of both tobacco and marijuana showed a 79% increase in total theophylline clearance.[4,5]

Mechanism: Smoking is thought to enhance theophylline metabolism by inducing hepatic microsomal enzymes.[3,6-8,11-13] The primary causal agents thought to be responsible for this enzyme induction are the polynuclear aromatic hydrocarbons found in cigarette smoke.[4,6,7,11] It has been suggested that cytochrome P-448 or cytochrome P-450 is the specific enzyme system that undergoes induction by polynuclear aromatic hydrocarbons.[6,7]

Recommendations: Patients who currently smoke and use theophylline and who quit smoking may require an adjustment of their theophylline dosage. Alterations in theophylline disposition may return to normal when smoking is stopped; however, this may require an extended period of time.[2,3]

References

1. Pfiefer, H.F., and Greenblatt, D.J.: Clinical toxicity of theophylline in relation to cigarette smoking, Chest **73:**455, 1978.
2. Powell, J.R., and others: The influence of cigarette smoking and the sex on theophylline disposition, Am. Rev. Resp. Dis. **116:**17, 1977.
3. Hunt, S.N., and others: Effect of smoking on theophylline disposition, Clin. Pharmacol. Ther. **19:**546, 1979.
4. Jusko, W.J., and others: Enhanced biotransformation of theophylline in marijuana and tobacco smokers, Clin. Pharmacol. Ther. **24:**406, 1978.
5. Jusko, W.J., and others: Factors affecting theophylline clearance: age, tobacco, marijuana, cirrhosis, congestive heart failure, obesity, oral contraceptives, benzodiazepines, barbiturates, and ethanol, J. Pharm. Sci. **68:**1358, 1979.
6. Jusko, W.J.: Influence of cigarette smoking on drug metabolism in man, Drug Metab. Rev. **9:**221, 1979.
7. Jusko, W.J.: Role of tobacco in pharmacokinetics, J. Pharmacokinet. Biopharm. **6:**7, 1979.

8. Cusack, B., and others: Theophylline kinetics in relation to age: the importance of smoking, Br. J. Clin. Pharmacol. **10:**109, 1980.

9. Grygiel, J.J., and Birkett, D.J.: Cigarette smoking and theophylline clearance and metabolism, Clin. Pharmacol. Ther. **30:**491, 1981.

10. Ogilvie, R.I.: Smoking and theophylline dose schedules, Ann. Intern. Med. **88:**263, 1978.

11. Jenne, J., and others: Decreased theophylline half-life in cigarette smokers, Life Sci. **17:**195, 1975.

12. Talseth, T., and others: Aging, cigarette smoking and oral theophylline requirement, Eur. J. Clin. Pharmacol. **21:**33, 1981.

13. Horai, Y., and others: Bioavailability and pharmacokinetics of theophylline in plain uncoated and sustained-release dosage forms in relation to smoking habit. I. Single dose study, Eur. J. Clin. Pharmacol. **24:**79, 1983.

14. Gardner, M.J., and others: Effects of tobacco smoking and oral contraceptive use on theophylline disposition, Br. J. Clin. Pharmacol. **16:**271, 1983.

15. Gisclon, L.G., and others: Pharmacokinetics of orally administered dyphylline, Am. J. Hosp. Pharm. **36:**1179, 1979.

16. Simons, K.J., and Simons, F.E.K.: Urinary excretion of dyphylline in humans, J. Pharm. Sci. **68:**1327, 1979.

Theophylline–Verapamil

Summary: In a case report the addition of verapamil to a patient on a stabilized dosage regimen of theophylline caused a doubling of theophylline serum concentrations and clinical manifestations of theophylline toxicity (tachycardia, nausea, vomiting, etc.). When theophylline was discontinued and subsequently modified to offset the apparent interaction, the theophylline concentration was very near the accepted therapeutic concentration and symptoms subsided.[1]

Related Drugs: Documentation is lacking regarding a similar interaction between theophylline and the other calcium channel blockers (diltiazem and nifedipine) and between verapamil and the other theophylline derivatives (aminophylline and oxtriphylline). However, based on a similar metabolic fate an interaction may be expected to occur. Dyphylline, a theophylline derivative not converted to theophylline in vivo, is not metabolized by the liver and is rapidly removed from the blood by glomerular filtration, active secretion, or both, and approximately 82% is excreted unchanged in the urine.[2,3] This is in contrast to theophylline, which is extensively metabolized by the liver. Therefore, if the mechanism involves competition for the N-demethylation metabolic process, dyphylline may not be expected to interact similarly with verapamil.[1]

Mechanism: The mechanism is unknown. However, both theophylline and verapamil have at least one metabolic process in common, N-demethylation. Also, theophylline clearance has been shown to be affected by substances that may compete with it for metabolism. It has been suggested that this is the mechanism of this interaction.[1]

Recommendations: Although further studies are needed, it is important to be aware of the possibility of this interaction occurring. Patients should be closely monitored for increased theophylline levels, and the dose of theophylline may need to be decreased.

References

1. Burnakis, T.G., and others: Increased serum theophylline concentrations secondary to oral verapamil, Clin. Pharm. **2:**458, 1983.
2. Gisclon, L.G., and others: Pharmacokinetics of orally administered dyphylline, Am. J. Hosp. Pharm. **36:**1179, 1979.
3. Simons, K.J., and Simons, F.E.K.: Urinary excretion of dyphylline in humans, J. Pharm. Sci. **68:**1327, 1979.

CHAPTER EIGHTEEN

Miscellaneous Drug Interactions

TABLE 18. Miscellaneous Drug Interactions

Drug Interaction	Significance Code	Potential Effects	Recommendations	See Page
Cimetidine–Aluminum Hydroxide	3	Aluminum hydroxide alone and in combination with other antacids reduces peak cimetidine blood concentrations and GI absorption by one-third.	Separate the administration of these 2 drugs by as much time as possible, regardless of the presence or absence of food.	664
Cimetidine–Metoclopramide	3	Metoclopramide reportedly decreases bioavailability of cimetidine, with no changes in half-life.	Cimetidine dosage may need to be increased.	666
Dihydroergotamine–Nitroglycerin	2	Nitroglycerin substantially increased the bioavailability of dihydroergotamine and significantly increased the mean standing systolic blood pressure.	Monitor patients for symptoms of ergotism and reduce the dihydroergotamine dosage if needed.	667
Ergonovine–Dopamine	2	Concurrent use of these agents may increase the incidence of gangrene, probably due to the synergistic peripheral vasoconstriction activity of both drugs.	Avoid concurrent use if possible. Chlorpromazine has successfully treated the hypertension that may result.	668
Hydrocortisone–Cholestyramine	3	Cholestyramine reduced the hydrocortisone plasma concentration area-under-curve, but the clinical significance was not determined.	An increased hydrocortisone dosage may be needed.	669
Levodopa–Papaverine	2	Papaverine has antagonized the pharmacologic effect of levodopa, which worsened rigidity, tremor, and bradykinesia.	Avoid concurrent use if possible. Higher levodopa doses may be necessary.	670
Metoclopramide–Atropine	3	When metoclopramide is given first, atropine reversed the metoclopramide elevation in lower esophageal sphincter pressure. Conversely, when atropine is given first, metoclopramide reverses the atropine-induced depression of lower esophageal sphincter pressure.	Avoid concurrent use, or give metoclopramide 2 hours before atropine.	671
Metoclopramide–Levodopa	3	Levodopa may reverse some pharmacologic activities of metoclopramide, including effects on prolactin secretion, lower esophageal sphincter pressure, and gastric emptying rate. When given before levodopa, meclopramide increased the bioavailability of levodopa.	Monitor patients for this interaction and adjust the levodopa dosage if necessary.	672

Abbreviation: GI, gastrointestinal.

TABLE 18. Miscellaneous Drug Interactions—cont'd

Drug Interaction	Significance Code	Potential Effects	Recommendations	See Page
Prednisolone–Oral Contraceptive Agents	2	Oral contraceptives decrease the clearance, increase plasma concentrations, double the area-under-curve, and prolong the half-life of prednisolone. This may lead to increased therapeutic and toxic effects of prednisolone.	The prednisolone dosage may need to be reduced.	673
Prednisone–Aluminum Hydroxide	3	Aluminum hydroxide may decrease the oral bioavailability of prednisone, although other studies fail to show any effect.	The prednisolone dosage may need to be reduced.	674
Pyridostigmine–Methylprednisolone	3	Concurrent use of these agents may result in decreased muscle strength, sometimes necessitating mechanical ventilation.	Ventilatory assistance may need to be provided. It may be necessary to discontinue methylprednisolone.	675
Thyroid–Cholestyramine	2	Cholestyramine may decrease the absorption of thyroid hormones.	Administer these agents as far apart as possible (optimally 4-6 hours) and observe for symptoms of hypothyroidism.	676

Cimetidine–Aluminum Hydroxide

3

Summary Concomitant, acute administration of aluminum hydroxide alone and in combination with other antacids has been shown to reduce peak cimetidine blood concentrations and reduce its gastrointestinal absorption by approximately one-third.[1-5] However, 2 other studies failed to show this effect when cimetidine was used concurrently with combination antacids.[4,6] Antacids given 1 hour before or after cimetidine in the fasting state, or 1 hour after the drug taken with a meal, did not affect cimetidine absorption.[5]

Related Drugs: Magnesium hydroxide alone, as well as in combination with other antacids, has also been shown to decrease cimetidine absorption.[1-5] A formulation of magnesium carbonate and calcium carbonate with a moderate neutralizing capacity did not influence cimetidine absorption,[6] and this was also seen when the formulation was used concurrently with magnesium trisilicate, magnesium hydroxide, and aluminum hydroxide.[4]

An antacid containing aluminum and magnesium hydroxide reduced both the maximum plasma ranitidine concentration and the area-under-curve by one-third; however, elimination of ranitidine was not changed.[7] However, 2 other studies reported that an antacid containing aluminum/magnesium hydroxide[8] and another antacid containing aluminum hydroxide and magnesium carbonate[9] had no effect on the absorption of ranitidine.

Mechanism: The exact mechanism is unknown; however, several mechanisms have been postulated. It has been suggested that some component of antacids interferes with the absorption of cimetidine. Aluminum hydroxide is a well known binding agent and has been reported to interfere with the bioavailability of several drugs, and magnesium hydroxide is also known to interfere with drug kinetics.[5] Other studies suggest that the total neutralizing capacity of the antacid is responsible for the interaction.[4,6] However, it has been shown that doubling the neutralizing capacity did not further inhibit cimetidine absorption. It is possible that magnesium and aluminum ions complex maximally to cimetidine at a neutralizing capacity between 50 and 72 mmol, have no further inhibition over 72 mmol, and may not maximally bind cimetidine below 50 mmol.[5]

Recommendations: The clinical significance of the reduction in cimetidine bioavailability has not been studied. If the concomitant use of antacids and cimetidine is selected, the administration of these agents should be separated by as much time as possible. It may be advisable to administer antacids one hour before or after cimetidine dosing in the fasting state. Another recommendation would be to administer cimetidine with meals, followed by the antacid 1 hour later.[5]

References

1. Gugler, R., and others: Impaired cimetidine absorption due to antacids and metoclopramide, Eur. J. Clin. Pharmacol. **20**:225, 1981.
2. Boedemar, G., and others: Diminished absorption of cimetidine caused by antacids, Lancet **1**:444, 1979.

3. Steinberg, W.M., and Lewis, J.H.: Mylanta II inhibits the absorption of cimetidine, Gastroenterology **78:**1269, 1980.
4. Bodemar, G., and others: Effects of antacids on the absorption of cimetidine, Gut **19:**A990, 1978.
5. Steinberg, W.M., and others: Antacids inhibit absorption of cimetidine, N. Engl. J. Med. **307:**400, 1982.
6. Burland, W.L., and others: Effect of antacids on absorption of cimetidine, Lancet **2:**965, 1976.
7. Mihaly, G.W., and others: High dose of antacid (Mylanta II) reduces bioavailability of ranitidine, Br. Med. J. **285:**998, 1982.
8. Eshelman, F.N., and others: Effect of antacid and anticholinergic medication on ranitidine absorption, Clin. Pharmacol. Ther. **33:**216, 1983.
9. Frislid, K., and Berstad, A.: High dose of antacid reduces bioavailability of ranitidine, Br. Med. J. **286:**1358, 1983.

Cimetidine–Metoclopramide

3

Summary: Concurrent metoclopramide and cimetidine administration has been reported to result in a decrease in the bioavailability of cimetidine by 22% to 27%.[1,2] There was no change in the half-life of cimetidine and the reported reductions were associated with significantly reduced excretion of cimetidine in urine.[1] This effect may be even greater when metoclopramide is given for an extended period or administered intravenously.

Related Drugs: There are no drugs related to metoclopramide. There is a lack of documentation concerning a similar interaction between the other H_2 antagonist (ranitidine) and metoclopramide.

Mechanism: The mechanism has been attributed to decreased cimetidine absorption, which may be related to metoclopramide's ability to increase gastric emptying time.

Recommendations: If metoclopramide is administered concurrently with cimetidine, the dose of cimetidine may need to be increased depending on the therapeutic outcome of the combination.

References

1. Gugler, R., and others: Impaired cimetidine absorption due to antacids and metoclopramide, Eur. J. Clin. Pharmacol. **20:**225, 1981.
2. Kanto, J., and others: The effect of metoclopramide and propantheline on the gastrointestinal absorption of cimetidine, Br. J. Clin. Pharmacol. **11:**629, 1981.

Dihydroergotamine–Nitroglycerin

2

Summary: Concurrent nitroglycerin substantially increased the bioavailability of dihydroergotamine by 56% to 370% and significantly increased the mean standing systolic blood pressure by 27%.[1] The 6 patients studied, who ranged in age from 51 to 82 years, had been receiving dihydroergotamine to treat autonomic insufficiency and postural hypotension.

Related Drugs: The other ergot alkaloid that is rapidly metabolized by the liver (ergoloid mesylates) may be expected to interact with nitroglycerin in a similar manner. However, the other ergot alkaloids (ergonovine, ergotamine, and methylergonovine) are slowly metabolized in the liver and would not be expected to interact to as great an extent, if at all. Other nitrates (e.g., amyl nitrite, erythrityl tetranitrate, isosorbide dinitrate [see Appendix]) may be expected to interact similarly with the ergot alkaloids based on pharmacologic similarity.

Mechanism: The absolute bioavailability of dihydroergotamine was found to be about 1%,[1] suggesting an almost complete first-pass metabolic effect. Nitroglycerin, by increasing splanchnic blood flow, decreased the first-pass metabolism of dihydroergotamine and subsequently increased its bioavailability.

Recommendations: Patients should be monitored for symptoms of ergotism (e.g., cold, pale, and numb feet and legs, muscle pain, headache, nausea, vomiting) when these agents are used concomitantly. The dosage of dihydroergotamine may need to be reduced in some patients.

Reference

1. Bolik, A., and others: Low oral bioavailability of dihydroergotamine and first-pass extraction in patients with orthostatic hypotension, Clin. Pharmacol. Ther. **30:**673, 1981.

Ergonovine–Dopamine

2

Summary: An isolated case report suggested that the vasoconstrictive properties of ergonovine and dopamine may be additive, leading to an increased incidence of gangrene.[1] The patient was admitted for a routine surgical procedure in which ergonovine was given postoperatively to control bleeding. After treatment for a severe hypotensive episode, a laparotomy was perfomed and dopamine infusion began. Two days later there was symmetric incipient gangrene in both hands and feet.

Related Drugs: In a retrospective study, approximately 5% of 741 women who received concurrent methoxamine and either ergonovine, methylergonovine, or oxytocin during continuous caudal block anesthesia developed severe hypertension.[2] Other reports are lacking of similar interactions between the other mixed acting sympathomimetic amines (metaraminol and phenylephrine) and the other ergot alkaloids (ergoloid mesylates, dihydroergotamine, and ergotamine); however, based on pharmacologic similarity an interaction may be expected to occur.

Mechanism: The interaction probably results from the synergistic peripheral vasoconstriction activity of both agents.

Recommendations: Although limited documentation is available, it indicates that concurrent use of these agents should be avoided if possible. Hypertension that resulted from the use of these agents was successfully treated with chlorpromazine.

References

1. Buchanan, N., and others: Symmetrical gangrene of the extremities associated with the use of dopamine subsequent to ergometrine administration, Intensive Care Med. **3:**55, 1977.
2. Casady, G.N., and others: Postpartum hypertension after use of vasoconstrictor and oxytocic drugs, J.A.M.A. **172:**1011, 1960.

Hydrocortisone–Cholestyramine

Summary: After a single dose of hydrocortisone in 10 healthy volunteers, cholestyramine caused a reduction in the hydrocortisone plasma concentration area-under-curve. The clinical significance of the interaction was not determined.[1]

Related Drugs: One study found no influence on the bioavailability of prednisolone after cholestyramine administration.[2] No documentation exists regarding an interaction between cholestyramine and the other corticosteroids (e.g., betamethasone, prednisone, triamcinolone [see Appendix]), and it would be difficult to determine if a similar interaction would occur because of conflicting data. Documentation is also lacking regarding an interaction with the other anion exchange resin (colestipol).

Mechanism: Cholestyramine has been demonstrated to bind hydrocortisone and prednisolone in vitro. The in vivo study failed to confirm this.[3] It has been suggested that cholestyramine also decreases and delays the absorption of hydrocortisone.[1]

Recommendations: Patients should be observed for a change in their clinical response to the corticosteroid, and an increase in the dose may be necessary.

References

1. Johansson, C., and others: Interaction by cholestyramine on the uptake of hydrocortisone in the gastrointestinal tract, Acta Med. Scand. **204:**509, 1978.
2. Audetat, V., and others: Beeintrachtigt cholestyramin die biologische verfugbarkeit von prednisolon? Schweiz. Med. Wochenschr. **107:**527, 1977.
3. Ware, A.J., and others: Influence of sodium taurocholate, cholestyramine, and Mylanta on the intestinal absorption of glucocorticoids in the rat, Gastroenterology **64:**1150, 1973.

Levodopa–Papaverine

Summary: Concurrent administration of papaverine in patients receiving levodopa therapy has resulted in the antagonism of levodopa's pharmacologic effect.[1,2] The loss of the therapeutic effect of levodopa results in worsening of rigidity, tremor, and bradykinesia, which may occur gradually over several weeks. After papaverine is discontinued, the effects of this interaction reverse in 7 to 10 days.

Related Drugs: There is no documentation regarding an interaction between levodopa and the peripheral vasodilator ethaverine, although because of pharmacologic similarity, a similar interaction may be expected to occur. There are no drugs related to levodopa.

Mechanism: The mechanism has not been determined in humans. The observed antagonism suggests that papaverine blocks the dopamine receptors in the striatum.

Recommendations: Papaverine should not be administered to patients concurrently receiving levodopa. Should co-therapy be chosen, higher doses of levodopa may be required in patients receiving this combination to achieve the same therapeutic effect.

References

1. Duvoisin, R.C.: Antagonism of levodopa by papaverine, J.A.M.A. **231:**845, 1975.
2. Posner, D.M.: Antagonism of levodopa by papaverine, J.A.M.A. **233:**768, 1975.

Metoclopramide–Atropine

3

Summary: The effect of metoclopramide on the lower esophageal sphincter pressure is opposite that of atropine.[1-3] When metoclopramide is given first, subsequent atropine administration slightly[2] or significantly[1] reveresed the metoclopramide-induced elevation in lower esophageal sphincter pressure. When atropine was given first, subsequent metoclopramide slightly[1] or significantly[2] reversed the atropine-induced depression of lower esophageal sphincter pressure.

Related Drugs: There appear to be no studies that document an interaction between metoclopramide and other anticholinergics (e.g., dicyclomine, propantheline, scopolamine [see Appendix]) although since they are pharmacologically related a similar interaction may be expected. There are no drugs related to metoclopramide.

Mechanism: Because many factors influence the tone of the lower esophageal sphincter, including cholinergic, adrenergic, and a reflex mechanism, it is difficult to document the mechanism of this interaction. However, it is postulated that because metoclopramide acts as a dopamine receptor antagonist, and dopamine is known to decrease lower esophageal sphincter pressure, the blockade of these receptors leads to an increase in pressure that may in turn be antagonized or potentiated by effects on cholinergic receptors.[1]

Recommendations: Since these agents antagonize the pharmacologic effect of one another, their concurrent use should be avoided. If the 2 drugs are to be used, it has been suggested that metoclopramide precede atropine by 2 hours.[3]

References

1. Cotton, B.R., and Smith, G.: Single and combined effects of atropine and metoclopramide on the lower esophageal spincter pressure, Br. J. Anaesth. **53:**869, 1981.
2. Brock-Utne, J.G., and others: Effect of metoclopramide given before atropine sulfate on lower esophageal sphincter tone, South Afr. Med. J. **61:**465, 1982.
3. de Villiers, F.: Metoclopramide and atropine as premedication, South Afr. Med. J. **61:**772, 1982.

Metoclopramide–Levodopa

3

Summary: There is evidence that the concurrent use of levodopa will reverse some of the pharmacologic activities of metoclopramide. Levodopa antagonizes the effect of metoclopramide on prolactin secretion,[1,2] lower esophageal sphincter pressure,[3] and gastric emptying rate.[4] Metoclopramide, when given before levodopa, increased the relative bioavailability of levodopa approximately 2-fold in 12 healthy subjects and in 1 patient with parkinsonism.[5] However, the pharmacologic activity of levodopa may not be increased because of the antidopaminergic effect of metoclopramide.

Related Drugs: There are no drugs related to metoclopramide or levodopa.

Mechanism: The exact mechanism is unknown. However, metoclopramide is a dopaminergic antagonist,[3,4] and administration of levodopa, the precursor of dopamine, apparently overcomes such antagonism by inhibiting the action of metoclopramide.[3]

Recommendations: The evidence suggests that a competitive antagonism is possible with the coadministration of these 2 agents. Therefore, patients should be monitored for such an interaction, with an appropriate adjustment in the dosage of levodopa if necessary.

References

1. McCallum, R.W., and others: Metoclopramide stimulates prolactin secretion in man, J. Clin. Endocrinol. Metab. **42:**1148, 1976.
2. Judd, S.J., and others: Prolactin secretion by metoclopramide in man, J. Clin. Endocrinol. Metab. **43:**313, 1976.
3. Baumann, H.W., and others: L-dopa inhibits metoclopramide stimulation of the lower esophageal sphincter in man, Dig. Dis. Sci. **24:**289, 1979.
4. Berkowitz, D.M., and McCallum, R.W.: Interaction of levodopa and metoclopramide on gastric emptying, Clin. Pharmacol. Ther. **27:**414, 1980.
5. Mearrick, P.T., and others: Metoclopramide, gastric emptying and L-dopa absorption, Aust. N.Z. J. Med. **4:**144, 1974.

Prednisolone–Oral Contraceptive Agents

Summary: The elimination of prednisolone was found to be inhibited in women taking oral contraceptive agents concurrently compared to women not on oral contraceptives. Decreased prednisolone clearance and increased plasma concentrations were reported as well as a doubled area under the plasma concentration-time curve and a prolonged half-life.[1,3] These changes in the prednisolone pharmacokinetic parameters suggest an increase in the therapeutic and toxic effects of prednisolone may be expected.

Related Drugs: There appears to be no documentation regarding an interaction between oral contraceptive agents and the other corticosteroids (e.g., hydrocortisone, prednisone, triamcinolone [see Appendix]) although an interaction may be expected to occur based on a similar metabolic fate.

Mechanism: The mechanism is unknown. However, it has been postulated that oral contraceptives inhibit the hepatic metabolism of prednisolone and other corticosteroids.

Recommendations: Patients should be monitored for corticosteroid toxicity during concurrent use of these agents. It may be necessary to reduce the dose of the corticosteroid.

References

1. Legler, U.F. and Benet, L.Z.: Marked alterations in prednisolone elimination for women taking oral contraceptives, Clin. Pharmacol. Ther. **31:**243, 1982.
2. Boekenoogen, S.J., and others: Prednisolone disposition and protein binding in oral contraceptive users, J. Clin. Endocrin. Metab. **56:**702, 1983.
3. Kozower, M., and others: The effect of prednisolone in oral contraceptive users, J. Clin. Endocrinol. Metab. **38:**407, 1974.

Prednisone–Aluminum Hydroxide

3

Summary: The concurrent administration of a single dose of prednisone and an aluminum hydroxide antacid preparation resulted in a decrease in the oral bioavailability of prednisone in a study involving 5 healthy volunteers and 12 patients with chronic liver disease.[1] Three other studies failed to show any effect of similar antacid preparations (either alone or in combination) on the oral bioavailability of prednisone or prednisolone.[2-4]

Related Drugs: The oral bioavailability of prednisone was also decreased when given concurrently with an antacid preparation containing aluminum and magnesium hydroxide.[1] Concurrent administration of magnesium trisilicate and dexamethasone reduced the suppressive effects of dexamethasone in 1 study involving 6 healthy volunteers.[5] Documentation is lacking regarding similar interactions between other corticosteroids (e.g., betamethasone, hydrocortisone, triamcinolone [see Appendix]) and other antacid preparations (e.g., calcium carbonate, magaldrate, magnesium oxide [see Appendix]), although based on the mechanism an interaction may be expected to occur.

Mechanism: Because of conflicting results, the exact mechanism has not been fully elucidated. However, it has been suggested that antacid preparations physically adsorb prednisone.[1,2] One study reports that this interaction is not related to delayed gastric emptying or to intestinal transit time abnormalities.[1]

Recommendations: Patients should be observed for a change in their clinical response to the corticosteroid, and the dose of the corticosteroid may need to be increased.

References

1. Uribe, M., and others: Decreased bioavailability of prednisone due to antacids in patients with chronic active liver disease and in healthy volunteers, Gastroenterology **80:**661, 1981.
2. Tanner, A.R., and others: Concurrent administration of antacids and prednisone: effect on serum levels of prednisolone, Br. J. Clin. Pharmacol. **7:**397, 1979.
3. Lee, D.A.H., and others: The effect of concurrent administration of antacids on prednisolone absorption, Br. J. Clin. Pharmacol. **8:**92, 1979.
4. Bergrem, H., and others: Glucocorticoids: absorption of prednisolone. I. The effect of fasting, food and food combined with antacids, Scand. J. Urol. Nephrol. **64**(suppl.):167, 1981.
5. Naggar, V.F., and others: Effect of concomitant administration of magnesium trisilicate on GI absorption of dexamethasone in humans, J. Pharm. Sci. **67:**1029, 1978.

Pyridostigmine–Methylprednisolone

Summary: In an uncontrolled study involving 9 patients receiving therapeutic doses of pyridostigmine, the concurrent administration of methylprednisolone resulted in a decrease in muscle strength in 71% of treatment courses. During 57% of treatment courses, severe muscle weakness occurred, necessitating mechanical ventilation. Improvement in muscle strength and response to pyridostigmine above baseline levels occurred after methylprednisolone was discontinued.[1] Other clinical observations have indicated that the concomitant use of these agents can affect muscle strength, although each agent alone has been used successfully in treating myasthenia gravis.[2,3]

Related Drugs: In the previous 9 patients, neostigmine was also used in place of pyridostigmine resulting in the same interaction with methylprednisolone.[1] The muscle single-twitch tension produced by neostigmine and pyridostigmine was increased by hydrocortisone in an animal study.[4] Documentation is lacking regarding an interaction between the other anticholinesterases (ambenonium and edrophonium) and the other corticosteroids (e.g., dexamethasone, prednisolone, prednisone [see Appendix]).

Mechanism: The mechanism of this interaction is unknown.

Recommendations: If severe muscle weakness occurs during concurrent use of these agents, ventilatory assistance should be provided. It may also be necessary to discontinue the corticosteroid.

References

1. Brunner, N.G., and othes: Corticosteroids in management of severe, generalized myasthenia gravis, Neurology **22:**603, 1972.
2. Millikan, C.H., and others: Clinical evaluation of ACTH and cortisone in myasthenia gravis, Neurology **1:**145, 1951.
3. Grob, D., and others: Effect of adrenocorticotropic hormone (ACTH) and cortisone administration in patients with myasthenia gravis and report of onset of myasthenia gravis during prolonged cortisone administration, J. Hopkins Med. J. **91:**125, 1952.
4. Patten, B.M., and others: Adverse interaction between steroid hormones and anticholinesterase drugs, Neurology **24:**442, 1974.

Thyroid–Cholestyramine

2

Summary: Cholestyramine may cause a clinically significant decrease in the absorption of thyroid hormones when these drugs are given simultaneously.

Related Drugs: Since all thyroid compounds are structurally similar, (e.g., liothyronine, liotrix, thyrotropin [see Appendix]), they may be expected to interact with cholestyramine. This conclusion is supported by evidence that levothyroxine sodium[1] and thyroxine[2] interact with cholestyramine.

Colestipol, another anion-exchange resin similar to cholestyramine, might also bind thyroid if administered concurrently.

Mechanism: Cholestyramine reportedly forms very strong ionic bonds with thyroid in the gastrointestinal tract, which results in decreased absorption of orally administered thyroid. Thyroid is excreted in the bile and reabsorbed into the body via the enterohepatic recirculation. Cholestyramine may bind thyroxine in the gut and prevent its absorption and enterohepatic circulation, which would increase the amount of thyroxine appearing in the feces.[2]

Recommendations: Thyroxine and cholestyramine should be administered as far apart as possible (optimally 4 to 6 hours). When these drugs are used concurrently, the patient should be observed for symptoms of hypothyroidism (e.g., weakness, fatigue, cold intolerance, and dry, puffy skin).[3]

If possible, before cholestyramine is added to the drug regimen of a patient maintained on a thyroid preparation, baseline thyroid status should be determined. Periodic evaluation of thyroid status should be performed to detect changes in thyroid response.

References

1. Northcutt, R.C., and others: The influence of cholestyramine on thyroxine absorption, J.A.M.A. **208:**1857, 1969.
2. Bergman, F., and others: Influence of cholestyramine on absorption and excretion of thyroxine in syrian hamster, Acta Endocrinol. **53:**256, 1966.
3. Haynes, R.C., and Murad, F.: Thyroid and antithyroid drugs. In Gilman, A.G., Goodman, L.S., and Gilman, A., editors: The pharmacologic basis of therapeutics. New York, 1980, MacMillan Publishing.

APPENDIX

Related Drugs

For the purpose of uniformity and consistency, the following groups of drugs have been arranged based on pharmacologic and chemical relationships. This appendix contains a complete list of the agents in a specific related drug class. If any of these agents are specifically implicated in a monograph by documentation or the mechanism of action of the primary drug interaction, a statement discussing their involvement appears in the related drug section of the monograph (see Introduction). Only three representative agents of a class are listed in parenthesis followed by "[see Appendix]," which refers the user to this section, enabling the user to locate the remaining agents that may be in that class. Unless specifically stated otherwise, all of the agents in a list may be expected to interact in a manner similar to the three agents listed.

Agents to Treat Shock
Dobutamine
Dopamine
Ephedrine
Epinephrine
Isoproterenol
Mephentermine
Metaraminol
Methoxamine
Norepinephrine
Phenylephrine

Aminoglycosides
Amikacin
Gentamicin
Kanamycin
Neomycin
Netilmicin
Paromomycin
Streptomycin
Tobramycin

Androgen Derivatives
All Inclusive
Danazol
Dromostanolone
Ethylestrenol
Fluoxymesterone
Methandriol
Methyltestosterone
Nandrolone
Oxandrolone
Oxymetholone
Stanozolol
Testolactone
Testosterone

C-17 Alkylated
Danazol
Ethylestrenol
Fluoxymesterone
Methandriol
Methyltestosterone
Oxandrolone
Oxymetholone
Stanozolol

Anorexic Agents
Benzphetamine
Diethylpropion
Fenfluramine
Mazindol
Phendimetrazine
Phenmetrazine
Phentermine
Phenylpropanolamine

Antacids
Aluminum Carbonate Gel, Basic
Aluminum Hydroxide Gel
Aluminum Phosphate Gel
Calcium Carbonate
Dihydroxyaluminum Aminoacetate
Dihydroxyaluminum Sodium Carb.
Magaldrate
Magnesia (Magnesium Hydroxide)
Magnesium Carbonate
Magnesium Oxide
Magnesium Trisilicate
Sodium Bicarbonate

Anticholinergics
Anisotropine
Atropine
Belladonna
Benztropine
Biperiden
Clidinium
Cycrimine
Dicyclomine
Ethopropazine
Glycopyrrolate
Hexocyclium
Hyoscyamine
Isopropamide
Mepenzolate
Methantheline
Methixene
Methscopolamine
Oxybutynin
Oxyphencyclimine
Oxyphenonium
Procyclidine
Propantheline
Scopolamine
Thiphenamil
Tridihexethyl
Trihexyphenidyl

Anticholinesterases
Ambenonium
Demecarium
Edrophonium
Neostigmine
Physostigmine
Pyridostigmine

Anticoagulants, Oral
Coumarins
Dicumarol
Phenprocoumon
Warfarin

Indandione
Anisindione
Phenindione

Antihistamines
Azatadine
Bromdiphenhydramine
Brompheniramine
Buclizine
Carbinoxamine
Chlorpheniramine
Clemastine
Cyclizine
Cyproheptadine
Dexbrompheniramine
Dexchlorpheniramine
Diphenhydramine
Diphenylpyraline
Meclizine
Phenindamine
Pheniramine
Phenyltoloxamine
Pyrilamine
Tripelennamine
Triprolidine

Antineoplastic Alkylating Agents
Nitrogen Mustards
Chlorambucil
Cyclophosphamide
Mechlorethamine
Melphalan

Nitrosoureas
Busulfan
Carmustine
Lomustine
Pipobroman
Streptozocin
Thiotepa
Uracil Mustard

Antineoplastic Antimetabolites
Cytarabine
Floxuridine
Fluorouracil
Mercaptopurine
Methotrexate
Thioguanine

Antiparkinsonism Anticholinergics
Belladonna
Benztropine
Biperiden
Cycrimine
Ethopropazine
Orphenadrine
Procyclidine
Trihexyphenidyl

Antipsychotics, Miscellaneous
Chlorprothixene
Haloperidol
Loxapine
Molindone
Thiothixene

Barbiturates
General
Amobarbital
Aprobarbital
Butabarbital
Butalbital
Mephobarbital
Metharbital
Pentobarbital
Phenobarbital
Secobarbital
Talbutal

Anesthesia
Methohexital
Thiamylal
Thiopental

Benzodiazepines
Alprazolam
Chlordiazepoxide
Clonazepam
Clorazepate
Diazepam
Flurazepam
Halazepam
Lorazepam
Oxazepam
Prazepam
Temazepam
Triazolam

Beta-Blocking Agents
Atenolol
Labetalol
Metoprolol
Nadolol
Pindolol
Propranolol
Timolol

Bulk Producing Laxatives
Hemicellulose
Malt Extract
Methylcellulose
Psyllium

Calcium Channel Blockers
Diltiazem
Nifedipine
Verapamil

Carbonic Anhydrase Inhibitors
Acetazolamide
Dichlorphenamide
Methazolamide

Central Nervous System Depressants
Acetylcarbromal
Alcohol, Ethyl
Chloral Hydrate
Ethchlorvynol
Ethinamate
Glutethimide
Meprobamate
Methyprylon
Paraldehyde
Triclofos

Cephalosporins
Cefaclor
Cefadroxil
Cefamandole
Cefazolin
Cefonocid
Cefoperazone
Ceforanide
Cefotaxime
Cefoxitin
Ceftizoxime
Cefuroxime
Cephalexin
Cephaloglycin
Cephalothin
Cephapirin
Cephradine
Moxalactam

Corticosteroids
Beclomethasone
Betamethasone
Corticotropin
Cortisone
Cosyntropin
Desoxycorticosterone
Dexamethasone
Fludrocortisone
Flunisolide
Fluprednisolone
Hydrocortisone
Methylprednisolone
Paramethasone
Prednisolone
Prednisone
Triamcinolone

Digitalis Glycosides
Deslanoside
Digitalis
Digitoxin
Digoxin

Ergot Alkaloids
Dihydroergotamine
Ergoloid Mesylates
Ergonovine
Ergotamine
Methylergonovine
Methysergide

Estrogenic Substances
Chlorotrianisene
Conjugated Estrogens
Diethylstilbestrol
Esterified Estrogens
Estradiol
Estrone
Estropipate
Ethinyl Estradiol
Polyestradiol
Quinestrol

Hydantoin Anticonvulsants
Ethotoin
Mephenytoin
Phenytoin

Inhalation Anesthetic Agents
General
Cyclopropane
Ether
Ethylene
Nitrous Oxide

Halogenated
Enflurane
Halothane
Isoflurane
Methoxyflurane

Local Anesthetics
Benzocaine
Bupivacaine
Chloroprocaine
Dibucaine
Etidocaine
Lidocaine
Mepivacaine
Piperocaine
Prilocaine
Procaine
Propoxycaine
Tetracaine

Loop Diuretics
Bumetanide
Ethacrynic Acid
Furosemide

Macrolide Antibiotics
Erythromycin
Oleandomycin
Troleandomycin

Monoamine Oxidase Inhibitors
Furazolidone
Isocarboxazid
Pargyline
Phenelzine
Procarbazine
Tranylcypromine

Narcotics
Alphaprodine
Butorphanol
Codeine
Fentanyl
Hydrocodone
Hydromorphone
Levorphanol
Meperidine
Methadone
Morphine
Nalbuphine
Oxycodone
Oxymorphone
Pentazocine
Propoxyphene
Sufentanil

Neuromuscular Blocking Agents
Depolarizing
Succinylcholine

Nondepolarizing
Atracurium
Gallamine
Metocurine
Pancuronium
Tubocurarine
Vecuronium

Nitrate Derivatives
Amyl Nitrite
Erythrityl Tetranitrate
Isosorbide Dinitrate
Pentaerythritol Tetranitrate
Nitroglycerin

Nonsteroidal Anti-inflammatory Agents
Fenoprofen
Ibuprofen
Indomethacin
Meclofenamate
Mefenamic Acid
Naproxen
Oxyphenbutazone
Phenylbutazone
Piroxicam
Sulindac
Tolmetin

Penicillins
Amoxicillin
Ampicillin
Azlocillin
Bacampicillin
Carbenicillin
Cloxacillin
Cyclacillin
Dicloxacillin
Hetacillin
Methicillin
Mezlocillin
Nafcillin
Oxacillin
Penicillin G
Penicillin V
Piperacillin
Ticarcillin

Phenothiazines
Acetophenazine
Carphenazine
Chlorpromazine
Fluphenazine
Mesoridazine
Methdilazine
Perphenazine
Piperacetazine
Prochlorperazine
Promazine
Promethazine
Thiethylperazine
Thioridazine
Trifluoperazine
Triflupromazine
Trimeprazine

Polypeptide Antibiotics
Bacitracin
Capreomycin
Colistimethate
Colistin
Polymixin B

Potassium-Sparing Diuretics
Amiloride
Spironolactone
Triamterene

Progestins
Hydroxyprogesterone
Magestrol
Medroxyprogesterone
Norethindrone
Norgestrel
Progesterone

Propanediol Derivatives
Carisoprodol
Chlorphenesin
Mephenesin
Meprobamate
Methocarbamol

Rauwolfia Alkaloids
Alseroxylon
Deserpidine
Rauwolfia serpentina
Rescinnamine
Reserpine

Salicylates
Aspirin
Choline Salicylate
Diflunisal
Magnesium Salicylate
Salicylamide
Salsalate
Sodium Salicylate
Sodium Thiosalicylate

Sulfonamides
Sulfacytine
Sulfadiazine
Sulfadoxine
Sulfamerazine
Sulfamethazine
Sulfamethizole
Sulfamethoxazole
Sulfapyridine
Sulfasalazine
Sulfisoxazole

Sulfonylureas
Acetohexamide
Chlorpropamide
Glipizide
Glyburide
Tolazamide
Tolbutamide

Sympathomimetics

Direct Acting
Albuterol - b
Dobutamine - a, b
Epinephrine - a, b
Ethylnorepinephrine -b
Isoetharine - b
Isoproterenol - b
Metaproterenol - b
Methoxamine - a
Norepinephrine - a, b
Terbutaline - b

Indirect Acting (All have alpha and beta agonist activity)
Amphetamine
Benzphetamine
Dextroamphetamine
Diethylpropion
Ephedrine
Fenfluramine
Mazindol
Mephentermine
Methamphetamine
Methylphenidate
Phendimetrazine
Phenmetrazine
Phentermine
Phenylpropanolamine
Pseudoephedrine
Tyramine

Mixed Acting
Dopamine - a, b
Metaraminol - a, b
Phenylephrine - a, b

---

a = alpha agonist activity
b = beta agonist activity

Tetracyclines
Chlortetracycline
Demeclocycline
Doxycycline
Methacycline
Minocycline
Oxytetracycline
Tetracycline

Theophylline Derivatives
Aminophylline
Dyphylline
Oxtriphylline
Theophylline

Thiazide Diuretics
Bendroflumethiazide
Benzthiazide
Chlorothiazide
Cyclothiazide
Flumethiazide
Hydrochlorothiazide
Hydroflumethiazide
Methyclothiazide
Polythiazide
Trichlormethiazide

Thiazide Related Diuretics
Chlorthalidone
Indapamide
Metolazone
Quinethazone

Thyroid Drugs
Dextrothyroxine
Levothyroxine
Liothyronine
Liotrix
Thyroglobulin
Thyroid

Tricyclic Antidepressants
Amitriptyline
Amoxapine
Desipramine
Doxepin
Imipramine
Nortriptyline
Protriptyline
Trimipramine

Guide to the Proper Use of the Index to Drug Interactions

The significance coding applied to each drug interaction monograph is applicable only to the drugs mentioned in the monograph title. Therefore, there is no significance code in the index for other drugs that may be mentioned within the monograph. This code appears in the index after each title entry only and will be noted by a white number in a black square. The significance coding is as follows: **1**, highly clinically significant; **2**, minimally clinically significant; **3**, minimally clinically significant; **4**, not clinically significant. For further discussion of the significance coding, refer to the User's Guide on p. xxix.

Trade names are listed in the index for single-ingredient products only, and the trade name entry will refer the user to the generic name of that product.

In some cases, specific drug names will not appear on the page number listed in the index. This indicates that the drug in question may be a member of a pharmacologically and/or chemically related class that is referred to within the body of the monograph. The complete listing of that related drug class may be found in the Appendix of Related Drugs. Also, other drugs may be referred to within a monograph that are not a member of a related drug class. These drugs may be mentioned in other sections of the monograph (e.g., Recommendations) and are indexed as well.

Drugs that are not available in the United States are not included as index entries unless (1) the drug is in the title of the monograph or (2) the drug is specifically documented within the monograph as a related drug.

Index to Drug Interactions

Aluminum hydroxide, magnesium hydroxide—cont'd
  chlorpromazine **3**, 426t, 431
  chlorprothixene, 431
  choline salicylate, 36
  diflunisal, 36
  divalproex sodium, 274
  fluphenazine, 431
  haloperidol, 431
  ketoconazole **3**, 343t, 377
  loxapine, 431
  magnesium salicylate, 36
  mesoridazine, 431
  methdilazine, 431
  molindone, 431
  perphenazine, 431
  piperacetazine, 431
  prednisone, 674
  prochlorperazine, 431
  promazine, 431
  promethazine, 431
  ranitidine, 664
  salicylamide, 36
  salsalate, 36
  sodium salicylate, 36
  sodium thiosalicylate, 36
  sodium valproate, 274
  thiethylperazine, 431
  thioridazine, 431
  thiothixene, 431
  trifluoperazine, 431
  triflupromazine, 431
  trimeprazine, 431
  valproic acid **3**, 218t, 274
Aluminum hydroxide, magnesium hydroxide, magnesium trisilicate
  cimetidine, 664
  deslanoside, 509
  digitalis, 509
  digitoxin, 509
  digoxin **2**, 496t, 509
Aluminum ions–tetracycline, 399
Aluminum oxide, sodium bicarbonate–ketoconazole, 377
Aluminum phosphate, 680
  beclomethasone, 674
  betamethasone, 674
  corticotropin, 674
  cortisone, 674
  cosyntropin, 674
  desoxycorticosterone, 674
  dexamethasone, 674
  fludrocortisone, 674
  flunisolide, 674
  fluprednisolone, 674
  hydrocortisone, 674
  isoniazid, 369
  methylprednisolone, 674
  paramethasone, 674
  prednisolone, 674
  prednisone, 674
  triamcinolone, 674
Aluminum trisilicate, magnesium trisilicate–valproic acid, 274
Alupent; *see* Metaproterenol
Alurate; *see* Aprobarbital
Amantadine
  amiloride, 548
  bendroflumethiazide, 548

Amantadine—cont'd
  benzthiazide, 548
  chlorothiazide, 548
  chlorthalidone, 548
  cyclothiazide, 548
  flumethiazide, 548
  hydrochlorothiazide, 548
  hydrochlorothiazide, triamterene **3**, 536t, 548
  hydroflumethiazide, 548
  indapamide, 548
  methyclothiazide, 548
  metolazone, 548
  polythiazide, 548
  quinethazone, 548
  spironolactone, 548
  trichlormethiazide, 548
Ambenonium, 681
  beclomethasone, 674
  betamethasone, 675
  corticotropin, 674
  cortisone, 675
  cosyntropin, 674
  desoxycorticosterone, 675
  dexamethasone, 675
  fludrocortisone, 675
  flunisolide, 674
  fluprednisolone, 675
  hydrocortisone, 675
  methylprednisolone, 675
  paramethasone, 675
  prednisolone, 675
  prednisone, 675
  succinylcholine, 91
  triamcinolone, 675
Amcil; *see* Ampicillin
Americaine; *see* Benzocaine
Amid-Sal; *see* Salicylamide
Amikacin, 680
  amoxicillin, 363
  ampicillin, 363
  atracurium, 102
  azlocillin, 363
  bacampicillin, 363
  bacitracin, 367
  bumetanide, 375
  capreomycin, 367
  carbenicillin, 363
  cefaclor, 365
  cefadroxil, 365
  cefamandole, 365
  cefazolin, 365
  cefonicid, 365
  cefoperazone, 365
  cefotaxime, 365
  cefoxitin, 365
  ceftizoxime, 365
  cefuroxime, 365
  cephalexin, 365
  cephaloglycin, 365
  cephalothin, 365
  cephapirin, 365
  cephradine, 365
  cloxacillin, 363
  colistimethate, 367
  cyclacillin, 363
  cyclopropane, 67
  dicloxacillin, 363
  ethacrynic acid, 375
  ether, 67
  furosemide, 375

Amikacin—cont'd
  gallamine, 102
  halothane, 67
  methicillin, 363
  methotrexate, 421
  methoxyflurane, 67
  mezlocillin, 363
  moxalactam, 365
  nafcillin, 363
  nitrous oxide, 67
  oxacillin, 363
  pancuronium, 102
  penicillin G, 363
  penicillin V, 363
  piperacillin, 363
  polymyxin B, 367
  succinylcholine, 102
  ticarcillin, 363
  tubocurarine, 102
  vecuronium, 102
Amikin; *see* Amikacin
Amiloride, 684
  amantadine, 548
  anisindione, 201
  aspirin, 549
  captopril, 309
  dicumarol, 201
  digitoxin, 507
  digoxin, 507
  guanethidine, 322
  indomethacin, 551
  lithium carbonate, 453
  phenindione, 201
  phenprocoumon, 201
  potassium, 550
  sulindac, 537
  warfarin, 201
Aminodur; *see* Aminophylline
Aminoglycosides, 680
Aminophylline, 685
  allopurinol, 642
  atracurium, 79
  busulfan, 413
  carbamazepine, 643
  carmustine, 413
  charcoal, 644
  chlorambucil, 413
  chlortetracycline, 657
  cimetidine, 645
  cyclophosphamide, 413
  demeclocycline, 657
  doxycycline, 657
  enflurane, 635
  erythromycin, 647
  furosemide, 650
  gallamine, 79
  halothane **1**, 632t, 635-636
  hydrocortisone, 651
  influenza virus vaccine, 652
  isoflurane, 635
  ketamine **3**, 632t, 637
  lithium carbonate, 466
  lomustine, 413
  mechlorethamine, 413
  melphalan, 413
  methacycline, 657
  methoxyflurane, 635
  metocurine, 79
  minocycline, 657
  nadolol, 656

Anisindione—cont'd
rifampin, 200
secobarbital, 192
sodium salicylate, 156
spironolactone, 201
stanozolol, 185
sucralfate, 202
sulfacytine, 203
sulfadiazine, 203
sulfadoxine, 203
sulfamerazine, 203
sulfamethazine, 203
sulfamethizole, 203
sulfamethoxazole, 203
sulfapyridine, 203
sulfasalazine, 203
sulfinpyrazone, 205
sulfisoxazole, 203
sulindac, 206
talbutal, 192
testolactone, 185
testosterone, 185
tetracycline, 207
thiamylal, 192
thiopental, 192
thyroglobulin, 208
thyroid, 208
tolbutamide, 587
triamterene, 201
vitamin E, 210
vitamin K, 196
vitamin K$_3$, 196
Anisotropine, 680
deslanoside, 523
digitalis, 523
digitoxin, 523
digoxin, 523
metoclopramide, 671
nitrofurantoin, 384
propoxyphene, 57
Anorexic agents, 680
Anspor; see Cephradin
Antabuse; see Disulfiram
Antacids, 680
Antepar; see Piperazine
Antianxiety and antipsychotic drug interactions, 425-468
Antiarrhythmic drug interactions, 111-130
Antibiotics
macrolide, 683
polypeptide, 684
Anticholinergics, 680-681
Anticholinesterases, 681
Anticoagulant drug interactions, 131-210
Anticoagulants, oral, 681
Anticonvulsant drug interactions, 211-278
Anticonvulsants, 683
Antidepressant drug interactions, 279-302
Antidepressants, tricyclic, 685
Antihistamines, 681
Antihypertensive drug interactions, 303-338
Anti-infective drug interactions, 339-406
Anti-inflammatory agents, non-steroidal, 684

Antilirium; see Physostigmine
Antimetabolites
antineoplastic, 681
antiparkinsonism, 681
Antineoplastic alkylating agents, 681
Antineoplastic antimetabolites, 681
Antineoplastic drug interactions, 407-424
Antiparkinsonism antimetabolites, 681
Antipsychotic and antianxiety drug interactions, 425-468
Antipsychotics, 681
Antivert; see Meclizine
Antrenyl; see Oxyphenonium
Anturane; see Sulfinpyrazone
Apogen; see Gentamicin
Apresoline; see Hydralazine
Aprobarbital, 681
acetazolamide, 271
alcohol, ethyl, 610
alseroxylon, 98
amitriptyline, 298
amoxapine, 298
anisindione, 192
azatadine, 611
beclomethasone, 612
betamethasone, 612
bromodiphenhydramine, 611
carbamazepine, 223
carbinoxamine, 611
chloramphenicol, 358
chlorcyclizine, 611
chlorpromazine, 439
chlortetracycline, 360
clemastine, 611
clonazepam, 226
corticotropin, 612
cortisone, 612
cosyntropin, 612
cyclizine, 611
cyproheptadine, 611
demeclocycline, 360
deserpidine, 98
desipramine, 298
deslanoside, 504
desoxycorticosterone, 612
dexamethasone, 612
dexbrompheniramine, 611
dexchlorpheniramine, 611
dichlorphenamide, 271
dicumarol, 192
digitalis, 504
digitoxin, 504
digoxin, 504
diphenhydramine, 611
diphenylpyraline, 611
divalproex sodium, 229
doxepin, 298
doxycycline, 360
ethoxzolamide, 271
fludrocortisone, 612
flunisolide, 612
fluprednisolone, 612
griseofulvin, 368
hydrocortisone, 612
imipramine, 298
isocarboxazid, 604

Aprobarbital—cont'd
lidocaine, 118
maprotiline, 298
meclizine, 611
methacycline, 360
methazolamide, 271
methoxyflurane, 77
methyldopa, 332
methylprednisolone, 612
metoprolol, 476
metronidazole, 382
minocycline, 360
nortriptyline, 298
oral contraceptive agents, 614
oxyphenbutazone, 53
oxytetracycline, 360
paramethasone, 612
pargyline, 604
phenelzine, 604
phenindamine, 611
phenindione, 192
pheniramine, 611
phenprocoumon, 192
phenyltoloxamine, 611
phenytoin, 262
prednisolone, 612
prednisone, 612
promazine, 439
protriptyline, 298
pyrilamine, 611
quinidine, 123
rauwolfia serpentina, 98
rescinnamine, 98
reserpine, 98
rifampin, 607
sodium valproate, 227
sulfacytine, 100
sulfadiazine, 100
sulfadoxine, 100
sulfamerazine, 100
sulfamethazine, 100
sulfamethizole, 100
sulfamethoxazole, 100
sulfapyridine, 100
sulfasalazine, 100
sulfisoxazole, 100
tetracycline, 360
theophylline, 654
tranylcypromine, 604
triamcinolone, 612
trimipramine, 298
tripelennamine, 611
triprolidine, 611
valproic acid, 227
warfarin, 192
Aquamephyton; see Phytonadione
Aquasol A; see Vitamin A
Aquasol E; see Vitamin E
Aquatag; see Benzthiazide
Aquatensen; see Methyclothiazide
Aralen; see Chloroquine
Aramine; see Metaraminol
Arfonad; see Trimethaphan
Aristocort; see Triamcinolone
Artane; see Trihexyphenidyl
Arthropan; see Choline salicylate
Ascorbic acid
anisindione, 155
aspirin ◼, 617t, 619-620

Cyclacillin—cont'd
propranolol, 473
sisomicin, 363
streptomycin, 363
sulfacytine, 398
sulfadiazine, 398
sulfadoxine, 398
sulfamerazine, 398
sulfamethazine, 398
sulfamethizole, 398
sulfamethoxazole, 398
sulfapyridine, 398
sulfasalazine, 398
sulfisoxazole, 398
tetracycline, 387
timolol, 473
tobramycin, 363
Cyclapen; *see* Cyclacillin
Cyclizine, 681
alcohol, ethyl, 599
amobarbital, 611
aprobarbital, 611
atenolol, 481
butabarbital, 611
butalbital, 611
labetalol, 481
mephobarbital, 611
metharbital, 611
methohexital, 611
metoprolol, 481
nadolol, 481
pentobarbital, 611
phenobarbital, 611
phenytoin, 239
pindolol, 481
propranolol, 481
secobarbital, 611
talbutal, 611
thiamylal, 611
thiopental, 611
timolol, 481
warfarin, 165
Cyclobenzaprine–guanethidine, 318
Cyclobenzpyrine
furazolidone, 297
isocarboxazid, 297
pargyline, 297
phenelzine, 297
procarbazine, 297
tranylcypromine, 297
Cyclophosphamide, 681
allopurinol [2], 408t, 411
aminophylline, 413
atracurium, 86
gallamine, 86
metocurine, 86
oxtriphylline, 413
pancuronium, 86
succinylcholine [2], 65t, 86
theophylline, 413
tubocurarine, 86
warfarin, 183
Cyclophosphamide, fluoro-uracil, methotrexate
bendroflumethiazide, 412
benzthiazide, 412
chlorothiazide, 412
chlorthalidone, 412
cyclothiazide, 412
flumethiazide, 412

Cyclophosphamide—cont'd
hydrochlorothiazide [3], 408t, 412
hydroflumethiazide, 412
indapamide, 412
methyclothiazide, 412
metolazone, 412
polythiazide, 412
quinethazone, 412
trichlormethiazide, 412
Cyclophosphamide, prednisone, vincristine, bleomycin
deslanoside, 511
digitalis, 511
digitoxin, 511
digoxin, 511
Cyclophosphamide, prednisone, vincristine, cytarabine
deslanoside, 511
digitalis, 511
digitoxin, 511
digoxin, 511
Cyclophosphamide, prednisone, vincristine, doxorubicin
deslanoside, 511
digitalis, 511
digitoxin, 511
digoxin, 511
Cyclophosphamide, prednisone, vincristine, procarbazine
deslanoside, 511
digitalis, 511
digitoxin, 511
digoxin, [2], 497t, 511
Cyclophosphamide, prednisone, vincristine, vinblastine
deslanoside, 511
digitalis, 511
digitoxin, 511
digoxin, 511
Cyclopropane, 683
alseroxylon, 337
amikacin, 67
deserpidine, 337
epinephrine, 70
gentamicin, 67
neomycin, 67
rauwolfia serpentina, 337
rescinnamine, 337
reserpine, 337
tobramycin, 67
Cycloserine–phenytoin, 257
Cyclosporine
amphotericin B, 378
ethotoin, 243
ketoconazole [2], 343t, 378
mephenytoin, 243
phenytoin [3], 215t, 243
sulfacytine, 297
sulfadiazine, 397
sulfadoxine, 397
sulfamerazine, 397
sulfamethazine, 397
sulfamethazine, trimethoprim [3], 345t, 397
sulfamethizole, 397
sulfamethoxazole, 397
sulfapyridine, 397
sulfasalazine, 397
sulfisoxazole, 397
Cyclothiazide, 685

Cyclothiazide—cont'd
amantadine, 548
captopril, 309
cephaloridine, 353
chlorpropamide, 565
colestipol, 539
cyclophosphamide, fluoroura-cil, methotrexate, 412
deslanoside, 515
digitalis, 515
digitoxin, 515
digoxin, 515
fenfluramine, 547
fenoprofen, 537
guanethidine, 322
ibuprofen, 537
indomethacin, 537
lithium carbonate, 453
meclofenamate, 537
mefenamic acid, 537
naproxen, 537
oxyphenbutazone, 537
phenylbutazone, 537
piroxicam, 537
probenecid, 540
sulindac, 537
tolmetin, 537
tubocurarine, 101
Cycrimine, 680, 681
chlorpromazine, 434
deslanoside, 523
digitalis, 523
digitoxin, 523
digoxin, 523
metoclopramide, 671
nitrofurantoin, 384
propoxyphene, 57
Cyproheptadine, 681
alcohol, ethyl, 599
amobarbital, 611
atenolol, 481
butabarbital, 611
butalbital, 611
labetalol, 481
mephobarbital, 611
metharbital, 611
methohexital, 611
metoprolol, 481
nadolol, 481
pentobarbital, 611
phenobarbital, 611
phenytoin, 239
pindolol, 481
propranolol, 481
secobarbital, 611
talbutal, 611
thiamylal, 611
thiopental, 611
timolol, 481
warfarin, 165
Cystospaz; *see* Hyoscyamine
Cytarabine, 681
methotrexate [3], 408t, 417-418
warfarin, 183
Cytarabine, cyclophosphamide, prednisone, vincristine
deslanoside, 511
digitalis, 511
digitoxin, 511
digoxin, 511

Methdilazine—cont'd
amitriptyline, 285
amoxapine, 285
amphetamine, 432
bacitracin, 391
benztropine, 434
butorphanol, 43
capreomycin, 391
clonidine, 450
codeine, 43
colistimethate, 391
desipramine, 285
diazoxide, 436
disulfiram, 468
doxepin, 285
ethotoin, 240
fentanyl, 43
guanethidine, 316
hydrocodone, 43
hydromorphone, 43
imipramine, 285
insulin, 570
levodopa, 437
levorphanol, 43
lithium carbonate, 467
maprotiline, 285
meperidine, 43
mephenytoin, 240
methadone, 43
methyldopa, 329
morphine, 43
nalbuphine, 43
nortriptyline, 285
oxycodone, 43
oxymorphone, 43
pentazocine, 43
phenindione, 152
phenobarbital, 439
phenytoin, 240
piperazine, 440
polymyxin B, 391
propoxyphene, 43
propranolol, 482
protriptyline, 285
succinylcholine, 94
trimipramine, 285
Methergine; see Methylergonovine
Methicillin, 684
allopurinol, 348
amikacin, 363
atenolol, 473
chloramphenicol, 386
chlortetracycline, 387
demeclocycline, 387
doxycycline, 387
erythromycin, 388
gentamicin, 363
heparin, 149
kanamycin, 363
labetalol, 473
methacycline, 387
metoprolol, 473
minocycline, 387
nadolol, 473
neomycin, 363
netilmicin, 363
oral contraceptive agents, 349
oxytetracycline, 387
paromomycin, 363
pindolol, 473

Methicillin—cont'd
probenecid, 390
propranolol, 473
sisomicin, 363
streptomycin, 363
sulfacytine, 398
sulfadiazine, 398
sulfadoxine, 398
sulfamerazine, 398
sulfamethazine, 398
sulfamethizole, 398
sulfamethoxazole, 398
sulfapyridine, 398
sulfasalazine, 398
sulfisoxazole, 398
tetracycline, 387
timolol, 473
tobramycin, 363
Methimazole
digoxin, 531
metoprolol, 493
propranolol, 493
Methixene, 680
deslanoside, 523
digitalis, 523
digitoxin, 523
digoxin, 523
metoclopramide, 671
nitrofurantoin, 384
propoxyphene, 57
Methocarbamol, 684
alcohol, ethyl, 608
imipramine, 609
warfarin, 182
Methohexamine–insulin, 573
Methohexital, 682
acetazolamide, 271
alcohol, ethyl, 610
alphaprodine, 96
alseroxylon, 98
amitriptyline, 298
amoxapine, 298
anisindione, 192
azatadine, 611
beclomethasone, 612
betamethasone, 612
bromodiphenhydramine, 611
brompheniramine, 611
buclizine, 611
butorphanol, 96
carbamazepine, 223
carbinoxamine, 611
chloramphenicol, 358
chlorcyclizine, 611
chlorpheniramine, 611
chlorpromazine, 439
chlortetracycline, 360
clemastine, 611
clonazepam, 226
codeine, 96
corticotropin, 612
cortisone, 612
cosyntropin, 612
cyclizine, 611
cyproheptadine, 611
demeclocycline, 360
deserpidine, 98
desipramine, 298
deslanoside, 504
dexamethasone, 612
dexbrompheniramine, 611

Methohexital—cont'd
dexchlorpheniramine, 611
dichlorphenamide, 271
dicumarol, 192
digitalis, 504
digitoxin, 504
digoxin, 504
diphenhydramine, 611
diphenylpyraline, 611
divalproex sodium, 227
doxepin, 298
doxycycline, 360
ethoxzolamide, 271
fentanyl, 96
fludrocortisone, 612
flunisolide, 612
fluprednisolone, 612
griseofulvin, 368
hydrocodone, 96
hydrocortisone, 612
hydromorphone, 96
isocarboxazid, 604
levorphanol, 96
lidocaine, 118
maprotiline, 298
meclizine, 611
meperidine, 96
methacycline, 360
methadone, 96
methazolamide, 271
methoxyflurane, 77
methyldopa, 332
methylprednisolone, 612
metoprolol, 476
metronidazole, 382
minocycline, 360
morphine, 96
nalbuphine, 96
nortriptyline, 298
oral contraceptive agents, 614
oxycodone, 96
oxymorphone, 96
oxytetracycline, 360
paramethasone, 612
pargyline, 604
pentazocine, 96
phenelzine, 604
phenindamine, 611
phenindione, 192
pheniramine, 611
phenprocoumon, 192
phenyltoloxamine, 611
phenytoin, 262
prednisolone, 612
prednisone, 612
probenecid, 97
promazine, 439
propoxyphene, 96
protriptyline, 298
pyrilamine, 611
quinidine, 123
rauwolfia serpentina, 95
rescinnamine, 98
reserpine, 98
rifampin, 607
sodium valproate, 227
sulfacytine, 100
sulfadiazine, 100
sulfadoxine, 100
sulfamerazine, 100
sulfamethazine, 100

781